A CONCISE REPERTORY
OF
HOMOEOPATHIC MEDICINES
Alphabetically Arranged

Dr. S.R. Phatak, M.B.B.S.

Fourth Edition
Revised & Corrected

by
Dr. C. Jeevanandam

B. JAIN PUBLISHERS (P) LTD.
USA — EUROPE — INDIA

A CONCISE REPERTORY OF HOMOEOPATHIC MEDICINES

Fourth Edition: 2005
18th Impression: 2024

All rights reserved. No part of this book may be reproduced, stored in a retrieval system or transmitted, in any form or by any means, mechanical, photocopying, recording or otherwise, without any prior written permission of the publisher.

© Dr D.S. Phatak

Published by Kuldeep Jain for
B. JAIN PUBLISHERS (P) LTD.
B. Jain House, D-157, Sector-63,
NOIDA-201307, U.P. (INDIA)
Tel.: +91-120-4933333 • Email: info@bjain.com
Website: www.bjain.com

Printed in India

ISBN: 978-81-319-0200-4

To my friend
Late Mr. S.L. KAPADI

PREFACE
To the First Edition

Prescribing in Homoeopathy is both Science and Art. But it is a difficult Art. Good case taking, sound knowledge of Materia Medica and skilful use of the reference books are the three prerequisites.

This repertory is intended to serve as a handy and useful reference book. It is an attempt to lessen the difficulties of the prescriber. No originality can be claimed in a book of this type, except that of presentation. There are advantages and disadvantages in the traditional type of repertory. The author feels that the present arrangement will minimize the disadvantages. Remedies for a particular rubric are reduced to minimum possible by a careful selection. No drug is given unless the author has used it in his own practice or unless there is strong justification provided for it, by authorities like Dr. Boger, Dr. Kent, Dr. Clark's Dictionary etc.

A concise repertory cannot take the place of exhaustive repertories of Kent, Boeninghausen and others. It is aimed at reducing the burden of the prescriber, in every sense of the word.

Plan of the Book & How to Use it

In this repertory, the headings mentals, generals, modalities, organs, and their sub-parts are all arranged according to their alphabetical order. All the physiological and pathological conditions such as appetite, aversions, desires, nausea, vomiting, thirst, fever, pulse etc. are also included in alphabetical order. Cross references are given wherever necessary. In such arrangement there will be no difficulty in finding the appropriate rubrics. In each such rubric all important symptoms, their concomitants and their modalities are given. But the prescriber should not entirely depend on the particulars, for finding out the correct remedy. If he cannot find the correct remedy, according to the totality of symptoms, under the particular organ or sub-part of it, so much the better, otherwise he has to find the remedy considering the general conditions and general modalities. For all the general modalities, the words Agg. and Amel. are printed AGG. and AMEL. For the modalities under particular rubric only, there should be no difficulty in finding out as to which modality is general and which is particular. For example "Eyes closing Agg". Though this modality is given under eyes, it modifies the general symptoms as well as those of the eyes.

Dr. Boger has a remarkable knack of coining a general rubric from some particular symptom. (Those who have used his Synoptic Key must have noticed it). For example, take the rubric 'Awkwardness'. This symptom is given by Dr. Kent in his repertory under, 'Extremities'. There it shows that the patient either drops things from his hands or walks stumbling. But when Dr. Boger made it a general rubric, it means that the patient's mental and/or physical behaviour may be awkward. All such headings coined by Dr. Boger are included in this repertory. Not only that but the author himself has coined a few new headings from his own experience. For example the rubric "unsteady sensation". Once a patient consulted the author for this sensation. This patient, whenever he used to stand for more than a few minutes, used to feel unsteady, not giddy, but as if he was not standing firmly on the ground. The author found for him the remedy from those given under unsteady gait.

Every homeopathic practitioner is aware that modalities and concomitants are the most important factors for finding a correct remedy. The author has garnered all useful modalities from different standard repertories and has included those in this book. The modality "Holding the breath Amel", is given only by Dr. Boenninghausen in his Therapeutic Pocket Book. This modality gave the author, once an opportunity to cure remarkably an ulcer on the dorsum of the foot due to Thromboangitis obliterans.

The repertories are compiled for finding out as far as possible a correct remedy by referring to the various symptoms given under various organs; along with the circumstances, conditions and timing which modify them. In order to arrive at the suitable remedy, the remedies given under a particular symptom are graded according to their importance. The prescriber, however, should bear in mind that every remedy—high grade or low grade becomes equally important when it is connected with peculiar concomitant or with and unusual condition or circumstance. **Repertorization does not mean mechanical repertorization. Totality of Symptoms does not mean numerical totality, but qualitative totality.** One peculiar concomitant or an unusual condition may determine the totality of the case.

Patients do not always tell their symptoms according to the rubric used in the repertory. Nor do they give all the information required by the prescriber. The prescriber has to find much of the information regarding modalities and concomitants by appropriate questioning and confirm it by cross-questioning. After this, the prescriber with his logical mind has to sift, evaluate and interpret the meaning of the symptom or symptoms correctly, to enable him to refer to the appropriate rubric in the repertory. All the modalities in a case are not equally important. The modality regarding the position or posture of a patient may sometimes be more valuable. If a patient says that he feels better only when he assumes some strange position, this condition should be considered first. This modality is not given in any standard repertory, though some positions in sleep are given. But Dr. Boger with his remarkable knowledge of behaviour of drugs has coined a heading, "Attitudes bizarre" given under generalities. The meaning is obvious. The patient's disposition whether mental or physical is bizarre, i.e. strange or unusual. Again some modality may be common, but when associated, with the diseased condition, with which it has absolutely no connection, becomes uncommon or unusual. Once the author was consulted by a patient who was suffering from what is known as peripheral neuritis. He was not suffering from diabetes, nor were there any untoward incidents preceding that condition. The patient felt pain in both the legs, below the knees. The pain was better by moving the legs, while walking and by hard pressure. But the patient told the author that when he belched or passed flatus, he felt much relief. If the prescriber will try to find a remedy for this group of symptoms from any other repertory, he is probably liable to miss the mark. But Dr. Boger has given the modality "Passing flatus up and down, Amel" under the rubric "Flatulence". The author has elevated the rank of this particular to the general rubric.

The aversions, desires, mental attitudes, causation, have their own place in the selection of the remedy, when they are very marked. Causations will be found under Agg's either general or particular. Mental attitudes will be found under mental conditions. Sometimes the appearance of symptoms on one side, or going upwards or downwards etc., give a right clue to the selection of remedy, when they are very marked. All these conditions are given under 'Directions' of symptoms. The prescriber should be alert; he should look everywhere to arrive at the correct remedy.

Everything cannot be explained in the preface. But the author hopes, that the few instances given about will enable the prescriber to understand what to look, where to look, and how to look. As said in the beginning, prescribing in homoeopathy is an Art. And one can only achieve sort of proficiency in this Art by constant and diligent study of the remedies given in various standard materia medica, with reference to their place value given in the repertory.

Story of This Book

The author conceived the idea of preparing and arranging the repertory in one alphabetical order when he used to discuss the uses of various repertories with the doctors who came to him for guidance in the study of Homoeopathy. The repertory had also to be a concise and handy one. Though this idea took root, the author on account of his indifferent health was reluctant to undertake this task. But his friend Mr. S. L. Kapadi, who knew about the idea, unexpectedly came to his help. One day he came to the author will a skeletal copy of this work and asked the author to fill up the gaps, check and recheck it. This skeleton work was prepared by Mr. Kapadi from author's rough draft, notes etc. of Marathi repertory. The author was surprised. This was more than what was expected from a layman.

The author had to consent. He arranged the work properly, rewrote it and made many additions. Dr. (Miss) Homai A. Merchant who used to come to the author for guidance in the study of Homoeopathy saw this hand-written copy. She herself very kindly offered to type it. The typed copy was lying with the author for nearly ten years. During this interval, many useful additions were made. But on account of various reasons, the author did not consider getting it printed. Mr. Kapadi induced my son to get it printed. When it was decided to publish it, my son approached Mr. D. P. Datay, who promised all help and undertook the composing work. The author had no choice left.

Dr. (Miss) Merchant again came to the rescue. When requested, very willingly she typed the whole work again for the press and made some valuable suggestions.

No work is ever complete. But it can be rightly claimed that considering the object of writing a compact, handy repertory useful for prompt reference, no effort was spared to make this work as complete as possible.

Thanks giving
Thanks are due to Dr. (Miss) Merchant of her neat typing. My son Dr. D. S. Phatak did the preliminary spadework. He went through all the cross references, looked the final proof carefully and deserves all praise.

The author does not know how to thank Mr. Kapadi, without whose preliminary help and persistence later, the book may not have seen the light of the day. Prescribers who find this book useful owe a great deal to this interest in it.

Finally the author is gratefully indebted to all those masters of Homoeopathy from whose works he has drawn freely to make this book as useful as possible.

The author is well aware of the mistakes which have crept in, inspite of careful proof reading. Lines under some rubrics are misplaced while printing. The prescriber is requested to correct the book as per errata and refer to the list of abbreviations when necessary.

Sept. 1963   **S.R. Phatak**

PREFACE
To The Second Edition

While compiling a Materia Medica as a companion volume to my repertory, I have had to go through different materia medicas written by various authors like Hering, Clarke, Boger, Boericke, Kent and many others.

While doing this I found many new clinical and pathological symptoms. So I have taken this opportunity to add these symptoms in this edition of my repertory. Very few changes were found necessary while revising the book.

My repertory was well received not only in India, but even abroad in America and England. The demand for it was persistent and increasing, but if my colleague Dr. P. Sankaran had not undertaken the responsibility of publishing it, the book in this second edition would not have seen the light so soon. Not only I thank him but users of this book must thank him also for this.

My friend Dr. (Miss) Homai Merchant has been kind enough to offer her services and type out the whole manuscript without a single murmur. For this I am grateful to her.

No repertory, whether exhaustive or concise, is ever complete. Yet, I hope this book will be more useful to prescribers to find the correct remedy in most of their daily routine cases. And if they know the techniques of Dr. Boger, they will have occasion to refer to the exhaustive repertories very rarely.

Lastly I must thank God for preserving me in spite of my old age and poor health to see this edition published.

Bombay, 21 Oct. 1977   **S. R. Phatak**

PREFACE

To The Third Edition

I am happy that after about 23 years this third edition is being published. The total period for the revision was about seven years.

The number of pages have increased partly because of bigger type, still the book remains handy. New additions are marked with '+' mark.

B. Jain Publishers deserve my thanks for the publication.

June 2000   **Dr. D. S. Phatak**

Carb-v	Carbo Vegetabilis
Card-m	Carduus Marianus
Cast-eq	Castor Equi
Castr	Castoreum
Caul	Caulophyllum
Caus	Causticum
Cean	Ceanothus
Cedr	Cedron
Cench	Cenchris Contortrix
Cep	Allium Cepa
Cham	Chamomilla
Chel	Chelidonium
Cheno	Chenopodium Anthelminticum
Chim	Chimaphila Umbellata
Chin	China Officinalis
Chin-ar	Chininum Arsenicosum
Chin-s	Chininum Sulphuricum
Chio	Chionanthus
Chlo-hyd	Chloral Hydrate
Chlor	Chlorum
Choles	Cholesterinum
Cic	Cicuta Virosa
Cimex	Cimex Acanthia
Cimi	Cimicifuga
Cina	Cina
Cinb	Cinnabaris
Cist	Cistus Canadensis
Clem	Clematis Erecta
Coca	Coca
Cocain	Cocaina
Coc-c	Coccus Cacti
Cocl	Cocculus Indicus
Codei	Codeinum
Cof	Coffea Cruda
Colch	Colchicum Autumnale
Coll	Collinsonia
Colo	Colocynthis

- Scapula, to: Merc.

Left: Bor; Bov; *Lil-t; Lyc; Phel.*

- Arms to fingers: Ast-r.
- Below: Ap; Bry; Bur-p; Cimi; Pho; Sul; Ust.
- Pain

Level 4   - Cough, with: Mos.

- drawn back, as if+: Croc.
- dysmenorrhoea, with: Caus.
- head, to: Glo.
- jumping: Croc.
- meals, after: Rum; Stro.
- menses

Level 5   at: Grap.

between: Ust.

2. An important change is that now with successive levels, the symptoms of the previous level is fully repeated. For instance, one fourth level symptom in the above extract reads:

Mammae, left, pain, head to

In the original arrangement, only a few words from the higher level should be considered in constructing the symptom at a lower level. Sometimes the exact meaning of the symptom was difficult to construe. For instance, in the original version:

COUGH:

Walking, Fast Agg: Sep.

    Amel: Canc-fl; Dros.

Could mean

    Cough, amel by walking fast: Canc-fl; Dros.

This now appears as:

    COUGH

        Walking

- Amel: Canc-fl; Dros.
- Fast Agg: Sep.

3. In order to retain the natural language as far as possible, after the head word in a symptom, the sequence of the rest of the words have been rearranged, as far as possible.
4. Although the repertory is based on alphabetical arrangement, for major organs, rubrics on locations are arranged first followed by complaints and sensations. Among the locations, the right side is followed by the left. Wherever this arrangement was not followed, it has been corrected.
5. Similarly, in certain modalities pertaining to stools, menses, etc., the order of appearance, viz., before, during and after, has been consistently followed.
6. There are two types of alternating symptoms - (i) alternating sides within the same organ/location, and (ii) symptoms alternating with other organs. The first category comes under locations and the second under complaints. This has been uniformly followed.
7. Additions made by Dr. D.S. Pathak have been placed at appropriated places and duplications avoided. The additions are indicated by placing '+' after the symptoms. Addition of remedies to the existing rubrics have also been indicated similarly.
8. Gradations of remedies have been restored to those of the original edition, wherever they differed.

9. The abbreviations follow those of Boger. In order to avoid confusion, a full list of abbreviation of remedies has been provided.

10. The cross reference within the same first level rubric is indicated by romans; where they refer to a different first level rubric, they are indicated by CAPITALS.

11. Indication of general agg and amel in capitals and particular agg and amel in romans has been consistently followed.

12. Each column begins with full details of the rubric. Where a rubric is broken between two columns, the continuation on the second column is indicated by the rubric head followed by two dots.

13. The header indicates the beginning and ending first level rubric word in each page.

14. In few cases, more than one abbreviation was found for the same remedy. This has been corrected.

Kuldeep Jain
C.E.O., B. Jain Publishers (P) Ltd.

ABBREVIATIONS
And their Remedies

Ab-c	Abies Canadensis
Ab-n	Abies Nigra
Abro	Abrotanum
Abs	Absinthium
Acaly	Acalypha Indica
Acet-ac	Acetic Acid
Aco	Aconite
Act-sp	Actea Spicata
Adon	Adonis Vernalis
Aesc	Aesculus Hippocastanum
Aeth	Aethusa Cynapium
Agar	Agaricus Muscarius
Agn	Agnus Castus
Agrap	Agraphis Nutans
Ail	Ailanthus Glandulosa
Alet	Aletris Farinosa
Alfalfa	Alfalfa
All-s	Allium Sativum
Alo	Aloe
Alu	Alumina
Alum	Alumen
Alu-sil	Alumina Silicata
Amb	Ambra Grisea
Am-br	Ammonium Bromatum
Ambro	Ambrosia
Am-c	Ammonium Carbonicum
Am-caus	Ammonium Causticum
Am-m	Ammonium Muriaticum
Am-ph	Ammonium Phosphoricum
Amy-n	Amyl Nitrosum
Anac	Anacardium
Ang	Angustura Vera

Ant-c	Antimonium Crudum
Anthr	Anthracinum
Ant-t	Atntimonium Tartaricum
Ap	Apis Mellifica
Ap-g	Apium Graeolens
Apoc	Apocynum Cannabinum
Aral	Aralia Racemosa
Aran	Aranea Diadema
Arg-m	Argentum Metallicum
Arg-n	Argentum Nitricum
Arn	Arnica Montana
Ars	Arsenicum Album
Ars-io	Arsenicum Iodatum
Ars-s-fl	Arsenicum Sulphuratum Flavum
Art-v	Artemisia Vulgaris
Aru-t	Arum Triphyllum
Asaf	Asafoetida
Asar	Asarum Europoeum
Ascl	Asclepias Tuberosa
Ast-r	Asterias Rubens
Atrop	Atropinum
Aur	Aurum Metallicum
Aur-m	Aurum Muriaticum
Avena	Avena Sativa
Bacil	Bacillinum
Bad	Badiaga
Bap	Baptisia Tinctoria
Bar-c	Baryta Carbonica
Bar-io	Baryta Iodata
Bar-m	Baryta Muriatica
Bell	Belladonna
Bels	Bellis Perennis
Benz	Benzenum
Benz-ac	Benzoicum Acidum
Benz-n	Benzinum Nitricum
Berb	Berberis Vulgaris
Berg-aq	Berberis Aquifolium

Bism	Bismuthum
Bor	Borax
Bor-ac	Boricum Acidum
Both	Bothrops Lanciolatus
Bov	Bovista
Brach	Brachyglottis Repens
Bro	Bromium
Bry	Bryonia Alba
Buchu	Buchu (Barosma Crenulatum)
Buf	Bufo
Bung	Bungurus Fasciatus
Bur-p	Bursa Pastoris
Cact	Cactus Grandiflora
Cadm	Cadmium Sulphuratum
Calad	Caladium Seguinum
Calc	Calcarea Carbonica
Calc-ac	Calcarea Acetica
Calc-ar	Calcarea Arsenica
Calc-f	Calcarea Fluorica
Calc-hyp	Calcarea Hypophosphorosa
Calc-io	Calcarea Iodata
Calc-p	Calcarea Phosphorica
Calc-pic	Calcarea Picrica
Calc-ren	Calculus Renalis
Calc-s	Calcarea Sulphurica
Calc-sil	Calcarea Silicata
Calend	Calendula
Cam	Camphora
Cam-ac	Camphoricum Acidum
Canc-fl	Cancer Fluviatilis
Cann	Cannabis Indica and Sativa
Canth	Cantharis
Caps	Capsiculm
Carb-ac	Carbolicum Acidum
Carb-an	Carbo Animalis
Carb-s	Carboneum Sulphuratum
Carb-tetra	Carboneum Tetramuriaticum

PUBLISHERS NOTE

To The Fourth Edition

A Concise Repertory of Homoeopathic Medicines by Dr. S.R. Phatak is an alphabetized re-working of Boger and Boenninghausen. The book is very popular and that is the reason that we keep on receiving a lot of suggestions for improvement of the book. Dr. C. Jeevanandam is one such intelligent reader who has been constantly advising us on corrections and change in style of presentation to make the next edition more user friendly. Impressed by his avid interest in the book we requested him to Revise and Correct the Third Edition. Dr. C. Jeevanandam is a great lover of homoeopathy and has tremendous admiration for Dr. Phatak's Repertory and it was the same spirit that he went through the book word by word to point out all the mistakes and design the new user-friendly format. The DTP and Editing of the Fourth Edition has been done under his able supervision. We at B. Jain are very grateful for his services which he did on voluntary basis.

The Changes Made for the Current Fourth Edition are as follows:

1. The text takes a new format, with distinctive style for each level of symptoms. The symptoms go up to five levels as the following illustration shows:

   Level 1 **MAMMAE:** Bell, Bry: Carb-an; Cham; *Con;* Hyds; Iod; Lac-c; Merc; Oci-c; *Pho; Phyt;* Sabal; Sil; Urt.

   Level 2 **Right:** Ign; Kali-bi; *Phel;* SIL.

   Level 3 • Below: Carb-an; Caust; Chel; CIMI; *Grap;* Laur; Lil-t; Merc-i-r; *Pho; Sul;* Ust.

   • Jumping alive, as if+: Croc.

Como	Comocladia
Con	Conium Maculatum
Conval	Convallaria Majalis
Cop	Copaiva
Corn	Cornus Circinata
Cor-r	Corallium Rubrum
Cratae	Crataegus
Croc	Crocus Sativa
Crot-c	Crotalus Cascavella
Crot-h	Crotalus Horridus
Crot-t	Croton Tiglium
Cub	Cubera
Culex	Culex Musca
Cund	Cundurango
Cup	Cuprum Metallicum
Cup-ac	Cuprum Aceticum
Cup-ar	Cuprum Arsenicum
Cup-ox	Cuprum Oxydatum Nigrum
Cur	Curare
Cyc	Cyclamen
Daph	Daphne Indica
Dict	Dictamnus
Dig	Digitalis
Dios	Dioscorea Villosa
Diph	Diphtherinum
Dol	Dolichos
Dros	Drosera
Dul	Dulcamara
Echi	Echinacea
Elap	Elaps Corallinus
Elat	Elaterium
Epip	Epiphegus
Equi	Equisetum
Erig	Erigeron
Eucal	Eucalyptus
Euon	Euonymus Atropurpurea
Euphor	Euphorbrium Officinarum

Euphr	Euphrasia
Eupi	Eupion
Eup-p	Eupatorium Perfoliatum
Eup-pur	Eupatorium Purpureum
Fago	Fagopyrum
Fer	Ferrum Metallicum
Fer-ar	Ferrum Arsenicosum
Fer-io	Ferrum Iodatum
Fer-p	Ferrum Phosphoricum
Fer-pic	Ferrulm Picricum
Flu-ac	Fluoricum Acidum
Form	Formica Rufa
Frax	Fraxinus
Gal-ac	Gallicum Acidum
Gamb	Gambogia
Gel	Gelsemium
Glo	Glonoin
Gnap	Gnaphalium
Goss	Gossypium
Gran	Granatum
Grap	Graphites
Grat	Gratiola
Grind	Grindelia
Guai	Guaiacum
Gymn	Gymnocladus
Ham	Hamamelis
Hecla	Hecla Lava
Helin	Helianthus
Hell	Hellebore
Helo	Helonias
Helod	Heloderma
Hep	Hepar Sulphuris Calcareum
Hura	Hura Brasiliensis
Hyd-ac	Hydrocyanic Acid
Hydroc	Hydrocotyle
Hyds	Hydrastis
Hyo	Hyoscyamus

Hyo-hydro	Hyoscyamine Hydrobromate
Hypr	Hypericum
Iber	Iberis
Ichthy	Ichthyol
Ign	Ignatia
Ind	Indigo
Iod	Iodum
Iodf	Iodoformum
Ip	Ipecacuanha
Iris	Iris Versicolor
Jab	Jaborandi
Jal	Jalapa
Jat	Jatropha
Just	Justicia
Kali-ar	Kali Arsenicum
Kali-bi	Kali Bichromicum
Kali-br	Kali Bromatum
Kali-c	Kali Carbonicum
Kali-chl	Kali Chloricum
Kali-cy	Kali Cyanatum
Kali-io	Kali Iodatum
Kali-m	Kali Muriaticum
Kali-n	Kali Nitricum
Kali-p	Kali Phosphoricum
Kali-per	Kali Permanganatum
Kali-s	Kali Sulphuricum
Kalm	Kalmia Latifolia
Kob	Kobaltum
Kre	Kreosote
Lac-ac	Lacticum Acidum
Lac-c	Lac Caninum
Lac-d	Lac Defloratum
Lach	Lachesis
Lachn	Lachnanthes
Lact-v	Lactuca Virosa
Lap-alb	Lapis Albus
Lapp	Lappa

Lathy	Lathyrus
Latro	Latrodectus Mactans
Laur	Laurocerasus
Lecith	Lecithin
Led	Ledum Palustre
Lept	Leptandra
Lil-t	Lilium Tigrinum
Lith	Lithium Carbonicum
Lob	Lobelia Inflata
Lol-t	Lolium Temulentulm
Lyc	Lycopodium
Lycoper	Lycopersicum
Lycps	Lycopus Virginicus
Lyss	Lyssin
Mag-c	Magnesia Carbonica
Mag-m	Magnesia Muriatica
Mag-p	Magnesia Phosphorica
Mag-p-aus	Magnetis Polus Australis
Mag-s	Magnesia Sulphurica
Maland	Malandrinum
Manc	Mancinella
Mang	Manganum
Mar-v	Marum Verum
Med	Medorrhinum
Meli	Melilotus
Menis	Menispermum Canadense
Meny	Menyanthes
Meph	Mephitis
Merc	Mercurius
Merc-c	Mercurius Corrosivus
Merc-cy	Mercurius Cyanatus
Merc-d	Mercurius Dulcis
Merc-i-f	Mercurius Iodatus Flavum
Merc-i-r	Mercurius Iodatus Ruber
Merc-sul	Mercurius Sulphuricus
Mez	Mezereum
Mill	Millefolium

Morph	Morphinum
Mos	Moschus
Mur-ac	Muriatic Acid
Murx	Murex
Myg	Mygale Lasiodora
Myr	Myrica Cerifera
Naj	Naja
Naph	Naphthaline
Nat-ar	Natrum Arsenicum
Nat-c	Natrum Carbonicum
Nat-m	Natrum Muriaticum
Nat-p	Natrum Phosphoricum
Nat-s	Natrum Sulphuricum
Nat-sal	Natrum Salicylicum
Nic	Niccolum
Nit-ac	Nitricum Acidum
Nit-m-ac	Nitro Muriatic Acid
Nux-m	Nux Moschata
Nux-v	Nux Vomica
Oci-c	Ocimum Canum
Oenan	Oenanthe Crocata
Ol-an	Oleum Animalis
Old	Oleander
Ol-j	Oleum Jecoris
Onos	Onosmodium
Op	Opium
Orig	Origanum
Osm	Osmium
Ox-ac	Oxalicum Acidum
Oxytr	Oxytropis
Paeon	Paeonia
Pall	Palladium
Par	Paris Quadrifolia
Passif	Passiflora Incarnata
Par-b	Pareira Brava
Petr	Petroleum
Petros	Petroselinum

Phel	Phellandrium
Pho	Phosphorus
Pho-ac	Phosphoricum Acidum
Phys	Physostigma
Phyt	Phytolacca
Pic-ac	Picric Acid
Pip-m	Piper Methysticum
Pit-ext	Pituitary gland
Plant	Plantago Major
Plat	Platinum
Plb	Plumbum Metallicum
Pod	Podophyllum
Polyg	Polygonum
Pop-c	Populus Candicans
Poth	Pothos Poetidus
Pru-sp	Prunus Spinosa
Psor	Psorinum
Ptel	Ptelea
Pul	Pulsatilla
Pulex	Pulex
Pyro	Pyrogen
Radm	Radium
Ran-b	Ranunculus Bulbosus
Ran-sc	Ranunculus Scleratus
Raph	Raphanus
Rat	Ratanhia
Rhe	Rheum
Rhod	Rhododendron
Rhus-r	Rhus Radicans
Rhus-t	Rhus Toxicodendron
Rob	Robinia
Rum	Rumex Crispus
Rut	Ruta Graveolens
Saba	Sabadilla
Sabal	Sabal Serrulata
Sabi	Sabina
Sal-ac	Salicylicum Acidum

Salix	Salix Nigra
Samb	Sambucus Nigra
Sang	Sanguinaria Canadensis
Sanic	Sanicula
Sant	Santoninum
Sarr	Sarracenia Purpurea
Sars	Sarsparilla
Scil	Scilla Maritima
Scop	Scoparius
Scut	Scutellaria Lateriflora
Sec	Secale Cornutum
Sele	Selenium
Senec	Senecio
Seneg	Senega
Sep	Sepia
Sil	Silicea
Sinap	Sinapis Nigra
Solid	Solidago Vigra
Sol-n	Solanum Nigrum
Spig	Spigelia Anthelmintica
Spo	Spongia Tosta
Stan	Stannum Metallicum
Stap	Staphysagria
Stic	Sticta Pulmonaria
Stil	Stillingia Sylvatica
Stram	Stramonium
Stro	Strontia Carbonica
Strop	Strophanthus Hispidus
Stry	Strychninum
Stry-a	Strychninum Arsenicosum
Stry-p	Strychninum Phosphoricum
Succi	Succinum
Sul	Sulphur
Sul-ac	Sulphuricum Acidum
Sulfo	Sulfonal
Sul-io	Sulphur Iodatum
Sumb	Sumbul

Symp	Symphytum Officinale
Symphor	Symphoricarpus Racemosa
Syph	Syphilinum
Tab	Tabacum
Tarn	Tarentula Hispania
Tarn-c	Tarentula Cubensis
Tarx	Taraxacum
Tell	Tellurium
Terb	Terebinthina
Thal	Thallium
Ther	Theridion
Thu	Thuja Occidentalis
Thymol	Thymol
Thyr	Thyroidinum
Til	Tilia Europa
Trif	Trifolium Pratense
Tril	Trillium Pendulum
Tromb	Trombidium
Tub	Tuberculinum
Uran-n	Uranium Nitricum
Urt	Urtica Urens
Ust	Ustilago Maydis
Uva	Uva Ursi
Vacci	Vaccininum
Val	Valeriana Officinalis
Vanad	Vanadium
Vario	Variolinum
Ver-a	Veratrum Album
Verb	Verbascum
Ver-v	Veratrum Viride
Vesp	Vespa Crabro
Vib	Viburnum Opulus
Vinc	Vinca Minor
Vio-o	Viola Odorata
Vio-t	Viola Tricolor
Vip	Vipera Torva
Visc	Viscum Album

Xanth	Xanthoxylum Fraxineum
X-ray	X-ray
Zin	Zincum Metallicum
Zin-ar	Zincum Arsenicum
Zin-chr	Zincum Chromatum
Zin-cy	Zincum Cynatum
Zing	Zingiber
Zin-io	Zincum Iodatum
Zin-p	Zincum Phosphoricum
Zin-s	Zincum Sulphuricum
Zin-val	Zinc Valerianate
Ziz	Zizia

ABDOMEN

Affections in general: Aeth; Arg-n; ARS; Bry; *Calc*; Carb-v; *Chin*; Colo; Ip; Lach; LYC; NUX-V; PHO; PUL; Sep; Sil; SUL; Ver-a.

Upper: Caus; *Cham*; Chin; Cocl; Nux-v; Pul.
- Drawn in: Thu.

Lower: See HYPOGASTRIUM

Sides: Asaf; Carb-v; Chin; *Ign.*
- Right: Ars; Lach; Lyc; *Rhus-t.*
- heavy: Tab.
- left, to: Sep.
- Left: Alu; Arg-m; Asaf; Bro; Dul; Flu-ac; Hep; Plb; Rhe; *Sil*; Sul; Tarx.
- right, to: Nux-v.
- heavy objects in, as if: Lyc.
- rigidity: Nat-m.
- Alternating: Arn; *Pul*; Sul.
- Distension: Caus; *Nat-m.*
- Flowing towards genitals, from: Colo.
- Sticking, in: Ign.
- running, when: Tub.

Backward: Arn; ARS; BELL; Bor; Carb-v; Chel; Con; Cup; Fer; Kali-p; Lyc; Nux-v; PHO; Plb; Pul; Sep; Sul; *Tab.*

Chest, to: Aeth; *Cham*; Lach.

Forward, into: Thu.

Groins, to: Pul.

Ileo-caecal region: See APPENDICITIS.

Scrotum, to: Ver-v.

Thighs, to: Lil-t; Mag-p; Sabal; Sabi; *Stap*; Thyr.

Transversely, across: *Chel.*

ABDOMEN

Upward: Aco; ARS; Calc; Carb-v; Kali-bi; Kali-c; Lac-ac; Saba.
- Right: Aco; Kali-c; Mag-m; *Murx*; Seneg; Sep.
- Left: Alu; Ign; *Naj*; *Nat-s*; Spo; Zin.
- Diagonally: Lach.

Afternoon
- Agg: Am-m.
- Amel: Nat-s.

Alternating with
- Head: Alo; Bry; Calc; Cina; Pod; Thu.
- Chest: Radm; Ran-b.
- Ear: Radm.
- Eye: Euphr.
- Other organs: Bry; Colo; Nux-v; Radm; Ran-b.

Anxiety, emotions, felt in: *Ars*; Aur; Carb-v; Cham; Cup; Kali-c; Mez; Nux-v; Pho; Ver-a.

Ball: See Lump.

Band, about: Caus; *Chel*; Chio; Lyc; Nux-v; Plb; *Pul*; Sul.

Bandaging amel: Cup; Flu-ac; Nat-m; Nit-ac.

Breath holding agg: Dros; Spig.

Breathing deep
- Agg: *Arg-n*; Caus; Kre; Pul.
- Amel: Card-m; Flu-ac; Thu.

Bubbling: *Lyc*; Pul; Sul-ac; Tarx.

Burning in (See STOMACH): Caps; *Caus*; Iris; Manc; Terb; Ver-a.

ABDOMEN

ABDOMEN, burning in
- Digestive tract, whole: *Iris.*
- Hot coals, as from: Ver-a.
- Steam passing through, as if: Ascl.
- Water running down: Chin.

Changing about, in: Dios; Mur-ac; Nux-v.

Clawing: Bell; Lyc.

Coition, after agg: Caus; Pho-ac; Ther.

Coldness, in: Amb; *Ars*; Cadm; Calc; Colch; Grat+; Kali-br+; Kali-c; *Meny*; Pho; Sec; Sep; Sul-ac; *Ver-a*; Zin.
- Burning, with: Pho.
- Colic, with: Calc; Kali-s.
- Eating, after: Pul.
- Icy: Colch; Crot-h+.
- Pressure agg: Meny.
- Throat, rising to: Carb-an.

Concussion agg: Bry.

Contracted: Mag-p.

Contraction, hour-glass: Rhus-t.

Convulsive motions, spasms, after: Buf.

Coughing agg: Anac; Ant-t; Bry; Dros; Lyc; *Nux-v*; Pall; Pho.

Covers, but lifts clothes: Bell; Lac-c; *Lach*; Lil-t; Pho; Sec; Stap; Tab.

Diarrhoea, sense of: Bry; Dul; Hyds; NUX-V; Pul; Ran-sc.

Distended, tympanitic, inflated, etc: *Abro*; *Aco*; Agar; Alo; ARG-N; Ars; CALC; CARB-V; Cham; CHIN; Cic; Cocl; *Colch*;

ABDOMEN, distended..
Colo; *Grap*; Hep; Hyo; KALI-C; Lach; Lil-t; LYC; Mag-c; *Merc*; *Nat-c*; *Nat-m*; Nat-p; Nux-m; NUX-V; *Pho*; Pho-ac; Raph; Rhus-t; Stram; Sul; *Terb*; Vario; *Ver-a*.
- Children, in: Bar-c; Calc; Caus; Sul.
- Clothes
  - feel tight: Mos.
  - loosening amel+: Onos.
- Contracts, when touched: Colch.
- Epilepsy, before: Cup; *Lach*.
- Fontanelles open, with: Sil.
- Hard: *Kali-c*.
- Hot: Merc-d.
- Hysterical: Tarx.
- Legs, cannot stretch: Colch.
- Lying agg: Carb-v
- Menses, during: Chin; *Cocl*; Kali-c; Nat-c; *Sul.*
- Milk, after: *Con.*
- Operation, after: Carb-an; Hypr.
- Painful: Aco; Ars; Bry; Caus; Lach; Merc; Rhus-t.
  - amenorrhoea, with: Castr.
- Parturition after: Lyc; *Sep.*
- Pregnancy, as if+: Vario.
- Sides+: Caus; *Nat-m.*
- Stools
  - after: Carb-v; Grap; *Lyc.*
  - amel: Hypr.
- Sudden: Nat-m.
- Whooping cough, with: Kali-s.

Drawing, as if: Caps; Pul: Sep.

ABDOMEN

Drawn, involuntarily: *Val.*
Drinking Water
- Agg: Ars; Pho; Zing.
- Ice-cold
  - agg: Calc-p; Nux-m; Rhus-t.
  - amel: Elap.
- impure+: Zing

Dropsy, ascites (See DROPSY): Acet-ac+; Ap; Apoc; Ars; Aur; Hep+: Lyc; Mur-ac; Scil: Terb.
- Cirrhosis of liver, from: Mur-ac.
- Diarrhoea, frequent attacks, with: Sil.
- Menses, suppressed, from: Senec.
- Pelvic region, fold on, with: Colch
- Suffocation, lying on left side: Ap.
- Urination scanty, with: Scil.

Eating
- Amel: Anac: Bov; *Chel*; *Grap*; Hep; Ign; Kali-p; Lach; Mag-m; Med; Petr; *Zin.*
- Fruits agg: Lyc.
- Too much agg: Ant-c; Cof; Ip; Nux-v; *Pul.*

Empty: See Hollow.
Eructation
- Amel: Amb; Bar-c; Rat.
- No amel from: *Chin*; Lyc.

Eye symptoms, with: Arg-n.
Fasting amel: Caus; Sil.
Fat: Am-m; *Chel.*
Fats agg: Carb-v; *Pul.*

Fist of a child moving, as of: Conval; *Nat-c*; *Sul*; THU.
Fermentation in: Chin; Lyc.
Fever, in agg: Ip; Ver-a.
Flabby: See Weak.
Flatus passing
- Agg: Aur; Canth; Flu-ac; Scil.
- Amel: Hep; Nat-m; Tarn.

Food, stale agg: Ars.
Formication: Plat.
- Voluptuous: Plat.

Fullness: *Carb-v*; *Chin*; Dig; Grap; *Kali-c*; Kali-m; LYC; NUX-V; Pho; Pho-ac; SUL.
- Food, small quantity+: Mur-ac.
- Full of water, as if: Crot-t; Hell; Pho-ac.
- Gurgling in: ALO; *Crot-t*; Gamb; Old; *Pod*; Pul; SUL.
- Stools, gushing, then: Alo; *Crot-t*; GAMB; Iris; Jat; *Nat-s*; Pho; Pod; Sec; *Sul*; Thu; Ver-a.

Hand, placing on agg: Psor; Zin-chr.
Hanging or falling down, as if: Acet-ac; Laur; Nat-m; Pho; Pod; *Sep.*
- Walking, when: Nat-m.
- Walks, therefore
  - bent: Carb-v.
  - carefully: Nux-v.

Hard: Bar-c; Bar-m; Calc; *Grap*; Merc; *Sil.*
- Body, moving in, as if: Bor; Lyc.

ABDOMEN

Heart, with: Merc-i-f.
Heavy: *Alo*; Am-m; Cup; *Grap*; Kali-c; Lyc; *Nux-v*; *Pul*; Sep; *Spig*; Stap.
- Right: Tab.
- Left: Lyc.
- Menses, during: Kali-s.

Holds: Agn; Lil-t; Merc; Rhus-t; Sep; Stap.

Hollow, empty, sinking sensation: Arg-n; Cocl; Ip; Old; PHO; *Pod*; Pul; Sec; SEP; *Stan*; Stap; Sul-ac; *Tab*.
- Bowels, knotted feeling with: Cham.
- Gnawing: Ox-ac.
- Stools, after: Petr; Pho; Pod; Sul-ac.
  - Amel: Mur-ac.

Hot food and drink amel: Lyc; Mag-p; *Nux-v*; Sul-ac.

Inactive: See Paralysis.

Inflammation, peritonitis: Aco; *Ant-t*; ARS; Bell; *Bry*; Colch; Hyo; *Ip*; Lach; Laur; Lyc; *Nux-v*; PHO; *Pul*; Pyro; Rhus-t; Terb; Til.
- Cold application amel: Calc.
- Tuberculous: Abro.

Kneading by hand amel: Nat-s.

Knots, lumps, felt in: Abro; Ars; Bism; Ign; Plb; Saba; Sec.

Laparotomy, after: Bism; Hep; *Nux-v*; Op; Raph; Stap.

Legs, extending amel: Phys.

Lifting agg: Bry.

Limbs, with: Aeth.

Lime boiling in, as if: Caus.

ABDOMEN

Lumps, balls in, as if: Anac; Kre; *Nux-v*; *Rhus-t*; Sul; Thu; Ust; Verb.
- Moving rapidly in: Saba.
- Rising, to throat: ARG-N; Raph.
  - coughing when: Kali-c.

Lying on
- Back, with knees drawn up amel: Bry; Lach; Rhus-t.
- Left side, amel; Scil.
- Stomach, amel: Rhus-t.

Milk
- Amel: Grap; Merc; Mez; *Nux-v*; Rut; Ver-a.
- Hot amel: Crot-t.

Motion amel: Chin; Petr.

Moving up and down, something in: Lyc.
- Convulsions, after: Buf.

Numb: Aco; Bry; *Plat*; *Pul*; Sars.

Pain
- Boring, grinding: Flu-ac; Plb; Polyg; Sars; Stan.
- Cutting: Bell; *Bry*; Chin; Colo; Dios; Ip; *Mag-c*; Merc; Nit-ac; Nux-v; *Polyg*; *Pul*; Rhe; *Sul*; Ver-a.
- Flatus passing on: Con.
- Gnawing, eating, ulcerative: Bell; *Carb-v*; Colo; Lyc; Pho; Sep.
- Griping, cramp, colic: *Bell*; *Cham*; Cocl; COLO; Cup; *Dios*; Ign; Kre; *Mag-m*; NUX-V; OP; *Plb*; Polyg; Radm; Rat; Sul; Val; *Ver-a*; Zin.

ABDOMEN, pain, griping
- arms, raising agg: Cup.
- associated symptoms, with: Plb.
- backache, with: Sars.
- cold drinks agg: Manc.
- coryza, stopped, after: Calc.
- diarrhoea agg: Phys.
- eating
  amel: Psor.
  after+: Val.
- eructations, with: Mag-p.
- habitual, in children: Bar-c.
- nightly: Calc; Cham; Chin; Lyc.
- riding in carriage agg: Carb-v.
- stools, hard amel: Ust.
- trembling and chattering of teeth with: Bov; Meph.
- yellow hands and blue nails, with: Sil.
• Hysterical: Stan.
• Indefinite, dull, aching: Ars; Colo; Cup; Lept; *Nux-v*; Plb; Pod; Pul; Rhus-t; Sep; Ver-a; Ver-v.
• Menses, instead of: Spo.
• Nausea, after: Latro.
• Paralytic+: Grat.
• Pinching: Ran-b; Tell.
• Radiating: Ip; *Mag-p*; Plb.
• Smarting, rawness: *Ars*; Bell; Canth; Nux-v; Ran-b.
• Sore spot in: Arg-n; Bar-c; Bism; *Kali-bi*; Pho; *Rhus-t*.
- Menses
  after:Pall.
  with: Ham.

ABDOMEN, pain
• Spasmodic: Caus.
• Stitching: *Bry*; Ip; *Sul.*
• Tearing, shooting: Ars; Cham; Colo.
• Uncovering agg: Rhe.
Paralysis of intestines: Bry; Con; Lyc; Mag-m; Nux-v; Op; Pho; PLB; *Rhus-t*; Tab; Thu.
• Laparotomy, after: Op.
Pressure
• Agg: Ars; Bry; Calc; Chel; Merc-c.
• Amel: Arg-n; Castr; COLO; Cup; Plb; Stan.
• Clothes, of agg: Arg-n; Bov; Calc; *Lach*; *Lyc*; *Nux-v*.
• Right hand on stomach, left hand on lumbar region amel: Med.
Protrudes, here and there: Thu.
Pushing: Thu.
Quivering, in: Calc; Con; Iod; *Nux-v*; Sabi; *Sul-ac*.
Restlessness, uneasiness: Ars; Calc; Ip; Pho; Sep.
Retracted, sunken: Ap; *Calc-p*; Cup; *Hyds*; Kali-br; PLB; *Ver-a*; Zin.
• Cholera, in: Kali-br.
• Constipation with: Carb-ac.
Retraction
• Agg: Ant-t; Asar; Nux-v; Zin.
• Amel, distending agg: *Ign.*
• Involuntary: Val.
• Vomiting, during+: Ver-a.
Rolling something, in: Lyc.

ABDOMEN

Rubbing
- Amel: Nat-s; Pall; Pho+; *Pod.*
- Gently with warm hand amel: Lil-t.

Rubs: Aran; Kali-c; Mag-c; Nat-c; *Pho*; Plb.

Rumbling, in: See FLATULENCE, noisy.

Shocks, in: *Agar*; Bry; Nux-v.

Singing agg: Pul.

Sitting crooked amel: Sul.

Sneezing agg: Pul.

Squeaking, in+: Kali-io.

Squeezing, in: Ant-t; Cocl; *Colo*; Scop: Stap.

Standing
- Agg: Nat-p.
- Amel: Thu.

Stiff: Lil-t; *Rhus-t.*

Stones in, as if: Ant-t; *Calc*; Cocl; Colo; Hyds; Nux-m; Osm; Pul; Scop; Sep.
- Sharp: Cocl; Colo.

Stools
- Amel: Colch; *Colo*; Gamb; Mag-c; NUX-V; Stan; Ver-a.
- After, agg: Petr; Pho; Pod; Sul-ac; Ver-a.
- Hard, amel: Ust.

Stream of fire, passing through during stools+: Ascl.

Stretching, with: Plb. ----

String, about: Chel.

Sugar agg: *Arg-n*; Ign; Ox-ac; SUL.

ABDOMEN

Summer agg: Guai.

Sunken: See Retracted.

Swashing in, as if: Rhus-t.

Sweet things agg (See Sugar Agg): Zin.

Talking unbearable: Caus; Helin; Kali-c; Laur.

Tension: Ap; *Arn*; Bar-c; Calc; *Caps*; CARB-V; Chin; Colch; COLO; Cup; Hep; Lil-t; Lyc; Mos; Plb; *Rhus-t*; Scop; Sep; *Sil*; Sul.
- Menses, during: Colo; Grap; *Nux-m.*

Thread, moving rapidly in: Saba.

Throbbing, pulsations: *Ant-t*; Calc; *Nux-v*; PUL; *Sele*; Sep.
- Aneurism, from: Bar-m.
- Deep in: Aesc.
- Eating agg: Sele.
- Here and there: Cann.
- Pregnancy, during: Sele.
- Sleep, preventing: Sele.

Tight clothes
- Agg: Caus.
- Amel: Flu-ac; Nat-m; Nit-ac.

Tobacco smoking amel: Colo.

Trembling in: See Quivering.

Tumour: Con.

Ulcer, ulcerative feeling: Kali-bi; Pho; Ran-b.

Uncovering:
- Amel: Cam; Med; Sec; Tab; Vip.
- Arms or legs Agg: Rhe.

Uneasiness: See Restlessness.

ABDOMEN
Urination
- While agg: Cham; Colo; Ip; Merc.
- After agg: Eup-pur.
- Amel: Carb-an; Dios; *Sep*; Tarn.

Urine, diminished secretion of, during pain: Arn; Grap.

Vomiting
- Agg: Grap; Merc; Stap; Ver-a.
- Amel: Arg-n; Ars; Asar; Hyo; Plb; Tab; Tarn.

Water
- Cold, flowing through: Kali-c.
- Full of, as if: Crot-t; Hell; Pho-ac.
- Hot, flowing or pouring in: Chin+; Sumb; Sang.

Weak: Arg-n; *Ign*; Merc; Pho; Sul-ac.
- Eructations amel: Kali-m.

Weight, load, pressure: Agar; Arn; Ars; *Bry*; Calc; Cham; Chin; Hyo; Lyc; *Nux-v*; Pul; Sep; Sil; *Sul.*

Yawning
- Agg: *Ars*; Phyt.
- Amel: Lyc; Nat-m.

ABDOMEN EXTERNAL: Ap; Bry; Merc; Nux-v; Plb; Sele; Sul.

Brown spots on: Lyc.

Bruised, sore: Aco; *Ap*; Ars; *Bell*; Bry; Chin; *Lach*; Lyc; Merc-c; NUX-V; Ran-b; Stan; Sul; Terb.

Cold to touch: Kali-s; Merc.

Cracks on skin: Sil.

ABDOMEN EXTERNAL
Hard: Sil.

Hot: Sil
- Clothes on as from: Nit-ac.

Motions, spasmodic: Cup.

Muscles
- Emaciation of: Plb.
- Twitching : Sec.

Pendulous, enlarged: Alu; *Calc*; Carb-v; Caus; Colch; Sanic; *Sep*; Sil; Sul; Syph; Tub; Vario.
- Children, of: Alu; Bar-c; Calc; Sanic; Sil.
- glands, swelling of, with: Mez.
- Girls, at puberty: Calc; *Grap*; Lach; Sul.
- Mothers, of: *Iod*; Nat-c; *Sep*.
- Navel: See NAVEL, inflated.

Red: Sang.
- Spots on: Hyo.

Sweat on: Amb; Anac; Cic.

Yellow spots on: Kob; Pho

ABORTION: Ap; *Bell*; Cham; Croc; Erig; Gel; *Ip*; Nux-m; Pul; SABI; SEC; SEP; VIB.

After
- AGG: Helo; Kali-c; *Lil-t*; Murx; Pyro; Rut; Sabi; Sec; Sep.
- Haemorrhage: Sabi.
- Urinary troubles: Rhe.

Exertion, from: *Erig*; Rhus-t.

Habitual: Alet+; Ap; Bacil; *Caul*; Fer; Lyc; *Plb*; Sil; *Syph*; Thu.
- Second month: Ap; Cimi; Kali-c; Vib.

ABORTION, habitual
- Third month: Bell; Plb; Sabi; Sep; Thu; Ust.
- Fourth to seventh month: Sep.

Mental shock or depression, from: Bap.
Preventive: Rat; Vib+.
Sexual frequency, from: Cann.
Tenesmus recti agg: Bell; Calc; Cocl; Con; Ip; Lyc; Merc; Nux-v; Rhus-t; Sep; Sul.
Threatened+: Asar.
- Falls, from+: Arn.

Weakness, from sheer: Merc; Sil.

ABRUPT: Cham; Med; Nat-m; Plat; *Tarn*.

ABSCESS (Suppuration): Arn; Ars-io; Bell; *Calc*; Calc-io; CALC-S; *Calend*; Cist; Echi; HEP; Kali-s; LACH; Lyc; MERC; Pho; Pul; Pyro; Rhus-t; SIL; Sul; Sul-ac; Sul-io; Syph; *Tarn*.

Blind: Lyc.
Bloody: Crot-h.
Bluish: Tarn-c.
Bones
- About: Asaf; *Aur:* Calc-f; Calc-hyp; Calc-p; Flu-ac; Guai; *Pho*; Pul; Sec; Sil; Stap; Symp.
- In: Guai.

Burning: ANTHX; ARS; *Pyro*; TARN-C.
Chilly, within: Merc.
Chronic: Calc-f; Iod; Merc; Sil; Stram; Sul.

ABSCESS
Cold: Ol-j.
Deep: Calc; Caps; Tarn.
Exertion physical, from: Carb-ac.
Fibrinous parts, of : Mez.
Glands of: Bell; CALC; *Calc-s*; Carb-an; Dul; HEP; Kali-io; Lyc; MERC; Nit-ac; *Pyro*; *Rhus-t*; SIL; *Sul*; Syph; *Tub*.
Impending, suppressed: Ars; Bell; Calc; *Hep*; Kre; Lach; Lyc; Merc; Sil.
Joints, about: Calc-hyp; Merc; Pho; Psor; Sil.
Menses, at: Merc.
Multiple, during fever: Ars; Hep; Sil.
Psoas: Chin; Sul; Symp.
Recurrent: Anthx; Calc-s; *Pyro*; *Syph*.
- Fever, after: Pho-ac.

Slow: Hep; *Merc*; Sil.
Submental: Stap.
To Hasten: Guai; *Hep*; *Merc*; Phyt; Sil.
Vesicles, on: Rhus-t.

ABSENTMINDED, absorbed, buried in thought: Aco; *Ap*; Arn+; *Asar*; Bov+; Calc-p; Cann; CAUS; CHAM; Hell; *Lac-c*; Lach; *Laur*; Mez; Nat-m; Nux-m; *Old*; Pho; *Plat*; PUL; SEP; Sul; Ver-a.

As if in dream+: Anac.
As to what will become of him: Nat-m.
Menses, during: Mur-ac.

ABSENT, parts of body were: Cocain.

ABSORBENT ACTION: Arn; Kali-io; Merc-d; *Sul*; Sul-io.

ABUSIVE, scolding, quarrelsome: *Aur*; CHAM; Dul; Hyo; *Ign*; Kali-io; LYC; Merc; Mos; Nit-ac; *Nux-v*; *Petr*; Plat; Ran-b; Rat+; Rut+; Sep; Sil; Stap; Sul; *Tarn*; Ver-v+.

Angry, when not+: Dul.

Children and family, to: Kali-io.

Himself and his family with+: Kali-c.

Husband, to : Thu.

Menses, before: Cham.

Mother, to: Thu.

Pains, at his+: Cor-r.

Person, absent+: Lyc.

Somebody on the road, to: Con.

Until the lips are blue, eyes stare, and she falls fainting: Mos.

ACHING : See PAIN, aching.

ACIDITY : See SOUR.

ACIDOSIS : Nat-p; Pho.

ACNE : See ERUPTIONS.

ACRIDITY : See DISCHARGES, acrid.

ACROMEGALY: Pit-ext; Thyr.

ACTINOMYCOSIS: Hecla; Kali-io; Nit-ac.

ACTIVE, agile: Ap; Cof; Lach; Nux-v; Stram, Tarn; Val.

Mentally: COF; OP.

Restless, hence agile+: Chel.

ACTIVE

When, amel: Con; Cyc; Helo; *Lil*-t.

ACTIVITY FRUITLESS: Ap; Arg-n; Bor; Calc; Kali-br; Lil-t; Stan; Tarn; Ther.

ACTS as if born tired: Onos.

ACUMINATE, conical, growth, eruptions etc: Ant-c; Ant-t; *Ars*; Hyds; Pul; *Sil*; Syph.

ADDISON'S DISEASE: Calc; Calc-p; Iod; Nat-m; Pho; Sil.

ADENOIDS: Agrap; Calc; Cal-io; *Calc-p*; Iod; *Merc*; Tub.

Post nasal : Mez.

Removal after: Kali-s.

ADHERENT, internal sensation: Berb; *Bov*; *Bry*; Calc; Colo; Hep; Ign; Kali-bi; Kali-io; Merc-c; Nux-v; Ol-an; Osm; Pho; Plb; Pul; RHUS-T; Rum; SEP; Ust.

ADMONITION AGG: Bell; Kali-c; Nit-ac; Plat.

ADYNAMIA: See WEAKNESS.

AEROPLANE, flying in AGG: Ars; Bell; Bor; Coca; Petr.

AFFECTATION: Stram.

AFFECTIONS, stifled: Sep.

AFTERPAINS: Arn; Cham; Cimi; Cup; Hypr; Kali-c; PUL; Rhus-t; Sabi; Sec; Vib; Xanth.

Child nurses, when: Arn; Cham; Sil.

Fear of death, with: Cof.

Frequent: Rhus-t.

Headache, with: Hypr.

• **Intolerable :** Cham; Cimi.

• **Lochia, with+:** Xanth.

AFTERPAINS

Violent, persistent: Vib.

Women, who had borne many children, in: Cup.

AGILITY: See ACTIVE.

AGITATION: See EXCITEMENT.

AGONY, anguish: Aco; Ars; Aur; Bell; Calc; Caus; Cann; Dig; Hep; Lach; Plat: Stram; Ver-a.

Cannot rest in any place: Ars.

AGORAPHOBIA: Aco; Arg-n; Arn; Calc; Hyd-ac; Nux-v; Sep.

AGUE: See FEVER, intermittent.

AIR

Blowing on part, through hole as if, or fanned as if: Aur; Cam; Chel; Chin; Cor-r; Croc; Culex; FLU-AC; Helod; HEP; Lac-d; Laur; Lil-t; Med; Mos; Náj; Nat-m; Nux-v; Petr; Sele; Sep; Sul; Syph; Ther; Thu; Thyr; Zin.

Clear, dry or cold weather AGG: ACO; Ars-io; Asar; Bry; Carb-an; CAUS; Cham; Hep; Ip; Kali-ar; Kali-c; Med; NUX-V; Samb; Sep; Spo.

Close, too, as if: Sars.

Cold, as if: Benz-ac; Chin; Lac-d; Laur; Lyss; Mez+; Mos; Thyr.

Draft agg: See WIND agg.

Hot, as if: Ast-r; Bry; Kali-c; Pul; Sul; Ver-a.

Hunger: See Open air amel.
- **Flatulency, with:** Kali-io; Zin.

Impurities, full of, as if: Trifo.

Inspiring cold
- **AGG:** Aesc; Am-c; Ars; CAUS; Cimi; Cist; Hep;

AIR, inspiring cold, agg .. Hyds; Hyo; Ign; Merc; Nux-v; Psor; Rum; Saba; Seneg; Sep; Syph.
- **AMEL:** Sele
- **Feels:** Lith.

Night or evening AGG: Aco; Am-c; Carb-v; MERC; Nat-s; Nit-ac; Sul.

Open Cool
- **AGG:** Am-c; Aran; Calc; Calc-p; Cam; Caps; Caus; Cham; Chin; Cist; Cocl; Cof; Colch; Cyc; Dul; Guai; Hep; Ign; Kali-bi; Kali-c; Mag-p; Merc; Nat-c; Nit-ac; Nux-m; NUX-V; Petr; Pho; Rum; Saba; Seneg; SIL; Sul; Urt; Vio-o.
- **AMEL:** Bap; Bry; Nit-ac; Plat; Radm.
- **And in house, both AGG:** Ars; Aur; Iod; Mez.

Open amel, in room agg, air hunger etc: Alu; Ap; Arg-n; Ars; Ars-io; AUR; Cann; Carb-v; Cep; CROC; Fer; Glo; Grap; Iod; Kali-io; LACH; Lil-t; Lyc; Mag-c; Mag-m; Med; Nat-s; Op; Pru-sp; PUL; Radm; Rhus-t; Saba; Sabi; Seneg; Sul; Tab; Tarn; Tub.
- **Riding in carriage, amel:** Arg-n; Naj.

Penetrating, too: Calc; Cimi; Colo.

Smoky, as if: Berb; Bro.

Thick and heavy, as if: Agn.

Too much enters the chest, as if: Chlor; Ther.

AIR Castles: Arg-n; *Cann*; Chin; Cof; Sul.

AIR HUNGER: See AIR, open, amel.

AIR PASSAGES
Burning: Ars-io; Sang; Seneg.
Numb: Sil.

AIR-SICKNESS: See AEROPLANE flying agg.

ALBUMINOUS, glairy: See DISCHARGES.

ALBUMINURIA: Ant-c; *Ap*; *Ars*; Aur; Bry; Calc-ar; *Canth*; *Fer*; Glo; Hell; Kali-c; Lac-d; Lach; Lyc; *Merc-c*; Nat-c; Nat-p; *Pho*; Pho-ac; Phyt; *Plb*; Pul; Rhus-t; *Sul*; Terb; Thu; Val.

Alcohol, after abuse of: Ars; Carb-v.

Diphtheria, after: Phyt.

Heart disease, from: Calc-ar.

Periodical: Pho.

Pregnancy
• During: Ap; Bur-p; Helo; Merc-c; Pho.
• During and after delivery: Merc-c; Pyro.

Septic: Carb-v.

ALCOHOLIC DRINKS
Abolishes taste for+: Strop.

AGG: See under FOOD & DRINKS.

ALCOHOLISM
Acute: Aco; Bell; *Op*.

Delirium tremens: Agar; Ars; Caps; *Cimi*; HYO; Lach; Nat-m; Nux-m; Nux-v; *Op*; STRAM; Stry.

ALCOHOLISM
Later: Carb-v; Nux-v.
• Recurrent: Anac; Aur; Bell; *Chin*; Hyo; Nux-v; Op; Stram; Thu.

ALIVE
Sensation as if something in: Calc-p+; *Cann*; *Caus+*; Cocl; CROC; Cyc; *Ign*; Op; Pul; *Sabi*; Sil; *Sul*; THU.

Walls, floor, etc, on: Cocl.

ALL-GONE sensation: See EMPTY.

ALONE, WHEN AGG: See COMPANY Amel.

ALTERNATE DAYS on agg: See DAY, alternate Agg.

ALTERNATIONS
Mental: Alu; Aur; *Bell*; Croc; Con; Fer; IGN; NUX-M; *Plat*; Stram; Sul-ac; Val; *Ver-a*; Zin.
• With physical: Arn; Cimi; Croc; Ign; Lil-t; *Murx*; Plat.

Nervous, with physical: Saba.

ALTERNATING effects, states, sides, metastasis: Abro; Agar; Alo; *Amb*; Ant-c; Arn; Ars; Bell; Berb; *Cann*; *Cimi*; *Cocl*; Croc; Cup; Fer-p; Glo; *Ign*; Iris; LAC-C; Lach; LYC; *Pho*; Psor; *Pul*; Sep; Stram; SUL; Sul-ac; Val; Xanth; Zin.

Contradictory: *Ign*; Nat-m; *Pul*.

Digestive and Skin+: Grap.

Rapidly: Croc.

Reaction, want of, with: Val.

AMAUROSIS: See VISION, paralysis of optic nerve.

AMBITION, loss of (See INDOLENCE): Arg-n; Caus.
Disappointment, from: Nux-v.
AMENORRHOEA: See MENSES, absent.
AMMONIACAL ODOUR: See DISCHARGES.
AMNESIC APHASIA: See APHASIA
AMOROUS, amative, erotic, lascivious: Agn; *Canth*; HYO; Lach; Lil-t; Lyc; Murx; Orig; *Pho*; Pic-ac; *Plat*; Scil: *Sele*; Senec; Stan; Stap; Stram; *Ver-a*.
Menses, before: Stram.
ANAEMIA: ARS; CALC; *Calc-p*; CHIN; FER; Fer-ar; *Grap*; *Kali-c*; Lac-d; Lyc; Mang; Med; Nat-c; NAT-M; *Nit-ac*; *Nux-v*; *Pho*; Pic-ac; Plat; Plb; *Pul*; Senec; Sep; SUL; Sul-ac.
Grief, from: Nat-m; Pho-ac.
Haemorrhage, after: *Chin*; *Fer*.
Pernicious: *Ars*; *Pho*; Pic-ac; Thyr.
ANALGESIA: See NUMBNESS.
ANASARCA (See DROPSY): Ant-c; Ap; Ars; Bell; Bry; Chin; Colch; Dig; Dul; Fer; Hell; Kali-c; Led; Lyc; Merc; Op; Pho; Pul; Rhus-t; Sabi; Samb; Sars; Scil; Sul.
Sudden : Kali-n.
ANEURISM: Aur; Bar-c; Cact; Calc-f; Carb-v; Kali-io; Lach; *Lyc*; Pul; Sul; Thu.
Anastomosis, from: Thu.
Aorta, of: Spo.
Pains, of: Gal-ac; Sec.

ANEURISM
Small, all over body: Plb.
ANGEL when well, devil when sick+: Bell.
ANGER, vexation, irritability, fretfulness, bad temper: Aco; Anac; *Ant-c*; Ant-t+; Aru-t; Aur; *Bry*; Calc; CHAM; *Cina*; Cocl+; *Colo*; Hep; *Ign*; Iod; Ip+; Kali-c; Kali-io; Kali-m; *Kre*; LYC; Mag-c+; Nat-c; *Nat-m*; *Nit-ac*; NUX-V; Op+; Petr; Pho; Rut; Saba; Samb; Senec; *Sep*; *Stap*; *Sul*; Sul-ac; Syph; Tarn; *Thu*; Thyr; Tub; Val; Zin.
Always+: Stap.
Bright light agg: Colch.
Consolation agg: Ign; Nat-m; Sep; Sil.
Easy+: Ab-c; Dros; Radm.
Fits of violent: Mos+; Stro; Tub.
• **Beats anything in way+:** Stro.
Menses, before: Cham.
Odours agg: Colch.
Pain agg: Ant-t.
Self, about+: Elap.
Sympathy agg: Sabal.
Touched, when: Ant-c; Sanic; Tarn.
Trifles, at: Dros; Kali-m; Pho; Sanic; Sep; Tub.
Understood , when not: Laur.
Waking on: Kali-c; LYC; Pho; Sanic; Tub.
ANGINA PECTORIS: Agar; Am-c; *Amy-n*; Ap; *Arn*; ARS; Arg-n; *Cact*; Chin-ar; Cimi; Cup;

ANGINA PECTORIS ..
Glo; Kalm; *Lach*; *Latro*; Lil-t; Naj; Nux-v; *Ox-ac*; Pho; Pru-sp; Rhus-t; *Spig*; *Spo*; *Tab*.

Constriction of throat, with+: Tab.
Hot Drinks amel: Spig.
Lies on knees, with body bent backwards: Nux-v.
Pain, excessive: Agar.
ANGLES: See SKIN, folds.
ANIMATION: See CHEERFUL.
ANKLES: Caus; Led; Lyc; Nat-m; Rhus-t; Rum; Sep; Sul.
Break: Pho.
Burning: See Heat.
Calf, to: Meny.
Caries of bones: Guai; Pul.
Cold: Calc-f; Ign; Mag-m; Med.
Cracking, in: *Canth*; Nit-ac+.
Cramp: Meny; Plat; Rum; Zin-io.
• Feet pressed on floor, amel: Zin-io.
• Toes, into: Nat-c.
Eruptions, on: Calc; Chel; Nat-p; Psor.
Fistulous opening: Calc-p.
Give way, afternoon+: Cham.
Heat: Kali-bi; Nat-c.
Heavy: Ant-c; Crot-t; Cup; Led; Nit-ac; Sec; *Sul.*
• Painful: Cup.
Inflammed: Mang.
Itching: Nat-p; Led; Sele.
Jerking: Calc.
Lameness: *Rut.*
Nervous: Mag-m.

ANKLES
Night agg: Mag-m.
Numbness: Lac-c.
Paralysis: Abro.
• Sensation of: Dros.
Sprain: Anac; *Led*; Nat-c; Rut; Stro.
• As if: Pru-sp.
Stiffness: Caus; Chel; Lathy; Sil; Sul.
Sweat, on: Crot-h; Naj.
Swelling: Ap; Arg-m; Arg-n; Asaf; Chel; Med; Stan; Stro.
• Cold+: Asaf.
• Diabetes, in: Arg-m.
• Evening: Kali-chl.
• Foot, cannot use: Asaf.
• Painful: Led.
• Sitting long, after: Rhus-t.
Tension: Caus; Merc; Pho.
Toes, to: Nat-c.
Tumours: Cup-ar.
Turned easily: Med.
Ulcers: Calc-p; Hyds; Syph.
Upwards: Guai.
Walking
• Agg: Lith; Med; Nit-ac.
• Amel: Caus.
Weak: Calc; Carb-an; Mang; Nat-c; Nat-s; Nit-ac; Pho-ac; Sec; *Sil*; Stro.
• Children, while learning to walk: *Carb-an*; Mang; Nat-s.
ANNOYED easily+: Ant-t.
ANOREXIA: See APPETITE Lost.
ANSWERS
Aversion to: See AVERSION.

ANSWERS
  Hastily+: Rhus-t.
  Imaginary questions: Pho.
  Irrelevently: Hyo; *Pho*; Stram; Sil.
  Monosyllable: Pho-ac; Pul; Sep.
  Nods by: Pul.
  Refuses to: Cam; Pho; Sul.
  Reluctantly+: Rhus-t.
  Repeats question, then: Zin.
  Slowly: Arn; Bap; Cocl; Gel; Hyo; Lyc; *Merc*; *Pho*; *Pho-ac*; Rhus-t; Thu; Zin.
  Then sleeps: Arn; *Bap*; *Hyo*; Pho-ac.
ANTAGONISM WITH SELF: Anac; Bar-c; Cann; Kali-c.
ANTHRAX: Anthr; Ars; Echi; Lach; Sec.
ANTHROPOPHOBIA, bashful (See SHY): Amb; Anac; BAR-C; Cocl; HYO; Iod; Kali-io; Kali-p; *Lyc*; Nat-c; Nat-m; PUL; *Rhus-t*; Sil.
ANTICIPATIONS
  And agg from: *Arg-n*; Ars; Carb-v; *Gel*; Lyc; Med; Nat-m; Pho-ac; Plb; *Sil*.
  Diseased conditions of: Ap; *Ars*; Bry; Chin; Chin-s; Nat-m; Nux-v.
ANTISOCIAL: Syph.
ANUS: Aesc; Carb-v; Grap; Kali-c; Lach; Mur-ac; Nit-ac; Nux-v; Paeon; Pho; Saba; Sep; *Sul*.
  Aphthous: Sul-ac.
  Ball, sensation of a: *Sep*.

ANUS
  Bubbles: Colo; Nat-m.
  Bug crawling, as if: Aesc; Fer-io; Sul.
  • Stools, after: Kali-m.
  Burning: Scop; Sul-ac.
  Contracted, painfully: Plb.
  • Prolapse, after: Mez.
  Cramps, when sitting: Mang.
  Crusts: Paeon; *Petr*.
  Desire to draw in: Agar.
  Discharge black, with or without stool: Merc-i-f.
  Drawn up: Plb.
  Dry: *Aesc*; Rat.
  Eruptions: Merc; NAT-M; *Nit-ac*; PETR; Polyg.
  • Eczema: Berb.
  • Hard, small: Caus.
  Excoriated: Carb-v; Caus; Grap; Lyc; Sul.
  Fissure: Alu; Caus; Cham; GRAP; *Ign*; Led+; Nat-m; NIT-AC; Paeon; *Rat*; Sep; Sil; Syph; *Thu*.
  • Bleeding: Grap.
  • Children, tall, in: Calc-p.
  • Deep+: Arn.
  • Infants, in: Kali-io.
  • Ulcerate: Grap.
  Fistula: Aur-m; Berb; Calc; Calc-p; Carb-v; Kali-c; Nit-ac; Paeon; Sil.
  • Itching, with: Berb.
  • Palpitation, with: Cact.
  • Pulsating: Caus.
  Fluid, warm, escaping from: Aco.

ANUS

Formication: Calc; Calc-s; Kali-c; Kali-m; Saba; Sul.
- Worm, as from: Cinb.

Hammering: Lach.
- Menses, with: Lach.

Itching: Carb-v; *Caus*; Coll; Flu-ac; Grap; *Lyc*; Mar-v; Med; *Nit-ac*; *Saba*; *Sul*; Vio-o.
- Alternating with itching in nose and ears: Saba.
- Around: Petr; Sul.
- Coition, after: Anac.
- Eczematous: Nit-ac.
- Menses, before: Grap.
- Pain, ending in: Zin.
- Pimples: Polyg.
- Pinworms, from+: Urt.
- Sleep, preventing: Mar-v.
- Stick, as if, with a: Rum.
- Sticking and+: Aco.
- Stools, after: Kali-m; Tell; Zin.
- Stooping, on: Arg-m.

Liver, to: *Dios*; Lach.

Long after stool: Nit-ac; Paeon.

Loose: See Open.

Moisture, at: ANT-C; *Caps*; *Carb-an:* Carb-v; Caus; Grap; Hep; NIT-AC; *Op*; PHO; *Sep*; Sil; *Sul*; Sul-io.
- Bloody: Ap.
- Constant: Sep.
- staining yellow: Ant-c
- Flatus, from: Ant-c; Carb-v.
- Foul: *Ant-c*; Hep; Paeon: Sul-io.
- Menses, during: Lach.

ANUS, moisture
- Mucus from
  - bloody: Op.
  - foul: Hep.
  - staining yellow: Ant-c.
  - urinating when: Carb-ac.

Navel, to: Colo; Lach.

Open, inactive, powerless: Ail; ALO; Alu; *Ap*; Ign; Kali-c; Op; PHO; Sec.
- As if: Ap; Pho.
- and stools pass right through: Apoc.

Plug in, as if+: Kali-bi.

Pricking: Cact.

Pouting, swollen and: Cham.

Pustules, small, hard: Caus.

Raw: See Sore.

Red: Med; Petr; Sul.
- Fiery: Med.

Retracted: Kali-bi; Nat-p; Op.

Sore: Kali-m; Lyc.
- Menses, during: Mur-ac.
- Stools, from: Kali-m.
- Walking, when: Kali-m.

Sweat: Sep.

Torn, as if: Erig.
- Warm cloth amel: Pho.

Trembling, in: Con.

Ulcer: Carb-v; Cham; *Kali-bi*; *Nit-ac*; *Sul*.

Warts, around+: Aur.

Wiping agg: Grap.

ANXIETY: See FEAR.

Others, for: Ars; Cocl; Pho; Sul.

APATHETIC: See INACTIVE.

APATHETIC

Unequal struggling, adverse circumstances, with: Pho-ac.

APATHY: See INDIFFERENCE.

All Pervading+: Bry.

APHASIA: See SPEAKING, lost.

Amnesic: Kali-br; Plb.

APHONIA: See VOICE, Lost.

APHTHAE: See MOUTH

APOPLEXY: ACO; Ant-c; Ant-t; ARN; Ars; Aur; Bar-c; *Bell:* Calc; COCL; Cof; Fer; *Gel*; *Glo*; HYD-AC; Hyo; Ip; Kali-m; *Lach*; Lyc; Nux-v; OP; Pho-ac; Pul; Rhus-t; Samb; Sep; Stram; Thu; Ver-a; Ver-v.

Pulse
- Irritable, with: Aco.
- Slow, full, face red, pupils small: Op.
- Small, weak, face bluish, pale: Lach.

Subarachnoid: Gel.

Waves of congestion, burning, throbbing, holds head: Glo.

APPARITION: See VISION, fantastic.

APPENDICITIS (Ileo-caecal region): ARS; *Bap*; Bell; BRY; Carb-v; *Chin*; COLO; LACH; Lyc; *Merc-c*; Mur-ac; *Nux-v*; *Pho*; Pho-ac; Plb; Pul; RHUS-T; SEP; SUL; THU.

APPETITE

Affected in general: Ant-c; Ars; *Calc*; CHIN; *Cina*; Grap; Iod; *Lyc*; Merc-cy; *Nat-m*; NUX-V; Petr; Pho; PUL; Sil; Strop; SUL; Ver-a.

APPETITE

Capricious, variable: Calc; *Cina*; *Coc-c*; Fer; Grap; *Iod*; Lach; Merc; Nat-m; Petr; *Pho*; Syph.

Easy satiety: Chin; Cyc; Lyc; Plat.

Increased, hunger: Ab-c; Arg-m; Ars; *Calc*; *Chin*; CINA; Grap; Iod; *Lyc*; *Nat-m*; *Nux-v*; Old; Petr; Pho; Psor; Pul; *Saba*; Sep; Stan; Stap; *Sul*; Ver-a.

- 11 A.M.: Hyds; Pho; SUL; Zin.
- Alternating with loss of appetite: Anac; Calc; Cina; *Fer*; Pho.
- Attacks of sickness, before: Bry; Calc; Hyo; Nux-v; Pho; *Psor*; Sep.
- Chill:
  - before: Cina.
  - during: Ars; Sil.
  - after: Ars.
- Cough, during: Nux-v.
- Diarrhoea, with: Nux-v; Petr.
- Digestion weak, with: Merc.
- Eating:
  - after: Chin-ar; CINA; Iod; Kali-p; *Lyc*; Murx; PHO; Phyt; Sars; Sil.
  - no desire, for: Op.
- Epilepsy, before: Calc; Hyo.
- Fever
  - during: Chin; Cina; *Pho*.
  - after: Ign.
- Headache
  - before: Epip.

APPETITE

APPETITE, increased, headache
- with: Bry; Kali-c; Kali-s; *Pho*; PSOR; Sele; Sep.
- Knows not, for what: Mag-m; Pul.
- Menses, during: Spo
- Nausea, with: Petr; Val; Ver-a.
- Navel, from: Val.
- Nightly: Chin; Lyc; *Pho*; *Psor*.
- Pain in stomach, with: *Lach*; Lyc; Sil.
- Ravenous: Ars; *Calc*; Cann; CHIN; CINA; Grap; IOD; *Lyc*; Nat-m; *Nux-v*; Old; Petr; PHO; PSOR; Pul; Rum: Saba; Sil; Spig+; SUL; *Ver-a*; Zin.
  - meals, 2 hours after: Calc-Hyp.
  - more he eats, more he craves: Lyc.
- Refuses to eat, but: Bar-c.
- Relish, without; NAT-M; Old; Op; *Rhe*; *Rhus-t*.
- Sleep, prevents: Chin; Ign; Lyc; Pho.
- Spine, from: Lil-t.
- Stomach full, when: Stap.
- Stool, after: Alo+; Kali-p; *Petr*.
- Sudden: Sul.
- Sweat, after: Cina.
- Sweets only, for: Kali-p.
- Vanishes
  - attempting to eat, on: Sil.
  - drinking water, after: Kali-m.
  - food, sight of: Caus; Pho; *Sul*.
  - smell or thought of, during pregnancy: Caus.

APPETITE, increased
- Vomiting
  - during: Caus.
  - after: Cina.
- Wait for food, cannot: Lach
- Weakness, with: Pho; *Sul*; Zin.

Loathing, after first bite: Caus; Cyc; Lyc; Plat; Pru-sp; Rhe.

Lost, diminished, wanting: Alu; Ars; Calc; Cham; Chel; CHIN; Cocl; Cyc; Fer; Kali-bi; Lyc; Nat-m; *Nux-v*; Pho; Pic-ac; Psor; *Pul*; Rhus-t; Sep; Sil; Sul.
- Brain troubles, in: Hell.
- Coition, after: Agar.
- Complete and early: Merc-cy.
- Day, only in: Arn
- Drinking water, after: Kali-m.
- Food, at the sight of: Colch; Kali-p; Pho; Sul.
  - pregnancy, during: Caus.
  - until it is tasted, then ravenous: Lyc.
  during pregnancy: Saba.
- Habitual: Kali-m.
- Hunger, with: Chin; Cocl; Nat-m; Nux-v.
- Illness, severe, after: Ant-c; Psor.
- Lifting agg: Sep.
- Months, for: Syph.
- Neither eats nor drinks for weeks+: Ap.
- Overwork, from: Calc.
- Returns
  - eating mouthful, after: Calc; *Chin*; Saba.

APPETITE, lost, returns
- thinking of food after: Calc-p.
• Sadness, from: Plat.
• Suddenly, eating, when: Bar-c.
• Thirst, with: Psor; Rhus-t.
• Tobacco, from: Sep.
• When desired thing is offered: Ign.

Nibbling: *Aeth*; Calc; Mag-c; Mag-m; Nat-c; Petr; Rhus-t.

ARMS (Upper limbs): Am-m; Ars; Bell; *Calc*; *Caus*; Cocl; Fer; Kali-c; Lyc; Merc; Nux-v; Pho; Pul; RHUS-T; Sep; *Sil*; SUL.

Right: Bell; Bism; Bry; Calc; Caus; Colo; Grap; Nat-c; Ran-sc; Sars; Sec; Sil; Stro.
• Dead: Scop.
• Heart affections, in: Ars; Kalm; Merc-i-f; Merc-i-r.
• Holds, during palpitation: Aur.
• Longer than body, as if: Cup.
• Motion, involuntary: Cocl.
• Numb: Lach; Mur-ac.
  - aphasia, with: Mur-ac.
  - neuralgia, over left eye, with: Mur-ac.
  - then left: Zin-io.
• Writing agg: Merc-i-f.

Left: Anac; Arn; Asaf; Cact; Cimi; Kali-c; Nit-ac; Rhus-t; Sabi; Scil; Stan; Stram; Sul.
• Bound to the side, as if: Cimi.
• Jerking all day: Cic; Cimi.
• Numb: Cact.
• Pinching: Kali-c.
• Shakes, epilepsy, before: Sil.

Alternating between: Aco;

ARMS, alternating between ..
Alu; *Calc*; Caus; Cham; Chin; *Cocl*; Colch; *Lac-c*; Lyc; Mag-m; Mang; Plat; Sep; *Zin*.

Upper: Cocl; Fer; Nat-m.
• Bone: See HUMERUS.
• Burning: Ther.
• Coldness: Ign.
• Contraction: Nat-m.
• Cramps, writing while: Val.
• Drawing: Lyc.
• Electirc shocks, as if: Agar; Val.
• Emaciated: Nit-ac.
• Fluttering in, while resting on table: Phyt.
• Heavy: Alu; Latro.
• Numb: Cact; Latro; Mag-m.
• Raise, cannot: Sang.
• Singing agg: Stan.
• Thumping pain in middle: Anac.
• Weak: Stan.
• Writing agg: Val.

Fore: Calc; Caus; Merc; Phyt; Rhus-t; Stap.
• Blue: Bism.
• Bone, exostosis of+: Dul.
• Cold: *Grap*; Med; *Pho.*
  - icy: *Bro.*
  - menses, during: Arg-n.
• Crushed, as if: Guai; Gymn.
• Drawing: Calc; Card-m; Caus; Rhus-t.
• Heavy: Arg-n; Mur-ac; Pho-ac; Strop.
• Hip, left, with: Merc-i-f.
• Moving the fingers, agg: Asaf.

ARMS, fore
- Numb: Grap.
- Paresis, contraction of fingers, with: Arg-m.
- Pronated: Cup; Plb.
- Trembling:
  - coition after: Nat-p.
  - writing while: Caus; *Merc*.
- Writing agg: Merc-i-r; Ran-b.

Alternting with lower limbs: Cocl; Fago; Kali-bi; Kali-m; Kalm; Nat-c; *Sil*; *Val*; Visc.

Bend, irresistable desire to: *Fer*.

Boils: Bro; Petr.

Bones: Asaf; Chin; Rhus-t; Sil; Stap.

Breathing deep agg: Cann.

Burning: Ver-a.

Chest, keeping on agg: Psor.

Clawing: Lach.

Cold: Bell; Kali-chl; Pho; Pul.
- Diarrhoea, during: Pho.

Cough agg: Dig.

Cramp: Am-c; Calc; Colo; Old.

Emaciated: Iod; Lyc; Plb.

Extended
- As if he has intended to take hold of something: Dul; Pho.
- Flexed and, alternately: Cic; Cup: *Lyc*: Tab.

Fall, helpless: Colch.

Floating, as if: Pho-ac.

Formication: Aco; Sec.

Fuzzy (R): Phyt.

Grasping amel: Lith.

Hairy: Med.

ARMS

Hanging down:
- Amel: Aco; Arn; Bar-c; CON; *Fer*; Led; Lyc; Mag-m; Pho; Rhus-t; *Sang*; Sil; Sul.
- Forceless+: Aco.

Has many, as if: Pyro.

Heaviness: Arg-n; Caus; Con; Gel; Kali-p; Nat-m; Plb; Pul; Strop.
- Right: Am-c.

Hot water flowing on, as if: Rhus-t.

Itching: Bov; Caus; Sul; Tell.

Jerking up: Cic; Cina; Saba; Stram; Sul.
- Outwards: Arg-n.
- Towards each other: Ip.
- Upwards: Arg-n.

Lameness: Bell; Calc; Sil.
- Right: Fer; Sang.
- Left: Bro.

Laughing agg: Carb-v.

Lifting weight amel: Spig.

Light, as if: Pho-ac.

Motion of
- Agg: Anac; Dig; Led; Nat-m; Ran-b; Rhus-t; Sep; *Spig*; Sul.
- Behind him agg: Fer; Ign; Kali-bi; Mar-v; Pul; *Sanic*; Sep.
- Clutching: Hyo.
- Constant, of one: Bry.
- Involuntary, of arm and leg+: Cocl.
- To and fro: Op.

Nervous: Rhus-t.

Numb: Aco; Ap; Cocl; Grap;

ARMS, numb ..
Kali-c; Kali-m; Lyc; Ox-ac; Plat; Rhus-t; Zin.
- Right: phyt; Scop.
  - then left: Zin-ar.
- Left: Aco; Cact; Dig; Lach; Naj; Rhus-t; Spig; Sul.
  - heart diseases, in: Aco; Cact; Latro; Rhus-t.
- Carrying anything, when: Amb.
- Grasping, anything firmly: *Cham*.
- Holding anything, in the hand: Ap.
- Lain, on: Carb-v; Kali-c; Nat-m; *Pul*; *Rhus-t*.
  - not lain on: Flu-ac; Mag-m.
- Lying agg: Sul.
- Raising them upright amel: Ars; Pul.
- Shoulder to fingertips: Ox-ac.

Paralysis
- Right: Am-c; Cup; LYC; *Sul*; *Zin*.
- Left: Calc; *Dig*.
- Tongue paralysis of, with: Caus.
- Writing, from+: Agar.

Pronation, agg: Petr.
Purring: Sep.

Raising
- Laterally agg: Syph.
- Up agg: Ap; Arg-n; Bar-c; Berb; Bry; Cocl; CON; Dig; Fer; Grap; Led; Mag-c; Nit-ac; Ran-b; Rhus-t; Sanic; *Sang; Spig; Sul;* Sul-ac; Tell.

Rat running upwards: *Bell*; Calc; Sul.

ARMS
Red spots on: Saba.
Restless: Agar; Ant-t; Caus; Kali-br; Mur-ac; Samb; Tarn.
- Sleep, during: Caus.

Separated from body, as if: Bap; Daph; Psor.
Shocks: Cic.
Short, as if: Aeth; Alu.
Sinking down: Nat-m
Sleeps, with arms apart: *Cham*; Psor.
Sticky: Cam; Carb-v; Pic-ac.
Stiff, become, before convulsions: Buf.

Stretched
- Palpitation, with: Cocl.
- Right angle, at: Op.
- Spasmodically, clenched fingers, with: Chin.

Supination agg: Cinb.
Sweat amel: Thu.
Swinging: Cina.
- To and fro amel: Sang.

Swollen+: Ver-a.
Tension: Dig.
- Writing, while: *Mag-p*.

Thighs, puts on, when coughing: Nic.
Throws widly: Kali-br.
Tingling: Grap; Pho; Sil.
Trembling: Merc; Nit-ac; Op; Plb.
- Concomitant, as a: Calc-p.
- Lain on: Cam.
- Taking hold of anything: Ver-a.
- Urinary difficulty, with: Dul.

ARMS

ARMS, trembling
- Writing, while: *Merc.*

Turning
- Agg: *Sang.*
- Amel: *Spig.*

Twisting sensation: Bell.
Twitching: Cic; Thu.
Ulnar nerves, along, both+: Pod.
Veins: Nux-v; Plb; *Pul*; Thyr.
Weakness: Aesc; Anac; *Bell*; Calc; *Cic*; Con; Dig; Elap; KALI-C; Stan; Sul; Val.
- One of, after apoplexy: Cadm; Pho.
- Right: Am-c.
- Taking hold of something: *Ars.*

Wind
- Blowing, as if, shoulders to fingers: Flu-ac.
- Cold, blowing on, as if: Ast-r.

Writing agg: Merc-i-f.
- Amel: Zin-ar.

ARROGANCE: See PRIDE.
ARTERIO SCLEROSIS+: Sumb.
ARTHRALGIA (See JOINTS): Arg-m; Plb; Symp.
ARTHRITIS DEFORMANS: Arn; Ars; Aur; Caus; Cimi; Colch; Cup; Guai; Hep; Iod; Kali-io; Merc; *Pul*; Radm; *Sabi*; Sul.

ASCENDING
AGG: Ars; Aur; Bor; *Bry*; *Calc*; Iod; Merc; Nat-m; Nit-ac; Nux-v; Pho; Pul; Sep; *Spo*; Sul.
AMEL: Con; Fer; Rhod; Val.

ASTHMA

ASCENDING
Steps AGG: Stan.
ASCITES: See ABDOMEN, dropsy.
ASKS FOR NOTHING: Bry; *Op*; Pul; Rhe.
ASLEEP SENSATION: See NUMBNESS.
ASPHYXIA
Charcoal fumes, from+: Bov.
Neonatorum: Ant-t; Cam; Laur.
- Loss of blood, in mother from: Chin.

ASSOCIATED EFFECTS: Ars; Cham; *Merc*; *Nux-v*; Pho; *Pul*; Sep; Sul; Tarn; Ver-a.
ASTHENOPIA: See under VISION.
ASTHMA (Bronchial): Aco; Amb; Arg-n; ARS; Ars-io; Cup; *Ip*; Kali-ar; *Kali-c*; Kali-n; *Lach*; *Lob*; Merc-i-r; *Nux-v*; PUL; *Samb*; *Sil:* SPO; Stan; Stram; Sul; Tab; Terb; Thu; Tub; Visc.

Bed, turning in agg: Ars.
Bending
- Head backwards amel: *Spo*; Ver-a.
- Shoulders backward amel: Calc-ac.

Cardiac (See RESPIRATION difficult): Cact; Chin-ar; Laur; Naj; Psor; Spo; Sumb.
Catarrhal: Calad; Caps.
Coition agg: Amb; Asaf; Kali-bi.
Cold, preceded by+: Sul.
Constitutionally: Calc; Iod; Sul.

ASTHMA

Consumptives, of: Meph.
Coryza
- With: Arg-n; Just; Nat-s; Spo.
- After: Just; Naj.
- - summer, in: Ars.

Cough
- With: Calad; Nat-m.
- After: Pho.

Diarrhoea
- After: Kali-c.
- Alternating, with: Kali-c.
- Then: Nat-s.

Digestion disturbed, after: Sang.
Drunkards, of: Meph.
Dust, inhalation of+: Poth.
Dysuria at night, with: Solid.
Eating
- Amel: Amb; *Grap.*
- Satisfying agg: Asaf.

Eructation amel: Carb-v; Nux-v.
Eruptions, alternating with: Calad; Hep; Kalm; Sul.
Exertion excessive, from: Sil.
Expectoration amel: Ant-t; Calad; Hypr; Ip; Stan; Zin.
Fog agg: Hypr.
Foot sweat, suppressed, from: Ol-an.
Fright, after: Samb.
Full moon+: Spo.
Goitre, in: Spo.
Hay fever, of: Ars; Aru-t; Chlor; *Iod*; *Naj*; Sep.
Hives, from: Ap; Pul.
Humid: Cann; Dul; Kali-bi; Nat-s; Seneg; Sul.

ASTHMA, humid

- Weather agg: Bar-c; Syph+.

Hysterical: Cocl; Ign; Lob; Mos; *Nux-m*; Nux-v; *Pul.*
- Tears, ending in flow of: Anac.

Ice water agg: Meph.
Infantile: Med; Vib.
Injury to spine, from: Hypr.
Itching, with: Calad; Cist; Saba.
Laughing agg: Ars.
Menses
- Absent, with: Spo.
- During, waking from sleep: Cup; *Iod*; *Lach*; Spo.
- Scanty, wth: Arg-n.

Miner's: Card-m; Nat-ar.
- Coal: Sul.

Nervous: Cham; Kali-p; Mag-p; Stram.
Night from 1 a.m. to 4 a.m.: Syph.
Odours, from: Asar; Sang.
Old people, in: Amb; *Ars*; Bar-c; Bar-m; Carb-v; Coca+; Con; Seneg.
Overheated, after being: Sil.
Rheumatism, with: Benz-ac; Visc.
Rocking amel: Kali-c.
Sailors, on shore: Bro.
Sexual excitation, with: Nat-c.
Sitting up, amel+: Naj.
Skin disease, with: Ip.
Spasmodic: Val.
Stools amel+: Poth.

ASTHMA
Summer
- During: Arg-n; Syph.
- Amel: Carb-v.

Suppressions, from: Hep.
Sycotic: Med; Nat-s; Sil.
Talking agg: Dros.
Throat, choking of, with: Hyd-ac.
Thunderstorm, during: Pho; Sep; *Sil*; Syph.
Tobacco smoking amel: Merc.
Uraemic: Solid.
Urinating, when: Chel; Dul
Urticaria, alternating with: Calad.
Vertigo, with: Kali-c.
Vomiting, alternating with: Cup.
Weather
- Cold, agg: Arg-n.
- Damp amel: Caus; Hep.
- Damp cold agg+: Ver-a.
- Dry agg: Cham.

Weekly: Chin; Ign; Sul.
Winter agg: Carb-v; Nat-m; Nux-v.

ASTIGMATISM: See Under VISION.
ATHLETE'S FOOT: Grap; Sanic
ATHEROMA: See CALCULI.
ATHETOSIS: Lathy; Stry; Ver-v.
ATONY: *Op*; Passif+.
ATROPHY: See EMACIATION.
ATTACKS RECURRENT: See RELAPSES.

ATTENTION
AGG: Ign.
AMEL: Cam; Gel; Hell.
ATTITUDE BIZARRE: *Cina*; Cocl; *Colo*; Gamb; Lyc; Merc; Nux-v; *Plb*; Zin.
AMEL: Rhe.
As if in: Nat-s.
AURA: (See different sensations)
Abdomen to head: Ind.
Arms, in: Calc; *Lach*; Sil; Sul.
Brain, wavy sensation in: Cimi.
General nervous feeling: Arg-n; *Nat-m*.
Genitals: See Solar plexus.
Glow, from foot to head: Visc.
Heart, from: *Calc-ar*; Lach; Naj.
Heels to occiput: Stram.
Knees to hypogastrium: Cup-ac.
Mouse running: See CREEPING.
Solar plexus or genitals from: Buf; Cic; *Nux-v*; Sul.
Various symptoms: Buf.
AUTOMATIC acts, motion: Bell; Calc; Hell; Hyo; Lyc; Mag-c; Nux-m; Pho; Sil; *Stram*; Zin.
Hand, right, towards mouth: Nux-v.
One arm and leg, head, etc: Apoc; Bry; Hell; Iodf; Myg; Pyro; Zin.
AUTUMN AGG: Chin; Colch; Dul; Lach; *Merc*; Merc-c; RHUS-T; Ver-a.
AVARICIOUS, greedy, miserly: Ars; Lyc; Med; Pul; Sep; Sul.

AVERSIONS, dislikes
Acids, sour things: Bell; Cocl; Dros; Fer; Saba; *Sul.*
Alcoholic stimulants: Hyo; Ign; Rhus-t; Strop.
Ale: Nux-v.
Amusement: Bar-c; Hep; Lil-t; Old; Sul.
Answer, to: *Glo*; *Hyo*; *Nux-v*; Sul-ac.
Apples: Lyss.
Approached, or being touched: ANT-C; Arn; CHAM; Cina; Con; Cup; Ign; Kali-c; Lyc; Tarn; Thu.
Bananas: Bar-c; Elap.
Bathing to: See BATHING.
Bed: Cedr; Grap.
Beef: Merc; Ptel.
Beer: Chin; Cyc+; Fer; Lyc; Nux-v.
Black things: Tarn.
Brandy: Ign; Merc.
• **Brandy drinkers, in:** Arn.
Bread: Chin; Con+; Cyc; Kali-c; Lil-t+; Lyc; NAT-M; Nit-ac; Pul; Sul; Tarn.
• **Butter, and:** Mag-c; Meny; Nat-p.
Brilliant objects: Buf.
Business: See Work.
Butter: Ars+; Chin; Cyc; Hep; *Pul*; Sang.
Cheese: Arg-n+; *Chel*; Old.
Children: Lyc; Plat.
Chocolate: Osm; Tarn.
Cocoa: Osm.
Coffee: CALC; Cham; Chel+;

AVERSIONS, coffee ..
Flu-ac; Lil-t+; Merc+; Nat-m+; NUX-V; Sul-ac.
• **Smell of:** Sul-ac.
Coition, to: See COITION and FEMALES.
Colours
• **Black, red, yellow, green:** Tarn.
• **Red:** Alu
Company: See COMPANY agg.
Conversation: Chel.
Covers, to: Aco; Cam; Iod; Pul; Sec; Sul.
Disturbed being: Bry; Gel.
Drinks
• **Hot:** Kali-s.
• **Thirst, with:** Hell.
Education: Sul.
Eggs: Fer; Kali-s.
• **Odour, of:** Colch.
Everything, for: Ant-c; Canth; Merc; Pul.
Farinacious food: Ars; Pho.
Fats: Ars+; Chin; Cyc; Kali-m; Merc+; Nat-m; *Petr*; Ptel; *Pul.*
Fish: Colch; *Grap*; Pho; Zin.
• **Salted :** Pho.
Fluids, all+: Stram.
Food: ARS; Chin; Cocl; Colch; Fer; Ip; Lil-t; NUX-V; Pul; Senec; Tub.
• **Best and digestible:** Carb-v.
• **Boiled:** Calc.
• **Certain:** Pul.
• **Every kind, of:** Kali-io+; Plat; Tub+.
• **Fried:** Plb.

AVERSIONS, food
- Hot: *Chin*; Merc-c; Sil.
- Hunger, with: Cocl; Nat-m; Nux-v.
- Diarrhoea, chronic, in: Ant-c; Ars; Chin; Nux-m; Pho; Pul.
- Loathing, disgust, with: *Ant-c*; Arn; Ars; Cham; *Colch*; Cyc; Ip; *Kali-c*; Nux-v; Op; Pul; Sep.
  - all+: Asaf; Cocl.
  - animal food: Sil.
  - convalescence, during: Kre.
  - eating, when: Nux-m.
      suddenly: Bar-c; Pul; Rut.
  - first bite, after: Rhe.
  - rich: Kali-m.
  - sadness, from: Plat.
  - salty: Sele.
  - seen, if: ARS; Colch; Nux-v; Pho; Sil.
  - smell of: Ant-c; Ars; Cocl; Colch; Ip; Nux-v; Pho.
  - solid: Coca: Fer; Stap.
  - thinking, of: Ars; Carb-v; Nux-m; Zin-chr.
  - warm: Chin; Grap; Ign; *Pho*; *Pul*; Sil.

Friends: Colo; Led.
- Pregnancy, during: Con.

Fruits: Bar-c; Ign.
- Sour: Fer.

Fuss, to: Nat-m.
Garlic: Saba.
Going out: Cyc.
Green things: Mag-c.
Gruel: Ars; Calc.
Herring: Pho.
Herself: Lac-c.

AVERSIONS
Ice cream: Radm.
Liquids: Grap; Hyo; Nux-v.
Literary persons: Sul.
Marriage: See MARRIAGE.
- Females: Nat-m.

Meat: Arn; Ars+; Calc; Calc-s; Chel+; Chin; Cyc; Fer; *Grap*; Hell; Manc+; Merc+; *Mur-ac*; Nit-ac; Nux-v; PETR; PUL; *Sep*; *Sil*; SUL; Syph; Tarn; Tub.
- Fond of, was+: Cact.
- Fresh: Thu.
- Salted: Card-m.

Members of the family: Crot-h; Flu-ac; Iod; Kali-p; Lyc; Pho; Plat; Senec; *Sep*.
- Children, one's own: Lyc; Pho; Plat.
- Husband: Glo; Nat-c; *Sep*; Thu.
- Mother: Thu.
- Talks, pleasantly to others: Flu-ac.
- Wife: Ars; Nat-s; Plat; Stap.

Men (Females): Nat-m; Sep.
Milk: Ant-t+; Arn; Bry; Fer-p; Guai+; *Ign*; Lac-d; Nat-c; Pul; Sep; *Sil*.
- But relishes it: Bry.
- Mother's: Cina; *Sil*.

Music (See MUSIC agg): Nux-v; Sep; Vio-o.
- Violin: Vio-o.

Night, of: Buf.
Noise (See NOISE, agg): Asar; Bor; Con; Kali-c; Op.
Nourishment, all kind of+: Ant-t.

AVERSIONS

Onions: Saba.
Oysters: Pho.
Persons, to certain: Am-m; Calc; Hep; Nat-c.
- **Sight, of:** Cic.
- **Who do not agree, with him:** Calc-s.

Pickles: Ab-c.
Places: Hep.
Play (child): Hep.
Plums: Bar-c.
Pork: Colch; Dros; Psor; Pul.
Potatoes: Alu; Cam; Thu.
Puddings: Pho; Ptel.
Religious, to opposite sex: Lyc; *Pul*; Sul.
Riding in carriage: Psor.
Salt food: Carb-v; Cor-r; *Grap*; Nat-m; Sele; Sep.
Saurkraut: Hell.
School, to: Calc-p; Nat-m.
Sitting: Iod; Lach.
Snuff: Spig.
Society: Anac; Nat-c; Stan; Syph.
Soup; Arn; Grap; Lyc; Rhus-t.
Sour things: See Acids.
Spoken to: Cham.
Sweets: Ars+; Bar-c; CAUS; *Grap*; Lac-c; Nit-ac; Radm; Senec; Sul.
Talk, to: See TACITURN.
Tea: Pho.
Thinking: Pho; Pho-ac.
Tabacco: Arn; *Calc*; IGN; Lob; Nat-m; *Nux-v*.
- **To his accustomed cigar:** Bro; Fer; *Ign*.

AVERSIONS

Touched: See Approached.
Veal: Zin.
Vegetables: Hell: Mag-c.
Water (See THIRSTLESS): Am-c; *Hyo*; *Nux-v*; *Stram*.
- **Cannot bear touch of it:** Am-c.
- **Pregnancy, during:** Pho.
- **Thinking of it agg:** Ham.
- **Thirst, with:** Hell.

Wine: LACH; Manc+; Merc; *Saba*; Sul.
Women: Dios; Lach; Pul.
- **Men, to:** Nat-m; Sep.
- **To her own sex:** Raph.

Work, for: Alo; Arg-n; Bap; Carb-v; Chel; *Chin*; CON; Cyc; GRAP; Ham; Lach; Meph+; Mill+; NAT-M; *Nux-v*; *Pho*; Pul; Psor; Rhod+; Rhus-t; Sul; Zin-chr.
- **Customary:** Sep.

Writing, for: Hyds; Scil.

AWAKES

Anger, in: Cham; *Lyc*.
Anxious: Lyc; Spo.
Bed moving, as if from: Lac-c.
Brain, shock in, with: Coca.
Called, as if: Rhod; Sep.
Coldness of hands and feet, from: *Carb-v*.
Confusion, in: Bov; Chin; Gel; Petr; Pho; Pul.
- **Children:** Aesc.

Cough, from: Hyo; Pul; Samb; Sul.
Dreams, from: Bell; Lach; Sil; *Sul*.

AWAKES

Erection with, and desire to urinate: Hep.
Exact hour: Sele.
Falling, as if: Guai.
Fever from: Bar-c; Nit-ac; Pho.
Frequently (cat naps): Alu; Bar-c; *Calc*; *Hep*; Mur-ac; Op; Pho; *Pul*; Rut+; *Sep*; *Sul.*
Fright, nightmare, etc. in: Arn; Bell; Bor; Cact+; Carb-v; *Cina*; Hyo; *Ign*; Lach; Lyc; Nat-m; Paeon; Sep; Sil; *Stram*; SUL; Thu; Tub; Zin.
• Menses, before: Sul-ac.
Heart
• Burning at, with: Benz-ac.
• Tremor, with: Merc.
Hunger, from: Lyc; Pho-ac; Psor.
Jerk, with a: Bell.
Nervous: Rhus-t.
Noise, from very slight: Asar; Calad; Nux-v; Sele.
Palpitation, with: Benz-ac; Calc; Merc; Merc-c; Nat-c; Radm; Sep.
Panting, with: Radm.
Perspiration, from: Ars; *Con.*
Pulse slow, with, at 11 p.m.: Ther.
Sad: Lyc.
Screaming: Stram; Sul.
Shocks, through body, from: Dig; Mag-m.
Singing: Sul.
Sleep, cannot again: Nux-v.
Someone were in room, as if, from: Mag-p.

AWAKES

Stupor, then: Hyo.
Suffocating: Kali-io; Samb; Spo; Val.
• Menses, during: Spo.
Tired (See SLEEP, unrefreshing): *Nat-m*; Pul; Rhus-t; *Syph.*
Too early: *Kali-c*; *Nat-c*; Nit-ac; Nux-v; Pic-ac; *Ran-b*; Sul.
Too late: *Calc*; Calc-p; Grap; *Nux-v*; Sep; Sul.
Trembling: Ign; Ver-a.
• Heart of, with: Merc.

AWAKENING

AGG (Mental symptoms): Calc; LACH; *Lyc*; *Stram*; Zin.
After AGG (General): Amb; Am-m; *Ap*; *Ars*; *Bell*; Calc; *Chin*; Caus; Hep; Hyo; Kali-bi; LACH; Lyc; Lycps; Nat-m; Nit-ac; *Nux-v*; Onos; *Op*; *Pho*; *Pul*; Sele; Sep; Spo; Stram; *Sul*; Tarn; Tub; Val.
AMEL: Pho; Radm; Sabal; Sep; Val.
And falling to sleep, both AGG: Stan.

AWKWARDNESS (mental, physical) drops things etc: Aeth; *Agar*; *Amb*; Anac; AP; Bar-c; *Bov*; Calc; Cam+; CAPS; Caus; *Hell*; Ign; Ip; Lach; Lol-t; Mos; Nat-m; Tarn.
Pregnancy, during: Calc.

AXILLAE: Carb-an; Carb-v; *Hep*; Pho; Sep; Sil; Sul.
Abscess: Hep; *Lyc*; Merc; Nit-ac; *Pho*; Rhus-t; Sil.
• Delivery, after: Rhus-t.

AXILLAE

Ache, in: Latro.
Acne: Carb-v.
Alternately: Colch.
Boils: Lyc; Pho; Sep.
Bubbling: Colch.
Burning, pressure: Grap.
Cancer: Ast-r.
Eruptions, in: Elap; Lyc; Nat-m; Psor; Sep.
Excoriation: Carb-v; Grap; Mez; Sep; Sul.
Glands, enlarged: Ast-r; Bar-c; Hep; Lach; LYC; *Nit-ac*; Pho-ac; *Sil*; Sul.
- Breast, pain in, with: Lact-ac.
- Hard: Ast-r; Carb-an; Iod; Sil.

Herpes: Carb-an.
Itching: Pho; Sang; *Sul*.
Lump, bluish, hard, in: Calc-p.
Menses before, agg: Sang.
Scurfs, scabs, in: Nat-m.
Stitches: Caus; Dros; Lyc; Sul.
- Below, left: Stan.

Sweat: Bry; Calc; Dul; Kali-c; *Lapp*; Nat-m; Petr; Rhod; Sele; *Sep*; Sil: Sul.
- Brown: Lac-c.
- Cold: Lapp.
- Garlicky: Lach; Sul.
- Offensive: Hep; Lapp; Lyc; Nat-s; Nit-ac; Petr; Sil; Sul.
- Onions like: Bov; Kali-p.
- Red: Lach; Nux-m.

Tumours: Ars-io; Bar-c.
Ulcers: Bor.

BACK

BACK: AGAR; Ars; Aur; *Bell*; CALC; Chin-s; *Cimi*; Cocl; Gel; Hypr; Kali-c; *Lach*; Nat-m; Nat-s; *Nux-v*; PHO; Pho-ac; *Pic-ac*; *Rhus-t*; Sec; SIL; *Sul*; Zin.

Right: Calc; Cic; Flu-ac; *Sul*; Zin.
- To left: Calc-p; Cocl; Kali-p; Sul; Tell.

Left: Dros: Glo; Sil.
- To right: Bell; Cund; Nat-c; Ox-ac.

Alternating sides: Agar; Bell; *Berb*; Calc; Calc-p; Kali-bi; Kalm.

Abdomen, to: Vario.
Changing, here and there: Berb; Cimi; Kali-bi.
Chest, into: Arn; Berb; Cam; Kali-n; Laur; Petr; Samb; Sars.
- Right: Aco; Calc-p; Kali-c; Lyc; Merc; Sep.
- Left: Bar-c; *Bry*; Mez; Plat; Zin.

Downward: Agar; Pul; Stram.
Forward from
- Scapular region: Bry.
- Left: Pho; Sul; Zin.
- Lumber region: *Berb*; Cham; Kali-c; Kre; SABI.
- Pelvis, around: Sabi; Sep; Vib.

Genitals, to: Kre; Sul.
Stomach, to: Berb; Cup.
Thighs, down: Berb; Caus; Cimi; Hep; Kali-c; Vib.
- Stools agg: Rhus-t.

Upward: Ars; Gel; Lach; Lil-t; Nit-ac; Pho; Radm; Sul; Zin; Val.

BACK

BACK, upward
- Occiput to, from sacrum: Ol-j.

Uterus, to: Sep; Vib.

Ache: *Eup-p*; *Phyt*; Pic-ac; Sanic; Stap; Vario; Zin.
- Chill, with: Caps.
- Colic in abdomen, with: Sars.
- Feet, to: Kob.
- Leucorrhoea
  - amel: Eupi.
  - with: Alet.
- Menses
  - before: Asar.
  - start, at: Jab.
  - with: Mag-m.
- Palpitation, with: Tub.
- Prostraction, with: *Berb*.
- Sexual excess, from: Symp.
- Stools, hard, after: Fer.
- Takes the breath away: Asar.
- Work, cannot: Aesc+; Asaf.
- Wrestling, from: Symp.

Acne: Carb-v; Rum.

Air, warm, streaming up to head, as if: Ars.

Alternating, with headache: Aco; Alo; Alu; Bro; Ign; Meli; Sep.

Bandaged, as if: Pul.

Bar on, as though a: Ars; Lach.

Bed early in, agg: Nat-m; Stap.

Bending
- Backward
  - agg: Calc-p; Chel; Cimi; PLAT.
  - amel: Ign; Petr; Rhus-t.
- Forward agg: Pic-ac.

BACK

Blood boils: Carb-an; Caus; Grap; Thu.

Blow or sudden shock: Bell; Cic; *Sep*; Stan.

Boiling water along: Ust.

Breaking, broken, pain as if: Arn; *Bell*; *Eup-p*; Ham; *Kali-c*; Lyc; Mag-s+; Nat-m; *Pho*; Senec.
- Piles, with: Bell.

Breathing deep agg: Colo.

Bubbling sensation: Lyc; Petros; Tarx.

Burning, heat: Agar; Alu; *Ars*; Bap; Carb-an; Mag-m; *Pho*; Sec; Sil; *Sul*.
- Coition, after: Mag-m; Merc.
- Downward: Calc-p.
- Upward: Bap; Pho.
- Walking in open air agg: Sil.

Catching, in: Dios.

Chair, leaning on
- Agg: *Agar*; *Plb*; *Ther*.
- Amel: Eupi; Sarr.

Chill, coldness: Cact; Caps; *Eup-p*; Gel; Lach; Merc; Nat-m; Nat-s; Nux-v; *Pul*; *Sil*; *Sul*; *Ver-a*.
- Down: *Agar*; Canth; Eup-p; Lac-c; Pho; *Pul*; Stram; Val.
- Up: Arg-n; Calc-p; *Lach*: Ol-j; Ox-ac; *Sul*.
  - and down: Eup-p; Gel; Ip; Pul; Sul.
- Itching, then: Am-m.
- Sudden: Croc.
- Urinating, after: Sars.

BACK

Coition, emission
- Agg: Fer: Kob; Mag-m; Nat-m; *Nit-ac*; Sabal; Stap; Sul+.
- Amel: Zin.

Cold
- Air spreading on: Agar.
- Water trickles down or spurts: Caps; Lyc; *Pul*; Vario.

Colic, with: Sars.

Contraction: Cimi; Hyd-ac; *Rhus-t*.

Coughing agg: *Bell*; *Bry*; Kali-bi; Nat-m; Sep.

Cramps: Arg-n; Caus; *Chin*; Led; Mag-m; Mag-p.
- Rising from sitting agg: Led.
- Walking agg: Mag-m.

Crawling: Euon; Lac-c; *Pho*; Sec.
- Cold: Ars; Lac-c.

Cyst, on: *Pho*.

Draft of air agg: Sumb.

Drawing: Card-m; Cimi; Nux-v; Stram.

Drinking agg: Caps.

Eating
- Agg: Kali-c.
- Amel: Kali-n.

Emaciated: Nux-v; Plb; Tab+; Thu.

Eructation amel: Sep; Zin.

Everything affects or agg: Kali-c; Lach; Sep.

Flatus
- Felt in+: Rhod.
- Passing amel: Berb; Pic-ac; Rut.

Heaviness: Bar-c; Cimi; Kali-c.
- Stooping, after: Bov.

Itching: Ant-c; Caus; Mez; Nit-ac; Sul.

Jarring agg: *Grap*; Thu.

Kidneys agg: Cadm; Senec; Solid.

Laughing agg: *Cam*; Con; Pho.

Lifting agg: Ant-t; *Grap*; Lyc.

Lying on
- Abdomen Amel: Acet-ac; Nit-ac; Sele.
- Back
  - agg: Colo; Pul.
  - amel: Kali-c; Nat-m; Pho; Rut.
- Hard surface, amel: Kali-c; *Nat-m*; *Rhus-t*; *Sep*.
- Pillow, amel: *Carb-v*; Sep.

Menses
- Amel: Senec.
- During, agg: Bry; Caus; Sul.
- Start of+: Jab

Mental exertion agg: Cham; Con; Nat-c; *Pic-ac*.

Motion, walking
- Agg: Aesc; Agar; *Kali-c*; Mur-ac; Ran-b; Rut.
- Amel: Arg-m; Arg-n; Dul; Pho-ac; Tab.

Move must, but no amel: Lach; Pul.

Muscles
- Atrophy: See EMACIATION.
- Paralysed: Cup; Gel; Led.

Night agg: Abro.

Numbness: Aco; Agar; *Berb*; Bry; Kali-bi; *Ox-ac*; Plat; Sep.
- Prickling: Ox-ac.

BACK

Nursing, while agg: Cham; Crot-t; Pul; Sul.

Pain
- Palpitation, with+: Tab.
- Spreads like a fan upwards: Lach; Nat-s.
- Takes the breath: Asar.

Plug, lump, nail, etc. sensation: Anac; *Arn*; Berb; *Carb-v*; Cinb; Pho.

Pressure
- Agg: Agar; *Bell*; *Chin-s*; Cimi; Pho.
- Amel: *Bry*; *Dul*; KALI-C; *Nat-m*; Rhus-t; Rut; *Sep*.
- By the end of stick amel: Sep.

Pulling agg: Dios.

Raising arm agg: Grap; Nat-m; Rhus-t; Sanic.

Rat running up, as if: Sul.

Riding in carriage agg: Calc-f: *Nux-m*; Petr.

Rising, from sitting agg: Led.

Sharp, darting, shooting: Kali-c; Nat-m; Ox-ac.

Short, as if: Agar; Aur; Hyo; Lyc; Sul.

Sit must, while turning in bed: Bry; *Nux-v*.

Sitting
- Agg: Agar; *Arg-m*; Arg-n; Calc; Kob; Rhus-t; *Sep*; Sul; Val; *Zin*.
- Down, when, agg: Zin.
- Erect agg: Kali-c; Lyc; Sul.

Spasms: Sec.

Spots, in agg: Agar; *Alu*; Caus;

BACK, spots, in agg ..
Chel; Chin; Kali-bi; *Lach*; Nit-ac; Ox-ac; *Pho*; Pho-ac; Plb; Rhus-t; Thu; Zin.

Sprained, easily as if: Calc; Grap; Lyc; Rhus-t.

Standing amel: Arg-n; Caus; Mur-ac; Sul.

Stiff: Agar; BERB; CAUS; Cimi; Dul; Kali-c; Led; Lyc; *Nux-v*; Pul; Rhus-t; Sanic; SEP; Sil; Stram; SUL.
- Ascends: Ars.
- Bend backwards, cannot: Stram.
- Menses, before: Mos.
- Painful: Caus; Rhus-t; Sanic.
- Side, One: Guai.
- Stools
  - agg: Fer.
  - amel: Asaf.
- Turns whole body to look around: Sanic.

Stooping
- Agg: Agar; Sep.
- Inability: Bor.
- Prolonged agg: Nat-m.
- Straightening, after agg: Nat-m.

Struck with hammer, as if: See Blow.

Stumbling agg: Sep.

Swallowing agg: Caus; Kali-c; *Rhus-t*.

Threads, extending to limbs (arms, legs), as if: Lach.

Throbbing, pulsating: Bar-c; Bell; Lyc; Nat-m; Pho; Sep; Sil; Thu.

BACK

Throwing shoulders backward amel: Cyc.

Tumour, peduncle, with: Con.

Turning, least, agg: Sanic.

Urination
- Before agg: Grap; *Lyc*.
- During agg: Ant-c; Ip; Kali-bi; Sul.
- After
  - agg: Caus; *Syph*.
  - amel: *Lyc*; Med.
- Delayed agg: Grap; Nat-s.

Walking: See Motion

Weak: Arg-n; Ars; Bar-c; Calc; *Cocl*; Grap; Kali-c; Nat-m; Nux-v; Pho; Pho-ac; Pic-ac; Sele; Sep; Sil; Zin.
- Coition after: Nat-p.
- Leucorrhoea, during: Con; Grap.
- Ovarian pain, with+: Abro.
- Too, to hold body: Ox-ac.
  - whooping cough, in: Ver-a.

Wrestling agg: Symp.

Writing, while or continuous agg: Lyc; Mur-ac; Sep.

Yawning agg: Calc-p; Plat.

BAD

Feels good and bad by turns: Alu; Psor.

Inheritance: Buf.

News, ailments from: Alum; Ap; *Calc*; Calc-p; Cic; *Gel*; Ign; Lyss; Med; Nat-m; Pall; Pho-ac+; Pul; Sul; Tarn.
- Fear of+: Ast-r.
- Tremors, nervous, from: Alum.

Part takes everything in: Anac; Bov; Caps; Cocl; Nat-m; Nux-v; Pul; Sanic+; Stap; Ver-a.

BALDNESS: See HEAD.

BALL, lump, knot, etc: *Arn*; Asaf; *Bry*; Cham; Chin; Con; Gel; *Ign*; Kali-c; Kali-m; Kob; Lac-c; LACH; Lil-t; Lyc; Mar-v; Merc-d; Merc-i-r; Mos; Nat-m; Nat-s; Nit-ac; Nux-m; *Nux-v*; Plant; Pho; *Pul*; Rhus-t; Senec; SEP; Ust; *Val*; Zin.

Cold, running through bowels: Buf.

Hard: Nux-m.

Hot: Carb-ac; Lyc; Phyt; Raph.
- Cold, alternating with: Lyc.

BAND: See CONSTRICTION.

BANDAGED feeling: Pic-ac; Plat; Tril.

BANDAGING AMEL: *Arg-n:* Bry; Lac-d; *Mag-m*; Pic-ac; Tril.

BARBER'S ITCH: See under ITCH.

BARKING (like a dog): Bell; Canth.

BAROMETER: Merc; *Pho*; *Rhod.*

BASHFUL: See ANTHROPOPHOBIA.

BATHING

Aversion, to or from AGG: *Am-c*; *Ant-c*; Calc; Calc-s; Clem; Phys; Psor; Radm; Rhus-t; Sep; Sil; Spig; SUL.

AMEL: Aco; Ap; *Ars*; *Asar*; Buf; Bur-p; Calc-s; Caus; Cep; Euphr; *Pul*; Spig.

BATHING
Cold
- AGG: *Ant-c*; Bels; Clem; Dul; Mag-p; Nux-m; *Rhus-t*; Sil; *Tub*; Urt.
- AMEL: Ap; Asar; Bels; Bry; Buf; Coc-c; Flu-ac; Hypr; Iod; Led; *Meph*; Nat-m; Phyt; Pul; Rat; Sep; Sul.

Eyes closes, when: Pho.
Face AMEL: Asar; Calc-s; Pho.
Hot AMEL: Anac; Chel; Lyss; Mag-p; Mez; Pyro; Radm; Rat; Stro.
Rivers, summer, in agg: Caus.
Sea, in
- AGG: *Ars*; Bro; *Mag-m*; *Rhus-t*; Sep.
- AMEL: Med.

Steam AGG: Lyss.
BEADS like, swelling etc: Aeth; Am-c; Ap; Iod; *Nat-m*; Pho.
Glands: See GLANDS.
BEARING down: See PAIN, pressing
BEAUTIFUL, things look: Sul.
BECLOUDED: See DULL.

BED
Aversion, to: See AVERSION.
Desire to remain in: Arg-n; Hyo.
- Trifle indisposition from+: Arg-n.

Falling out of, as if: Arg-n; Ars.
Getting out of
- AGG: Am-m; *Bry*; Calc; CARB-V; Cimi; Cocl; Con;

Ign; *Lach*; *Pho*; *Pul*; *Rhus-t*; Sul.
- AMEL: Aur; Dul; Ign; Pul; Sep.

Hard, sensation: ARN; *Bapt*; Con; Dros; Gel; Kali-c; Nux-v; Pho; Plat; *Pyro*; *Rhus-t*; *Sil*; Til.
Heat of AGG: Dros; *Merc*; Op; Psor; Pul; Sabi; Sec; *Sul*.
Hot, as if: Op.
Leaves: Cham; Grap; Lac-c; Led; Merc; Ver-a.
Lumps in: Arn; Mag-c.
Lying, in
- AGG: Alu; AMB; Calc; Carb-an; *Chel*; Chin; *Dros*; *Fer*; Hell; *Hep*; Hyo; *Iod*; Kali-c; LACH; *Lyc*; *Merc*; *Nit-ac*; PHO; PUL; Rum; Sang; SEP; SIL; SUL.
- AMEL: Am-m; *Bry*; Caus; Cic; Cocl; Kali-c; Hep; Mag-m; Mang+; NUX-V; Pyro; Scil; Stan.

Moving, as if: Lac-c.
Occupied by whole body, as if: Pyro.
Rising from AMEL: Pho-ac; Pul.
Sinking under him, as if: Bap; Bell; *Bry*; Calc-p; Chin-s; Kali-c; Lach; Lyc; Rhus-t.
Sitting up in AMEL: *Kali-c*; Samb.
Sliding down, in: Ap; Ars; Bap; Chin; Colch; Hell; *Hyo*; *Mur-ac*; Tab; Zin.
Small, too, to hold him: Sul.

BED

Sores (See ULCERS): Arn; Chin; *Flu-ac*; Grap; Lach; Petr; Sep; Sil; Sul-ac.
- Children, in: Cham; Sul.
- Early: Val.

Turning over in
- AGG: Bell; Cact; Calad; Carb-v; Con; Lac-c; NUX-V; *Pul*; Sang; Stap; *Sul*; Zin.
- AMEL: Nat-m.
- Rises for: Bry; NUX-V.

Wetting: Ap; Arg-n; Arn; Ars; BELL; *Calc*; *Caus*; Cina; Equi; Fer; Grap; Lac-c; Kre; Mag-p; *Merc*; Nat-m; Nit-ac; PUL; *Rhus-t*; Sabal; Sec; Sep; *Sil*; SUL; Syph; Tab; Tub; Verb; Vio-t.
- Adults, of: Kali-c.
- Catheterisation, from: Mag-p.
- Cause, without any, except habit: Equi.
- Children, weakly, in: Chin; Kali-p; Thyr.
- Exertion, from any+: Sabal.
- Head, blow on, from: Sil
- Menses, during+: Hyo.
- Moon, full agg: Cina; Psor.
- Morning: Carb-v.
- Old men: Apoc; Benz-ac; Kali-p; Sec.
- Pregnancy, in: Pod.
- Sleep, during
  - first: *Caus*; Kre; Pho-ac; Sep.
  - later part: Chlo-hyd.
- Waking difficult: Bell; Chlo-hyd; *Kre*.
- Worms, from+: Sil.

BEES STINGING
- AGG: Led; Urt.
- As if: Ap; Gel.

BEHIND, as if

Abyss: Kali-c.

Someone is, or desire to look: Anac; Bro; Crot-h; Led; Med; Sanic; Tub.

Someone whispering: Med.

BENDING

Backwards, stretching limbs
- AGG: Aco; *Calc*; CHAM; Chel; Cinb; COLCH; Iod; Kalm; Merc-c; PLAT; PUL; Radm; *Ran-b*; RHE; RHUS-T; *Sep*; STAP; *Sul*; *Thu*.
- AMEL: Alet; *Alu*; ANT-T; Arn; Bell; *Calc*; Cham; Chel; Cocl; *Dios*; Flu-ac; *Guai*; Hep; Hypr; *Ign*; Lach; Lyss; *Nux-v*; Plb; Pul; Rhus-t; Sabi; Sec; Seneg.

Forwards, or doubling up AMEL: Aco; *Calc*; Caps; Caus; Cham; Chin; Cimi; *Colo*; Grap; *Kali-c*; Lil-t; Lyc; Mag-m; *Mag-p*; Merc-c; Par-b; Plat; Pul; *Rhe*; *Rhus-t*; Sec; *Sep*; *Sul*; Thu; Tril.

Forward and backwards
- AGG: *Chel*; Cof.
- AMEL: Tril.

Prolonged AMEL: Pul; Rhus-t; Scil.

Sideways AGG: Bell; Calc; Kali-c; Nat-m.

BEREAVEMENT: *Amb*; Plat.

BERI BERI: Ars; *Elat*; Rhus-t.

BESIDES HIMSELF
Frantic, madness, from pain etc: ACO; Aur; Calc; CHAM; *Cof*; Hep; Hyo; Lyc; Nat-m; *Nux-v*; Stram; Ver-a.

Walking, someone : Calc.

BEWILDERED, things look strange, loss of sense of location:
Apoc+; ARG-N; Bap; Bell; *Bry*; *Calc*; *Cann*; Carb-v; *Cocl*; Crot-h; Flu-ac; *Glo*; Grap; Hell; Hyo; *Lach*; Med; Merc; Nat-m; *Nux-m*; Onos; *Op*; PETR; PLAT; Rhus-t; *Sep*; *Sil*; Stram; Stry; Tub; Val.

Children+: Aesc.

Washing face amel: Ars; Pho.

BILATERAL: See SYMMETRICAL.

BILE DUCTS: Am-m; Chel; Gel; Merc-d; Nat-p; Rhe.

BILHARZIASIS: Ant-t.

BILIOUS (See YELLOWNESS):
Chio; Eup-p; Nat-s; Sang; Tarx.

BIRTHMARK, naevi: Arn; Ars; Calc; Calc-f; Carb-an; Carb-v; Flu-ac; Lach; *Lyc*; Pho; Plat; Radm; *Sep*; *Sul*; Thu; Ust.

Flat+: Mur-ac.

Smooth, mottled: Con; Pho; Sep; Sul.

Spidery: Carb-v; Lach; *Plat*; Sep; Thu.
- Red; Med.

BITE, impulse to: *Bell*; Buf; Cup; Hyo+; Lyss+; Phyt; Pod; Sec; Stram.

BITES
Cheeks, or tongue
- Chewing or talking
  - when not: Dios.
  - while: Buf; Caus; *Cic*; Hyo; *Ign*; *Nit-ac*; Ol-an.
- Night, sleep in: Cic; Pho.

Fingers, hand, etc: Aco; Aru-t; Med; Op; Plb.
- Sleep, in: Elap.

Objects, any: Buf.

Pillow: Lyc; Pho.

Spasms, in: Art-v; Buf; Caus; Cup; Oenan; Op.

Spoons, pots etc: Ars; Bell; Hell.

Tongue, tip of, during sleep: Ther.

BITING, chewing
AGG: Alo; *Am-c*; Am-m; Bry; Chin; Euphr; Hep; Ign; Meny; *Merc*; *Mez*; Nat-m; Nit-ac; Pho; Pod; Pul; RHUS-T; *Sep*; *Stap*; *Verb*; Zin.

AMEL: Bry; Cocl; Cup-ac; Seneg; *Stap*.

Bug like: Kali-bi; Syph; Tell

Fleas as of: Mez; Stap; Syph; Tab; Visc.

BLACK, dark (discharges, discolouration of skin, etc):
Ant-t; Arn; *Ars*; Bap; Carb-ac; Carb-v; *Chin*; Crot-h; Cyc; Elap; Fer; Gel; Hell; Kre; *Lach*; Mag-m; *Merc*; Merc-c; Nux-v; Op; Pho; Plb; *Sec*; Stap; Stram; Sul-ac; Ver-a.

Blue: See ECCHYMOSIS.

Spots: Ars; Crot-h; Lach; Vip.

BLACKWATER FEVER: *Ars*; Crot-h; Lyc.

BLADDER (Urinary)

Affections in general: Aco; Ap; Bell; Benz-ac; *Canth*; *Caus*; Colo; *Dul*; Equi; *Hyo*; Lach; *Lyc*; *Merc-c*; *Nux-v*; PUL; *Rut*; *Sabal*; Sars; Sep; Stap; *Sul*; Uva.

Aching: Caps; Terb.
- Heavy: Sabal.

Atony: Ars; CAUS; Mur-ac+; Op; Plb; Stan.
- Old age: Ars+; Stram.
- Retention long, from: Canth.

Back, to: Sars.

Bleeding: Terb.

Burning: Berb; CANTH; *Caps*; Cep; *Merc-c*; Pul; Rhe; Senec; Terb; Zin-ar.
- Neck: Canth; Zin-ar.

Bursting: Par-b; Sanic+; Zin.

Calculi: Benz-ac; Berb; Calc; Canth; Lyc; Sars; Sep.

Cancer: Crot-h.

Chill, spreads from: Sars.

Coition, after: Cep.

Colds agg: Caus; Dul; Pul; Sul.

Cold, sensation, in: Lyss; Sabal.
- Genitals, extending, to: Sabal.

Coughing agg: Caps; Ip.

Cramp: Berb; Caps; Carb-v; Mez; Nux-v; Pru-sp; Pul; Sars.
- Operation after: Colo; Hypr.

Crawling, in: Sep.
- Urination, after: Lyc.

Cutting: Aeth+; Pall; Terb; Thu.
- Stools, amel: Pall.

BLADDER

Desire for urination postponed, if agg: Pul; Sul-ac.

Empty, sensation, in: Stram.
- Distended, when: Lycps.
- Involuntary urination after: Helo.
- Pain, with: Calc-p.

Falls to side lain on, sensation: Pul; Sep.

Fullness, sensation: Dig; Equi; Pall; Rut.
- Desire to urinate, without: Ars; Caus.
- Motion, up and down, with: Rut.
- Sensation, without: Lac-d.
- Urination
  - after: Dig; Eup-pur.
  - scanty, with: Pall.

Griping: Canth.

Heaviness: Canth; Lyc; Nat-m; Pul; Sep.

Inflamed: Aco; Ap; Bell; Canth; Cub+; Equi; Lach; Lyc; Polyg; Sars; Solid; *Terb*.
- Prostate hypertrophy, from+: Sabal.

Injury, operations, after: Arn; Calend; *Stap*.

Insensible: Stan.

Irritable: Bell; Buchu; Nux-v; Sabal; Stap.

Itching in, with urging to urinate at night: Sep.

Lump in: Kre; Lach.

Lying on abdomen amel: Chel.

BLADDER

Navel, alternating with: Terb.
Neck of: Bell; Canth; Merc-c.
Paralysis: *Ars*; Caus; Dul; *Gel*; Hyo; *Nux-v*; Op; Plb; Stram; Zin.
- Hysterical: *Zin*.
- Laparotomy, after: Op.
- Old people: Ars.
- Parturition after: Ars; Caus.

Pelvis and thighs to, after urination: Pul.
Rectum, with: Amb.
Retention of urine: See Under URINE.
Sitting
- Agg: Card-m.
- Amel: Con.

Sore: Ap; *Canth*; *Equi*; *Terb*.
- Urination, profuse, with: Stic.

Spermatic cord, to: Lith.
Stabbing in region of: Chel.
Stone rolling sensation: Pul.
Tenesmus: Agar; Ars; Bell; Cann; CANTH; *Dig*; Dul; Equi; Lil-t; MERC-C; *Par-b*; Plb; Pru-sp; Sul; *Terb*; Thu.
- Menses during: *Tarn*.
- Rectum, with: Erig; Canth; Caps; Merc-c.
- Stool, during: Caps; Nux-v.
- Vomiting, purging, micturition, with: *Crot-h*.

Thick: Dul.
Throbbing, pulsating: Dig.
Ulceration, suppuration: Petr; *Pul*; Sep; *Sul*.
Urging to urinate, when not attended to agg: Pul; Sul-ac.

BLADDER

Walking
- Agg: Con; Pru-sp; Pul.
- Amel: Ign; Terb.
- Open air in, amel: *Terb*.

Weakness: Caus; Hep; Mag-m; Mur-ac; Op.
- Parturition, after: Ars; Caus.

Worm sensation, in: Bell; Sep.
BLAMES himself: Op.
BLAND: See DISCHARGES.

BLEEDING

AGG: *Chin*; Fer; Ip; Nat-m; Pho-ac; Stic; Sul-ac.
AMEL: Ars; Bov; Buf; Calad; Card-m; Fer; Fer-p; Ham; Lach; Meli; Sars; Sele.
Nose, from AMEL: Bro.
Prolonged AGG: Plat.
Sequelae, chronic+: Stro.
Slight, causes great AGG: Buf; Carb-an; *Chin*; Ham; Hyds; Sec.
Suppression, of AGG: Bur-p.
BLINDLESS: See under VISION.
Day: See under DAY.
Night: See NIGHT, blindness.
BLISTERS: See ERUPTIONS, vesicles.
BLOATED: See PUFFINESS.
BLONDES: Bro; *Calc*; Pul.

BLOOD

Boils: Anthx; Arn; Crot-h; Lach; Pho; Pyro; Thu+.
Blisters: Sec.
Cannot look at: *Alu*; Nux-m; Plat.

BLOOD

Circulation stands still: Aco; Lyc; *Saba*; Sep; Zin.

Clot would not, and wound would not heal: Visc.

Cold, as if: Ver-a.

Gushing, as if: Ox-ac.

Hot, as if: Med; Sec.

Restlessness in: Iod.

Rushes of: Bell; Fer; Glo; Lach; Sang; Spo; Sul.
- Downward: Aur; Meph; Thyr.
- Upward: Aco; Arn; Bell; Bry; Fer; Glo; Kali-io; Meli; Pho; Sang; Stro.

Stagnated, as if: Carb-v; Lyc.

Stasis: Carb-v; Ham; Pul; Sep; Sul.

Streaked: See DISCHARGES, blood streaked.

Watery and mixed with clots: See HAEMORRHAGES.

BLOOD PRESSURE

High: Aur; Bar-c; Bar-m; Cof; Con; Cratae; Glo; Iod; Lycps; Scop; Stro; Sumb; Tab; Uran-n+; Ver-v; Visc.
- Diastolic low, and: Bar-m.

Low: Cact; Gel; Naj; Radm; Ther.

Sudden rise of: Cof.

BLOOD SEPSIS (septic conditions, fevers etc): Ail; Am-c; Anthx; *Arn*; ARS; *Bap*; *Bell*; Bry; Calc; *Carb-v*; *Chin*; Colch; Crot-c; *Crot-h*; Echi, Elap; *Fer*; Gel; Hyo; *Kali-c*; Kali-p; Kre; LACH; Lyc; *Merc*; Merc-cy; *Mur-ac*; Naj; *Nat-m*;

BLOOD SEPSIS ..
Nit-ac; Nux-v; *Pho*; *Pul*; Pyro; *Rhus-t*; Sec; Stram; *Sul*; Sul-ac; Tarn-c; Vario; Ver-a; Ver-v; Zin.

Adynamic: Elap; Pyro.

BLOOD VESSELS

Affections in general: Aco; Amy-n; Ap; *Arn*; *Bell*; CARB-V; Fer; *Flu-ac*; Gel; Glo; *Ham*; Hyo; *Lach*; Lyc; Nat-m; *Pho*; PUL; Sang; *Sec*; Sep; Sul; Sul-ac; *Thu*; Vip; Zin.

Bubble rolling through: See Shot rolling through.

Calcareous, deposit, in: Vario.

Cold feeling, in: ACO; ARS; Pyro; RHUS-T; Sul-ac; *Ver-a*.

Distended, full, varicose (See VEINS): Arn; *Ars*; Bell; Bels+; Calc; Calc-f; Carb-v; Card-m; *Flu-ac*; *Ham*; Lach; Lyc; Lycps; Plat; *Pul*; Sang; Sec; *Sep*; Stap; Sul; Vip; Zin
- Fever, during: Chin; Hyo; Led; Pul.
- Insanity
  - with: Arn; Ars; Flu-ac; Lach; Lyc; Sul; *Zin*.
  - followed, by: Anac; Ant-c; Arn; Ars; Bell; Caus; Hyo; Ign; Lach; Lyc; Nux-v; Pho; Sep; Sul; Ver-a.
- Knots and enlargements in: Sabi.
- Menses agg: Amb; Fer.
- Pregnancy, during: Fer; Mill; Pul; Tril; Zin.
- Tenderness, with: Ham; Merc-cy.

BLOOD VESSELS, distended
- Ulceration: Card-m+; Caus; Clem+; Ham; Lach; Lyc; *Pul*; Sec; Vip.

Heat, burning, in: *Ars*; Bry; Calc; Med; *Rhus-t*; Syph.

Inflamed, phlebitis: Aco; Ap; *Ars*; Chin; Kali-c; Ham; *Lach*; PUL; *Spig*; *Sul*; Vip.

- Forceps delivery, after: Cep.

Painful: *Ham*; *Pul*; Thu; Zin.

Shot rolling through the arteries, sensation: Nat-p.

Swelled: Ap; Paeon; *Pul*.

Vascular: Lach; Lyc; Thu; Tril; Zin.

Vibrate, as if: Phel.

Writhing in: Bell; Hyd-ac.

BLOODY: See DISCHARGES, bloody.

BLOWING NOSE
AGG: Arn; *Aur*; Calc; CHEL; Grap; HEP; Iod; Kali-bi; Lach; *Merc*; Pho; Pho-ac; *Pul*; Spig; SUL; Zin.

AMEL: *Mang*; Merc; Sil.

Inability in children: Am-c.

BLOWS, shocks, thrusts, crash, explosions, as from: Alo: Ap; Arg-m; Bell; CANN; Chin; Cic; Croc; Cup; Dig; *Glo*; Hell+; *Naj*; Nat-m; Pho; Spig; Sul+; Sul-ac; Tab; Tarn; Zin.

BLUISH, purple (discharges, discolouration of skin) etc: Aco; *Arn*; *Ars*; Bap; Cam; Carb-an; *Carb-v*; *Crot-h*; CUP; DIG; Elap; *Fer-p*; Kre; LACH; Laur; Mang; Merc-cy; *Mur-ac*; *Nux-v*; *Op*; Ox-ac; Rhus-t; Sec;

BLUISH PURPLE ..
Sil; Sul; *Tarn-c*; Thu; *Ver-a*; VER-V.

Affected parts: Carb-an; Lach; Sec.

Burning, with: Anthx; Ars; Lach.

Injury, from: *Arn*; Bell; Con; Lach; Pul; Sul-ac.

Spots: Arn; Ars; Crot-h; Hell; Lach; Led; Nux-m; Nux-v; Op; Pho; Pho-ac; Sec; Sul-ac.

- Red: Plb; Phyt.

BOARD
Like sensation or feel: Bap; Carb-an; Dul; Nux-m; Rhus-t; Tarn-c.

Lying on, as if: Bap; Sanic.

BOILING
As if: Am-m; Led; Ust.

Tea seems cold+: Cam.

Water, side lain on: Mag-m.

BOILS: Arn; *Bell*; Bels; Hep; *Lach*; *Lyc*; *Merc*; *Petr*; *Psor*; *Rhus-t*; Sil; Sul.

Blind: Fago; Lyc.

Blood: See BLOOD.

Body, all over: Bels+; Vio-t.

Crops, of: Echi; Sil; Sul; Syph.

Impotency, with: Pic-ac.

Injured places, on: Dul.

Mature, do not: Sanic.

Menses, at: Merc.

Periodical: Ars.

Receding: Lyc.

Recurring: Calc.

- Spring, every: Bell.

Scars, leave: Kali-io.

BOILS
Small and sore: *Arn*; Lapp; Pic-ac; Sec; Tub.
- Green: Sec.
- Menses, during: Med.

Succession of: Anthx; Arn; Sul.

BOLDNESS, daring, courageous:
Agar; *Ign*; Op; Tub.

Foolish: Calad.

BONES
Affections in general: Arg-m; ASAF; *Aur*; CALC; *Calc-f*; CALC-P; Chin; Cocl; Cup; Eup-p; Flu-ac; Hep; Kali-io; Lyc; MERC; Mez; *Nit-ac*; *Pho*; PHO-AC; Phyt; PUL; Pyro; Rhod; Rhus-t; *Rut*; Sil; Stap; *Sul*; Syph.

Band sensation: Con.

Bare, become: Ars; Asaf; Aur; Calc; Chin; Con; Hep; Lach; Lyc; Merc; Mez; Nit-ac; Pho-ac; Pul; Rut; Sabi; Sep; Sil; Stap; Sul.
- Necrosis, with: Both.

Breaking, bruised pains: *Arn*: Cocl; *Eup-p*; Hep; Nit-ac; Pul; Rut; Thu; Val.

Brittle, fractured, etc: Asaf; Buf; *Calc*; Calc-f; Calc-p; *Lyc*; *Merc*; Par; Pho-ac; Rut; SIL; *Sul*; Symp; Thu.

Burning: Euphor; Mez; Zin.

Caries: Ang+; Ars; *Asaf*; *Aur*; Calc; Calc-f; Con; *Flu-ac*; HEP; Kali-io; Lach; *Lyc*; Mang; MERC; Mez; Nit-ac; Pho; Pho-ac; Pul; Radm; SIL; Stap; Syph; Tell; *Ther*; Tub.

BONES, caries
- Sweat, profuse, with: Chin.

Cold, chilly feeling: *Aran*; Berb; Calc; *Eup-p*; Kali-io; Pyro; Ver-a.

Condyles, prominences: Arg-m; Cyc; Rhus-t; Sang; Ver-v.

Curvature, soft, etc: ASAF; CALC; Calc-io; CALC-P; Hep; *Lyc*; *Merc*; PHO; Pho-ac; Pul; Sep; *Sil*; *Sul*.

Cutting: Anac; Aur; Dig; Kali-m; Lach; Osm; Saba.

Deep, in long: Rut.

Exostoses: Arg-m; *Aur*; Aur-m; Calc; CALC-F; Hecla; Merc; Mez+; PHO; Pho-ac; *Sil*; Stap; Sul-io; Syph.
- Injury, after: Calc-f.
- Painful: Aur; Daph; Kali-io; Merc; Syph.
- Suppression of itch, after: Sul.
- Syphilitic: Flu-ac; Hep; Merc.

Fracture: See Brittle.
- Often: *Merc*.
- Union dealayed: Thyr.

Gnawing: *Bell*; Stro.

Growth defective: Agar; Calc; *Calc-p*; Fer; Pho-ac; Sil.

Heavy: Sul.

Inflammation: Sil.

Injury to: See under INJURIES.

Itching: Caus; Cocl; Cyc; Kali-m; Pho; Ver-a.

Jerk in: Asaf; Chin; Sil; Sul.

Large, as if: Mez.

Marrow: Am-c; Chel; Chin; Kali-c; *Lyc*; Mag-m; Naj; Ol-an; Op; Stro; Sul.

BONES, marrow
- Pain in: Chin.

Night agg: Aur; Kali-io; *Lyc*; MERC; Nit-ac; Pho-ac+; Sil+; *Syph*.

Non union: *Calc*; *Calc-p*; Pho-ac; Sil; Symp.

Ossification slow: Calc-p.

Painful, in general: Asaf; *Eup-p*; Kob; *Merc*; Nit-ac; Pho-ac; *Phyt*; Pul; *Pyro*; Rut; Zin.

Periosteum: Asaf; Flu-ac; Kali-io; Kali-n; Mang; Merc; Mez; Pho; *Pho-ac*; Phyt+; Rhod; Rut; Sul.
- Inflammation: Ars; Asaf; Aur; Calc; Calc-f; Con; Hep; Lach; Merc; Mez; Nit-ac; Pho-ac; Pul; Sep; Sil; Stap; Sul; Tell.
- Painful: *Merc*; Rhus-t.

Pinching: Pho-ac; *Verb*.

Pricking: Thu.

Rent asunder, tearing, shattered: Aur; Chin; Kali-c; Lach; Merc; Rhod; Spig.

Sawing: Pho; Sul; Syph; Tarn.

Scraping: *Chin*; *Pho-ac*; *Rhus-t*; Saba; Thu.
- Night, at: Pho-ac.

Sensitive: Mang; Nit-ac.

Skin near, pain: Cyc; Merc; Sang.

Spongy: Guai.

Squeezed, as if+: Alu.

Sticking, in: Arn; *Symp*.

Swashing, like a wave: Bell.

Tension: Bell.

BONES

Torn loose from flesh, as if: Ap; Bry; Dros; Lach; Nat-c; Ol-an; Pho-ac; *Rhus-t*; Rut.
- Blow, from: Ign.

Tuberculosis of: Dros; Pho; Pul; Stan.

Ulceration, deep+: Asaf.

Walk, must: Rut.

Weather changes agg: Am-c.

BOOKWORMS+: Cocl.

BOOTS, drawing of, AGG: Calc; Grap.

BORBORYGMY: See FLATUS, noisy.

BORING, grinding: See PAIN.

BORING into parts (nose, ears) AMEL: Aru-t; Chel; *Nat-c*; Pho; Spig; Thu.

BORROWS TROUBLE: Acet-ac; Ap; Bar-c; Calc; Sang.

BOUNDING internal (See ALIVE sensation): Croc; Ther; Thu.

BOWELS: See ABDOMEN and INTESTINES.

BRAIN: Aco; Arg-n; Bell; Bov; Calc; Dul; Hyo; Lach; *Nux-v*; Pho; Pic-ac; Stram; Sul; Syph; Tub; Zin.

Air, cold, blowing on, as if: Cimi.

Bandaged, as if: Bry; Lac-c; Nat-m; Nit-ac; Sul.

Bruised: Bap; *Chin*; Gel; Mur-ac; Phyt.

Burning heat: Aco; Bell; Canth; Glo; Med; *Pho*; Ver-a.
- Boiling water, as if: Aco.

BRAIN, burning heat
- Fiery: Hyd-ac.

Cloth, cold, around, as if: Glo; *Sanic*.

Cloud was going over: Hyd-ac.

Coldness: Mos; Pho.

Concussion: *Arn*; *Cic*; Hell; Hyo; *Hypr*; Nat-s; Op; Sul-ac; Zin.
- Headache, from: Kali-br.
- Knocking foot against anything, when: Bar-c.
- Mis-step, from: Led.

Contracted, hard, painful, as if: Laur.
- Relaxed, and, as if+: Lac-c.

Crazy feeling: Vario.

Degeneration, softening of: *Arg-n*; Aur; Bar-c; Caus; *Pho*; Plb; *Sil*; *Stry*; Syph; Zin; Zin-p.

Fag, weak, tired: Anac; Ap+; Bar-c; Bell; Calc; *Caus*; Gel; Kali-p; Lach; Lyc; *Nat-c*; *Nux-v*; PHO-AC; *Pic-ac*; *Plb*; *Psor*; Pul; Sil; Stap; Sul; *Zin*; Zin-p.
- Grief, from: Kali-br.
- Occiput, cold, with+: Pho.

Falls
- Down: Laur.
- Forehead from as if: Rat.
- Side lain on: Amb+; Phys.

Forehead and, empty space between, as if+: Caus.

Formication: Hyp.

Frozen, as if: Ind.

Full of fluid, as if: Cur.

Haemorrhage in: Aco; Bell; Calc; Gel; Ip; Lach; Op.

Heavy: Form; Hypr; Mag-c.

BRAIN

Hot vapour coming from below, as if: Ant-t; Sars; Sul.
- Swallowing, when: Form.

Humming, roaring in: Kre; Lach; Pho.

Knocking against skull, as if: Chin.

Large, as if: Cimi; Form; *Glo*.

Liquid, as if: Mag-p.

Loose, as if: Aco; Amb+; Am-c; Bar-c; *Bell*; *Chin*; Glo; Guai+; Hyo+; Hypr+; Kali-c; Kali-m; Laur; Nux-m; NUX-V; Rhus-t; *Spig*; Sul; Sul-ac; Tub.
- Sitting quiet amel+: Sul-ac.
- Stooping, on: Nat-s.
- Walking, on: Cyc.

Lump on right side, as if: Con.

Marble, feels as if changed to: Cann.

Metal striking on, as if+: Phel.

Needles at: Tarn.

Numb: Ap; Buf; Calc; Con; Grap; Hell; Kali-br; Plat.

Paralysis of, incipient: Am-m+; LYC; Zin.
- Sensation of, after emission: Sil.

Parts were changing, as if: Mag-p.

Pressed out of forehead, as if: Bell; Lach.

Raised several times in succession, as if: Thu.
- Stooping, on: Kob.

Rolling over: Plant.

Shattered, as if: Rhus-t.

BRAIN
 Softening, of: See Degeneraion.
 Spoon, stirred with, as if: Arg-n; Iod.
 Stitches, at: Alu.
 Swashing
  • To and fro, as if: Chin; Hell.
  • Water, as of: Hyo.
 Torn, as if: Cof; Stap.
 Tumour: Arn; *Bar-c*; Bell; Calc; *Con*; Glo; Grap; *Kali-io*; *Plb*; Sep.
 Turned over, as if+: Plant.
 Waving in, as if: Cimi; Glo; Phys.
 Wrapped, as if: Cyc; Op.
BRANNY: See DESQUAMATION.
BREAKFAST
 AGG: Carb-v; CHAM; Nat-m; *Nat-s*; NUX-V; PHO; Sep; Thu; Zin.
 AMEL: Calc; Croc; Iod; Myr; Nat-s; Stap.
BREAKING
 Broken: See PAIN.
 Things: Ap; Stram; Tub.
BREATH
 Cold: *Cam*; *Carb-v*; Chin; Cist; Pho; VER-A.
 Desire to take deep: See RESPIRATION, Deep.
 Holding
  • AGG: Cact; *Kali-n*; Led; Merc; *Spig*.
  • AMEL: *Bell*.
 Hot: *Bell*; Cham; Cof; Med; Nat-m; Rhus-t; Saba; Stro; Zin.

BREATH, hot
 • As if: Radm
 • Burns, nostrils: Ptel; Rhus-t.
 Loss of, when standing in water: Nux-m.
 Offensive: Ail; Anac; ARN; *Ars*; *Aru-t*; Aur; Bap; CARB-V; *Cham*; Crot-h; Hell; Kali-chl; Kali-p; Kre; *Lach*; Meph; MERC; Merc-cy; *Nit-ac*; NUX-V; Plb; Pod; Pul; Pyro; Rhe; Spig; Sul; Tub; Ver-v.
 • Cheese, like rotten: Mez.
 • Constipation, with: Carb-ac.
 • Ether or chloroform like: Ver-v.
 • Garlicky: Petr; Tell.
 • Girls, at puberty: Aur;
 • Onion like : Asaf; Sinap.
 • Palpitation with: Spig.
 • Sour: Grap.
 • Unnoticed by himself: Bar-c.
 • Urine like: Grap.
 Stops
 • Coughing or drinking, on: Am-m; Anac.
 • Children in, when they are lifted: Calc-p.
 • Swallowing, when: Anac.
BREATHE AGAIN, cannot: Ap; Bell; Coca; Dros; Helo; Latro; Laur; Rum.
BREATHING
 Deeply
 • AGG: *Aco*; Arn; Ascl; *Bor*; BRY; Calc; Caus; Grap; *Kali-c*; Lyc; Merc; *Pho*; Ran-b; Rhus-t; Rum; Sabi; Sang; Scil; Spig; Sul.

BREATHING, deeply
- AMEL: Aco; Cann; *Colch*; Cup; *Ign*; Lach; Nat-m; Osm; Ox-ac; Seneg; Spig; *Stan*; Verb.

Hot air
- As if: *Trif.*
- Takes the breath away: Arg-n.

Irregular agg: Cact; Rum.

Sponge, dry, as if through: Spo.

Tube, metallic, as if through: Merc-c.

BREGMA: Ars; *Merc*; Zin-chr.

BRINY: See SALTY and FISHY.

BRITTLE, broken, feeling: Chel; Cup; Flu-ac; Par; Radm; Thu.

BRONCHIECTASIS, bronchorrhoea: All-s; *Ars*; Bacil; *Calc*; Cep; Cop; Eucal; Grind; *Hep*; Kali-bi; Kali-c; *Lyc*; Phel; *Pul*; Sil; STAN; Tub.

Senile+: Eucal.

BRONCHITIS: Ant-t; Ars; Bry; Calc; Dros; *Fer-p*; Hep; Hyds; Ip; Lyc; Nat-s; *Pho*; Pul; Sang; Senec; Sil; Spo; Stan; Stic; Sul.

Capillary: Ant-t; Bell; Carb-v; *Fer-p*; *Ip*; Seneg; Terb.

Children, drowsiness, with+: Tub.

Cold, from every: Mang.

Senile: Am-c; Ant-c; Ant-t; Ars; Cep; Kre; Seneg.

BROWNISH, rusty (discharges, discolouration of skin) etc: *Ars*; Bap; Berb; *Bry*; Carb-v; Chel; Hyo; Iod; Kre; Lyc; Lycps; Manc; *Nit-ac*; Op; Petr; Pho; *Rhus-t*; Sec; SEP; Stap; *Sul*; Thu; Ver-a.

BROWNISH
Spots: Crot-h; Iod; Lach; Lyc; Merc; Petr; Pho; Sanic; Sep; Sul; Thu.

BROWS: Bell; Caus; Kali-c; Nat-m; Par; Sele.

Aching: Stro.

Dandruff: Sanic.

Hair falling: *Kali-c*; Med; Plb; Sele.

Knits: Vio-o.

Outward, along: Cinb; Echi; Kali-bi; Mez; Vio-o.

Quivering between: Ang.

Swelling, hard, over: Sang.

Twitch: Cina; Echi.

Warts, on: Caus.

BRUISED: See PAIN, sore.

BRUNETTES: Nit-ac; Plat.

Firm-fibred+: Nux-v.

BUBBLES, sensation of: *Berb*; Nux-v; *Pul*; Rhe.

Air suppuration, with: Sul.

Bursting: Sul.

BUBO: Bad+; Bell; Carb-an; Cinb; Hep; Kali-io; Merc-i-r; Nit-ac; Phyt.

Neglected+: Carb-an.

Suppuration, stubborn: Merc-i-r.

BULLAE: Manc; Ran-sc; Syph.

BUNIONS: Agar; Benz-ac; Grap; Paeon; Rhod; Sil.

Pressure, amel+: Grap.

BURNING (See HEAT): ACO; AP; ARS; *Aru-t*; BELL; BRY; Buf; *Canth*; Caps; *Carb-v*; Caus; Euphr; Grap; Iod; *Iris*; Lyc;

BURNING ..

Mag-m; *Med*; Mez; *Nat-m*; *Nit-ac*; *Nux-v*; PHO; Pho-ac; Pic-ac; Pru-sp; PUL; Rat; RHUS-T; Saba; *Sang*; *Sec*; *Sep*; *Sil*; Spig; Spo; Stan; SUL; *Terb*; Zin.

Bathing, washing agg: Rhus-t; Sul.

Cold parts, in: Sec; Ver-v.

Dry, all symptoms agg: Bry.

Fiery: *Ap*; *Ars*; *Bell*; Carb-an; Guai; Kali-c; Kre; Mez; Pho; Radm; Spig; *Tarn-c*; *Tub*; Vesp.

Heat
- Agg: Rat; Zin-val.
- Amel: Alu; *Ars*; Caps; Carb-v; Lyc; Sec.

Hot iron: See under HOT.

Internal: Euphor; Merc-c; Mez.
- External coldness with: Ars; Kali-n; Ver-a.
- Itching, with: Mez.

Intolerable: Sabi.

Painful: Aco; ARS; Canth; Carb-v; *Caus*; Merc; Pho; Sul.

Parts
- Grasped with hand: *Caus*.
- Lain, on: Sul

Pepper like: Coc-c; Lach; Mez; Nat-s; Xanth.

Pricking: Ver-v.

Pungent, glowing: Cep; Rut; Tarn-c.

Raw, smarting, biting: Am-c; Aru-t; Berb; *Canth*; Caps; Carb-v; Erig; Hyds; Lyc; Manc; Ran-sc; Sinap; Sul; Sul-io.

BURNING

Shivering, with: Aco; Ars; Bry; Chin; Ip; Samb; Ver-v.

Spot, local: Agar; Glo; Ran-b; Sang; Sele; Sul; Ver-v.

Steam over, like: Pulex.

Stinging: Ant-c; AP; *Ars*; Berb; *Con*; *Dul*; *Glo*; Iris; Lyc; Mez; Nux-v; *Pho*; Pho-ac; Rhus-t; Sil; Urt.

BURNS and scalds: Ars; *Canth*; Carb-v; *Caus*; Ham; Kali-m; Kre; Pic-ac; Stram+; Urt.

Granulations, unhealthy: Petr; Plant+.

Ill effects of: Carb-ac; Caus.

Radium: Pho.

Sun: Bov; Cam; Canth; Kali-c; Ver-a.

Suppuration, with: Calc-s.

Vapour, hot, from: Kali-bi.

X-ray: Calc-f; Pho; Radm; X-ray.

BURNT, scalded, as if: ARS; Canth; Cyc; *Hyds*; *Hyo*; Iris; Lyc; *Mag-m*; Phyt; Plat; PUL; Ran-b; Sang; *Sep*; *Ver-a*; *Ver-v*.

BURROWING, digging: See PAIN.

BURSAE: See GANGLIA.

BURSTING: See PAIN.

BUSINESS

Failure: Amb; Cimi; Kali-br.

Worry: Acet-ac; Amb+; Caus; Kali-p; Lil-t; Nux-v; Pod.
- Though, prosperous: Psor.

BUSY, when (See OCCUPATION)

AMEL: Con; Cyc; Helo; Ign; Iod; Lil-t; Nat-c; Nux-v; *Sep*.

BUSY

Forgets, everything: Ant-c.
Restlessness: Ver-a.
BUTTOCKS: Grap; Pho-ac; Stap; Sul.
Abscess: Sul.
Boils: Pho-ac.
Burning: Merc.
Cold: Agar; Daph.
• Numb, and: Calc-p.
Cramp: Grap.
• Leg stretching agg: Sep.
Emaciated: Lathy.
• Infants, in; Nat-m.
Hot: Colch.
Jerking up: Cup.
Large: Am-m.
Nodes on: Ther.
Numb: Alu.
Pimples on: Kob.
Red: Carb-v; Cham; Sul.
• **Spots:** Mag-c.
Sitting agg: Stap.
Sore: Ars.
Stitching: *Calc-p*; Guai.
Swelling: Pho-ac.
Upwards, lumbar region to: Stap.
Warty growth, small, flat: Con.
BUZZING: See HUMMING.
CALCULI, urinary, biliary etc, formation of, in general: *Bell*; Benz-ac; *Berb*; *Bry*; *Calc*; *Chin*; Coc-c; *Colo*; Dios; Dul; Hyds; Lach; LYC; Merc; *Nux-v*; Oci-c; Par-b; Pod; Pul; *Sars*; Sep.
Deposits: Vario.

CALCULI

Operations, after: Mill.
CALF: Alu; Arg-n; Ars; CALC; Cam; *Cham*; *Cup*; *Grap*; Ign; *Lyc*; Nit-ac; *Nux-v*; Pul; Rhus-t; Sep; Stan; Stap; SUL; Val; VER-A.
Boils: Sil.
Bruised, as if: EUP-P; Stap.
Cold: Con.
• Spots, on: Stro.
Cord, as if bound by: Lol-t.
Cramps: Arg-n; Ars+; *Calc*; Cam+; Caus; CHAM; Colo; CUP; Grap; Hep; *Ign*; *Lyc*; NUX-V; *Plat*; *Plb*; *Sec*; *Sep*; Sil; Stro; SUL; *Ver-a*; Vib; Vip; Zin-io.
• Bed in
  - left, at night: Phys.
  - turning over on: Mag-c.
• Coition agg: Cup; Grap.
• Colic, with: Colo; Plb.
• Crossing legs, on: Alu.
• Dysentery, in: Merc-c.
• Fear, from: Lach.
• Foot, turning, sitting, while: Nat-m.
• Heels, to: Val.
• Menses, before: Vib.
• Muscles become flat: Jat.
• Pressing foot on floor amel: Zin-io.
• Soles, and: Stro.
• Standing amel: Cup-ar.
• Stools, during: Ap; Pod; Sec; Ver-a.
• Stretching legs in bed: Calc; Sul.

CALF, cramps, stretching leg
- amel: *Cup*.
• Tailors: Anac; Mag-p.
• Walking, while: Anac; Calc-p; Cinb; Lyc; Sul.
- amel: Ver-a.
Crossing, legs agg: Val.
Drawing, when walking: Carb-an.
Itching: Caus.
Jerking: Op.
Lumps in: Merc; Nit-ac.
Numb: Plat.
• Aching, with: Lapp.
Rigid, stiff: Arg-n; Mag-m.
Rising from seat agg: Anac.
Sacrum, to: Merc-i-r.
Short, as if: Arg-m; Sil.
Swelling: Dul.
Tense: See Rigid.
Twitching: Grap.
Weariness of: Bor.
• Palpitation, with: Calc-p.
Wind, cool up from: Helo.
CALLOSITIES, corns: ANT-C; Bry; *Calc*; Cist; *Grap*; Ign; *Lyc*; Pho; Phyt+; Radm; Rhus-t; SEP; SIL; Sul; Symp.
Burning: Arg-m; Ign; Ran-sc; Sep.
Cracks, deep in: Cist; Grap.
Hanging, down agg: Ran-sc.
Inflamed: Sil; Sul.
Painful: Ign; Lyc; Nat-m+; Ran-sc; Sul.
Pressing: Lyc; Sul.
Pressure, slight, from: Ant-c.

CALLOSITIES
Shooting: Bov; Nat-m.
Soft: *Sil.*
Sore: Carb-an; Flu-ac; Ign; Lyc; Sil.
Stinging: Alu; Bry; Calc; Calc-s; Nat-c; Nat-m; Rhus-t; Sul.
Tearing: Lyc; Sil; Sul.
CANCER: ARS; Ars-io; Ast-r; Aur; Bels; *Bro*; Buf+; *Calc*; CARB-AN; Clem; CON; Cund; GRAP; Hyds; Iod; *Kre*; LYC; NIT-AC; Petr; Pho; *Phyt*; *Sec*; Sep; SIL; *Sul*; Symp; Thu.
Burning pain of, abdomen+: Calc-ar.
Cancrum oris, noma: Ars; Con; Kali-chl; Kali-p; Tarn-c.
Deposits, removal after: Kali-p; Maland.
Encephaloma: *Pho.*
Epitheliomo: *Ars*; Ars-io; Con; Kali-s; Lyc; Ran-sc; Sep; *Thu.*
• Flat: Cund.
Glands, of: *Aur-m*; CARB-AN; CON.
Lupus: *Ars*; *Calc*; *Grap*; *Lyc*; Merc; Nat-m; Rhus-t; Sep; *Sil*; Stap; Sul.
• Hypertrophicus: Ars; *Grap.*
• Vorax: Ars; Sep; Sil; *Stap*; Sul.
Retard progress to+: Trif.
Sarcoma (See FUNGUS GROWTH): Ars; Bar-c; Carb-an; Lach; Lap-al; Pho; Sil; Symp; Thu.
• Burning: Bar-c.
• Lympho: Ars; Ars-io.

CANCER, sarcoma
- Osteo: Calc-f; Hecla; Syph.

Scirrhus: Bels; Carb-an; Clem; Con; Petr; Sep; *Sil*; Sul.

Smoking, from: Con.

CANTHI (Eyes, of): *Agar*; Calc; Carb-v; Kali-n; Nat-m; Nux-v; Pho; *Pul*; *Sil*; SUL.

Inner: *Agar*; *Bell*; *Stap*; Zin.
- Itching: Rut.
- Swellling over: Kali-c; Pul.

Outer: Calc; Ran-b; Sul.
- Lump in: Sul-ac.
- Polypus: Lyc.
- Twitching, chewing, while: Kali-n.

Cracks: Ant-c+; Caus+; Grap; Lyc.

Gum, in: *Agar*; *Ant-c*; Calc; Grap; Lyc; Stap.
- Stickly: Euphr; Kali-bi.

Inflamed: Ant-c; *Arg-n*; Bor; Calc; Euphr; *Grap*.

Itching: Alu; Arg-m; Calc.

Raw+: Ant-c.

Red
- Dark: Rhus-t.
- Pale: Ap.

CAP SENSATION: *Carb-v*; *Cyc*; *Grap*; Lach.
- Tight+: Berb.

CAPRICIOUS: See CHANGING MOODS and APPETITE.

CARBUNCLE: Anthx; *Ars*; *Bell*; Echi; Hep; Lach; Led; Pyro; Sil; Sul-ac; Tarn-c.

Bluish, red: Lach.

Burning: Tarn-c.

CARBUNCLE

Bursting as if+: Vip.

Impotency, with: Pic-ac.

Scarlet: Ap; Bell.

Stinging: *Ap*; Nit-ac.

CARE AND WORRY: Acet-ac; Ambr; Anac; Ars; Calc; Chin; Con; *Ign*; Kali-br; Kali-p; Mag-c; Pho+; Pho-ac; Pul.

Causeless: Petr.

Trifles, about: Ars.

CARESSES

AGG: Bell; Calc; Chin; Ign; Plat.

Proof, against: Cina.

CARIES: See under BONES.

CARPHOLOGY, picking at bed clothes, nervous picking: *Ars*; Bell; Hell; HYO; Lyc; Mur-ac; *Op*; Pho; Pho-ac; Rhus-t; STRAM; Tarn; Ver-v; Zin.

One spot, lips, fingers etc: Ars; *Aru-t*; Cham; Con; Kali-br; Lach; Tarn; Thu.
- Bleeds, until: Arg-m; Aru-t; Cina; Con; Pho.
- Sore, until: Aru-t; Pho-ac; Zin.

CARRIED

Dislikes to be+: Bry.

Wants to be: Acet-ac; Ant-t; Ars; Benz-ac; CHAM; Cina; Kali-c; Lyc; Rhus-t; Ver-a.
- Caressed, and: Kre; Pul.
- Erect, wishes+: Ant-t.
- Fast: Aco; *Ars*; *Bro*; Ver-a.
- Shoulders, over: Cina; Pod; Stan.
- Sitting up: Ant-t.

CARRIED, wants to be
- Slowly: Pul
- Will not be laid down (children): Benz-ac.

CARRIES things from one place to another, and back again: Mag-p.

CARRYING BURDENS
 AGG: Cadm; Rut.
 Back, on AGG: Alu.
 Head, on AGG: Calc; Rut; Tarn.

CAR SICKNESS, sea sickness etc: Ars; Bor; *Cocl*; Colch; Con; Glo; Kre; Lyss; PETR; Sanic; Sele; *Sep*; *Tub*; Ther.
 Railway: Kali-io.
 Riding
 - AMEL: Ars; *Grap*; *Nit-ac*; Tarn.
 - Air open, in amel: Naj.
 - Downhill agg: Bor; Psor.
 Stomach, felt in, without nausea: Kali-p.

CARTILAGE: Arg-m; Calc-p; Nat-m; Rut; Sul; Symp.
 Ulceration: Merc-c; Merc-d.

CARUNCLE: See URETHRA.

CATALEPSY: Cic; Cof; Gel; *Grap*; Hyo; Ign; Lach; Op; Pho-ac; Plat.
 Limbs can be moved by others+: Stram.
 Menses, during: Plat.
 Sexual excitement, from: Con; Plat.

CATARACT: See LENS.

CATHETERISM: Aco; Mag-p; Nux-v; Petros.

CAUTION: Calc; *Ign*; Nux-v; *Pul*; Ver-a.

CELIBACY: *Con*; Pho.

CELLARS, vaulted places agg: Aran; Ars; Calc; Dul; Nat-s; Pul.

CELLULAR TISSUE (cellulities etc): Ap; Ars; Bry; Lach; Merc; Rhus-t; Sil; Tarn-c; Vesp.
 Indurated: Anthx; Kali-io; Merc-i-r; Rhus-t.
 Subacute: Mang; Sil.

CENSORIOUS: *Aco*; ARS; Guai+; NUX-V; Sul.

CEPHAL HAMEMATOMA: Calc-f; Merc; Sil.

CEREBRO-SPINAL
 Axis: Agar; Arg-n; Chin; Cocl; *Gel*; Ign; *Nux-v*; Pho.
 Fever (meningitis): *Ap*; Arn; *Bell*; Bry; Cup; *Gel*; Hell; Merc-d; Nat-s; Stram; Sul; Ver-v; Zin.
 - Basilar+: *Ver-v.*
 - Suppressed discharges, from: Stram.
 - Tubercular: Bacil; Calc; Iod; Iodof; Lyc; Merc; Sil; Sul; Tub.
 - Urine, pale, clear with: Bell; Hyo; Lach; Pho.

CERVIX (Uterus)
 Cancer (See UTERUS): Tarn.
 Cauliflower-like growth: Kali-ar.
 Erosion of: Arg-m; Hyds; Kali-bi; Kre; Phyt; Sul-ac; Thu.
 Indurated: Aur; Carb-an; Con; Nat-c; Sep.

CERVIX
Lower, in vagina: Calend.
Open, dilated, as if: Lach; Sanic.
Os rigid, contracted, during labour: Bell; *Caul*; *Cham*; *Cimi*; *Gel*; Ver-v.
Painful: Goss.
Spongy: Arg-m: Ust.
Ulceration: Buf+; Med; Mez.
- Prolapse of uterus with+: Arg-n.

Warts, on: Calend.

CHAGRIN: See MORTIFICATION.

CHANCRE
Hard: Carb-an; Cinb; Kali-io; Merc; Merc-c; *Merc-i-f*; Merc-i-r.
Soft: Cor-r; Merc; Nit-ac; Thu.

CHANGE OF POSITION
AGG: *Caps*; Carb-v; Chel; Con; *Euphor*; *Fer*; Lach; Lyc; Pho; *Pul*; Samb.
AMEL: Agar; Ars; Cham; IGN; *Meli*; *Nat-s*; Pho-ac; Pul; Pyro; RHUS-T; *Sep*; Syph; *Val*; Zin.
Legs drawn up, when: Hell.
Lying long in one, after agg: Nat-s.

CHANGE OF TEMPERATURE or weather, on-coming storms etc
AGG: Agar; *Ars*; Calc-p; Carb-v; *Dul*; *Gel*; Hypr; Lach; Mag-c; Mez; Nat-c; Nit-ac; Nux-m; Petr; *Pho*; *Psor*; Pul; Ran-b; *Rhod*; RHUS-T; Rum; Sabi; Sep; *Sil*; Sul-io; Tub; Verb.

CHANGE OF TEMPERATURE
AGG and AMEL: Mang.
Rapid AGG: Sep.
Wants and AMEL: Mang; Sep; Tub.

CHANGING MOODS, erratic, fitful, capricious:
Aco; ALU; Amb; Bry; Cham; Cina; Croc; FER; Grap; IGN; Ip; Kali-c; LACH; *Nux-m*; PLAT; PUL; Stap; Senec; *Stram*; SUL-AC; Tarn; *Val*; ZIN.
Menses, before: Cham.
Rapidly (disposition or symptoms): Asaf; Croc; Rhod; Sep; Tab; Tarn; Tub; *Val.*
- Touch, on: Asaf.

CHAPS: See CRACKS.

CHARCOAL FUMES, ill effects+:
Am-c; Op.

CHEEKS:
Bell; Caus; Ign; Merc; *Rhus-t*; Stap.
Bites, when chewing or talking (See BITES): Carb-an; Caus; IGN; NIT-AC; Ol-an.
Blisters inside: Med.
Cold: Colo.
Contraction, sudden: Eup-p.
Cyst: Grap; Thu.
Drawing, in bones: Caus; Chel; Colch; Plat; Verb.
Eruptions: Ant-c; *Euphr*; Kre; Rhus-t; Stap.
- Herpes: Con.

Flapping, heavy breathing, with: Cheno.
Hangs, down: Ap.
Heat: Sang; Tab.
- Affected side: Tub.

CHEEKS, heat
- Toothache, with: Fer-p.

Induration, inside: Caus.
Numb: Caps; Mez; Nux-v; Old; Plat.
Painful: Verb.
- Splinters, as if+: Agar.

Pale and hot, one+: Mos.
Purple (centre): Diph.
Red: *Aco*; Arn; Bell: CHAM; Chin; *Fer*; *Ign*; *Lyc*; Mos; Nux-v; Pho; *Pul*; Sang; Sul.
- Colic, during: Cham.
- Hot, in open air: Val.
- Left: Ver-a.
- One: Sep.
  - and cold+: Mos.
- Spot: Rhus-t.

Scabs, bran-like, covered with: Lith.
Swollen: Arn; Cham; *Merc*.
- Hard: Am-c; Calc-f.
  - growth over, with; Hep.
- Inside: Am-c; Caus.
- Menses, during: Ap; Grap.

Tearing, bones, in: Lyc; Merc.
Tubercles, small, in: Asaf.
Twitching (R): Mez.
CHEERFUL: Aur; Bell; CANN; COF; *Croc*; Hyo; Nat-m; *Op*; *Plat*; Spo; Stram; Tarn.
Coition, after: Nat-m.
Convulsions, after: Sul.
Fearful, but: Nat-c
Heart disease, with: Cact.
Menses
- Before: Coco; Flu-ac.
- During: Flu-ac.

CHEERFUL
Pains
- During: Spig.
- After: Form.

Sad, and alternately: Senec.
Stool, after: Bor; Nat-s.
Sudden crying+: Chin.
CHEESY ODOUR: Pho; Sanic; Sep.
Old: Bry; Hep; Sanic.
CHEST AND LUNGS
Affections in general: *Aco*; ANT-T; Arn: ARS; BRY; Calc; Chel; Chin; Dul; *Fer-p*; Guai; Iod; Ip; *Kali-c*; *Lyc*; Op; Phel; PHO; PUL; *Ran-b*; Ran-sc; *Rhus-t*; Sang; Scil; Senec; Seneg; *Spig*; Stan; Sul; Tub; *Ver-v*; Verb.
Right: Arn; Ars; *Bell*; Bry; Carb-an; Chel; *Colch*; Colo; Iod; *Kali-c*; Lach; *Lyc*; Mur-ac; Psor; Pul; Scil.
- Nail, deep, in: Chel.
- Right arm into: Hyds; Kre; Lob; Pho; Phyt; Plb; Sang.
- To left: Aco; Lach; Petr.

Left: Am-m; Arg-m; Calc; Con; Euphor; Flu-ac; Kali-c; Kali-n; Laur; Lyc; Nat-s; Nit-ac; *Nux-v*; Pho; Rhus-t; Seneg; Stan; Sul.
- Lower epigastrium, to: Ox-ac.
- Rumbling, audible: Cocl.
- To right: Ap; Calc; Grap; Kre; Pho; Plb; Zin.

Alternating sides: *Agar*; Ap; Ars; *Calc*; *Cimi*; Dul; Grap; Hypr; Lyc; Mang; Mos; PHO; Plb; Ran-b; Rum; Thu.

CHEST

Arms, into: Bry; Dig; Dios; Latro.
- Right: Pho.

Backward, extending: Ars; Bry; *Calc*; Caps; Carb-v; *Chel*; Con; Cup; Kali-bi; Kali-io; Lil-t; *Merc*; Nat-m; Pho; Sep; Spig; *Sul*; Ther.
- Right: Aco; Ars; *Carb-v*; *Chel*; Dul; Guai; Kali-bi; Nit-ac; Phel; Phyt; Sep; *Sul*.
- Left: Bry; Kali-n; Lil-t; *Lyc*; Mur-ac; Nat-m; Phys; Rhus-t; Spig; Sul-ac; Ther.

Changing about: *Aco*; Alu; Arg-n; Bell; Cact; Caus; Colch; Fer; *Lyc*; Mag-m; Merc; Nat-c; Pho; *Pul*; Seneg.
- Pressure amel: Caus.

Deep in: Arn; Bry; Cep; Dros; Eup-p; Kali-c; Kre.

Downward: Agn; Kali-bi.
- Right: Dul; Nit-ac; Sang; Sep.
- Left: *Kali-c*; Laur; Pho; Pul; Scil; Zin.

Epigastrum, to: Ox-ac.

Forward: Berb; Bor; BRY: Castr; *Kali-c*; Kali-n; Psor; Rat; *Sep*; Sul.
- Right: Aco; Colo; Merc.
- Left: Agar; Bar-c; *Bry*; Lac-c; Naj; Pho; *Sul*; Thu; Zin.

Middle: Calc; Dul; Kali-bi; Phel; Sep.

Upper: Calc; Iod; Mang; Pul; Stan.

CHEST

Upward: Ars; Calc; Caus; Lach; Mang; Mur-ac; Thu.
- Right: Arn; Plat; Thu.
 - to left: Petr.
- Left: Am-m; Bov; *Coc-c*; Kali-c; Laur; Med; *Scil*; Spig; Stan; Zin.
 - to right: Calc; Carb-v; Grap; Ign; Lil-t.

Transversely: Caus; Thu.
- Arms, to: *Alu*.

Throat, into: Ap; Bell; Calc; Laur; Pho; Sul; Thu; Zin.

Abscess of lung: Calc; Hep; Pho; Sil.

Air in, enters too much or forced, as if: Chlor; Sabi; Ther.

Alternating with abdomen: Radm.

Anxiety felt, in: Aco; Ars; Aur; Bry; Calc; Merc; Pho.

Apices, pain in: Guai; Pul.
- Left: Myr; Ther.

Arms
- Raising agg: Tarn; Tell.
- Using agg: Rhus-t.

Band, sensation of a: Aeth; Cact; Helo; Ign; Lob; Pho; Sul.
- Lower: Cocl; Cup; *Plat*.

Bar across: Kali-bi.

Bending
- Backwards amel: Flu-ac.
- Forwards amel: Ascl.

Blowing nose agg: Chel; Sumb.

Boots, putting on agg: Arg-n.

CHEST

Breathing deep
- Agg: Nat-p.
- Amel: Chel

Brown spots on: Carb-v.

Bubbles: Merc.

Burning, heat: *Aco*; Ap; *Ars*; Bell; Canth; CARB-V; Euphor; Kali-m; Lyc; Naj; *Pho*; Sang; Spo; *Sul*; *Tub*; Ver-v.
- Cold feeling in stomach, with: Polyg.
- Coughing agg: Iod; Pho; Seneg; Spo; Thu.
- Epistaxis, with: Thu.
- Expectoration bloody, with: Psor.
- Hands icy cold, with; Thu.
- Hot stream, as from: Kre; Merc; Sang.
- Inspiration, on: Laur.

Bursting: Bro.

Chloasmae: Card-m; Sep; Sul; Thu.

Clothing
- Agg: Ars; *Caus*; Chel; *Lach*.
- Seem too tight+: Chel.
- Wet, as if: Ran-b.

Cold
- Air, draft
  - agg: Act-sp; *Calc-p*; Petr; Pho-ac; Ran-b.
  - amel: Fer.
- Drinks agg: Pho; Psor+.
- Pain on coughing: Med.
- Water, washing with, amel: Bor.

CHEST

Coldness in: ARS; Bry; Carb-an; Kali-c; Lil-t; Med; Nat-c; *Old*; *Sul*.
- Cold air, breathing, on: Cor-r; Lith; *Ran-b*.
- Drinking, after: Elap.
- Expectoration, after: Zin.

Congestion: *Aco*; *Bell*; Bry; *Cact*; Cam; Dig; Fer; Fer-p; Ip; Lach; Nux-v; *Pho*; Rhus-t; Seneg; Sep; Spo; SUL; Terb; *Ver-v*.
- If desire for urination not attended to: Lil-t.

Contracted, with asthma: Cadm.

Coughing agg: Bor; BRY; Caus; Elap; Lyc; *Pho*; Scil; Seneg; Spo; Stan; Sul.

Cramp, constriction, spasm: Aeth+; Asaf; Cact; Fer; Grap+; Ign; Mos; Nux-m; Nux-v; Radm; Sul; Tab; Vip.
- As from sulphur fumes+: Kali-chl.
- Bends double: Hyo.

Dancing amel: Caus.

Desire to urinate if delayed agg: Lil-t.

Direction of pain, various: Thu.

Distension: Ars; *Lach*; Thu.

Dryness: Fer; Lach; Merc; Pho; Pul.
- Coughing, with: Pho.
- Left: Naj.

Emaciation: Kali-io; Petr; Senec.

CHEST

Emphysema: Am-c; Ant-t; Ars+; Coca+; Grind; Hep; Lach; Lob; Seneg.
- Senile: Lob.

Empty, hollow: Carb-an; Cocl; Med; Pho; Stan.
- Coughing, when: Sep; Stan.
- Eating, after: Nat-p; Old.
- Expectoration, after: Rut; Stan; Zin.
- Left: Naj.
- Singing, while: Stan.

Empyema: Arn; Ars; Calc-s; Kali-s; Merc; Sil; Sul.
- Pleurisy, after: Sil

Epistaxis amel: Bro; Carb-v.

Eructation amel: Amy-n; Bar-c; Canth; Lach; Pho; Sep.

Fasting agg: Iod.

Fixed, immmovale: Ox-ac; *Pho*; Stry.

Fluttering, in: Lil-t; Naj; Nat-m; Nat-s; Nux-m; Pho-ac; Spig.

Fulness: Aco; Ap; Glo; Lach; Pho; *Sul*.
- Heart, weak or dilated with: Chlo-hyd.

Gangrene of lung: *Ars*; Caps+; Carb-v; *Kre*; Lach.

Haemorrhage (See HAEMOPTYSIS): Chel; Stan.
- Menses, before: Dig.
- Parturition, after: Arn; Chin; Pul.
- Pneumonia, results of: Calc-s; *Sul-ac*.
- Puerperal fever, in: Ham.

Hawking agg: Calc; Rum; Spig. **Heavy:** See Load.

Hepatisation of lung: Pho; Sul.

Hiccough agg: Stro.

Hold, must: Arn; *Bry*; *Dros*; Eup-p; Nat-s.

Hollow: See Empty.

Hot
- Application amel: Pho.
- Drops, as of: Hep.

Hydrothrax+: Adon; Flu-ac; Lyc.

Injury, after: Rut.

Itching: Ant-c; Sul.
- Nose, up to: Con; *Ip*.

Laughing agg: Bry.

Legs, hanging amel: Sul-ac.

Lifting agg: Alu; Psor; Sul.

Load, heavy on, pressure: Am-c; Ant-t; Aur; Cact; Fer; Lach; Lil-t; *Nux-v*; *Pho*; *Pul*; Seneg; Stro; *Sul*; Ver-v.
- Motion amel: Seneg.

Lump, plug, sensation: *Amb*; Am-m; *Anac*; Bur-p; Cup; *Kali-m*; PHO; *Ran-sc*; Stic; Sul; Tarx; Zin.
- Behind+: Gel.
- Moving up and down, on swallowing empty: Lil-t.

Lung, apex (R): Elap.
- Bubbling in (R): Tell.
- Burning like fire: Buf.
- Constricted by wire, as if+: Asar.
- Distend, cannot: Asaf; Crot-t.

CHEST, lung
- Down, coated, with as if: Bro.
- Hard and small, as if (R): Ab-c.
- Hot, feel+: Aco.
- Moving, waves in, as if: Dul.
- Rivet, as of (L)+: Sul.
- Seperated forcibly, as if: Elap.
- Smoke, full of, as if: Bar-c.
- Sticking, ribs to, as if: Kali-c.
- Stuffed up cotton with, as if: Kali-bi; Med.

Lying
- Abdomen, on
  - agg: Ascl.
  - amel: Bry.
- Back, on amel: Bor; *Cact*; Pho; Sul.
- Painful side, on amel: Amb; *Bry*; Nux-v.
- With, arms, near chest amel: Lac-ac.

Morning agg: Calc; *Carb-v*; Sep.
Motion amel: Seneg.
Narrow, as if: Agar; Seneg.
Numb: Glo; Stic.
- Left arm, down: Glo.

Oedema, pulmonary: Ant-t; Ars; Lach; Merc; Sul.
- Sudden: Rhus-t.

Operation
- For fistula, after: Berb; Calc-p; Sil.
- Upon chest, after: Abro.

Paralysis of lungs: ANT-T; Ars; *Bar-c*; *Carb-v*; *Chin*; Ip; Kali-io; *Lach*; *Lyc*; Op; *Pho*.
- Old people, in: Bar-c; Chin.

CHEST
Pleurisy: Aco; Arn; Ascl+; Bry; Carb-an; Guai; Kali-c; Merc-d; Pho; Seneg; Sul.
- Adhesions, after: Ran-b.
- Breathing deep agg: Guai.
- Debility, paralytic, with: Saba.
- Exudation: Abro; Fer; Iod+; Kali-io+; Seneg.
- Neglected: Ars; Sul.
- Recurrent: Guai.
- Stitch, after; Carb-an.

Pneumonia: ACO; *Ant-t*; Ars; *Bry*; Carb-v; Chel; *Fer-p*; Hep; Iod; Kali-bi; Lob; *Lyc*; *Merc*; PHO; *Pul*; *Rhus-t*; Sang+; *Seneg*; *Sep*; *Sul*; Tub; Ver-v.
- Catarrhal: *Ant-t*.
- Cerebral type: Aco; Arn; Bell; Bry; Cann; Canth; Hyo; Lach; Merc; Nux-v; Pho; Pul; Rhus-t; Stram; Sul.
- Haemorrhage, after: Chin; Pho-ac.
- Infants: *Ip*.
- Influenza, after+: Tub.
- Neglected, unresolved: Ars-io; *Lyc*; Pho; Pyro; *Sil*; *Sul*; Sul-io.
- Secondary: Fer-p; Pho.

Pressure
- Amel: *Arn*; Bor; BRY; Caus; *Dros*; Eup-p; Nat-s.
- Clothes, of agg: Benz-ac.
- Hands, of amel+: Sep.
- Spine, on agg: Sec; Tarn.

Pulsation: Asaf; Bell; Cact; Seneg; *Sul*.

CHEST, pulsation
- Night: Pul.
- Right: Asar; Crot-t; *Dig*; Ign; Ind; Paeon; Pho.
- Left: Am-m; Cann; Gel; *Meny*.

Purring: Caus; Glo; Spig.

Rattling (See RESPIRATION, rattling): Hep; Lob; Pho; Sil; Sul; Tub.
- Coarse: Ant-t; Cup; Kali-s.
- Expectoration, without: Am-c; *Ant-t*; Carb-v; Caus; Con; Hep; Ip; Kali-s; Lob; Pho; Sep; Sul; Tub; Ver-a.
- Fine: Ip.
- Loose: Seneg.

Rushes of blood: Kali-n; Pho; Seneg; Sul.

Scraping: Seneg.
- Talking agg: Seneg.

Shocks, jerks: Agar; *Con*; Grap; *Lyc*; Plat; Sul.
- Coughing, when: Lyc; Seneg.

Shoulder, throwing back amel: Calc.

Shuddering in: Agar; Aur.

Singing agg: Am-c.

Small, too, as if: Ign.

Sneezing agg: Bry; Caus; Dros; Merc; Mez; Seneg.

Soreness: Alu; Calc; Chel; Chin; Kali-bi; *Pho*; Rhod; Seneg; *Stan*.
- Cold air agg: Pho-ac.
- Expectoration, after: Cist.
- Scapulae, between, with: Chin.
- Touch agg: Chin.

CHEST

Spot, in: Agar; Anac; Buf; Nat-m; Ol-j; Seneg; Thu; Tub.
- Brown: Lyc; Sul.
- Red: Guai; Saba; Sul.
- Yellow: Ars; Pho.

Sprain: Lyc; Rhod; Tell.

Squatting agg: Cadm.

Squeezed, by hand, as if+: Colch.

Stabbing: Kali-c; Nat-m.

Stitching: *Aco*; *Bry*; Kali-c; Myr; Ol-j; *Pho*; *Ran-b*; Rhus-t; Scil; Spig+; Sul.
- Right: Bor.
- Left: Pho.
- Bilateral: Ran-b.
- Breathing, impeding: Arg-m.
- Burning: Sang.
- Coughing agg: Merc.
- Flying+: Fer.
- Pleurisy, after: Carb-an.
- Pressure amel: Arn; Bor.
- Sneezing agg: Merc.

Stooping agg: Mez; Seneg.

Stuffed up, as if: Amb; Lach; Med; Radm+.

Talking agg: Alu.

Tickling: Rhus-t; *Rum*.

Tight: Ars; Asaf; *Aur*; Cact; Caus; Fer; Ign; Ip; Nat-m; *Nux-v*; PHO; Pul; Sul; Tab; Terb+.
- Right: Am-m; Cocl; Sul.
- Left: Grap; Lyc; Sul-ac; Sumb.
- Coition, close of, at: Stap.
- Coughing amel: Con.

CHEST, tight
- Motion, least agg: Ip.
- Stooping agg: Mez.

Trembling, in: Lapp; Spig+.
Ulcerative, pain: Ran-b.
Uncovering amel: Fer; Sars.
Uterine symptoms, with: Stan.
Vapour, as if, in: Merc.
Velvety feeling: Ant-t.
Vomiting, green amel: Cocl.
Weakness: Ant-t; Arg-m; *Calc*; *Carb-v*; *Kali-c*; LAUR; *Nit-ac*; Ran-sc; *Seneg*; STAN; SUL.
- Coughing, when: Pho-ac.
- Exertion, after: Spo.
- Expectoration, after: Stan.
- Singing, when: Stan.
- Sitting, when: Pho-ac.
- Talking, while: Pho-ac; *Stan*; Sul.
- Waking, after: Carb-v.
  - amel: Pho-ac.

Wandering pain: Seneg.
Water in, as if: Hep.
Wine agg: Bor.
Yawning agg: Bor; Grap; Nat-s; Sul.

CHEWING: See BITING.
Constant, with frothy saliva: Asaf.
Food escapes from mouth, during: Arg-n.
Motions: Aco; Amy-n; Bell; BRY; Calc; *Cham*; Cup; *Hell*; Lach; *Lyc*; Mos; *Ver-v*.
- Brain affections, in: Bry.
- Chorea, in: Asaf.
- Sleep, in: Calc+; Ign.

CHEWING, motions
- Spasms, before+: Calc.

Swallowing, and, sleep, in: Calc; Cina; Ign.

CHICKEN POX: Aco; Ant-c; Ant-t; Bell; *Led*; Pul; *Rhus-t*; Sul.

CHILBLAINS, FROSTBITE: Abro; AGAR; Ars; Carb-v; Hep; *Nit-ac*; Nux-v; Petr; *Pul*; Sul.

Unbroken+: Terb.

CHILDBED: See PREGNANCY.

CHILDISH, foolish: Aeth; *Alo*; Amb; ANAC; BAR-C; BELL: *Buf*; Cic; Con; *Hell*; HYO; Lach; Lyc; Merc-c+; *Nat-c*; Nux-m; Nux-v; *Op*; *Pho-ac*; Pic-ac; Plb; Rhod+; Sep; Sil; *Stram*; Sul; Thyr; Ver-a.

Body grows, but: Buf.

Epilepsy
- Before: Caus.
- After: Tab.

Furor, alternative, with+: Aeth.

Parturition, after: Ap.

CHILDREN, infants: *Aco*; Ant-t; *Bell*; *Bor*; CALC; CALC-P; *Cham*; *Cina*; Cof; Ip; *Merc*; Phyt; Pod; Pul; Rhe; Sep; SIL; *Sul*.

Afraid of everything: Calc.
Boils, disposition to: Mag-c.
Breath, loses, when angry: Arn.
Choke on swallowing liquids: Kali-br.

CHILDREN

Clumsy+: Asaf.
Crawl nervouly: Sil.
Cyanotic from birth: Bor; Cact; Dig; Lach; Laur.
Dragged on mother's arms: Sil.
Emotional, chat and laugh: Alo.
Fat, chubby: Bell; Seneg.
Fed, improperly: Aeth.
Fontanelles
- Depressed: *Ap*; Calc.
- Occipital bone, sinking: Mag-c.
- Open: *Ap*; CALC; CALC-P; *Ip*; *Merc*; *Pul*; *Sep*; SIL; Sul; Syph.
- Pulsate strongly: Gel.
- Reopening, of: Calc-p.

Fuss, likes+: Pul.
Hold on to mother's hand: Bism.
Jump, start, scream fearfully: Nat-c; Sul.
Lifting agg: Bor; Calc-p.
Nose, red, raw, dirty with: Merc.
Nurse, daytime only: Ap.
- All the time+: Calc-p.

Pale on running: Sil.
School, overtaxed with+: Zin.
Scream and cry, always: Lac-c+; Psor+; Rhe.
Sleep all day, cry all night+: Lyc.
Sour smelling+: Med.
Stammering: Bov.

CHILDREN

Suckling: Bor; Calc; Calc-p; Kali-bi; Mag-c; Pho-ac; Pul; Sul.
- Die, early, birth after: Arg-n.
- Few weeks old, shrivelled and old looking: Op.

Talk late: Agar; Bar-c; Calc-p; *Nat-m*; Sanic.
Tall, thin+: Calc-p.
Unhealthy+: Psor.
Walk
- Late: Agar; Calc; Calc-p; Caus; *Sil*; Sul.
- Unable to, from ankle affections: Mang.

Want to be nursed in arms, will not be laid down: Benz-ac.
Weak without cause: Sul-ac.
Weep, cry continuously, new born infants: Syph; Thu.

CHILL: Ant-c; Ant-t; *Aran*; *Arn*; Ars; *Aur*; CAM; Canth; *Carb-v*; Caus; Chel; *Chin*; *Chin-s*; *Eup-p*; Gel; Grap; Hep; Ign; *Ip*; Lac-d; LYC; Meny; Mez; MOS; NAT-M; Nit-ac; *Nux-m*; Nux-v; PUL; Rhus-t; *Saba*; Sep; *Sil*; *Stap*; Symp; Thyr; VER-A.

Abdomen, begins in: Amb; Ap; Ars; Ign; Pho; Sep; *Ver-a*.
Air, craves: Alu; Sep; Tub.
Alternating with
- Fever: *Am-m*; *Ars*; *Bell*; Bry; Calc; Cham; Chin; Cocl; Eup-p; GEL; *Hep*; Hyds; Ip; Kali-io; Lach; *Merc*; Nux-m; NUX-V; Ol-an; *Rhus-t*; Samb.

CHILL, alternating with
- Sweat: Ars; Chin; Mez; Nux-v; Spig.

Anticipates: Ap; ARS; *Bry*; *Chin*; Chin-s; *Nat-m*; NUX-V.
- Postponing, or: Bry; Ign.

Back, starts in: Bell; *Caps*; Caus; Cocl; Dul; *Eup-p*; *Gel*; Hyo; *Lach*; Lyc; *Nat-m*; Pul; *Rhus-t*; See; Sep; Stap; Stro; Sul.

Bed, putting hand out of: *Bar-c*; *Hep*; NUX-V; *Rhus-t*; Tarn; TUB.
- Turning over in: Nux-v; Pul.

Bladder, starts in: Sars.

Bones, felt in: Pyro.

Changing type: Ign; Pul.

Chest, starts in: *Ap*; Carb-an; Sep.

Coition, after: Nat-m.

Cold water
- Dashed over him, as if: Arn; Rhus-t.
- Poured over him, as if: Canth; Led; Merc; Pul.

Concomitant, as a: Saba.

Congestive: Aco; Arn; Gel; Nux-v; Psor; Ver-a.

Convulsions, after: *Cup*.

Coryza, with: Mag-c.

Coughing agg: Ap; Eup-p; Pul; Rhus-t; Thu.

Covers
- Agg: *Ap*; Calc-s; Cam; *Ip*; Led; *Pul*; *Sec*; *Sep*.
- Did not amel: Lyc.

Creeping: Merc.

CHILL

Desire to
- Held down, be: Gel; Lach.
- Talk: Pod.

Drinks
- Agg: *Ars*; Asar; Calc; *Caps*; Chel; *Chin*; *Eup-p*; Lach; *Nux-v*; Ver-a.
- Amel: *Caus*; *Cup*; Manc.
- Cold agg: Rhus-t.
- Warm agg: Alu; Bell; *Pul*.

Drowsiness, with: Ant-t; Cam; Chel; Gel; Nux-m; OP; Ver-a.

Dyspnoea, with: Ap.

Eating, after: Ars; Asar; Bell; Carb-an; Kali-c; Ran-b; Tarx.

Exertion, after: Zin-val.

Extremities, starts, in: Arn; *Bell*; *Carb-v*; Caus; Sec; Sul.

Fever, with: Aco; Ars; Bell; Cham; *Gel*; Hell; Ign; Nit-ac; Nux-v; Rhus-t; Sul.
- For a long time: Pod; Pyro.

Figner tips numb, with: Stan.

Fire, besides agg: Pulex.

Flower, smell of, from: Lac-c.

Fright, from: Gel.

Grief, from: Gel; Ign.

Head, to: Glo.

Heated, overheated, when: *Carb-v*; *Pul*; Samb; *Sil*; Ver-a.

Holding cold things in hand: Zin.

Irregular: Ars; Nux-v; Psor; Pul; Sep.

Itching, with: Mez.

Lips, begins in: *Bry*.

Lying, on: Pul.

CHILL, lying
- Back, on: Tell.

Menses
- Before: Lyc; Mag-c; Pul; Sil.
- During: Pul; Sep; Sil; Sul.
- Start, at: Jab.

Mental exertion, after: Nux-v; Zin-val.

Motion
- Arms of, agg: Rhus-t.
- Slight, after: Ars; *Nux-v*; *Spig*.

Moving bed clothes slightly, on: Arn; Nux-v.

Nervous: Gen; Zin-val.

Nightly: Pyro.

Noise, from: Ther.

Nosebleed, with: Thu.

Pain, with: *Agar*; Ars; Bov; Calc-p; *Cam*; *Colo*; Dul; Kali-n; *Mez*; *Pul*; SEP.

Palm and sole, starts from: Dig.

Partial: See COLDNESS.

Postponing: Chin; GAMB; Ign; *Ip*.

Pressure amel: *Bry*; Pho.

Rigours, shaking: Chin; Chin-s; Ign; Nat-m; Pyro.
- Inspiring, on: *Bro*.
- Skin, cold, with: Cam.
- Urinatin agg: Stram; Thu.
- Yawning, with: Thu.

Scapulae, starts between: Pyro.

Scratching agg: Agar; Mez; Petr.

Single parts, in: See COLDNESS, partial.

CHILL
Sitting amel: Ign; Nux-v.

Sleep
- First, after: Lyc.
- In: Bor.

Spine to arms: Lept.

Stone in abdomen, as if+: Aran.

Stools
- After: Canth; Med; Merc; Merc-c; Plat; Rhe.
- Urging, with: Dul.

Suffocated, as if: Arg-n; Mag-p.

Summer, in: Psor.

Sunset, after: Ars; Ign; Pul

Sunshine
- Agg: Nat-m.
- Amel: Anac; Con.

Sweat, with: Cham; Eup-p; Lach; Nux-v; Pul; Pyro; Tub.

Then heat, then chill: Thu.

Throat sore, with: Mag-c.

Through and through: Am-c; Aran; Calc; Cinb; Elap; Kali-bi; Mos.

Toothache, with: Mag-c.

Touch agg: *Aco*; *Chin*; Lyc; *Nux-v*; Spig.

Trembling and shivering with: Anac; Ant-t; Plat; Sil.

Uncovering
- Hands: Mag-c.
- Least: Hep; Nux-v; Rhus-t; Sil.

Urinating
- On: Gel; Nit-ac; Plat; Thu.
- Urging, with: Dul.

CHILL

Urticaria, with: Ap.
Vomiting, with: Dul.
Waking, on: Alu; Arn.
  • As often as he wakes: *Am-m.*
Walking, while: Chin.
Warm
  • Covering, in spite of: Asar.
  • Room, in: Pho.
Waves, in: Carb-an.
Wet, from: Lapp; Led; *Rhus-t*; Thu.
Wind, in: Sanic.
Writing, while: Agar.
Yawning, with: Carb-an; Kre; Meny; Thu.

CHILLED

From exposure to cold AGG: ACO; Ars; *Bell*; Bry; Cham; Clem; Cof; *Colch*; *Dul*; *Hyo*; *Ip*; MERC; NUX-V; PHO; *Pul*; RHUS-T; Sep; *Sil*; *Spig*; *Sul*; Ver-a.
While hot, sweating, by ices, exposure to cold of single parts etc. AGG: *Aco*; Ars; Bell; Bels; Bro; Bry; Dul; Fer-p; *Hep*; Kali-c; Merc-i-f; *Nux-v*; Pho; Psor; Pul; Rhod; RHUS-T; Sep; SIL; Zin.
CHIN: Caus; Plat; Sil.
  Cold: Aeth; Kali-n.
  Drawn to sternum: Phyt.
  Eruption: Nat-m; Rhus-t; Sep; Sil; Sul.
    • Between, lips and: Kali-chl.
    • Eczema: Merc-i-r.
    • Granular, honey coloured: Ant-c.

CHIN

Gland, under: Led; Stap.
Hair
  • Falling+: Grap.
  • On, in women: Ol-j.
Numb: Spo.
Sweat: Con.
Too long, as if: Glo.
Twitches, trembles: Agar; *Ant-t*; Gel.
Ulcer: Cund.

CHLOASMAE: Card-m; Caul; *Lyc*; Rob; *Sep.*
  Sun, exposure, from: Cadm.
CHLOROFORM AGG: Pho.
CHOKING (See THROAT, choking and RESPIRATION, difficult): Con; Grap; Lycps; *Meph*; Mos; *Tarn*; Terb; Thyr; Val.
  Coughing agg: Tarn.
  Drinking agg: Meph.
  Eating, when: Zin-val.
  Goitre, in: Meph.
  Head, bending backward amel: Hep; Lach.
  Nervous: Mos.
  Sleep agg: *Lach*; Spo; Val.
  Speaking agg: Meph.
  Sudden: Samb.
  Water agg: Stram.

CHOLERA: Ars; *Cam*; Carb-v; *Cup*; Cup-ars; Hyd-ac; Sec; *Ver-a.*
  Diarrhoea epidemic, during: *Ip*; Pho.
  Infantum: Aeth; Guai; Med; Psor; Stram+; Tab+; Zin+.

CHOLERA, infantum
- Body remains warm: Bism.
- Opisthotonos, with: Med.

Morbus: Ant-t; Crot-h; Guai; Iris; *Pod*; *Ver-a*.

CHORDEE: See ERECTION, painful.

CHOREA: Abs+; *Agar*; Art-v; Bell; Calc; CAUS; Chin; Cic; *Cimi*; Cina; *Cup*; Ign; LACH; Mag-p; Myg; Nux-v; *Stram*; *Tarn*; Ver-v.

Children, who have grown too fast: Pho.

Coition after (women): Agar; Cedr.

Colour, bright, sight of amel: Tarn.

Cordis: Cimi; Tarn.

Dancing, excessive: Bell; Hyo; Stram.

Ear piercing, from: Lach.

Eating agg: Ign.

Emission, seminal, with: Dios.

Emotions, from: Laur; Mag-p.

Exertion amel: Zin.

Face
- Cold, clammy, up to knee with: Laur.
- Of: *Caus*; Cic; Cina; Cup; Hyo; *Myg*; Nat-m; Zin.

Foot sweat suppressed, from: Form.

Fright or shock: *Caus*; Cup; Cup-ar; Nat-m; Visc; Zin.

Haemorrhages, after: Stic.

Hands, on: Cina.

Holding amel: Asaf.

CHOREA
Hysteria, and+: Croc.

Imitation, from: Caus; Cup; Tarn.

Jerks constant, cannot keep still: Laur.

Left arm, right leg: Agar; *Cimi*.

Long standing, obstinate+: Chlo-hyd.

Lying on back amel: *Cup*; Ign.

Menses
- Absent or difficult, with: *Pul*.
- During: *Zin*.

Misses, laying hold on anything: Asaf.

Muscles, local, of: Hyo.

Music amel: Tarn.

Old age+: Aeth.

Pocket, keeping hand in: Ast-r.

Pregnancy during: Bell; Caus; Cup; Gel.

Puberty, at: Asaf; Caul; *Cimi*; Ign; Pul.

Return at the same hour: Ign.

Rheumatic: *Caus*; Cimi; Rhus-t; Spig.

Right arm, left leg: Tarn.

Run
- better then walk: Tarn.
- Or jump must, cannot walk: Buf; Kali-br; Nat-m.

Side
- One: Calc; Cocl; Cup.
- Lain, on: Cimi.

Sleep
- Agg: Tarn; Ver-v; Ziz.

CHOREA, sleep
- Amel: *Agar*; Cup; Hell; Mag-p; Myg.

Stools at agg: Mag-p.
Swallow, cannot: Art-v.
Sympathetic: Caus.
Thunderstorm, approaching agg: Agar; Rhod.
Tongue, protrusion of, with: Sumb.
Weekly: Croc.
Wet, after getting: Rhus-t.
Wine agg: Zin.

CHOROID: Pho.

CHRONICITY: *Alu*; Arg-n; *Ars*; *Calc*; *Caus*; *Con*; Kali-bi; Kali-io; *Lyc*; Mang; Pho; Plb; Psor; *Sep*; *Sul*; Syph; Tub.
Stubborn: Kali-io.

CICATRICES: Calc-f; Caus; Flu-ac; *Grap*; Hypr; *Merc*; Naj; Petr; Phyt; Sil; Syph; Thiosin.
Absorption, aids+: Grap.
Blue, become: Sul-ac.
Burn: Carb-an; Grap; Tell.
Cancerous diathesis+: Grap.
Depressed, round: Kali-bi; Syph.
Discoloured, raised: Bad.
Green, become: Led.
Itch: Flu-ac; Iod; Led; Naj.
- Pimples, with: Iod.

Painful: Hypr; Nat-m; *Sil*.
- Weather, change of, during: Nit-ac.

Purple, become: Asaf.
Red, become: Lach; Nat-m; Sul-ac.

CICATRICES
Re-open: Carb-v; *Caus*; Croc; Grot-h; Flu-ac; Glo; *Graph*; Iod; Lach; Nat-m; PHO; SIL.
- Cracks and burns: Sars.
- Suppurate: Croc.
- Turn black: Asaf.

Shiny: Sil.
Tension, in: Kali-c.
Thick: *Grap*.
Ulcerate: Asaf: Calc-p.
Vesicles, around: Flu-ac.
White: Radm; Syph.

CIRCULATION: See BLOOD.

CLAIRVOYANCE: Aco; Lach; Lyss; Med; Nux-m; Op; Pho.

CLAUSTROPHOBIA: See FEAR, narrow places.

CLAVICLE
Air: Chlor; Rum.
Cold water running from, down to toes, along a narrow line, as if: Caus.
Emaciation, about: Lyc; Nat-m.
Hawking agg: Rum.
Painful: Lac-c; Tell; Pul.
Skin blue: Thu.
Stitch: Ol-an; Pul.
Tension: Lyc; Zin.
Under: Calc-p; Cratae; Rum.

CLAVUS: See PLUG.

CLIMAXIS: Aco; Amyl-n; Cimi; Con; Fer; Gel; Grap; LACH; Mang; Meli; Murx; Psor; Pul; Sabi; *Sang*; *Sep*; Stro; *Sul*; Sul-ac; Sumb; Vip; Xanth.
Hypertrophy, body, one side: Lyc.

CLIMAXIS
Premature: Abs.
Women, fat: Calc-ar.
CLITORIS: Am-c; Coll.
Erect, after urination, with sexual desire: Calc-p.
Stitching, stinging (night): Bor.
Swollen, as if: Colch; Coll.

CLOTHES
Cold, as if: Ars-io.
Damp, as if: Calc; Guai; Lac-d; Lyc; Pho; Ran-b; Sanic; Sep; Tub; Ver-v.
Fire on, as if: Ars-io.
Fit him, would not: Ver-v.
Heavy, too: Con; Euphor.
Large, too: Psor; Thu.
Packs and unpacks without consciousness+: Mag-c.
Pressure of
- AGG: Arg-n; Bov; Bry; *Calc*; Carb-v; Caus; Con; Glo; Hep; LACH; Lil-t; LYC; Nit-ac; *Nux-v*; Onos; Psor; Sec; Sep; Spo; Sul; *Tub*.
- AMEL: Psor; Saba.
- Chest on agg: Benz-ac.
- Groins, about agg: Hyds.
- Neck, about agg: Agar; *Ap*; Caus; Chel; Con; Glo; Kali-c; LACH; Merc; *Sep*.
- Pit of stomach agg+: Lith.
- Waist about agg: Ap; Bro; Carbo-v+; Grap; Lach.
- Tears+: Cam.

Tight, as if: Arg-m; Caus; Chel; Glo; Nux-v; Rum.
- Abdomen, about: Mos.
- Chest, about: Meli.

CLOTHES
Uncomfortable: Spo.
- Groins, about: Hyds.

Wear his best: Con.

CLOUDY WEATHER
AGG: Alo; Am-c; Arn; Ars-io; Aur; Bar-c; Cham; Chin; Hypr; Lach; Mang; Merc; Nux-m; Pul; *Rhus-t*; Sabal; Sabi; Sep; Stram; Vio-o.
AMEL: Bry; Kalm; Lapp.
Mental effects agg: Alo; Pho.

CLUTCHING SENSATION: *Bell*; Cact; Lil-t; Thyr.

COAL GAS AGG: Am-c; Arn; Bell; Bov; Carb-s; Cof; Op; Sec.

COAT, wears in summer, hot weather: Hep; Hyo; Kali-ar; Merc; Psor.

COATED or furred as if: *Alu*; *Caus*; Chin; *Cocl*; Colch; Dig; Dros; *Iris*; Kali-c; *Merc*; *Nux-m*; PHO; Pho-ac; PUL; Rhod; Ver-a.

COBWEB SENSATION: Alu; *Bar-c*; BOR; Bro; Calc; Con; GRAP; Ran-sc; Sumb.

COCCYX: *Ap*; Arn; Bels; *Caus*; *Hypr*; *Kre*; Rut; Sil; Zin.
Abscess just below: Paeon.
Bent back, as if: Mag-p.
Bruised, as if, preventing sitting: Am-m+; Cist.
Burning: Pho.
- Sitting, on: Ap; Cist.
- Touched, when: Carb-an; Cist.

Coition agg: Kali-bi.

COCCYX

Drawing: Caus.
Elongated, as if: Xanth.
Heavy: Ant-c; Ant-t; Arg-n.
Injury: Bels; Carb-an: *Hypr*; Mez; Sil.
Itching: Bov; Grap.
Jerks, during menses: Cic.
Motion, slight agg: Tarn.
Numb: Plat.
Painful: Carb-an; Cast-eq+; Caus; Con; Grat; *Hypr*; Petr; Sil; Tarn; Thu+; Xanth.
- Abdomen, pressing on amel: Merc.
- Fall, as from: Kali-io.
- Menses, during: Cic.
- Soles tender, with+: Thu.
- Stool
  - during: Pho; Sul.
  - after: Euphor; Grat.
- Urination, before+: Kali-bi.

Parturition, after: Tarn.
Pulling up, from: Lil-t.
Riding in carriage agg: Nux-m.
Rising from a seat
- Agg: Euphor; *Lach*; *Sil*; Sul.
- Amel: Kre.

Sitting
- Agg: Am-m; Ap; Kali-bi; Par; Petr.
- On something sharp, as if: Lach.

Sleep, during agg: Am-m.
Standing amel: Arg-n; Tarn.
Stitches: Pho-ac.
Swelled, as if: Syph.
Thighs, to: Rhus-t.

COCCYX

Ulcer: Paeon.
Up
- and down extending: Kali-bi.
- spine to arms: Hypr.
- spine to occiput: Pho.
  - stools
    during: Pho.
    after: Euphor.

Urination agg: Grap; Kali-bi.
Weight: See HEAVY.

COITION

AGG: AGAR; Buf; Calad; *Calc*; Canth; *Chin*; *Grap*; KALI-C; Kali-p; Kre; Lyc; *Nat-c*; *Nat-m*; Nat-p; Pho-ac; Sele; *Sep*; *Sil*; Spig; Stan; Stap; Sul.
AMEL: CON; Merc; *Stap*.
Aversion to (in males): Arn; Clem; *Grap*; *Lyc*; Rhod; Psor.
Fright, during agg: Lyc.
Incomplete+: Nat-c.
Interrupted agg: Bell.
Motions, as of: Caus; Pho.
Painful (males): Arg-n; Calc; Sabal.

COLD

AGG (easily chilled, lack of vital heat): *Agar*; Am-c; Ant-t; Aran; ARS; *Aur*; *Bar-c*; CALC; Calc-f; *Calc-p*; *Cam*; *Caps*; CAUS; *Chin*; Cimi; *Cist*; Cocl; Colch; *Dul*; *Eup-p*; *Fer*; *Grap*; Hell; Hep; Hypr; *Kali-bi*; KALI-C; Lac-d; *Lyc*; *Mag-c*; *Mag-p*; Merc; Mez; MOS; *Nit-ac*; *Nux-m*; NUX-V; Pho; Pho-ac; *Psor*; Pyro; Ran-b; Rhod; RHUS-T; *Rum*; SABA;

COLD

COLD, agg ..
Sep; SIL; Spig; *Stan*; STRO; Sul; VER-A.

AMEL (uncovering or cold application amel): *Aco*; *Ap*; Arg-n; Asar; *Aur*; Calc; Cam; *Cham*; Dros; Fer; Flu-ac; Guai; IOD; Kali-io; Kali-s; *Led*; *Lyc*; Merc; Mur-ac; *Op*; Psor; PUL; Rhus-t; Sabi; *Sec*; Spig; SUL; Syph; Tab; Thu.

Head to, agg: Ant-c; Bar-c.

Heat, and both AGG: Ant-c; Calc; *Caus*; Fer; *Flu-ac*; Grap; Hell; Kali-c; Lach; MERC; *Nat-m*; *Pho-ac*; Sep; Sil; Sul; Sul-ac; Syph; Tab; Thu.

Needles, as of: *Agar*; Ars.

Night, with hot days AGG: Aco; Dul; Merc-c; Rum.

Painful, is: Cist; Mez; Mos.

Pains: Arn; Med; Syph.

Place, entering AGG: *Ars*; Bell; *Ip*; Kali-ar; Nux-v; *Ran-b*; Sep.

Single part of, as hands in cold water, head, feet AGG: Agar; Am-c; Bell; *Calc*; HEP; *Nux-v*; *Pho*; Psor; RHUS-T; *Sep*; SIL; Tarn; Thu; Zin.

Sitting, lying on ground or a moist floor AGG: Ars; Calc; Caus; Dul; *Nux-v*; Rhod; Sil.

Sores: *Ars*; Hep; NAT-M; Pho; Rhus-t; Sep.

Tendency to take: Aco; Alu; Ars; *Ars-io*; Bacil; Bar-c; Bry; CALC; *Calc-p*; *Cham*; *Dul*; *Hep*; KALI-C; Kali-p; *Lyc*; Mag-c; Merc; *Nat-m*; *Nit-ac*;

COLD, tendency to take ..
NUX-V; Ol-j; Pho; Pho-ac; *Psor*; Rhus-t; *Sep*; SIL; *Sul*; *Tub*.

• Draft on chest agg: Pho-ac.
• Menses, first AGG: Calc-p.
• Overheated, after being: Kali-c.
• Sweating, after: Nit-ac.

Weather agg: See AIR, open cool and CHANGE OF TEMPERATURE.

COLDNESS

COLDNESS: *Aco*; Am-c; Aran; ARN; *Ars*; Aur; Bell; *Bry*; *Calc*; *Cam*; Caps; Caus; *Chin*; Dul; *Eup-p*; Fer; *Gel*; Grap; *Hep*; Ign; Ip; Kali-c; Kali-p; *Laur*; *Led*; *Lyc*; Mag-p; Merc; Mos; Nat-m; Nux-m; NUX-V; *Pho*; *Pho-ac*; *Psor*; Pul; *Pyro*; Rhus-t; Saba; *Sep*; *Sil*; Symp; VER-A.

Affected parts, of: Ars; Bry; Calc; Caps; Caus; Cocl; Colch; Lach; Led; *Meny*; *Mez*; *Rhus-t*; Sec; Sil.

Alternating or coinciding, heat in other parts with: Polyg.

Bed, in: Pho; Sil.
• Early A.M.: Mur-ac.

Bearing down, with: Castr; Sec; Sil.

Cold water, as if in: Led.

Coughing agg: Lyc.

Covers agg: *Ap*; Calc-s; Cam; Ip; Led; *Pul*; Sec; Sep.

Exertion, from: Plb; Sil; Zin-val.

External: Am-m; Ars; Cam; *Ign*; Kali-n; Nit-ac; *Nux-v*; Old; *Ver-a*; Zin.

COLDNESS, external
- Internal burning, with+: Sec.

Extremities, of: Amb; Ant-t; Ars; *Bell*; Calc; Cam; *Carb-v*; Caus; Pul; Sec; Sil; Stram; Ver-a.

Fanning, wants: Carb-v.

Flushes of: Lach.

Hot weather, in: Asar.

Icy: Agar; *Ap*; Cact; *Carb-v*; Elap; *Helod*; Hyd-ac; *Lyc*; Med; Meny; Nit-ac; Ol-an; Pho; *Sec*; *Sil*; Ver-a.
- Body, of+: Bar-m; Jat.
- Cramps, colic, with: Cup-ac.
- Fire, even near: Cadm.
- Menses, with: Sil.
- Nausea, vomiting, with: Val.
- Pain, with: Dul.

Internal: Anac; *Ap*; *Ars*; *Calc*; Caus; Cocl; Dig; Elap; Hep; *Laur*; Merc; Nux-v; Pho; Pul; *Sul*; Ther.

Menses
- At the start of: Jab.
- During: Led; Sil.

Night agg: Meny; Pho.

One part, other part hot: Ap; Bry; Cham; *Polyg*; Zin.

One sided: *Bry*; Carb-v; Caus; Con; *Dros*; Lyc; *Mos*; Nux-v; Par; *Pul*; Sil; Thu.
- Convulsion, during: Sil
- Right: Bar-c; Bry; Chel; Rhus-t; Saba.
- Left hot, as if: Par.
- Left: Carb-v; Caus; Dros; Lyc; Sul; Thu.
- epilepsy, before: Sil

COLDNESS

Pain, during: Agar; Alu-sil; Ars; Caus; Dul; Led; Mos; Sil.
- Nerve, along: Terb.

Partial, of single parts: *Ars*; Berb; Calc; Carb-v; Chel; Chin; Cist; *Dul*; *Ign*; Kali-c; Kali-chl; Lyc; Meny; Nat-m; Pho-ac; Plat; PUL; *Rhus-t*; Sec; *Sep*; Sil; *Spig*; Sul; VER-A.
- Burn, when become warm: Zin-val.

Parts lain, on: Arn; Mur-ac.

Rising from stooping, on: Merc-c.

Room, warm in: Sep.

Scratching, after: Agar; Mez; Petr.

Spots, in: Agar; Calc-p; Petr; Sep; Stro; Tarn; *Ver-a*.

Upper, parts: Ip.

COLDS: See CORYZA.

Taking AGG: Bell; Bry; Calc; *Cam*; Carb-an; Cham; Cist; Colo; Kali-n; Merc.
- Menses, during first agg: Calc-p.

COLIC: See PAIN, cramping, and FLATULENCE.

COLITIS MUCOUS: Asar; Colch; Cop; Kali-p; Rhus-t; Zin-val.

COLLAPSE (rapid, sudden, prostration): *Aco*; Aeth; *Am-c*; Ant-t; Arn; ARS; *Cam*; Carb-s; CARB-V; Colch; Con; Cup; Hyd-ac; Ip; Laur; Merc-cy; Naj; Pho; Sec; Sep; Tab; Sul; VER-A; Ver-v.

COLLAPSE

Diarrhoea, after: *Ars*; *Cam*; *Carb-v*; Sec; *Ver-a*.

Dry: Am-c; Cam; Phys.

Heart, of: Am-c.

Injury, from: Acet-ac; Sul-ac.

Moist: Colch.

Nervous: Am-c; Laur.

Paralysis, before: Con.

Photopsies, after: Sep.

Sudden: Ars; Crot-h; Grap; Hyd-ac; Pho; Sep.

Vomiting
- During: Ars.
- After: *Ars*; Ver-a.

COLLAR

AGG (See CLOTHES, pressure of around neck): Ant-c; Cench; Lach; Merc-c.

Tight, too, as if: Amyl-n: Sep.

COLOURS, bright

AGG: Sil.

AMEL: *Stram*; *Tarn*.

COMA: See UNCONSCIOUSNESS.

Vigil: Aco; Hyd-ac; *Hyo*; Laur; Mur-ac; Op; Pho.

COME AND GO: See PAIN, fleeting.

COMPANY, crowd

AGG: *Aco*; *Amb*; Anac; Ant-c; Aur; BAR-C; Bell; *Carb-an*; *Cham*; *Cic*; Fer-p+; GEL; IGN; Lyc; *Nat-c*; *Nat-m*; *Nux-v*; Sep; Thu.

- Menses, during agg: Con.

AMEL (deisre for): Arg-n; *Ars*; Bism; Bov; Dros; Hep; Hyo;

COMPANY, amel ..
Kali-c; Lac-c; Lyc; *Pho*; Radm; STRAM.

COMPLAINING, lamenting: Aur; *Cof*; Lyc; *Ver-a*; Ver-v.

Plaintive, sleep, in: Stan.

COMPLAINTS

Broods over imaginary: Naj.

Describe, cannot properly: Pul.

COMPLEXION clears+: Sars.

COMPREHENSION, difficult: See DULL.

What he reads or hears about: Sele.

COMPRESSION: See PAIN, squeezing.

CONCENTRATION, difficult: See DULL and DISTRACTION.

CONCUSSIONS: Arn; Bry; Cic; Con; *Rhus-t*; Sul.

CONDIMENTS: See FOOD AND DRINKS.

CONDYLES: See under BONES.

CONDYLOMATA (See FUNGUS GROWTH): *Med*; *Nit-ac*; Psor; *Thu*.

CONFIDENCE, want of self: Anac; Arg-n; Ars; *Lyc*; Old; Pic-ac; *Sil*; Ther.

CONFUSION, incoherence, muddled: BELL; *Bry*; Calc; *Caps*; *Carb-v*; *Gel*; HYO; Lyc; *Nux-v*; PHO; PHO-AC; RHUS-T; Sep; STRAM; Tab; Tub; *Ver-a*; *Zin*.

Daily affairs, about: Lyc.

Location, about: Cic; *Glo*; *Nux-m*; Petr.

CONFUSION

One's own identity: *Alu.*

Present, for the past: Cic.

Waking, on: Bov; Chin; Gel.

CONGESTION: *Aco*; *Alo*; Amyl-n; *Ap*; *Arn*; Aur; BELL; Bry; Cact; *Calc*; *Chin*; *Cup*; *Fer-p*; Gel; *Glo*; Lach; Lil-t; Meli; Mill; Nat-s; Nux-v; Op; *Pho*; *Pul*; Rhus-t; Sang; Sep; *Sul*; Terb; *Ver-v*; Vip.

Sudden: Aco; Bell; Glo; Ver-v.

CONICAL FORMATION: See ACUMINATE.

CONJUNCTIVA: *Aco*; Ap; ARG-N; Ars; *Bell*; *Cep*; EUPHR; Merc; PUL; Rhus-t; *Sul.*

Granular: Ap; Arg-n; Ars; Kali-bi.

Inflamed (conjunctivitis): *Aco*; *Ap*: *Arg-n*; Arn; *Ars*; BELL; Calc; Calc-s; CEP; EUPHR; *Merc*; PUL; *Rhus-t*. SUL.
- Gonorrhoeal: Arg-n; Kali-bi; Nit-ac; *Pul*.
- Menses absent, with: Euphr.

Phlyctaenae: Ars; Grap.

Pouting: Nit-ac.

Raw: Kali-io; Lyc.

Saccular: Ap; Ars.

Spots, yellow: Pho-ac.

Spring, in: Kob; Nux-v.

Ulcer: Alu; Caus.

CONSCIENCE

Terror of+: Cyc.

Troubled from, (anxiety)+: Dig.

CONSOLATION

AGG: Arg-n; Cact; Hell; *Ign*;

CONSOLATION agg..
Kali-s; Lil-t; *Nat-m*; *Sep*; *Sil*; Sul; Syph.

AMEL: Asaf; *Pul.*

Refuses, for one's own misfortune: Nit-ac.

CONSPIRACIES against him, suspects there were: Ars; Lach; Plb+; Pul.

CONSTIPATION

AGG: Alo; Arg-n.

AMEL: *Calc*; Merc; Psor; Ust.

Remedies in general: ALU; Alum; Anac; BRY; *Calc*; Caus; *Cocl*; Coll; Con; GRAP; *Hep*; Hyds; *Kali-c*; Lac-d; Lach; *Lyc*; Mag-m; *Nat-m*; Nux-m; NUX-V; *Op*; *Pho*; Plat; *Plb*; Rut; *Sanic*; *Sep*; SIL; *Stap*; *Sul*; Thu; Ver-a; Zin.

Absolute: Op.

Alternate days, on: Calc; Cocl; Con; Kali-c; Lyc; Nat-m.

Bowels action lost, as if: Aeth.
- Rectal atony+: Alet.

Chronic: Bry; Grap; Lac-d; *Nux-v*; Op; Plb; Sul; Sul-io; Tab+; Ver-a.

Cloudy weather agg: Alo.

Colds agg: Ign.

Debilitated, literary persons+: Nic.

Diarrhoea, alternating with: ANT-C; Calc; *Chel*; Fer; Kali-c+; Lyc; Nat-s; Nit-ac; *Nux-v*; Op; Pho; *Pod*; Pul; Sul+.
- Old people, in: Ant-c; Pho.

CONSTIPATION

Hard faeces, from: Alu; *Bry*; *Grap*; Mag-m; Nat-m; Nit-ac; Nux-v; Op; Plb; Sil; Sul; Verb.

Heart, weakness of, with: Phyt.

Heat of body, with: Cup.

Home, away from, when: *Lyc.*

Inactivity from, difficult stools: *Alu*; Alum; *Bry*; Chin; Grap; *Hep*; Kali-c; Mag-m; *Nat-m*; Nux-m; *Nux-v*; Op; Plb; Pyro+; Psor+; Rut; Sanic; Sele; Sil.

Infants of: Aesc; Alu; Bry; Coll; Lyc; Mag-m; Nux-v; Plb; Psor; Sele; Sep; Ver-a.
- Bottlefed, artificial food: Alu; Nux-v; Op.
- Newborn: Zin.

Lean far back, must to pass stool: Med.

Menses
- After: Kali-c.
- Amel: Aur.
- Instead of: Grap.

Mental shock, nervous strain, from: Mag-c.

Milk, cold, amel+: Iod.

Monday, every: Stan.

Neurasthenia, with: Ign.

Obstinate: Aeth; Ascl+; Hyds; Sul-io; Syph.
- Infants, in+: Croc.
  - nursing+: Ver-a.
- Old people+: Phyt.

Painful: Nit-ac; Tub.

Pregnancy, during: Hyds; Lach; Lyc; Nat-s; Nux-v; Plat; Plb; Sep.

CONSTIPATION

Purgatives or enema
- Amel: Lac-d.
- No relief from: Tarn.

Riding in carriage from: Ign.

Sea, going to, from: Bry; Lyc.

Standing amel: Alu; CAUS.

Stool
- difficult though soft: *Alu*; Anac; Chin; *Hep*; Ign; NUX-M; Plat; Psor; Pul; *Sep*; Sil; Stap.
- Recedes: Mag-m; *Op*; Sanic; *Sil*; Thu.
  - menses during: Sil.
- Removed must be: Lyc; Nat-m; Plat; Sanic; Sele; Sep; Sil.
- Scanty, with ' profuse urination at night: Alu; Bry; Caus; Grap; Hep; Kali-c; Kre; Lyc; Nat-c; Nux-v; Rhus-t; Sabi; Samb; Scil; Sep; Spig; Sul.

Strain, must: Alu; Chin; Coll; Nat-m; *Nux-v*; Rat; Sep; Sil.

Travelling, while: Alu; Lyc; Nux-v; Op; *Plat.*

Unable to pass the stool in presence of others: AMB.

Unsatisfactory, insufficient stools, from: Alo; *Alu*; Arn; Caps; Card-m; Cham; *Grap*; Kali-c; LYC; *Mag-m*; MERC-C; NAT-C; Nat-m; Nit-ac; NUX-V; Sele; *Sep*; *Sul.*

Urging
- Abortive: Anac; Con; Lyc; Mag-m; Nat-m; *Nux-v*; Pul; Sep; Sil; Sul.

CONSTIPATION, urging
- Absence, of: Alu; *Bry*; Grap; Hyds; *Op*.
  - for days+: Alum; Grap.
- Coition, after: Nat-p.
- Constant, not for stools: Lach.
  - urination amel: Lil-t.
- Crampy: Plb.
- Eating, on: Sanic.
- Erection, with: Ign; Thu.
- Ineffectual: Caps; Lac-d+; Merc; *Merc-c*; Rhe; Rhus-t; *Sul*.
- Irresistible: Alo; Nat-c.
- Neuralgia, with: Iris.
- Passes flatus only: ALO; Carb-v; Mag-m; Myr; Nat-c; *Nat-s*; Pho; Rut; Sep.
- Rectum, prolapse of, with: Rut.
- Sleep, in: Phyt.
- Stool, after: Merc.
- Urination amel: Lil-t.
- Walking agg: Kob.

Urine
- Frequent, with: Sars.
- Retention of, with: Canth.

Weather cold+: Ver-a.

Working days, after: See MONDAY.

CONSTRICTION, band, gathered together etc: Anac; Arg-n; Ars; Asar; BELL; CACT; Carb-ac; Carb-v; Chel; *Chin*; Cimi; Cocl; Con; Grap; Hyo; *Ign*; *Lach*; Lyc; Merc; Merc-c+; *Naj*; NIT-AC; Nux-v; *Plat*; *Plb*; *Pul*; Radm; Rat; Rhus-t; Sil; Stan; Stram; Sul.

CONSTRICTION
Hollow organs+: Tab.
Iron band encircled with, as if+: Colo.
Pain, during: Colo; Ign; Lyc.
Paralytic states, in: Alum.

CONSUMPTION, tuberculosis: Agar; Ars; CALC; CALC-P; *Dros*; *Hep*; *Iod*; KALI-C; Kali-s; Kre; Lach; LYC; Nit-ac; Ol-j; Phel; PHO; Psor; PUL; Sang; Senec; *Sep*; *Sil*; *Spo*; STAN; *Sul*; *Ther*; TUB; Zin.

Fever, in: Bap; Chin-ar; Fer-p.
Incipient: *Iod*; *Tub*.
Injury to chest, after: Mill; Rut.
Neglected+: Kre.
Recurring: Fer-p; Kali-n.
Stone-cutters: *Calc*; Lyc; Pul; *Sil*.
Weakness, in: Ars-io; Chin-ar.

CONTEMPT, holds everything in+: Ip.

CONTEMPTUOUS, scornful: Bry; Cham; Chin; Cic; Guai; Nux-v; Plat.

CONTINENCE AGG: Ap; Calc; *Con*; Flu-ac; Lyc; Plat.

CONTORTIONS, distortions: Agar; Bell; Caus; Cic; Guai; Hyo; Plat; Rut; Sec; Sil; Stram; Tarn.

CONTRACTION: *Am-m*; Anac; Calc; Caus; Colo; Grap; Guai; *Ign*; Lyc; Nat-c; Nat-m; *Plb*; Rut; Sec.

Pain, after: Abro.
Relaxation, and: See OPENING AND SHUTTING.

CONTRACTION

Sense of, general: Am-m; Cact; Guai; Kali-m; Nux-v; Pho.

Stiff, pain after: Pho.

CONTRACTURES: See STRICTURE.

CONTRADICT, disposition to: Hep; Rut+.

CONTRADICTIONS, intolerant of, AGG: Ast-r; Aur; Calc-s+; Cocl; Echi+; Fer; Helo; *Ign*; *Lyc*; Nux-v; *Sep*; Thyr+.

CONTRADICTORY and alternating states: Anac+; *Ign*; Nat-m; *Pul*; Tub.

CONTRARINESS: Alu; Anac; *Ant-c*; *Ant-t*; Arg-n; Ars; Bry; CHAM; Kali-c; Nux-v; Tarn.

CONTROL, lacks: Anac; Arg-m; Arg-n; Caus; Old; Stap; Tarn.

CONVERSATION

AGG: Amb; Helo; Ign; Nat-m; Sil; Stap.

AMEL: Aeth; Eup-p; Lac-d.

Imaginary beings, with: Chlo-hyd.

CONVULSIONS, spasms: Agar; Amb; *Ars*; Art-v; BELL; Buf; *Calc*; Cam; Castr; Caus; Cham; Chin; *Cic*; Cimi; Cina; CUP; *Gel*; HYO; Hypr; *Ign*; *Ip*; KALI-C; LACH; Med; Mez; Nux-m; *Nux-v*; Op; Plat; Plb; Pul; STAN; STRAM; Sul; Tarn; Thu; Ver-v; ZIN; Zin-val.

Right side: Bell; *Lyc*; Nux-v.
- Left paralysed: Art-v.

Left side: Calc-p; Ip; Sul.

CONVULSIONS

Brain tumour, from: Plb.

Cerebral softening, from: Caus.

Children, in: Art-v; Bell; Cina; Cof; Hell; Ip; Meli; Op; Stram; Ver-a; Zin.
- Attention thrust on them, from+: Ant-t.
- Dentition, during: *Calc*; *Cham*; Gel; Ign+; Terb; Passi+; Zin.
- Diarrhoea, with: Nux-m.
- Fear or Fright+: Ign.
- Holding, when amel: Nic.
- Hour, same, daily+: Ign.
- Nursing angry or frightened mother: Buf.
- Playing or laughing excessively, from: Cof.
- Strangers, approach from: Op.

Choreic: Stic.

Clonic and tonic, alternately: Ign; Mos; Stram.

Coition
- During, agg: Agar; Buf.
- After: Agar.

Coldness of body, with: Cam; Hell; *Oenan*; Ver-a.

Colic, during: Bell; Cic; Plb.

Consciousness
- With: Cina; Hell; *Ign*; Nux-m; *Nux-v*; Plat; *Stram*; *Stry*.
- Without: Arg-n; Buf; *Calc*; *Canth*; *Cic*; HYO; Oenan; *Plb*; Visc.

Coughing, with, after: Cina; Cup; Ip; Just.

Degenerative: Aur-m; *Pho*; Zin-p.

CONVULSIONS

Diarrhoea
- With: Nux-m.
- After: Mag-p; Zin.

Dysmenorrhoea, with: Caul; Nat-m.

Dyspnoea, alternating with: Plat.

Elbow, bending or stretching amel: Nux-v.

Emission, during: Art-v; Grat; *Nat-p.*

Emotional excitement, from: Cham; Cup; Nux-v; Op.

Epileptic: See EPILEPSY.

Eructation, amel: Kali-c.

Eruptions
- Fail to break out, when: Ant-t; *Cup*; *Zin*.
- Suppressed, from: Caus.

Falling, with: Bell; Cham; Cup; Hyo; Oenan.

Fear, from: Art-v; Calc; Hyo; Ign; Ind; Op.

Fever, during: Ars; Bell; Cam; Carb-v; Cina; Hyo; Nux-v; Op; Sep; Stram; Ver-a.

Goitre, suppression, after: Iod.

Grasping tight amel: Mez; Nux-v.

Grief, from: Art-v; *Hyo*; *op*.

Haemorrhage
- During: Chin; Plb; Plat; Sec.
- After: Ars; Bell; Bry; Calc; Cina; Con; Ign; Lyc; Nux-v; Pul; Sul; Ver-a.
- Suppression, from+: Mill.

CONVULSIONS

Head drawn back+: Tab.

Heart disease, from: Calc-ar.

Hysterical: Asaf; Cimi+; Con; Ign; Mos; Stan+; Zin-val.

Injuries
- After: Cic; Hep; Hypr; Nat-s; Op; Rhus-t; Val.
- Head, to: Art-v.
- Slight: Val.
- Spinal: Zin.

Internal: Caus; *Cocl*; *Hyo*; Ign; Ip; Mag-m; Nux-v; Pul; Stan.

Knocking body, from: Hypr.

Laughing, while: Cof; Grap.

Light, glare of, agg: Op.

Limbs, attempting to use, on: Cocl; PIC-AC.

Masturbation, after: Buf; Calc; Lach; *Plat*; Stram; Sul.

Menses
- Before: Buf; Caus; Cup; Hyo; Kali-br; Pul; Ver-v.
- During: Art-v; Cedr; Cup; Gel; Oenan; Plat.
- After: Syph; Ver-v.
- Instead, of: Cic; Oenan; Pul.
- Suppressed, from: Buf; Calc-p; Cocl; Gel; Glo; Mill; Pul.

Milk suppressed, from: Agar.

Miscarriage, after: Rut.

Night, at: *Cup*; Nit-ac.
- Vertigo, during day time: Nit-ac.

Noise amel: Hell.

One side: Art-v; Calc-p; Ip; Plb.
- Paralysis of other: Art-v.
- Speechlessness, with: Dul.

CONVULSIONS

Opisthotonos, with: Ver-v.

Pains
- During: *Bell*; Colo; Ign; Kali-c; Lyc; Nux-v.
- After: Chin; Plat.

Paralysis, with: *Caus*; Nux-m.

Pregnancy, during: See ECLAMPSIA.

Pressure on spine agg: Tarn.

Prodrome, as a: Ver-v.

Puberty at, in girls: Art-v; Caul; Caus.

Puerperal: See ECLAMPSIA.

Punishment, from: Agar; Cham; Cina; *Ign*.

Religious, excitement, from: Ver-a.

Rubbing, amel: Pho; Sec.

Runs in circle, before: Caus.

Sleep, during: *Ars*; BELL; Kali-c; Lach; Sep; *Sil*; *Sul*.

Sleeplessness and+: Alu; Bell; Bry; Calc; Carb-an; Carb-v; Cup; Hep; Hyo; Ign; Ip; Kali-c; Merc; Mos; *Nux-v*; Pho; Pho-ac; Pul; Rhe; Rhus-t; Sele; Sep; Sil; Stro; Thu.

Stomach, slight pressure on, from: Canth.

Stools, during: Nux-v.

Strange person, approach or sight of: Lyss; Op.

Sudden: Hyd-ac.

Suppression from: Abs; Caus; Mill.

Suppurative conditions from: Ars; Buf; Tarn.

CONVULSIONS

Tears and/or laughter with+: Alu.

Tobacco swallowing, from: Ip.

Tonic: *Bell*; Buf; Cam; *Cic*; *Ign*; *Ip*; *Op*; Petr; Plat; *Sec*; Sep.
- Single parts, of: Ign.

Touched, when: *Cic*.

Twiching, with: Ver-v.

Uraemic: Ap; Ars; Oenan+; *Ver-v*.

Vaccination, after: *Sil*.

Vertigo, after: Hyo; Tarn.

Vomiting
- With: Ant-c.
- Amel: Agar.

Wetting, from: Cup.

Whooping cough, with: Hyd-ac.

Worms, from: Cic; *Cina*; Ign; Stan.

Yawning, while: Grap.

COORDINATION, disturbed: *Agar*; *Alu*; Arg-n; Bar-c; Bell; Caus; Cimi; Cocl; Con; Echi; Fer; Gel; Glo; Grap; Hyo; Ign; Kali-p; Lach; Merc; Nux-v; Onos; Pho; Plat; *Rhus-t*; Sul.

COPPER COLOUR (discharge, skin, etc): Carb-an; Cor-r; Merc; Mez; Nit-ac; *Rhus-t*; Syph.

Eruptions: Hydroc; Merc-d; Sars.

Spots: Benz-ac; Lach; Med; Nit-ac.
- Remaining after eruptions: Med.

COPPER FUMES AGG: Ip; Merc; Pul.

CORNEA

Affections in general: CALC; *Cann*; Con; *Euphr*; Hep; Merc; Merc-i-f; *Pul*; Sul.

Herpes on: Ran-b.

Inflamed (keratits): Calc; Merc; Merc-c; Sul; Syph; Thu.
- Bathing cold amel: Syph.
- Recurrent+: Grap.

Injected: *Aur*; Grap; Ign; Merc.

Opacity: *Ap*; *Arg-n*; Cadm; *Calc*; CANN; Con; LACH; *Pul*; *Sil*; SUL; ZIN-S.
- Dense: Kali-bi.
- Injury, from: Euphr.
- Old age, in (arcus senilis): Calc; Kali-c; Merc; Pho; *Pul*; *Sul*; Vario.
- Small-pox vaccination, after: Sil.
- Spots, in: Calc-f.

Pustules, on: Kali-m.

Rough: Sil.

Scratched or chipped, as if+: Merc-i-f.

Spots, on: Ap; Calc; Con; Nit-ac.
- Yellow, with network of blood vessels around: *Aur*.

Sunken+: Aeth.

Ulcers: Arg-n; *Ars*; Calc; Euphr; Hep; *Kali-bi*; *Merc-c*; *Sil*; Sul.
- Pain and photophobia, without: Kali-bi.
- Perforating: Ap.

CORNS: See CALLOSITIES.

CORPULENCE: See OBESITY.

CORRODING: See DISCHARGES, acrid.

CORYZA

CORYZA: *Aco*; Amb; ARS; Bell; Calc; *Cam*; Carb-v; CEP; *Cham*; Chel; *Euphr*; Eup-p; *Fer-p*; GEL; *Hep*; Ign; Kali-io; Lac-c; Lach; MERC; *Merc-c*; Nat-m; Nit-ac; *Nux-v*; Pho; PUL; *Rhus-t*; Saba; Sele; Stap; *Sul*; Tell; Thu.

Aged, of: Am-c; Ant-c; Cam.
- Palpitation, with: Anac.

Air, open
- Amel: Calc-p; Calc-s; Cep; Nux-v; Stic+.
- And agg: Tell.

Alternate days: Nat-c.

Annual (hay fever): Ars; Ambro; Cep; Gel; KALI-IO; Kali-p; Nat-m; *Nux-v*; Pho; PSOR; Saba; Senec; Sep; SIL; Sinap; SUL.

Ascending: Aru-t; *Bro*; Lac-c; Merc; Sep.

Autumn, in: Merc.

Bloody, infants, in: Calc-s.

Changeable: Stap.

Change of season, temperature: Cep; Gel.

Children, in: Merc-i-r.
- Discharge, bluish+: Am-m.

Chill, with: Merc; Nux-v.

Chilled by snow or ice, from: Ant-c; Dros; Iod; Laur; Pul; Seneg; Ver-a; Verb.

Chronic: Bro; Cist; Hep; Kali-bi; Sil; Sul.
- Asthma, causing: Sil.

Cold bathing amel: Calc-s.

Coughing agg: Agar; Bell; Euphr; Ip; *Lach*; Nit-ac; *Scil*; Sul; Thu.

CORYZA

Day, by: Nux-v.
- Damp agg: Kali-io.

Descending: Ars; Bry; Carb-v; Iod; Kali-c; Lyc; Pho; Stic; Sul; Tub.

Diphtheria, in: Aru-t; Kali-bi; Nit-ac.

Diarrhoea, then: Alu; Calc; Sang; Sele; Tub.

Draft, least agg: Nat-c.

Dry: Calc; Caus; Chin; Mag-c; Nux-v; Pho; Samb; Stic.
- Indoors: Thyr.
- Nose, obstruction with: Mang.

Dyspnoea, with: Ars-io; Kali-io; Nit-ac.

Eating agg: Carb-an; Nux-v; Sanic; Tromb.

Epistaxis, with: Senec; Sil.

Exhausting: Arg-m.

Fever, in: Bry; Merc.

Flowers, odour of agg: Saba; Sang.

Fluent
- And dry alternately: Nat-m.
- Indoors: Calc-p; Cep; Nux-v.
- Thick and alternately: Stap.

Hair-cut, after: Bell; *Nux-v*; Sep.

Headache, then: Ant-c.

Hoarseness, with: Ars-io; Caus; Tell.

Hot: Cham; Iod.

Hunger, with: Ars-io.

Knees, hot, with+: Ign.

Lying
- Agg: Euphr; Spig.
- Amel: Merc.

Menses, at: Am-c; Bar-c; *Grap*; Kali-c; *Lach*; Mag-c; Pho; Senec; Sep; Zin.

Milk agg: Lac-d.

Newborn: Dul.

Nose stopped, with: Ars.

One side: Nux-v; Pho; Phyt.

Peaches, odour of agg: Cep.

Periodical attacks: *Bro*; *Grap*; Sil.

Polyuria, with: Calc.

Salivation, with: Calc-p; Kali-io.

Sea-bathing amel: Med.

Singer's: Cep.

Sleep, in: Flu-ac; Lac-c.

Smell acute, with: Kalm.

Sneezing
- With: Carb-an.
- Then: Naj.

Stooping agg: Laur.

Stopped, suppressed: Ars; *Aru-t*; Bell; Bro; Bry; Calc; Chin; LACH; *Lyc*; Mar-v; *Nit-ac*; NUX-V; Pul; Sil.
- As if: Osm.

Stubborn, lingering+: Saba.

Sudden attacks: Iod; Plant; Syph; Thu; Zin.

Summer, in: Dul; Gel.
- Diarrhoea, with: Dul.

Swallowing agg: Carb-an.

Tendency to recur: See COLD, tendency to take.

CORYZA

Throat, sore, with: Merc; Nit-ac; Nux-v; Pho.
Urination, burning, with: Ran-sc.
Violent attacks: Ars; Aru-t; Lyc.
- Palpitation, with (aged)+: Anac.

Warm room amel: Ars; Dul; Saba.
Yawning agg: Carb-an; Cup; Lyc.

COTTONY feeling: Onos.

COUGH

Remedies in general: Aco; Amb; *Ars*; *Bell*; Bry; Carb-v; Caus; Cham; Chin; Cina; Coc-c; Con; DROS; HEP; *Hyo*; *Ign*; Ip; *Kali-c*; *Lach*; Lyc; Merc; Nat-m; NUX-V; PHO; PUL; *Rum*; *Sang*; SEP; *Spo*; Stan; *Sul*.

Abdomen, stomach or epigastrium, from: *Ant-c*; Arg-n; Bell; BRY; Dros; Ign; Kali-bi; *Kali-m*; Lach; Nat-m; *Nit-ac*; Pho; Pho-ac; Pul; Rum; Sang; SEP.

Air, open
- Agg: Ars; Kali-n; Pho; Rum.
- Amel: Bry; Coc-c; Iod; Mag-p; Pul; Radm.

Alternate days agg: Lyc.
Anger, from: Ant-t; *Cham*; Saba.
- Children: Anac; Ant-t.

Arms
- Raising agg: Bry; Fer; Tub.
- Stretching agg: Lyc.

COUGH

Ascending stairs, when: Arg-n.
Auditory canal, touching agg: Kali-c; Lach; Mang; Sil.
Barking: Aco; Amb+; *Bell*; *Dros*; Hep; Lyss; Rum; *Spo*; Stic; Stram.
- Dry+: Clem.
- Eructations, with: Ver-a.

Bed
- Turning in agg: Kre.
- Warmth of
  - agg: *Caus*; Nux-m; *Pul.*
  - amel: Arg-n; Cham; Kali-bi.

Bends backwards, child+: Ant-t.
Bloody, taste, with: Ham.
Bouts
- One: Calc.
- Two or three: *Merc*; Pho; Plb; Pul; Stan; *Sul*; Thu.
- Three or four: *Bell*; Carb-v; Cup.
- First, more violent, but succeeding weaker and weaker: Ant-c.
- Isolated: Cor-r.

Brain complaint, in: Glo.
Breast, left, coldness of, with: Nat-c.
Breathing, interrupts: See Suffocating.
Cannot, deep enough: Caus; Rum.
Cardiac: See Heart complaints, with.
Causes distant pains: Caps.
Change of position agg: Kre.

COUGH

Chest
- Holds, during: Arn; *Bry*; *Dros*; Eup-p; Nat-s; Pho; Sep.
- Wetting amel: Bor.

Chill
- Before: *Rhus-t*; Samb; Tub.
- During: Pho; Rhus-t; Saba.

Coition, after: Tarn.

Cold
- Air, inspiring agg: Cep+; *Rum*; Sang.
- Drinks
  - agg: *Ars*; Calc; Carb-v; Coc-c; Hep; Manc; *Psor*; Rhus-t; Scil; Sil; Spo; Ver-a.
  - amel: Caps; *Caus*; Coc-c; *Cup*; Ip; Onos; Tab.
  - warm agg: Stan.
- From, every: Mang; Sang.
- Milk agg: Ant-t; Spo.
- Water, standing in agg: Nux-m.
- Wind on chest agg: Pho; Rum.

Company agg: *Amb*; Ars; Bar-c.
Condiments agg: Alu.
Consciousness, loss of with: Cup.
Consolation, agg: Ars.
Constipation agg: Con; Grap; Sep.
Convulsions, with: Cina; *Cup*; Lach; Meph; Stram.
Coryza, with: See CORYZA.
Coughing agg: Bell; *Ign*; Hep; Mar-v; Stic; Thyr.
Cries before: Arn; *Bell*; *Bry*; Cina; Hep; *Pho*.

COUGH

Dancing agg: Pul.
Daytime only: Rum; Thu.
- Long spells, with: Vio-o.

Deep: Dros; *Hep*; Lyc+; Spo; Stan; Ver-a; Verb.
- Breathing
  - agg: Bell; Bro; Con; Cup; Grap; Lyc; Stic.
  - amel: Pul; Verb.

Descending agg: Lyc.
Diarrhoea, amel: Buf.
Drinking
- Agg: Ars; Bry; Dros; Hyo; Meph; Psor.
- Amel: Op; Spo.

Drunkards, of: Coc-c+; Stram.
Dry (without expectoration): *Aco*; Alu; Ars; Bell; Bry; Calc; Hyo; Ign; *Ip*; Kali-c; Laur; Nat-m; Nat-s; *Nux-v*; Petr; *Pho*; Pho-ac; Pul; Rum; Sele; *Spo*; Stic; *Sul*; Tub.
- Day and night: Xanth.
- Diarrhoea, after: Abro.
- Emaciation, with: Lyc.
- Evening: Pul.
- Hand, laying on pit of stomach amel: Arg-n; Croc.
- Loose and dry, alternately: Ars.
- Menses, at: Zin.
- Night: Cimi; Hyo; Merc; Stic.
  - loose by day: Ars; Hep; Merc; Pul; Sil; Sul.
- Pining children, in: Lyc.
- Smoking, from+: Hell.
- Speaking+: Cimi.

COUGH, dry
- Spot, in larynx, from: Con; Hyo; Nat-m.
- Vomits, until: Mez; Stic.

Dust, feathers, as from: Chel; Ign; Rum.

Eating
- Agg: Bry; Chin; Cor-r; *Hyo*; Kali-bi; *Nux-v*.
- Amel: Euphr; Radm; Spo.
- Fatty food, from: Mag-m; Pul.
- Fish agg: Lach.
- Fruits agg: Arg-m; Mag-m.
- Hastily agg: Sil.
- Irritating things agg: Alu.
- Meat agg: Stap.
- Warm food agg: Bar-c.

Emaciation, with: *Acet-ac*; Amb; Lyc; *Nit-ac*.

Emotions, from: Amb; Caps; Ign; Spo; Verb.
- Evening to sunrise: Aur.

Empty tube, as if from: Osm.

Eructation
- Agg: *Amb*; Bar-c; Carb-v; Lob; Stap.
- Amel: Sang.
- With: Kali-bi; Lob.

Eruptions, receding, when: Dul; Led; Pul.

Evening
- Agg: Bry; Calc; Nux-v; Rhus-t; Sep; Tub.
- Midnight, to: Hep.

Exertion
- Agg: Dul; Stan; Pho.
- Amel: Radm; Stro.

Exhausting: Ars; Bell; *Carb-v*;

COUGH, exhausting .. Caus; Hyo; *Pho*; Sep; Stan; Ver-a.
- Sweat, with: Hyo.

Expectoration
- Agg: Coc-c; Tarn.
- Amel: *Ant-t*; *Ap*; Aral; Cist; *Coc-c*; Grind; Kali-bi; Sep; *Stan*; *Zin*.

Eyes
- Closing for sleep at night agg: *Hep*.
- Complaints, with: Nat-m.

Falls down: Nux-v; Pho.

Fatty food, from: Mag-m; Pul+.

Fever
- Before: Samb.
- During: *Aco*; Ars; Calc; Con; Ip; Kali-c; Nat-m; Nux-v; Pho; Saba.

Flatus passing amel: Sang.

Fluid gone wrong way, as if, from: Lach.

Fog agg: Sep.

Foul air, raises up: Calc; *Caps*; Culex; Dros; Guai; *Lach*; Mez; *Sang*; Sep; Sul.

Fright, form: Samb.

Futile: Kali-c.

Habitual: Calc.

Hair sensation in trachea, from: Sil.

Hands, puts on thighs, during: Nic.

Hawking agg: Am-m; Coc-c.

Headache, with: Carb-v; Sul+.

Heart complaints, with: Adon; Arn; Lach; Laur; Lycps; Naj; Nux-v; Spo.

COUGH

Hollow: Amb+; Bell; Carb-v; Caus; Lyc+; *Spo*; Ver-a.

Hot
- Applications
  - amel: Ars; Hep; Lyc; Nux-v; Pho; Rhus-t; Rum; Sil.
  - Abdomen, to amel: Sil.
- Things agg: Mez.

Hour, same: Lyc; Saba.

Incessant: *Aco*; ALU; *Caus*; Cham; Chin; *Cof*; Crot-h; Cup; DROS; HYO; Ip; Kali-c; Lach; Lyc; *Nux-v*; Pho-ac; Pul; *Rhus-t*; RUM; Scil; Sep; SPO; Ver-a.
- Sleep, preventing: Stic.

Influenza, after: Am-c; Sang.

Inspiration, every agg: Aco; Stic.

Jerking
- Lower limbs+: Stram.
- The body together: Agar; Ther.

Lachrymation, with+: Scil.

Lactation, during: Fer.

Lamenting+: Arn.

Larynx, pressure of agg: See Pressure.
- Spot, dry in, from+: Nit-ac.

Laughing agg: Arg-n; Chin; Con; Mang; Pho.

Lifting agg: Amb.

Liver symptoms with+: Am-m.

Looking at
- Fire agg: Ant-c; Stram.
- Light: Stram.

COUGH

Loose
- Expectoration, with: Ars; *Calc*; *Led*; Lyc; Nat-c; Pho; *Pul*; *Sep*; Stan.
- By day: *Ars*; Calc; *Cham*; *Hep*; *Merc*; *Pul*; *Sil*; *Sul*.
- Morning: *Bry*; *Carb-v*; *Hep*; *Par*; *Pho*; *Pul*; *Scil*; *Sep*; Sil; Stan; Sul; Sul-ac.
  - 9 to 11 A.M: Nat-c.
- Night, at: Sep.

Lying
- Agg: *Ap*; *Ars*; Caus; Con; Dros; *Hyo*; Kre; Psor; *Pul*; Radm; Rum; Sang; Sep.
- Amel: Calc-p; *Euphr*; Fer; *Mang*.
- Abdomen on, amel: Eup-p; *Med*.
- Back on, agg+: Am-m.
- Head on high pillow, amel: Carb-v; *Chin*.
- Knees on, with head on pillow amel: Eup-p.
- Right side, on agg: Am-m+; *Merc*; Seneg; *Stan*; Stap; Syph.
- Left side on agg: Sep.

Measles
- In: Dros; Ip; Pul.
- After: Cof; Stic.

Meat agg+: Stap.

Menses
- Amel: Senec.
- Before: Arg-n; Grap.
- During: Calc-p; Grap; Sep; Zin.
- Suppressed, agg: Dig.

Metallic: Kali-bi.

COUGH

Midnight, at: Aral; Dros; Lach.
- To morning+: Rhus-t.

Milk, cold agg: Ant-t; Spo.

Morning
- Agg: Ars; Euphr; Hep; *Lyc*; Mos; Pul; Rum; Sele.
- And evening agg: *Aco*; Bor; *Calc*; *Carb-v*; *Caus*; Cina; Fer; Fer-p; Ign; *Lyc*; Merc; Nat-m; Pho; *Rhus-t*; Sil; Ver-a.

Mouth
- Covering amel: Rum.
- Rinsing
  - when: Coc-c.
  - with cold water amel: Coc-c.

Muffled: Saba.

Music agg: *Amb*; Calc.

Neck, touch of agg: Bell; Bro; *Lach*.

Nervous: Amb; Caps; Cimi; Ign; Verb.

Night
- Agg: Bar-c; Bell; Calc; Cimi; Con; Dros; Hyo; Laur; Nux-v; Petr; Pho; Pul; Stic.
- Only: Amb; Caus; Petr.
- Urine, spurting, with: Colch.

Noise agg: Arn; Pho-ac; Tarn.

Occiput, pain in, with+: Anac.

Odours, strong, agg: Merc-i-f; Pho; Sul-ac.

Pain, in distant parts+: Caps.

Painful: *Aco*; Arn; BELL; BRY; *Caps*; *Caus*; Dros; Elap; Eup-p; Kali-c; *Nat-m*; NUX-V; *Pho*; *Rhus-t*; *Scil*; Seneg; Spo; Stan; Stic; Sul.

COUGH

People coming and going agg: Carb-v.

Piano playing agg: Calc.

Pregnancy
- During: Apoc; *Cham*; *Con*; Kali-br; Nux-m; *Pul*.
- Early, causing abortion: Rum.
- Reflex, from+: Kali-br.

Pressure on
- Abdomen amel: Con.
- Epigastrium amel: Croc; Dros.
- Larynx agg: Cina; *Lach*; Rum.
- Temples amel: Petr.
- Throat pit agg: Rum.

Prodrome, as a: Bry; Rhus-t; Saba; Samb; Tub.

Reading
- Loudly agg: Amb; Mang; Nux-v; Pho.
- Mind in, agg: Cina.

Repose amel: Ip.

Retching, gagging
- With: Pho.
- Amel: Lach.

Reverberating: Cor-r; Kali-bi; *Stram*; Verb.

Room
- Entering or leaving agg: *Pho*; Rum.
- Warm, entering, on: Bry; Nat-c; Thyr; Ver-a.

Rubs, face and eyes with hands, during (child): Caus; Pul; Scil.

Saliva runs: Am-m; Lach; Thu; Ver-a.

COUGH

Salty things agg: Alu; Con; Lach.
Sawing: Spo.
Sciatica, alternating with, in summer: Stap.
Shattering: Bry; Carb-v; Ign; Kali-c; *Mang*; *Nit-ac*+; Nux-v; *Pho-ac*; Rum; Stan.
Short: Aco; Ars; *Caus*; *Cof*; Ign; Lach; Laur; *Merc*; Nat-m; Pho; *Rhus-t*; Sang; *Sep*; Stan; Tub.
Singing agg: Alu; Arg-n; Dros; Hyo+; Kali-bi; Pho; Stan.
Sit up, must: Con; Hyo; Phel+; Pho; *Pul*.
Sitting
- Agg+: Nat-p.
- Bent amel: Iod.

Sleep, first, after: Aral.
Smallpox
- During: Plat.
- After: Calc.

Smoking
- Agg: Arg-n; Ars; Colo; Dros; Euphr; Hell; Merc; Radm; Stap+.
- Amel: *Arg-n*; Euphr; Hep; Ign; Merc; Sep; Tarn.

Sneezing
- With: Agar; Alu; Bell: Bry; Cina; Lob; Psor; *Scil*; *Seneg*.
- Amel: Osm.
- Then: *Agar*; Scil; Seneg; Sul.

Sour things agg: Alu; Con; Sul.
Speaker's: Coll.
Spine, from: *Agar*; Nux-m; Tell.
Spleen, enlarged or pain with: Scil.

COUGH

Standing
- While walking agg: Ign.
- Sitting, after: Alo.

Sternum, tickling behind with+: Rhus-t.
Stomach, pain in, with: Lob.
Stooping agg: Arg-n; Caus; Hep; Spig.
Stranger, at the sight of: *Ars*; Bar-c; Pho.
Student's: Nux-v.
Suffocating: Alu; *Ant-t*; *Bor*; Bro+; *Carb-v*; *Chin*; Cina; *Cup*; *Dros*; Hep; Hyo; *Ip*; Kali-c; *Lach*; *Meph*; Nux-v; Op; *Samb*; *Sang*; *Seneg*; *Spo*; *Stram*; SUL.
- Gurgling down in throat, then: Cina.

Sulphur fumes, as from: Ign; Lyc.
Sun, in: Ant-t.
Sunset to sunrise+: Aur.
Surprise, happy agg: Aco; Merc.
Swallowing
- Agg: Aesc; *Bro*; Cup; Nat-m.
- Amel: Ap; Spo.
- Empty
  - agg: Lyc; Nat-m.
  - amel: Bell.

Sweet things
- Agg: Bad; Med; Spo; Zin.
- Amel: Sul.

Talking
- Agg: Alu; Amb; Anac+; Con; Dros; Hyo; Meph; Rum; Sanic; Sil+; Stan+.
- Loudly agg: Coc-c.

COUGH

Taste, bloody with: Ham; Rhus-t+.
Tea agg: Spo.
Tearing: Rhus-t.
Teeth
- Ache with: Lyc; Sep.
- Cleaning agg: Carb-v; Coc-c; Dig; Euphr; Sep; Stap.

Temperature, change of agg: Kali-c; *Pho*; Rum; Sep; Verb.
Throat or larynx, from: *Aco*; Amb; Calc; CHAM; *Con*; Hep; IP; Kali-c; Lach; Nat-m; Nux-v; Pho; Rum; *Sang*; Sep.
- Right side, from: Agar; Dros; Stan; Stic.
- Left side, from: Caus; Hep; Lach; Lith; *Rhus-t*; Tell.
- Back of, from: Dul.
- Dry, with: Thu.
- Stretching Agg: Lyc.

Tickling: Aco; Ars; *Arn*; Bell; *Cham*; *Con*; DROS; *Hyo*; *Iod*; *Ip*; Kali-c; LACH; *Lyc*; Nat-m; NUX-V; PHO; Pho-ac; Pul; *Rhus-t*; RUM; Sang; Sep; Spo; *Stan*; Sul.
- Constant: Nat-c; Op.
- Dry, with fever but no thirst: Ars; Con; Pho; Pul; Saba; Scil.

Tight: Pho; Stan.
- Clothes agg: Stan.

Tired when, agg: Stic.
Tongue, protruding agg: Lyc.
Tonsils, enlarged: Bar-c; Lach.
Trembling, with: Pho.

COUGH

Tube, empty, as if from: Osm.
Uncovering, agg: Hep; Nux-v; Rhus-t; Rum.
Urination involuntary, with+: Ver-a.
Urine spurting, with+: Scil.
Uvula elongated+: Alu; Merc-i-r.
Vapour, as from: Bro; Lyc.
Violent: See Whooping.
Violin, playing on: Kali-c.
Voice, from excessive use of: Coll.
Vomiting
- Before: Sul-ac.
- With: *Alu*; ANT-T; *Bry*; Carb-v; Coc-c; Cor-r; *Dros*; Fer; Hep; IP; Kali-c; Laur; Nux-v; Pul; Rhus-t.
- Amel: Mez.

Wakes: Caus; Hyo; Pho; Pul; Samb; Spo; Sul.
- Does not: Arn; Bacil; Cham; Cyc; Lach; Lycps; Nit-ac; Verb.
- Midnight, after: Samb.

Walk, cannot, without: Stan.
Walking
- Amel: Canc-fl; Dros.
- Fast agg: Sep.

Warmth
- Amel: Hep; Ip; Lyss; Pho; Rum.
- Bed of, amel: See under Bed.

Weather
- Change: See Temperature.
- Cold, foggy amel: Spo.

COUGH, weather, cold
- to, warm and vice versa agg: Rum.
Weeping, crying agg: Arn; Bell; Hep; Ver-a.
Wetting the chest amel: Bor.
Whooping, violent, spasmodic: Agar; BELL; CARB-V; Caus; Cham+; *Cina*; *Coc-c*; Con; *Cor-r*; *Cup*; *Dros*; Hep; Ign; *Ip*; *Kali-c*; Kali-s; Lach; *Meph*; Mez; NUX-V; Pho; Pho-ac; *Pul*; Scil; Sep; Stan; Stic+; *Stram*; Tub; *Ver-a*; Ver-v.
- Air, cool, Amel+: Mag-p.
- Catarrhal phase: Aco; Dul; Ip; Nux-v; Pul.
- Defervescent stage: Ant-t; Pho; Pul.
- Drags on+: Sep.
- Facial herpes, with: Arn.
- Lachrymation, with+: Nat-m.
- Neglected, with complications: Ver-a.
- Obstinate: Calc-p.
- Spasmodic phase: Carb-v; Cina; Coc-c; Dros; Kali-c; *Nux-v*; Pul; *Ver-a*.
- Throws him down+: Nux-v.
- Torn loose feeling, with: Osm.
Winter agg: Ant-t; Cham; Kali-m; Nat-m; Nit-ac; Psor.
- Old people in, during entire season: Ant-c; Kre.
Writing, while: Cina.
Yawning
- Agg: Arn; Asaf; Bell; Mur-ac.
- And, consecutively: Ant-t; Nat-m.
Yawns and sleeps+: Anac.

COUGHING
AGG: Aco; Ars; *Bell*; BRY; Calc; Caps; Carb-v; Cina; *Dros*; *Ip*; Merc; NUX-V; *Pho*; *Pul*; *Rhus-t*; *Sep*; Spo; Stan; Sul; Tell.
AMEL: Ap; Stan.
Distant parts, pain in, when: Caps.
COUNTS CONTINUOUSLY: Phys; Sil.
COURAGEOUS: See BOLDNESS.
COVERS AGG (See also HEAT agg), cold application AMEL: Aco; *Ap*; Calc; *Iod*; Kali-io; Kali-s; *Lach*; Led; Lil-t; LYC; Op; Pul; Sanic; *Sec*; Spig; *Sul.*
Wants: Tub.
COWARDLY (See ANTHROPOPHOBIA): Amb; Anac; Bar-c; *Gel*; Kre; Lach; Lyc; Nux-m; Ol-an; Pul; Sil; STRAM.
CRACKING in joints: See JOINTS.
CRACKLING like tinsel: Aco; Calc; Cof; Hep; Rhe; Sep.
CRACKS, fissures, chaps (See also SKIN): Ant-c; Ant-t; Calc; Calc-f; Caus+; Cist; *Fer*; *Grap*; Flu-ac; Hep; *Ign*; Lyc; *Merc*; Merc-c; Mez; Mur-ac; Nat-m; NIT-AC; PETR; Pho; Pul; Rat; Rhus-t; Sars; *Sep*; *Sil*; *Sul.*
Small: Merc-i-r.
CRAFTY (See DECEITFUL): Tarn.
CRAMP : See PAIN, crampy.
Writer's (See FINGERS, working agg): Arg-m; Arn; Dros; Gel; Mag-p; Pic-ac; Sul-ac.

CRASH: See BLOWS.

CRAVINGS (See also DESIRES)

Alcoholic drinks for: Arn; *Ars*; Asar; *Calc*; Caps; Crot-h; *Lach*; Nux-v; *Op*; Sele; Stap; Sul; Syph.
- Beer: Aco; Mos+; Nat-p; Petr; Psor+; Stro; *Sul*.
- Brandy+: Mos; Sul-ac.
- Menses, before: Sele.
- Which she disliked: Med.
- Wine+: Hypr; Mez; Ther.

Almonds: Cub.

Appetite, without: Op.

Apples: Alo; Ant-t; Guai; Sul; Tell.

Ashes: Tarn.

Bacon: Calc; Calc-p; Mez; Radm; Sanic; Tub.

Bananas: Ther.

Bitter
- Drinks+: Aco.
- Things: Dig; Nat-m.

Bread: Fer; Grat; Stro.
- Butter and: Merc.
- Rye+: Ign.

Butter: All-s; Fer; Merc.

Buttermilk: Ant-t; Bur-p; Chin-s; Elap; Sabal.

Cabbages: Cic.

Chalk: See Lime.

Charcoal: Alu; Calc; Cic; Psor.

Cheese: Arg-n; Cist; Pul+.

Cherries: Chin.

Cloves: Alu; Chlor.

Coarse, raw food: Ab-c; Alu; Ant-c; Calc; Calc-p; Ign; Sil; Sul; Tarn.

CRAVINGS

Coffee: Ars; Aur+; Bry; Caps+; Con; Lach+; Mez; Mos; Nux-v; Strop.
- Black: Mez.

Cold things, for: Aco; ARS; Bism; *Bry*; Cadm; Cham; *Chin*; Cina; Diph; Eup-p; Flu-ac; Lept; Manc; Merc; *Merc-c*; Nat-s; Onos; PHO; Rhus-t; Thu; VER-A.

Condiments, spices, pickles: Ant-c+; *Ars*; Calc-p; Caps; Chel; *Chin*; Cist; Flu-ac; *Hep*; Lac-c; Nux-m; Nux-v; *Pho*; Pul; Sang; Stap; *Sul*; Tarn.

Cucumber: Ant-c; Ver-a.

Delicacies, dainties: Aur; *Chin*; *Ip*; Lil-t; Mag-m+; Petr+; Rhus-t; Saba; Spo; *Tub*.
- Sexual desire, with: Chin.

Different kinds: Rhe.

Dry: Alu.

Effervescent drinks: Colch; Pho-ac.

Eggs: *Calc*; Nat-p.

Farinacious food: Lach; *Nat-m*; Saba; Sumb.

Fats, fatty things: Calc-p; Mez; *Nit-ac*; Nux-v; Sul.

Finery, beautiful things: Aeth; Lil-t; Sul.

Fish: Nat-m; Sul-ac.
- Fried: Nat-p.

Fried things: Plb.

Fruits: Alu; Ant-t+; Mag-c+; Pho-ac; Sul-ac; Ver-a.
- Acid: Ars; Cist; Ther; *Ver-a*.
- Juicy: Ant-t; Pho-ac; Stap; Ver-a.

CRAVINGS

CRAVINGS, fruits
- Oranges: Cub; Med; Ther.

Green things: Calc-s; *Med.*
Ham+: Mez.
Herring: *Nit-ac*; Pul; Ver-a.
Honey: Saba.
Hot things: *Ars*; *Bry*; Chel; Fer; Lac-c; Lyc; Saba.
Ice: Ars; Elap; Lept; Med; Ver-a.
- Cream: Calc; Eup-p; *Pho*; Sil.
- Pain, during: Med.
- Water: Aco; Ars; Lept; Old+; Onos; Pho; Sil; Ver-a.

Indefinite things (knows not what): *Bry*; Chin; *Ign*; *Ip*; *Pul*; Ther; Zin-chr.
Indigestible things: Alu; Calc; Calc-p; Cyc.
Juicy things: See Fruits, juicy.
Lemonade: *Bell*; Cyc; Nit-ac; Pul; Sabi; Sec; Sul-io.
Line, chalk, clay, earth: Alu; Ant-c; *Calc*; Cic; Ign; *Nit-ac*; *Nux-v*; Psor; SIL; Sul; *Tarn.*
Liquids: Stap; Sul.
Many things: Cic; *Cina*; Stap.
- Pleased, with nothing: All-s.
- Refuses, when given: Stap.
  - to eat them: Rhe.

Meat: Kre; Lil-t; Mag-c; Vio-o.
Milk: *Ap*; Ars; Aur+; Chel+; Cist; Lac-c; Merc; Nat-m+; *Pho-ac*; *Rhus-t*; Saba; Sabal; Sanic; Stap; Sul.
- Boiled: Abro; Nat-s.
- Cold: Rhus-t; Pho; Pho-ac; Tub.
  - ice: Sanic.
- Sour: Ant-t; Mang.

CRAVINGS, milk
- Warm: Bry; Calc; Chel.
- Which
  - amel+: Ap.
  - he disliked: Sabal.
  - he drinks much: Lac-c.

More than he wants: Ars.
Mustard: Cocl.
Nuts: Cub.
Onions: Bels; Cep; Cub.
Oysters: Lach; Nat-m+; Rhus-t.
Particular thing: Rhe.
Pepper: Lac-c.
- Cayenne: Merc-c.

Pickles: See Condiments.
Pork: Crot-h; Radm; Tub.
Potatoes: Nat-c; Ol-an.
- Raw: Calc.

Pregnancy, during: Calc-p; Chel; Sep.
- Strange things: Chel; Lyss; Mag-c; Sep.

Rags, clean: Alu.
Refreshing things: Med; Pho-ac; *Pul*; Ver-a.
Relish, what cannot: Bry; Ign; Mag-m; Pul.
Salty things: Alo+; Arg-n; Calc-p; *Carb-v*; Caus; Con+; Lac-c; Med; Merc-i-r; NAT-M; Nit-ac+; *Pho*; Thu; Ver-a.
Sand: Sil; Tarn.
Sardines: Cyc.
Smoked things: *Caus*; Kre; *Tub.*
Snuff: Bell.
Sour things: *Aco*; Ant-t; *Arn*; Ars; Bell; Cham; Con+; Cor-r;

CRAVINGS, sour things ..
Hep; Mag-c+; Med+; Myr; Pod; Pul; Radm; Sec; Sep; *Sul*; Ther; Ver-a.

Spicy things: See Condiments.

Stimulants: Carb-ac+; Crot-h; Sele.
- Which agg+: Naj.

Strange things: Bry; Calc; Calc-p; Chel; Hep.
- Many, from inability to distinguish, edible from non-edible: Cic.

Sweet
- Drinks: Buf.
- Things: *Arg-n*; Calc; Carb-v; CHIN; Cina; Ip+; *Kali-c*; Kali-p; *Lyc*; Mag-m; Med; Merc; Saba; *Sul*; Thyr; Tub.
- Weakness, with: Thyr.

Tea: Alu; Hep; Sele.

Things
- That are refused, when offered: Bry; *Cham*; Dul; Hep; Kre; Pho; Phys; Stap.
- That disagree: Pul.

Tobacco: Asar; Carb-v; Daph+; Stap; *Tab*.
- Smoking: Calc-p; Carb-ac; Glo; Med; Ther.

Tomatoes: Fer.

Vegetables: Alu; Mag-c+; Mag-m.

Vinegar: Arn; Hep; Kali-p.

Wine: See Alcoholic drinks.

CRAWLING

As of insects, bugs, flies etc: Calad; Carb-an; Dul; Lac-c; Myr; Nat-c; Oenan; Osm; Pho-ac; Pic-ac; Stram; Tab; Tarn.

Bad news, after: Calc-p.

Body, all over: Cist.

Floor, on: Abs; Lach.

Outward: Chel.

Spider, as of a: Visc.

Waist, around: Oenan.

CRAZY: See INSANITY.

Feels like going: Syph.

CREEPING, running as of a mouse, etc: *Bell*; *Calc*; Cimi; Lyc; Nit-ac; Pho; Rhod; Sep; Stap; *Sil*; *Sul*.

Cold: Frax; Lac-c.
- Menses, before: Ant-t.

Left side: Nit-ac.

Nervous: Canc-fl.

CREPITATION: Aco; Calc; Cof; Rhe.

Skin, under: Carb-v.

Synovial: Nat-p.

CRETINISM: Aeth; Anac; Bar-c; Buf; Thu; Thyr.

Agile+: Calc-p.

CRIES, shrieks, screams (See also WEEPS, SORROWS): *Aco*; AP; BELL; Bor; Calc; Cam; *Cham*; Cic; Cina; *Cup*; Glo; Hyd-ac; Ign; Jal; Kali-c; *Lyc*; Mag-p; Pho; *Plat*; Pul; Rhe; *Stram*; Syph; Ver-a; Ver-v; Zin.

Anger from: Nux-v; Zin.

Calls someone, as if: Alo; Anac+.

CRIES

Cephalic: Ap; Bell; Hell; Lyc; Rhus-t; Zin.

Children: Bor; Lac-c; Rhe.
- Fist in mouth, with: Ip.
- Hernia, inguinal, congenital: Thu.
- Moved, when: Zin.
- Sob, and in sleep: Hyo.
- Stools
  - before: Bor; Kre.
  - during: Val.
- Sycotic taint+: Thu.
- Touched, when: Ant-t.
- Waking on, with trembling: Ign.

Convulsions before: Cic; Cup; Hyd-ac; Ver-v.

Cough agg: *Arn*; *Bell*; *BRY*; Cina; *Hep*.

Cramps in abdomen, during: Cup.

Desire, but cannot+: Am-m.

Feels as though she must cry: Anac; Calc; Elap; Lil-t; Sep.
- Reason, without+: Chel.

Genitals, grasping, with: Aco.

Hard to please: Ip.

Help, for: Cam; Ign; Plat.

Hiccough, with: Cic.

Holds on to something, unless she: SEP.

Involuntary: Hyd-ac.

Kindly spoken to, when: Sil.

Loudly: Hyd-ac.
- As if to call someone+: Anac.

Night, at: Kre.

Nursing, when, (children): Bor.

CRIES

Pains, with: Aco; Ap; Bell; Cact; Cham; Cof; Cup; Mag-p; Plb; Sep; Zin.

Plaintively in stupor, touch agg: Hyo.

Sleep, during: *Ap*; Bor; Cina; Hell; Hyo; Ign; *Lyc*; Pul; Rhe; Tub; *Zin*.
- Eyes fixed and trembling, with: Ant-t.

Suddenly: Chin; Plb.

Touch, on: Ant-c; Kali-c; Rut; Stram.

Trifles, at: *Kali-c*.

Urination, before: Aco; *Bor*; *Lyc*; Sanic; Sars.

Waking
- On: Zin.
- Without: Hyo.

CRIME committed, as if+: Caus.

CRITICAL, exacting: *Ars*; Lyc; Sil; Sul.

CROSSING LIMBS

AGG: Agar; Alu; *Asaf*; Aur; Bell; *Dig*; Lyc; Pho; *Rhus-t*; Val.

AMEL: Ant-t; Lil-t; Murx; Rhod; *Sep*; Thu.

CROSSNESS (See ANGER): Ant-c; Ant-t; Aru-t; *Cham*; Cina; Cratae+; Hep; Iod; Kre; Nat-c; Radm+; Sanic; Syph.

During day, merry at night+: Med.

Flatulence, with+: Cic.

CROUP: *Aco*; *Hep*; Kali-bi; Kali-io; Kali-s; Merc-cy; Pho; *Spo*.

Diphtheritic: Iod; *Lach*; Spo.

CROWD: See COMPANY.
  Fear of: See under FEAR.
  Room, in AGG: Lyc; Pho; Sep.
CRUELTY: Abro; *Anac*; Kali-io; Med; Plat.
  Hearing AGG: *Calc.*
CRUSHING: See PAIN, squeezing.
CRUSTA LACTEA: See HEAD EXTERNAL, eruptions.
CRUSTS, scabs: Ars; CALC; *Dul*; *Grap*; *Lyc*; Mag-m; Manc; *Merc*; *Mez*; Nat-m; Nit-ac; Petr; Psor; Radm; *Rhus-t*; Sil; SUL.
  Adherent: Arg-n; Lyc.
  Beneath, pus: Bov; Lyc; Mez; Thu.
  Body, over whole: *Dul*; Psor.
  Brown: Manc; Old.
  • **Yellow:** Dul.
  Burning: Ant-c.
  Conical: Sil; Syph.
  Cracked: Vio-t.
  Dirty: Psor.
  Falling: Nit-ac.
  Gummy: Vio-t.
  Horny: Ran-b.
  Humid: Merc; Nit-ac; *Stap*; Vinc; Vio-t.
  Shiny: Old.
  Tenacious fluid: Vio-t.
  Thick: Bov; *Calc*; Clem; Dul; Kali-bi; Mez; Petr.
  • **Foul:** Vinc.
  White: Ars.
  Yellow: Grap.

CUNNING (See DECEITFUL): Tarn.
CUPPED: Thu; Vario.
CURDY: See DISCHARGES.
CURSING: Anac; Lil-t; Nit-ac; Stram; Tub; Ver-a.
CURVATURE: See BONES and SPINE.
CUTTING: See under PAIN.
CYANOSIS: See BLUISH.
  Infants, in: See CHILDREN, Cyanotic.
CYNICAL: Lyc; Nit-ac; Tarn.
CYSTITIS: See BLADDER, Inflamed.
CYSTS: Ap; Ars; BAR-C; CALC; GRAP; *Lyc*; Nit-ac; PHO; Sabi; SIL; *Sul*; Thu.

DAMP
  Cold AGG: Bar-c; CALC; Carb-v; Cimi; DUL; Lach; *Merc*; Nat-s; Nux-m; *Rhod*; RHUS-T; Ver-a; Zin.
  Ground AGG: Dul; Rhus-t.
  Night AGG: Merc; Phyt; Rhus-t.
  Sheets were as if+: Lac-d.

DAMPNESS, wet weather, working in water
  AGG: Alu; *Am-c*; Ant-c; Ant-t; *Aran*; *Ars*; Bry; Cact; CALC; Calc-p; Card-m; Caus; Cham; Cimi; *Clem*; Colch; DUL; Gel; Kalm; Lyc; Mag-p; Med+; Merc; *Nat-s*; Nit-ac; Nux-m; Pho+; Phyt; *Pul*; Pyro; *Rhod*; RHUS-T; Sabal; Sabi; Senec; *Sep*; *Sil*; Sul; Terb; Tub.
  AMEL: See AIR, clear, dry Agg.

DANCING: Agar; Bell; Cic; Cocl; Croc; Hyo; Stic; *Tarn.*
AGG: Bor; Spo.
AMEL: *Ign*; SEP; Sil.
DANDRUFF: Ars; Canth; *Grap*; Lyc; Nat-m; *Pho*; Stap; Sul; Thu.
Itching: Med.
Scaly, profuse: Sanic.
White: Ars; Kali-m; Mez; *Nat-m*; *Thu.*
Yellow: Calc; *Kali-s.*
DARK: See BLACK.
DARKNESS
AGG: See LIGHT, amel.
AMEL: Con; *Euph*; Grap; Pho; *Sang.*
DARTING: See PAIN, darting.
DAY (periodicity)
Alternate on
- **AGG:** *Ars*; Canth; CHIN; Clem; *Ip*; Lyc; *Nat-m*; Nux-v; Pul; Rhus-t.
- **AMEL:** Alu.

Every fourth AGG: Ars; Lyc; Pul; Saba.
Every seventh (weekly) AGG: Ars; Canth; Chin; Gel; *Iris*; Lac-d; Lyc; Pho; *Sang*; Sil; *Sul*; Tell.
Every tenth AGG: Lach; Pho.
Every fourteenth
- **AGG:** *Ars*; Calc; Chin; Con; *Lach*; Nic; Pul; Sang; Sul.
- **AGG and every** fourteenth day amel: Mag-m.

Every twenty one (3rd week) AGG: Aur; Chin-s; Mag-c; Tarn; Tub.

DAY
Every twenty eighth (monthly, 4th week) AGG: *Nux-m*; NUX-V; Pul; SEP; Tub.
Every forty two, (6th week) AGG: Ant-c; Mag-m.
Every ninety (3 months) AGG: Chin.
Twice a day: Verb.
DAY
Break AMEL: Colch; Syph.
Hot with cold nights AGG: Aco; Dul; Merc; Rum.
Time only
- **AGG:** Agar; Euphor; Med; *Nat-m*; *Pul*; Rhus-t; SEP; STAN; SUL.
- **AMEL:** Kali-c; Syph.
- **Pain:** Ham

DAY-BLINDNESS: Both; Castr; Lyc; Pho; Ran-b; Sil; Stram.
DAZED: See BEWILDERED and DULL
DEAD
Look: Thu.
Thinks
- **Everything is:** Mez.
- **He is:** Agn; Ap; Ars; Grap; *Lach*; Mos; *Op*; Pho; Plat.

DEADNESS: Aco; Agar; Bar-c; Grap; Lyc; Rhus-t; Sec.
DEAFNESS: See HEARING.
DEATH
Agony: Ant-t; *Ars*; Carb-v; Tarn-c.
Apparent: Aco; Ant-t; Carb-v; Cof; Op; Petr; Plat.

DEATH

Believes she is going to die
- On certain day: Aco; Hell.
- Soon and that she cannot be helped: Agn.

Certain, is: Hyds.

Desires: *Aur*; Caus; Hyds; Kre; Lac-c; Lach; Ran-b+; Sep; Sul+.

Fear, of: See under FEAR.

Longs, for+: Aran.

Near, seems, must settle his affairs: Petr.

Premonition+: Ap.

Thoughts of: Aco; Grap.
- Calmly: Zin.

DEBAUCHERY:
Agar; Ant-c; Carb-v; Lach; *Nux-v*; Sele; Stram; Sul-ac.

DEBILITY:
See WEAKNESS.

DECEITFUL, tricky, duplicity:
Arg-m; Buf; Cup; Merc; *Op*; Plb; Tarn; *Ver-a*.

DECEIVED, always being:
Rut.

DECOMPOSITION:
Mur-ac; Pho; Pyro; Sec.

Rapid: Crot-h.

DECUBITUS:
See BED, sores.

DEEDS he could do great:
Hell.

DEFINANT:
Arn; Lyc.

DEGENERATION

Calcareous+: Flu-ac.

Fatty: See under FATTY.

DEJECTED:
See DESPAIR, SADNESS and SORROW.

DELICATE, tender, sickly, easily enervated:
Ars; Calc; Calc-p; Caus; Cimi; Colch; Con; Croc; Cup; *Ign*; Kali-p; Lyc;

DELICATE ..
Mar-v+; Nat-c; Nux-m+; Pho; Pic-ac; Psor+; Sep+; Sil; Stro; Sul; Tab; Ver-a; Zin.

DELIRIUM:
Aco; *Agar*; Ars; Aru-t; BELL; Bry; Cann; Chel; *Cup*; *Dul*; HYO; *Lach*; Lyc; Nit-ac; Nux-v; *Op*; Rhus-t; Sec; *Stram*; Syph; VER-A; Ver-v.

Abortion, after: Rut.

Anxious: Aco; Ap; *Stram*.

Colic, alternating with: Plb.

Easy: Agar; Dul; Ver-a.

Eyes brilliant, with: Ail.

Foolish: Bell; Op; Stram; Sul.

Frightful visions, with: Bell; Calc; Stram.

Haemorrhage, after: Arn; Ars; Bell; Ign; Lach; Lyc; Pho; Pho-ac; Sep; Scil; Sul; Ver-a.

Loquacious: See LOQUACITY.

Maniacal, furibund, wild, raving: *Aco*; Agar; Ail; Ap+; *Ars*; BELL; Bry; Canth; HYO; Lyc; Nit-ac; Op; Sec; STRAM; VER-A.
- Trifles, over+: Thu.

Mental or physical exertion, from: Lach.

Music, from hearing: Plb.

Muttering: Ail+; Ant-t+; Bry; *Hyo*; Lach; *Mur-ac*; Pho; STRAM.
- Himself, to: Tarx.
- Incessant+: Ver-v.

Night, at: Plb; Syph.

Pains
- With: Dul; *Ver-a*.
- Limbs, alternating with: Plb.

DELIRIUM

Picking lips, fingers, nose: See CARPHOLOGY.
Quarrelsome: Nit-ac.
Rolls on floor: Calc; OP.
Same subject all the time, talks: Petr.
Sleep, in: Ap; Bell.
Sleepiness, with: Bry; Pul.
Sleeplessness, and: *Aur*; Bell; Bry; Calc; Chin; Colo; Dig; Dul; Hyo; Ign; Lyc; Nat-c; Nux-v; Op; Pho; Pho-ac; Plat; Pul; Rhus-t; Saba; Samb; Sele; Spo; Sul; Ver-a.
Speaks in foreign language: Lach; Nit-ac; Stram.
Stares
  • At one fixed point: Ign.
  • Wild+: Ver-v.
Tremens, dipsomania: Agar; Ars; Caps; *Cimi*; HYO; Lach; Nat-m; Nux-m; Nux-v; *Op*; STRAM.
  • Hiccough, with+: Ran-b.
Variable: Lach; Stram.
Waking, on: HYO; Lach; Zin.

DELTOID
DELTOID: Bar-c; Fer; Fer-p; Syph; Urt; Vio-o.
Right: Colo; Kalm; Lycoper; Mag-c; Phyt; Sang; Stap.
Left: Fer.
Arms
  • Raising up agg: Zin.
  • Rotating inwards agg: Urt.
  • Turning agg: Sang.
Motion, violent amel: Phys.
Paralysis: Caus.
Reading agg: Stan.

Relaxed, as if: Merc-c.

DELUSIONS: See IMAGINATIONS and PERCEPTION CHANGED.

DEMENTIA: Anac; Bell; Lyc; *Nux-v*; *Pho*.
Business worry, from: Lil-t.
Sexual excess, from: Lil-t.

DENTITION: Calc; Calc-p; Cham; Cof; Kre; Mag-p; Rhe; Sil; Stap+; Sul; Tub.
Delayed+: *Tub*.

DEPRAVITY (See MORAL PERVERSIONS): *Buf:* Tarn.

DEPRESSION: See SADNESS.

DERMATALGIA: See SKIN, painful.

DERMOID: Calc; Nat-c; Nat-m; Nit-ac.

DESCENDING
AGG: Arg-m; *Bor*; Con; Fer; *Gel*; Phys; Rhod; RUT; STAN; Ver-a.
AMEL: Bry; Spo.
Misses steps of stairs, while: Stram.

DESIRES (See also CRAVING)
Beautiful things, finery: Lil-t; Sul.
Certain things, but opposes it if proposed by others: Caps.
Change, always: Tub.
Death: See DEATH, Desires.
Friend, but treats him outrageously: Kali-c.
More than she needs: Ars.
Respect due to him, shown: Ham.

DESIRES

Things, then throws them away: Sec.

To beat children: Chel; Ox-ac.

To be read to: Chin; Clem.

To cut others: Lyss.

To do
- Mental work: Aur; Tarn.
- Something great: Cocain.

To get drunk+: Sele.

To get into
- Country, away form people: Calc; Elap; Merc; Sep.
- Solitude to practise masturbation: Buf; Ust.

To go
- Home (thinking he is not there): *Bry*; Calc; Lach; Op.
- Place to place: Sanic.

To kill: See KILL.

To pull
- Her Hair: *Ars*; *Bell*; *Cup*; Dig; Lil-t; Med; Tarn; Tub; Xanth.
- Nose of strangers: Merc.

To remain in bed: Arg-n; Hyo.

To scratch: Arn.

To set things on fire: Hep.

To sing: Spo.

To talk: Arg-m; Arg-n; Stic.

To travel: *Calc-p*; Cimi; Iod; Merc; Tub.

To wear his best clothes: Con.

DESPAIR, hopelessness: Aco; Anac; Arn+; *Ars*; *Aur*; Calc; Caus+; Cof; Hell; *Ign*; Iod; Kali-io; Lept; Lyc; Nit-ac+; Pho-ac; PSOR; STAN; Syph; Tab; Ver-a.

DESPAIR

Anger, with: Tarn.

Heart disesae, in: Aur.

Liver affections, with+: Lept.

Position in society, about: Ver-a.

Recovery, of: Aco; Ars; Bry; Calc; Psor; Syph.

Salvation of+: Ver-a.

Trifles, over: Grap.

DESQUAMATION, branny, scaly, etc:
Am-c; *Ars*; Ars-io; Bell; Calc; Canth; Dul; *Grap*; Hep; KALI-C; Kali-m; Merc; Mez; Nat-m; Nit-ac; PHO; Pul; Rhus-t; Sars; Sele; Sep; Stap; SUL.

Branny: Radm; Tub.

Brown: Am-m.

DESPONDENT: See SADNESS.

DESTRUCTIVE:
Ap; Flu-ac; Pho; Stram; Tarn; Tub.

DETERMINED: See STUBBORN.

DEVELOPMENT: See GROWTH.

DIABETES

Insipidus: See URINE, profuse.

Mellitus: Arg-m; Ars; BOV; Carb-v; Chio; Colo; HELO; *Iris*; Kre; LYC; *Nat-m*; PHO; PHO-AC; PLB; Ran-b; Sep; Scil; *Sul*; TARN; TERB; Thu; URAN-N.

- Boils, successive, with: Nat-p.
- Children, in: Cratae.
- Lung affections, with: Calc-p.

DIAPHRAGM: Bry; Cact; Cimi; Cup; Ign; Stan; Stry.
Contracted: Mez.
Cord, bound tightly by, taking breath away: Cact.
High: Card-m.
Inflammation: Cact; Nux-v.
Neuralgia: Stan.
Viscera, drawn up against: Spo.

DIARRHOEA: Agar; *Alo*; Ant-c; Ant-t; *Ars*; Bap; Bar-c; Bry; Calc; Canth; Carb-v; *Cham*; *Chin*; *Cina*; *Colo*; *Con*; *Crot-t*; Dul; Fer; *Gamb*; Hell; Hep; Iod; Ip; *Iris*; Kali-bi; Lyc; *Merc*; Merc-c; Nat-m; *Nat-s*; Nit-ac; *Pho*; *Phos-ac*; POD; *Psor*; *Pul*; *Rhe*; *Rhus-t*; Sec; Sil; *Sul*; Thu; VER-A.
Acute disease, after: Carb-v; Chin; Psor; Sul.
Alternating with other complaints: Pod.
AMEL: Abro; Nat-s; Pho-ac; *Zin.*
Asthma, then: Kali-c.
Bathing agg: Pod.
Beer agg: Alo; Chin.
Bloody, in infants: Calc-s.
Breakfast
 • After: Nat-s; Thu.
 • Amel: Bov: Nat-s.
Burns, after: Ars; Calc.
Buttermilk agg: Pod.
Cancer of rectum, from: Card-m.
Care, domestic agg: Cof.
Children
 • Emaciated, of: Acet-ac; Tub.

DIARRHOEA, children
 • Summer, in+: Cup.
Chocolate agg: Lith.
Choleric: See CHOLERA.
Chronic: Ars; Calc; Nat-m; Petr; Pho; Psor; Sil; *Sul*; Tub.
Coffee agg: Cist; Cyc; Ox-ac.
Coldness with: Grat.
 • Children: Chin.
 • Old people: Bov.
Constipation, alternating with: See CONSTIPATION.
Cold drinks
 • Agg: Caus; Chin; Hep; Lyc; Stap.
 • Amel: Pho.
Cold water, in hot days from+: Ver-a.
Colds agg: Calc; Dul; Nux-m; Rum; Tub.
Cucumber agg: Ver-a.
Day only: Kali-c+; Nat-m; Petr; Phyt.
Debility
 • With: Ars; Ver-a.
 • Without: Ap; Calc; Grap; *Pho-ac*; Pul; Rhod; Sul; Tub.
Diuresis, with: Mag-s.
Drinking agg: *Arg-n*; ARS; Caps; Cina; CROT-T; Fer; Nux-v; Pho; Rhus-t.
Dropsy, in: Acet-ac; *Ap*; Apoc; Hell.
Eating agg: *Alo*; *Ars*; Calc; Calc-p; CHIN; Chin-ar; Cina; *Colo*; *Crot-t*; *Fer*; Grap; Iod; Kre; Lyc; Mag-c; *Nux-v*; *Pod*; Pul; Tromb.
Egg, from: Chin-ar.

DIARRHOEA

Exanthemata, in: Ant-t.
Fatigue agg: Fer.
Fever during
- Intermittent: Bap; *Cina*; Nux-v; Rhus-t.
- Puerperal: Pyro.

Fish agg: Chin-ar.
Flatus, passing after: Kali-ar.
Fright, from: Pho+; Pul.
Fruits agg: Calc-p; Cist; Chin; Lach; Lith; Lyc; Rhod.
- Acid, sour: Pod.
- Canned: Pod.
- Unripe: Pho-ac; Rhe; Sul-ac+.

Goitre, with: Cist.
Hair, washing agg: Tarn.
Hot bath amel: Sec.
Housewife, in: Cof.
Indiscretion of food, slightest, after: Grap+; Pho; Pul; Sul-ac.
Infants+: Sul.
Jaundice, with: *Chio*; Dig; Lycps; Nux-v; Pul; Rhe.
Lemonade agg: Phyt.
Lienteric: See Eating Agg.
Lumbar ache, with: Bar-c; Kali-io+.
Menses
- Agg: Am-m; *Bov*; Caus; Colo; Kre; Lach; Mag-c; Nat-s; *Pho*; Pho-ac; Pul; Sec; Sul; Ver-a; Vib.
- Appear, as if would+: Kali-io.
- Suppressed, from: Glo.

Mental exertion agg: Pic-ac.
Milk
- Agg: Calc; Chin; Mag-m; Nat-c; Pod; Sep; Sul.
- Boiled agg: Nux-m; Sep.

Morning agg: *Alo*; Bov; Bry; *Kali-bi*; Lil-t; Mag-c; *Nat-s*; Onos; Pho; *Pod*; Psor; Rum; SUL; Tub.
- Bed, driving out of: Dios; Nat-s; Psor; *Sul*; Syph+; Tub.
- Children, of: Cimi; Iod.
- Frothy: Stic.
- Muddy water: Lept.
- Offensive: Grap.
- Rising, after: *Bry*; Lil-t; *Nat-s*; Rum.
- Wait, cannot+: Lit-t.
- Watery: Colo.
- Weakness, with: Dios.

Motion agg: Ap; Bry; Fer; Ver-a.
Muscus, then weakness: Bor.
Nervous, emotions agg: Aco; ARG-N; *Cham*; *Cof*; Fer; GEL; Hyo; Ign; *Op*; Pho; Pod; *Pul*; *Ver-a*; Zin+.
Nightly: *Chin*; *Fer*; Psor; Rhus-t; Stro.
Old age: Ant-c; Ars; Bov; Gamb; Nit-ac.
- Painful: Carb-v.

Opium, after: Nat-m.
Oysters agg: Alo+; Bro; Sul-ac.
Painful: Ars; Bry; Cham; Colo; Merc; Merc-c; Rhe; Rhus-t; Sul.
Painless: *Ars*; Bap; Bism; Bor; *Chin*; FER; Hep; *Hyo*; Iris+; Kali-p; *Lyc*; Nat-m; PHO; PHO-AC; POD; *Pul*; Scil; *Stram*; *Sul*; Tub; VER-A.

DIARRHOEA, painless

- Urination frequent, with: Bism.

Parturition, after: Coll; Hyo; Rhe.

Periodical: Stro.
- Alternate days: Alu; *Chin*; Iris.
- Fourth day, every: Saba.
- Summer: Kali-bi.
- Weeks, every three: Mag-c.

Persistent+: Kali-bi.

Phthisis of: *Ars*; Bry; Carb-v; Chin; Fer; Hep; Nit-ac; Pho; Pho-ac; Pul; Rum; Sul.
- Early: Fer+; Kali-io.

Pregnancy, during: Ant-c; Chin; Dul; Lyc; Merc; Petr; Pho; Pul; Rhe; Sep; Sul; Thu.

Rheumatism
- Then: Cimi; Kali-bi; Dul.
- With: Stro.

School girls: Calc-p; Pho-ac.

Sea shore agg: Syph.

Sense of: Dul; *Nux-v*; Pul.

Sleep
- During: Sul; Tub.
- Amel: Pho.

Small pox, during: Ars; *Chin*.

Smoking agg: Bor.

Sour things
- Agg: Bro; Lach.
- Amel: Arg-n.

Spasms, tonic, with: Terb.

Standing amel: Merc.

Starches, from: Nat-c.

Stoppage, suddenly from agg: Mag-p; Zin.

DIARRHOEA

Sudden, with fever: Bap.

Summer: See Weather, hot.

Thin persons, in: Calc; *Sil*; Sul-ac.

Typhoid, in: Hyo; Pho.

Ulcers in intestines, from: Kali-bi; Merc-c.

Urinating agg: Alo; *Alu*; Hyo.

Vegetables agg: Lyc.

Vomiting, after: Manc.

Walking, only when: Rhe.

Warm drinks agg: Flu-ac.

Weakness, absent+: Rhod.

Weaning, after: Arg-n; CHIN.

Weather
- Change of: Dul; Pho-ac; Psor.
- Hot Agg: Aco+; *Bry*; Cam; Castr; Chin; Crot-t; Fer+; Fer-p; Gamb; Kre; Nux-m; Old; *Pod*.
  - cold drinks, from: Nux-m.
  - eruptions, with: Hypr.

DIGESTION affected: Aeth; Ant-c; Arg-n; Ars; *Bry*; *Calc*; CHIN; Fer; Lyc+; Merc; NUX-V; Old; Pho; PUL.

Brain exhausion, from: Aeth; Calc-f.
- Children: Calc-f.

Coition, after: Dig; Pho.

Dietetic errors, from: See ERRORS IN DIET.

Eating hurriedly, from: Anac; Cof; Old.

Masturbation, emission, from: Bar-c.

Over eating, from: Rut; Sep.

DIGESTION, disordered
Sprain, from: Rut.
Weak: Lyc+; Old.

DIGGING: See PAIN, boring.

DINNER
AGG: *Alo*; *Bry*; Grat; Mag-m; Merc-i-r; Sul-ac; *Zin*.
AMEL: Chel; Cinb.

DIPLOPIA: See VISION, double.

DIPSOMANIA: See DELIRIUM tremens.

DIPHTHERIA: AP; *Ars*; Bro; *Diph*; Kali-bi; Kali-chl; Kali-io; Lac-c; LACH; *Lyc*; MERC-CY; *Merc-i-f*; Merc-i-r; Mur-ac; Pho; *Phyt*; *Rhus-t*; Spo; Sul-ac.
Carrier: Lach.
Effects+: Pyro.
Fever, intense+: Tarn-c.
Laryngeal: *Bro*; *Iod*; *Kali-bi*; Lac-c; *Lach*; Merc-cy.
Nasal: Am-c; *Kali-bi*; Manc; Nit-ac.
Painless: Ap; Carb-ac; *Diph*.
Relapsing: Diph.

DIRECTION of symptoms
Alternating: See ALTERNATING effects etc.

Appear on one side, go to other, and there AGG: Arg-n; Fer; Iris; Lac-c; LYC; Mang; Nat-m; Tub.

Ascending: Aco; ASAF; *Bell*; Calc; Cimi; Con; Croc; Cup; Dul; Gel; Glo; IGN; Kali-bi; Kalm; Kre; LACH; *Led*; *Naj*; Op; PHO; *Pul*; Saba; SANG; SEP; SIL; Strop; *Sul*; Thu; Zin.

DIRECTION
Backward: Bar-c; *Bell*; *Bry*; *Chel*; Con; Crot-t; Cup; Gel; *Kali-bi*; Kali-c; Kali-io; Lil-t; Merc; Nat-m; Par; Pho; Phyt; Pru-sp; Pul; *Sep*; Spig; SUL.

Crosswise, across: *Bell*; Berb; Calc; *Chel*; *Chin*; Fer; Hell; Kali-bi; Kali-m; *Lac-c*; Sep; *Sil*; *Sul*; Val; *Ver-a*; Zin.

Diagonal: *Agar*; *Alu*; Amb; Ap; Bor; Kali-io; *Kalm*; Lach; Lyc; *Mang*; Murx; Nat-c; Nux-v; *Pho*; RHUS-T; Stic; Sul-ac; Tarx.

Downward: Alo; Arn; Aur; Bar-c; *Berb*; Bry; Caps; Cic; Cof; Hypr; KALM; Lach; Lyc; Pul; Rhod; Rhus-t; Sele; Zin.

Forward: Berb; Bry; Carb-v; *Gel*; Lac-c; *Sabi*; *Sang*; Sep; Sil; SPIG.

Here and there: Aco; Agar; *Am-c*; Bar-c; Calc; Chel; Chin; Cimi; Cina; COCL; Grap; IGN; Lyc; Mag-c; Mag-p; Op; Pho; Pho-ac; Rat; Rhus-t; Sec; Stan; Stap; *Sul*; *Thu*; *Val*; Ver-v; *Zin*.

Increase gradually
- Decrease gradually: Arg-n; Ars; Gel; *Glo*; Kali-bi; Kalm; Lach; *Nat-m*; Pho; PLAT; Pul; *Sang*; *Spig*; STAN; *Stro*; Sul; Syph.
- Decrese suddenly: *Arg-m*; Caus; *Ign*; *Pul*; *Sul-ac*.

Increase suddenly
- Decrease suddenly: Arg-n; *Bell*; *Kali-bi*; *Nit-ac*; Spig; Sul.
- Decrease gradully: Pul; Sabi.

DIRECTION

Increase with the sun: Kalm; *Nat-m*; *Sang*; Sele; Spig.

Outward: *Asaf*; Bell; Berb; Bry; Chin; Kali-bi; Kali-m; Kalm; Lith; Pru-sp; Sep; Sil; *Val*; Zin.

Radiating, spreading: Agar; Arg-n; Ars; Bap; *Berb*; Caus; Cham; Cimi; *Colo*; *Cup*; *Dios*; Kali-bi; Kali-c; Kalm; Mag-p; *Merc*; Mez; Nux-v; Phyt; Plat; Plb; Sec; Sil; Spig; Xanth.

- Distant parts to: Berb; Cup; Dios; Mag-p; Plb; Tell; Val; Xanth.

Side

- Lain on, go to: *Ars*; *Bry*; Calc; Hep; Kali-c; Mar-v; Merc; Mos; Nux-m; *Pho-ac*; PUL; Sep; Sil.
- Not lain on, go to: Bry; Cup; Flu-ac; Grap; *Ign*; Kali-bi; Kali-c; Mar-v; Pul; Rhus-t.
- Right: AP; Arg-m; Ars; Aur; Bap; BELL; Bor; *Bry*; CALC; *Canth*; *Chel*; Colo; Con; Crot-h; *Gel*; Iris; Kalm; LYC; Lyss; Naj; NUX-V; Psor+; PUL; Ran-sc; *Rat*; *Rum*; *Sang*; Sars; Sec; *Sil*; Sul-ac; *Tarn*.
  - left to: Aco; Amb; Am-c; *Ap*; *Bell*; Calc-p; Caus; Chel; Cup; Lil-t; LYC; Merc-i-f; Pho; Rum; *Saba*; Sang; *Sil*; Sul-ac; Syph; Ver-a.
  - paralysed, or weak as if: Elap.
  - upper, left lower: Amb; Pho; Sul-ac.

DIRECTION, sides

- Left: Arg-n; ASAF; Asar; *Calc-f*; Caps; *Cina*; *Clem*; Croc; EUPHOR; Grap; Kre; LACH; Lil-t; MEZ; Nat-s; Old; *Pho*; *Rhus-t*; Scil; Sele; SEP; Spig; *Stan*; SUL; Thu.
  - does not belong to her: Sil.
  - right, to: Ars; Bro; Calc; Cep; Fer; Lach; Merc-i-r; Nux-m; Pul; *Rhus-t*; Saba; Stan; Tarx.
  - upper, right lower: Agar; Led; Rhus-t; Tarx.
  - weak or paralysed as if: Lach; Pod.
- Up and down (rising and falling): Ars; Bap; Bar-c; Bry; Calc; Cimi; Echi; Eup-p; *Gel*; *Glo*; Kali-c; Lach; Lil-t; Lyc; Osm; *Pho*; *Plb*; Pod; Pyro; *Sul*; *Ver-a*.

Uppermost AGG: *Bry*; Grap; Ign; Rhus-t.

DIRTY: See GRAY.

Habits: Am-c; *Caps*; Chel; *Grap*; Lach; Merc; Nux-v; Pho; Psor; Sep; Sul.

He is: *Lac-c*; Lycps; Rhus-t; *Syph*.

DISAPPOINTMENT: Alu; Cocl; Nat-m.

Loss of ambition, from: Nux-v.

DISBEHAVIOUR of other+: See MISDEEDS.

DISCHARGES

Loss of vital fluids AGG: Aco; Agar; CALC; Calc-p; CARB-V; CHIN; Chin-s; Cimi; Grap; Ip; *Kali-c*; Lach; Pho; *Pho-ac*; Pul; Sec; Sele; Sep; *Stap*; Ver-a.

DISCHARGES

AMEL (suppression agg): Ars; Bell; Bry; *Calc*; Cam; Cham; Chin; Colch; Cup; *Dul*; Hell; *Ip*; LACH; Lyc; Mill; Nux-v; Op; Petr; *Pho-ac*; *Psor*; PUL; *Rhus-t*; *Sep*; *Sil*; Stic; Stram; SUL; Ver-a; *Zin*.

Increased in general, moistness increased: Ant-t; *Ars*; CALC; Carb-v; Cham; *Chin*; *Dul*; *Fer*; Grap; *Hep*; Ip; Iris+; *Jab*; Kali-io; Lyc; *Med*; MERC; Nat-m; *Nat-s*; Nux-v; Op; Pho; Pho-ac; *Pul*; *Rhus-t*; *Samb*; Scil; Sele; SEP; *Sil*; *Stan*; SUL; Sul-ac; *Tab*; Thu; *Ver-a*.

Acrid, excoriating: *Am-c*; ARS; Ars-io; Aru-t; *Bro*; Carb-an; Carb-v; Caus; Cep; Cham; Cist; Colch; Eucal+; Euphr; Flu-ac; *Grap*; Hep; Hyds; *Iod*; Iris; Kali-io; *Kre*; Lil-t; Lyc; *Med*; MERC; Merc-c; Mez; Mur-ac; *Nit-ac*; Pho; Pru-sp; Ran-sc; *Rhus-t*; Sabi; Sang; *Sep*; *Sil*; SUL; Sul-ac; Sul-io; Tell; Thu; Tub.

Albuminous: Alu; *Am-m*; Berb; BOR; Calc-p; Coc-c; Jat; *Nat-m*; Pall; Petr; Phyt; Seneg; Sep; Stan; Tarn.

Almond, bitter, smell like: Benz-ac.

Ammoniacal, odour of: Am-c; Asaf; Aur; Benz-ac; Iod; Lac-c; Lach; Mos; *Nit-ac*; Pho; Stro.

Black: See BLACK.

Bland: Euphr; Kali-m; *Hep*; *Merc*; *Pul*; Sil; Sul.

Bloody: See HAEMORRHAGE.

DISCHARGES, bloody

• **Water, like:** See Meat water like.

Blood streaked: Ars; Asaf; Bry; Chin; Crot-h; *Fer*; Hep; Ip; Lach; *Merc*; Nit-ac; *Pho*; Rhus-t; Sang; Senec; Seneg; Sil; *Sul*; Tub; Zin.

Briny, fishy odour: Bell; Calc; Grap; Iod; Med; Ol-an; Sanic; Sele; *Tell*; Thu.

Brown: See BROWN.

Burning: Ars; Calc; Cep; Kali-io; Kre; *Merc*; Merc-c; Pul; Sinap; Sul.

Curdy: Bor; Helo; Merc; Til.

Destroying hair: Bels; Lyc; Merc; Nat-m; Nit-ac; Rhus-t; Sil.

Excessive: Ars; Pod; Ver-a.

Foamy, frothy: Ap; Arn; Ascl; Chel; Elat; Grat; *Ip*; *Kali-bi*; Kali-c; Kali-io; Kob; Kre; Laur; Led; *Mag-c*; Merc; Nat-s; Oenan; *Pod*; Rhe; Rhus-t; Rum; Saba; Sep; VER-A.

• **Bloody:** Op.

Foul: Eucal; Kre+; Meph.

Gelatinous: Alo; *Arg-n*; Berb; COLCH; Colo; Dig; HELL; *Kali-bi*; Laur; Pod; *Rhus-t*; Sabi; Sele; Sep.

Gluey: Ars-io; Grap; Merc; Mez; Vio-t.

Green: See GREEN.

Gushing: Ars; Bell; Berb; Bry; CROT-T; Elat; *Gamb*; Grat; *Jat*; Kali-bi; Mag-m; *Nat-c*; Nat-m; *Nat-s*; Pho; Pod; Sabi; Stan; *Thu*; Tril; Ver-a.

DISCHARGES

Hot: Aco; *Am-c*; *Bell*; Bor; Cham; Euphr; Iod; Kre; Op; *Pul*; Sabi; Sul.

Involuntary: See INCONTINENCE.

Itching, causing: *Calc*; Flu-ac; Led; Mang; *Med*; Par; Rhod; *Rhus-t*; Sul; Tell.

Lumpy: Aeth; Alo; *Ant-c*; Calc-s; *Cham*; *Chin*; Coc-c; Croc; *Grap*; KALI-BI; Kali-m; Kre; LYC; Mang; *Merc*; *Merc-i-f*; PLAT; Rhus-t; Sep; Sil; Stan.

Meat water like: Ars; Calc; Fer-p; Kali-io; Kre; Mang; Merc-c; Nit-ac; Rhus-t; Stro.
• Acrid: Canth.

Milky: Calc; Kali-m; Kali-p; Nat-s; PHO-AC; *Pul*; Sep.

Molasses, like: Croc; Ip; Mag-c; Pho.

Mucous, altered: *Ant-t*; Arg-m; Arg-n; *Ars*; CALC; Calc-s; Caus; *Cham*; Grap; Hep; Hyds; KALI-BI; *Lyc*; *Merc*; NAT-M; *Nit-ac*; Nux-v; *Pho*; PUL; SEP; Sil; *Stan*; *Sul*.

Musty, mouldy: *Bor*; Carb-v; *Colo*; Crot-h; Mar-v; *Merc*; Nux-v; *Pho*; *Pul*; *Rhus-t*; Sanic; *Stan*; Stap; Thu; Thyr.

Offensive: See OFFENSIVENESS.

Persistent: Iod.

Red (See RED): Ars-io; Kre; Merc; Rhus-t.

Redden parts: Ars; Kre; Merc.

Retained, ceasing: Bur-p; Cam; Hyd-ac.

DISCHARGES

Scanty, bringing great amel: Ap; Arg-m; Lach; Scil.

Sexual excitement, from: Senec.

Slimy: Bor; Calc; Chin; *Kali-bi*; Lyc; Mag-c; Merc-d; Nat-m; Par; Pho; Pho-ac; *Pul.*

Stain indelibly, fast: *Bur-p*; Carb-ac; Lach; *Mag-c*; Mag-p; Med; Merc; Pulex; Sil; Thu; Vib.
• Yellow: Bell; Carb-an; Grap; Kre; Lach; Merc; Sele.

Sticky, pasty, stringy: Ant-t; Arg-n; Bov; Bry; Caus; Coc-c; Croc; *Grap*; Hyds; KALI-BI; Kali-c; Kali-m; *Lach*; Lapp; Lyc; Mez; Myr; Nat-m; Osm; *Pho*; Phyt; Plat; *Pul*; Rum; Stan; Sul-ac; Thu; Ust; Ver-a.

Suppressed: Hyd-ac; Stram; Ver-a.

Tarry: Lept; Mag-c; Mag-m; Nux-m; Plat.

Thick: Arg-m; *Ars*; Ars-io; Bor; *Calc*; Calc-s; Canth; Carb-v; Con; Croc; Dul; Grap; *Hyds*; *Kali-bi*; Kali-io; Kali-m; Merc; Merc-cy; Nat-m; Psor; PUL; Sil; Sul.

Turn grass green: Calc-f.

Urinous odour: Benz-ac; Canth; *Colo*; Nat-m; Nit-ac; Ol-an; Sec; Urt.

Vicarious: *Bry*; Con; Dig; Fer; Ham; *Lach*; Lycps; Mill; Nux-v; *Pho*; *Pul*; Sec; Senec; *Sep*; Sul.

Watery, thin: Ars; *Asaf:* Canth; *Caus*; Cham; Crot-h; Cup; Flu-ac; Gamb; *Grap*; Grat; Iod; Iris; Kali-io; Mag-m; *Merc*;

DISCHARGES, watery
Mur-ac; Nat-s; Pho; *Pod*; Rhus-t; Sabi; Sec; Sil; *Sul*; Ver-a.
White: See WHITE.
Yellow: See YELLOW.
• Green: See under YELLOW.
• Tenacious: Sumb.

DISCOLOURED: See under different colours, and MOTTLED

DISCONTENT, displeased, dissatisfied: Anac; Asaf; *Bism*; Calc-p; Cham; *Hep*; Kali-c; Kali-m; Kre; Led+; Lil-t; Merc; Nat-m; PUL; Rut; *Sul*; Tub.
Cause, without: Clem.
Easily+: Caul.
Everything, with: Kre; Nat-m.
Her own things, with: Lil-t.
Himself, with: Asaf; Con; Hep; Rut.
Others, with: Hep; Rut.
Weeping amel: Nit-ac.

DISCORDANT: See CONFUSION and CO-ORDINATION.

DISCOURAGED (See DESPAIR): Kali-m; Myr; Stan.

DISGUST (See AVERSION): Merc; *Pul*; *Sul*.
Body, one's own for: Lac-c.
• Odour, of: Pyro.

DISLOCATED, sprained, as if: Asaf; Arn; Calc; Cham; *Chel*; Grap; *Ign*; Nat-m; Petr; *Pho*; *Pul*; *Rhus-t*; *Sul*; Thu.
Parts, lain on: Mos.

DISLOCATION easy, spontaneous: Ars; *Calc*; Carb-an; Chel; Grap; Lyc; Nat-c; Pho+; Pru-sp; Rhus-t; Rut; Sep.

DISLOCATION
Ill effects+: Psor.
Lameness, after: Rhe.

DISOBEDIENCE: Chin; Tarn.

DISORDERLY: Stram.

DISPLEASED: See DISCONTENT.

DISPLEASURE, reserved: See under RESERVED.

DISSATISFIED: See DISCONTENT.

DISTENSION, feeling of (See ENLARGED as if): *Glo*; Mag-c; Ran-b; Rut.
Pain, during: Pul.

DISTORTIONS: See CONTORTIONS.

DISTRACTION, cannot collect ideas, concentration difficult: ACO; Aeth+; Agn+; Alu; Am-c; Anac; Cocl; Hell; Lach; Nat-c; Old; Pho-ac; Senec+; Sul; Thu; Zin.

DISTRUSTFUL: See SUSPICIOUS.

DIVERSION AMEL: Con; Hell; Helo; Ign; Lil-t; Nat-c; Orig; Pall; Pip-m; *Sep*.

DOMINEERING: Lil-t; Lyc; Pall; PLAT; Sul; *Ver-a*.

DOTAGE: Aeth: Ars.

DOUBLING UP AMEL: See BENDING, forwards.

DOUBTING PEOPLE: Alu; Calc; Sul-io.

DOWNWARD: See Under DIRECTIONS.

DRAFT agg: See WIND Agg.

DRAGGING SENSATION: Lil-t; Sep.
   Load, as from a+: Alo.
   Waist down: Visc.
DRAWING: See PAIN, drawing.
   Up limbs
     • AGG: Carb-v; Pul; Rhus-t; Sec.
     • AMEL: Calc; Merc-c; Ran-b; Sep; Sul; Thu.
DRAWN
   Back: See RETRACTION.
   Together: Carb-v; *Chin*; Merc; Naj; Nat-m; *Nux-v*; Par; Pul; *Rhus-t*; *Sele*; *Sul*.
DREAMINESS, revery, ecstasy: ACO; Agar; Amb; Anac; *Ant-c*; Cann; Cof+; *Lach*; *Nux-m*; Old; OP; PHO; Sep; Sul; Ver-a.
DREAMS: Am-m; Arn; Ars; Bry; Calc; *Chin*; *Grap*; Lach; Lyc; *Mag-c*; *Nat-m*; NUX-V; PHO; PUL; *Rhus-t*; *Sil*; *Sul*; Thu.
   Accidents: Ars; Grap.
   Affairs, household+: Bry.
   Agreeable, pleasant: *Calc*; *Nat-c*; *Nux-v*; OP; *Pul*; Sep; *Stap*; *Vio-t*.
   Amorous, erotic: Am-m; Arg-n; Bism; Cact+; Cam; Lach; Nat-c; Nat-p+; Nux-v; Op; Pho; Pho-ac; Senec; Stap; Vio-t.
     • Coition, of: Bor; Sumb.
     • Emission, with: Stap.
     • Leucorrhoea, with: Petr.
     • Menses, before: Calc; Kali-c.
   Animals, of: Arn; Merc; Nux-v; Op+; Pho; Pul.
     • Cats, black: Daph.

DREAMS
   Anxious, frighful: Am-m; Arn; Cact+; Calc; Chin; Cocl; Crot-h; Grap; Kali-c; Kali-m; Lach; Lyc; Nat-m; Nat-p+; Paeon; Pul; Ran-sc; Sil; Tub.
     • Menses, before and after: Sul-ac.
     • Same over and over again: Ign.
   Awake, on falling to sleep: Bell; Lach; Sil; Sul.
   Black forms+: Op.
   Blood, of: See FIRE.
   Bodies, mutilated+: Arn.
   Care and Toil+: Ap.
   Confused+; Rut.
   Day's work, difficulties: Am-m; Ars; *Bry*; Nux-v; Pul; RHUS-T.
   Dead
     • Bodies: Anac; Chel+; Ran-sc.
     • Funeral+: Chel.
     • Persons: Ars; Cann; Crot-h; Elap; Mag-c; Nat-p; Pho; Thu.
   Death, of: Ars+; Lach.
   Drinking, water: Med.
     • Emission, followed by: Merc-i-f.
   Drowning, of: Ver-v.
   Events
     • Previous day, of: Bry.
     • Long past: Sil.
   Falling: Bell; Cact; Dig; Sumb; Thu.
     • From high place+: Nux-m.
   Fantastic: Calc; Calc-io; Carb-an; Lach; Nat-m; Op.
   Fighting+: Nat-s; Ran-b.

DREAMS

Fire, blood, vivid: *Anac*; Aur; Cann; Carb-v; Grap; Hep; Hyo; Laur; Lyc; Mag-c; Mag-m; Manc+; Meny; *Pho*; Radm; *Rhus-t*; *Rut+*; *Sil*; *Sul*; Tub.
- Continued after waking+: Psor.
- Remembered well+: Mang.

Flying: Ap; Latro; Stic.
Frightful: See ANXIOUS.
Gloomy: Plant.
Horrible+: Adon.
Horrid+: Chlo-hyd.
Journey: Kali-n.
Jumps out of bed, in+: Calc-f.
Laborious, exhausting: Arn; Bry; Echi; Pul; Rhus-t.
Lachrymation, with: Plant.
Loathsome: Lach.
Lying left side, on: Sep.
Many: Ars; Senec.
Menses, during+: Nux-m.
Nausea, in+: Arg-m.
Piecing together bodies of her children: Dict; Pho.
Pursued, being+: Nux-m.
Quarrelsome+: Echi.
Shame: Con; Tub.
Sleep, first: Sil.
Snakes: Arg-n; Lac-c; Lach; Ran-sc.
Thieves, robbers: Alu; Mag-c; Nat-m; Sanic.
True, seem on waking: Arg-m; Radm.
Urinating, of: Kre; Lac-c; Seneg; Sep.

DREAMS

Vivid: See FIRE.
Water, being on: Ver-v.
Weeping: Calc-f; Glo; Kre; Plant; Sil; Stram.

DREAMY: See DREAMINESS.

DRINKING

AGG: *Arg-n*; Ars; Bell; *Canth*; *Chin*; *Cocl*; *Crot-t*; Fer; *Lach*; Merc-c; NUX-V; *Pho*; *Phyt*; Pod; *Pul*; *Rhus-t*; *Sil*; *Stram*; Sul-ac; VER-A.

AMEL: Bism; *Bry*; *Caus*; Cist; Coc-c; Cup; Lob; Nux-v; *Pho*; Sep; *Spo*.
- Little Amel: Lob.

Excites urination and stool: Caps.
Hastily: Anac; Bry; Hep.
Rapidly AGG: Ars; Nit-ac; *Nux-v*; *Sil*.

Sips, in
- AGG: Merc.
- AMEL: Bell; Cist; Kali-n; Scil.
- Difficulty, with: Spo.
- Milk Amel: Diph.

Warm AGG: Rhus-r.

Water
- Bad AGG: All-s; Zing.
- Seems to run outside, not going down oesophagus: Ver-a.
- Too much AGG: Grat.

DRINKS

Cold agg and amel: See under FOOD.
Agg, when over heated+: Bels.
As if: Elap.

DRINKS

DRINKS, as if
- Warm, seem: Nat-m.

Desire, for: See THIRST.

Hot
- AGG: Ap; *Bry*; Grap; Lach; *Pho*; *Pul*; Phyt.
- AMEL: Ail; Ars; Lyc; Nux-v; Sul-ac.
- Seem cold: Cam.

Little, eats much but seldom: Ars.

Much, eats little: Dig; Sep; Sul.

Neither, nor eats for weeks: Ap.

Offensive, as if: Arn.

Thirst, without: Calad; Cam; Cocl.

Urination, profuse, after: Lycps.

DRIVING: See RIDING.

DROPPING like water: See TRICKLING.

DROPS things: See AWKWARD.

DROPSY, oedema: Acet-ac; Agar; *Ant-c*; AP; ARS; Aur; Bell; Bry; Canth; Card-m; CHIN; *Colch*; *Como*; *Dig*; Dul; Fer; *Grap*; HELL; Iod; Kali-c; Kali-io; Led; Lyc; Med; MERC; *Old*; *Op*; *Pho*; Pul; Rhus-t; Samb; *Scil*; *Sep*; Sil; Stro; SUL; Terb; Til; Zin.

Alcoholism, from: Ars; Flu-ac; Sul.

Diarrhoea, with: Acet-ac; Ap; Apoc; Hell.

Exanthema, after: Ars; Hell; Rhus-t; Sul.

General: See ANASARCA.

DROPSY

Glands, pressure of, from: Kali-io.

Haemorrhage, after: Acet-ac; Apoc; Chin; Fer; Helo; Senec.

Heart, affection, with: Adon; Cact; Conval; Cratae: Dig; Iod; Lac-d; Pru-sp; Scop; Strop.

Jaundice, with: Merc-d.

Kidney affections, with: Apoc; Ars; *Dig*; Helo; *Merc-c*; Terb.
- And heart with: *Merc-d.*

Liver affection, with: *Apoc*; Card-m; Flu-ac; Lac-d; Lach; Lyc; Mur-ac.

Morning
- Agg: Ap; Aur; Kali-chl; Pho; Sep; Sil.
- Amel: Bry.

New born: Ap; Carb-v; Dig; Lach; Sec.

Numbness, with: Flu-ac.

Puberty or menopause, at: Pul.

Quinine, from: Apoc.

Saccular: Ap; Ars; Kali-c.

Serum exudes: Ars; Lyc; Rhus-t.

Skin, red, with: Como.

Spleen diseases, from: Lach.

Sprains, from: Bov.

Thirst
- With: *Acet-ac*; *Apoc*; Ars.
- Without: Ap; Hell.

Urination or secretion, profuse, with: Scil.

Urine suppressed, fever, and debility: Hell.

DROWSINESS: See SLEEPINESS.

DRUGS, abuse of

In general: Alo; Ars; Cam; *Carb-v*; Cham; Colo; Hep; *Hyds*; Kali-io; Mar-v+; Nat-m; Nit-ac; NUX-V; *Pul*; Sec; *Sul.*

Anaesthetic vapour: Acet-ac; Amy-n; Hep; Pho.

Antityphoid injections: Bap.

Aspirin and similar: Arn; Carb-v; Lach; Mag-p.

Bromides: Cam; Helo; Nux-v; Zin.

Castor oil; Bry; *Nux-v.*

Cod liver oil: Hep.

Cosmetics: Bov.

Digitalis: Chin; Laur; Nit-ac.

Disease, and AGG: Alo; Carb-v; Nux-v.

Heart remedies: Lycps.

Iodides: Ars; Bell; *Hep*; Hyds; Pho.

Iron: Chin; *Hep*; *Pul*; Sul; Zin.

Lead: *Alu*; Caus; Colo; Kali-io; Op; Plb.

Mercury: *Aur*; *Bry*; *Carb-v*; Chin+; Guai; *Hep*; Iod; Kali-io; *Lach*; Mez+; Nat-s; NIT-AC; Phyt; Sars; *Stap*; *Sul.*

Narcotis: Am-c; Bell; Carb-v; *Cham*; *Cof*; *Lach*; Merc; *Nux-v*; Pul.

Opium: Cham; Mur-ac; Nat-m; *Pul*; Ver-a.

Purgatives: Hyds; Lyc; *Nux-v*; Op; Sul.

Quinine: Arn; *Ars*; Carb-v; Fer; Ip; *Nat-m*; Nux-v; *Pul*; Sul; Ver-a.

Sulphur: Calc; Merc; *Pul.*

DRUGS, abuse of

Tar locally: Bov.

Terpentine: Nux-m.

Tetanus, antitoxin: Mag-p.

DRUNKARDS: Asar+; Caps; Cocl; Sul-ac.

DRY clear or cold weather Agg: See AIR, clear etc. agg.

DRYNESS: Aco; Alu; *Ars*; *Bell*; Bry; *Calad*; Calc; Canth; *Fer*; Iod; Lach; Lyc; Mag-m; Meli; *Nat-m*; Nat-s; NUX-M; *Pho*; Plb; Pul; *Rhus-t*; Sanic; Sang; Sec; Sep; *Sul*; Thyr; Tub; Ust; Visc.

Internal: Aesc; *Bell*; Bry; Grap; Op; Petr; Rum.

Partial, local: Aco; Alu; *Bell*; Bry; Grap; Kali-bi; *Lyc*; *Nat-m*; NUX-M; Petr; *Pho*; PUL; Rhus-t; Stram; SUL; Ver-a.

Profuse secretion, with: Euphr; Lyc; Merc; Nat-m.

DUALITY, in pieces, seperated as if

Divided into half and left side does not belong to her: Sil.

Someone else: *Anac*; Arg-n; BAP; Calc-p; Cann; Cyc; GEL; *Lach*; Lil-t; Nux-m; PETR; Pho; Pyro; Sil; *Stram*; Ther; Thu; Tril; Xanth.

DULL, beclouded, difficult comprehension, stupefied: Ail; Ant-t; Ap; Arg-n; Arn; *Bap*; *Bar-c*; BELL; BRY; CALC; Carb-v; Cocl; GEL; GLO; *Hell*; HYO; Kali-br; Kali-c; Lach; LAUR; LYC; NAT-C; *Nux-m*; NUX-V; Old; Op; Petr;

DULL ..
Pho; PHO-AC; Psor; Pul; RHUS-T; SEP; SIL; STRAM; *Sul*; Tub; *Ver-a*; Zin.

Children: Arg-n; Bar-c; Calc-p; Sul.

Emission, after: Caus.

Old people: Amb; Bar-c.

Puberty, at (girls): Ap.

Studying, reading: Aeth; Hell; Nux-v.

What he reads or hears, about: Sele.

DUODENUM
Affection of: Ars; Chin; Hyds; Kali-bi; Merc-d; Nat-p+; Pod; Uran-n.

Obstruction of: Canc-fl.

Ulceration: *Kali-bi*; Symp; Uran-n.

DUPLICITY: See DECEITFUL.

DUSK: See TWILIGHT.

DUSKY COLOUR (pale): Ail; *Ant-t*; Ars; *Bap*; Cam; Crot-h; *Gel*; *Hell*; Lach; *Nit-ac*; *Nux-v*; Op; Sec.

DUST, feathers
As of: Ars; Bell; CALC; Chel; Chin; DROS; Hep; Ign; *Lyc*; Pho-ac; Pul; Rum; Sul.

AGG: Am-c; Ars; Bell; *Bro*; CALC; Chel; Chin: DROS; Hep; Ign; Just; *Lyc*; Pho-ac; Pul; Rum; Sil; Sul.

Fine, in air, AGG: Bell.

DWARFISH: Amb; BAR-C; Bar-m; Calc; Calc-p; *Con*; Med; Ol-j; Sil; *Sul*; Syph; *Thyr*.

DYSENTERY: Aco; Alo; Ars; *Canth*; *Caps*; Carb-v; Colch; *Colo*; Gel; Ham; Ip; Mag-c; Merc; MERC-C; NUX-V; *Pho*; *Rhus-t*; Stap; *Sul*.

After, AGG: Alo; Colch+.

Autumnal: Arn; Colch.

Climaxis, at: Lit-t.

Diarrhoea, after: Lept.

Emaciated, undersized children: Bar-m.

Fever, with: Bap; Fer-p; Nux-v.

Food or drink, least, agg: Stap; Tromb.

Head hot, limbs cold, with: Ip.

High altitude+: Coca.

Old people, in: Bap.

Periodic (in summer): Arn; Kali-bi.

Pot bellied children+: Calc.

Rheumatic pain, with: Ascl.

Tenesmus+: Calc.

DYSMENORRHOEA: See MENSES, painful.

DYSPEPSIA: See DIGESTION affected.

DYSPHAGIA: See SWALLOWING.

DYSPNOEA: See RESPIRATION, difficult and ASTHMA.

DYSURIA: See URINATION, difficult.

EARS: Aur; *Bell*; *Calc*; Cham; FER-P; Grap; Hep; Lyc; Mang; MERC; Petr; Pho; Pho-ac; Plant; *Psor*; PUL; SIL; SUL; *Tell*; Zin-chr.

Right: *Bell*; Flu-ac; Iod; Kali-c; Kali-n; Nit-ac; Nux-v; Plat; Sil; Spo.

EAR, right
- Skin, stretched over, as if+: Asar.

Left: Anac; Asaf; Bor; Grap; Guai; Ign; *Old*; *Vio-o*.
- Right, to: Grap; Mur-ac.
- Tickling over: Zin-val.

Alternating: Bell; *Bry*; Caps; Caus; Chel; Cocl; Fer-p; Glo; Kali-c; *Mag-m*; Med; Mos; *Nit-ac*; Sul.
- Abdomen, with: Radm.
- Teeth, with: Plant.

Behind: Aur; Bar-c; Calc; Canth; *Caps*; Caus; Glo; *Grap*; Lach; Lyc; Merc; Old; Petr; *Pho*; Psor; Sanic; Sil; Stap; Zin-chr.
- Body, hard, as of: Grap.
- Cracks: *Grap*.
- Eczema: Tell.
- Herpes: Sep.
- Moisture: *Grap*; Lyc; *Petr*; *Psor*.
- Screw, sensation+: Ox-ac.
- Throbbing: Zin-chr.
- Tumour: Berb.

Below: Bell.

Between (ear to ear): Plant.

Everything affects: Cann; Gel; Mang; Plant.

External: Alu; Kali-c; Kre; Merc; Pho-ac; *Sep*; *Spig*.
- Blue: Tell.
- Boils on: Merc.
- Itching: Agar; Pul; Rhus-t; Sul; Tell.
- Painful: Petr.
- Red: *Aco*; Agar; Ap; Caus;

EARS, external, red ..
Chin; Ip; Nat-p; *Pul*; Pyro; Sul.
- left: Ant-c; Carb-v; Kre.
- menses, during: Agar.
- Swelling, sudden: Calc-p.
- Veins, distended: Dig.

Internal: *Calc*; Caus; Grap; Kali-c; Mang; *Nux-v*; *Pho*; *Psor*; *Pul*; *Sep*; *Spig*.

Glands, of: Bell; Cham; Con; Lach; *Merc*; Rhus-t; Sil.

Lobules: Bar-c; Caus; *Chin*; Kre; Pul.
- Cysts: Nit-ac.
- Herpes, on: Sep.
- Hot and red: Cam.
- Itching: Arg-m.
- Red: Cham.
- Ulceration of ring hole: Kali-m; Med; Stan.

Ossicles, sclerosis of: Thyr.

Outward in: Agar; Calc; Canth; Chel; Merc; Psor.

Tympanum, drum
- Burning: Ang.
- Calcareous deposit, on: *Calc-f*; Syph.
- Coated white: Grap.
- Exudation, serous, on: Jab.
- Injury, to: Tell.
- Perforated: Caps; Hep; Kali-bi+: Sil; Tub.
- Retracted: Merc-d.
- Scaly: Grap.
- Thickened: Ars-io; Merc-d; Mez.

Abscess: Calc-pic; *Merc*; Syph.

Aching: CHAM; Dul; FER-P; Nux-v; Plant: PUL; Sul; Tell.

EARS, aching
- Both, in: Phyt.
- Faints: Hep; Merc.
- Head, with: Psor; Sang.
- Hiccough, with: Tarn.
- Nausea, with: Dul.
- Swallowing agg: Gel.
- Throat, extending, to: Cep.
- Writing agg: Phyt.

Air
- As if, in: Grap; *Mez.*
  - cold: Kali-c; Mill.
- Hot, from: Aeth; Canth.
- Rushing out, as if: Chel; Stram.

Bleeding: Cic.
- Easy, polyp+: Calc.

Blood, hot, rushing in, as if: Lyc.

Blowing nose agg: See NOSE, blowing agg.

Body, between, as if: Plant.

Boil, in: Bov; Pic-ac.

Boring with fingers
- Amel: Chel; Colo; Lach; *Mez*; Nat-c; Spig.
- Tendency: Sil.
  - children, in: Cina; Psor; Sil.

Bubble bursting in: Nat-c.

Burning, in: Caus.

Chewing agg: Anac; Ap; Seneg; Sul.

Cold
- Agg: Caps; *Hep*; Sil.
- Amel: Bell.
- Heat, or Agg: Cic.

Cold taking Agg: Fer-p; Kali-m; Merc-d; Pho.

Coughing agg: Calc; Caps; Dios.

EARS
Crawling, out: Chel.
Crusts, on: Bar-c.
Discharge, from: Bar-m; *Calc*; Calc-p; Calc-s; Carb-v; Caus; *Con*; Grap; Hep; Kali-bi; Kali-c; Kali-s; LYC; MERC; Petr; PSOR; PUL; *Sil*; Sul; Tell; Vio-o.
- Birth, from: Vio-o.
- Black: Naj.
- Briny: Grap; Naj; Sele; *Tell.*
- Deafness, with: Asaf: Elap+; Lyc+.
- Diarrhoea, offensive, with: Psor.
- Eruptive disease, after: Cist.
- Green: Lac-c.
- Headache
  - with: Psor.
  - after: Abs.
- Itching, with: Crot-t; Elap+.
- Mastoid, swelling with: Carb-an.
- Polypus with: Kali-s.
- Pus: CALC; Calc-s; *Con*; *Hep*; Kali-bi; Kali-c; Kali-s; Lyc; *Merc*; Pho; Psor; *Pul*; *Sil.*
  - bloody: Rhus-t.
- Recurring: Vio-o.
- Stopped, suppressed: Aur; Carb-v; Merc; PUL.

Dryness: *Grap*; Lach; Petr.

Echo, in: Caus; Colo; Nit-ac; Pho.
- Peculiar noise with every: Lyc.
- Sneezing, on: Bar-c.
- Sounds unnatural+: Terb.

EARS, echo in
- Voices+: Caus; Pho.
- Words, one's own: Sars.

Eructation agg: Grap.

Excoriated, raw: *Ars*; Cep; *Kali-bi*; *Merc*; PSOR; Sul; Tell.

Eyes, and: Vio-o.

Fluttering, sudden: Merc-d.

Foetor, from: *Calc*; Carb-v; *Caus*; Hep; Kali-p; Nat-c; PSOR; *Sil*; *Sul*; Thu.

Foreign bodies in, as if: Pho; Plant.

Front, something in, as if: Pho.

Haematoma: Bell.

Head turning, agg: Carb-v; *Mag-p*.

Heat emanating, from: *Aeth*; Caus.

Hollow, as if: Nux-v.

Hot: Caps; Chin; Nat-p.

Inflamed: FER-P; Merc; Merc-c; Pho; Pul; Sul; Tell.
- Slap, after: Calc-s.

Inserting finger and drawing parts apart amel: Aeth.

Itching in: Aur; Hep; Kali-c; Mang; Nux-v; Petr; Sep; Sil; Sul.
- Boring with fingers amel: Bov; Colo; Zin.
- Cerumen, increased, with: Cyc.
- Laughing, when: Mang.
- Scratch, must, until it bleeds: *Arg-m*; Nat-p.
- Sneezing, with: Cyc.
- Swallowing amel: Nux-v.
- Talking, when: Mang.

EARS

Jerking: Plat.

Kidneys, and: Thu; *Vio-o*.

Laughing agg: Mang.

Leaf, sensation of a: Sul-ac.

Lying on face amel: Radm.

Mouth opening amel: Nat-c.

Music agg: Pho-ac; Tab.

Neck, down to: Tarx.

Nodes, on: Berb.

Noise
- Agg: Aco; *Bell*; Cof; Con; Nux-v; OP; Spig; Sul; *Ther*.
- Amel: Calend; Grap; Jab; Nit-ac.

Noises, in: See HEARING.

Nose, blowing agg: Act-sp; Calc; Dios; Pho-ac; Sul.

Numb: Plat; Verb.

Open and close
- As if: Bor.
- Cool air to, as if: Mez.
- Ear to ear: Alet.

Pregnancy agg: Caps.

Pressed
- Apart: Par.
- Out, something, from: Pul.

Puffy: Tell.

Pulsation: Lach; Mag-m; Med.

Quivering in: Bov; Kali-c.
- Bad news, from: Kali-c; Sabi.

Red: See under External.

Riding in crriage amel: Grap; *Nit-ac*; Pul.

Scabby: Grap; Radm.

Scarlatina, after: Mur-ac; Sul.

Singing agg: Pho-ac.

EARS

Sizzling or frying in, as if: Calc-hyp.

Skin stretched over, as if: Asar.

Slap after, agg: Calc-s.

Speaking
- Loudly agg: Mang; Terb.
- Painful: Terb.

Stitches: BELL; Caus; *Cham*; Chin; *Con*; Dul; Grap; KALI-C; Kali-io; *Merc*; *Nux-v*; PUL; SUL

Stopped, as if: Asar; Carb-v; *Con*; Kali-m; *Lyc*; *Merc*; PUL; Sil; Spig+.
- Blowing nose, on: Sul.
- Chewing, when: Sul.
- Full moon, at: Grap.
- Plug, as from: Asar; Led.
- Swallowing amel: Sil.
- Valve or membrance, with, as if: Bar-c; Iod; Nat-s.
- Yawning amel: Nat-m; *Sil.*

Surging, in: Kali-p.

Swallowing
- Agg: Ap; Bov; Gel; Lach; Mang; Nit-ac; Nux-v; Phyt.
- Moving, something, in: Nat-c.

Toothache, with: Glo; Plant; *Rhod.*

Trembling in, after sad news: Kali-c; Sabi.

Twitch, blowing nose or sneezing: Act-sp.

Urination, profuse agg: Thu.

Vertex, to: Mur-ac.

Voice
- Echoes in: Caus; Pho.
- One's own sounds unnatural: Terb.

EARS

Water
- Cold, coming out, as if: Merc.
- Drop of, as if, in: Aco.
- Falling from height, as if: Nat-p.
- Hot, coming out, as if: Aco; Cham.
- Sipping amel: Bar-m.
- Swashing in, as if: Ant-c; Grap; Merc; *Sul.*

Waves, in: Kali-p.

Wax
- Blackish: Pul.
- Chewed paper, like: Con; Lach.
- Dark, flowing: Calc-s.
- Decreased: Lach.
- Falling, small balls, in: Dios.
- Foul: Caus.
- Hardened: Lach; Pul.
  - black: Elap.
- Increased: Caus.
- Red: *Con*; Psor.
- Whitish: Lach.
- Yellow: Carb-v; Kali-c.

Wind Agg: *Cham*; Lach.

Worm, in, as if: Rhod.

EAT

Aversion, or refusal to: Anac; Kali-chl; Hell; *Hyo*; Pho-ac; Phyt; Tarn; Ver-a; Vio-o; Zin-chr.

Chokes, on attempting to: Zin-val.

Everything and anything: Plat; Sul.

Excreta, his own: Ver-a.

EAT
Greedily: Lyc; Zin.
Hunger, wihout: Calad.
Little, is sufficient: Rhe.
More than he drinks: All-sat.
Neither drink nor, for weeks: Ap.
Too tired to: Bar-c; Stan.
When asked, only: Ant-c.

EATING
AGG: *Alo*; Am-c; Anac; ARS; Bell; Bry; CALC; Calc-p; CARB-AN; CARB-V; CAUS; *Chin*; *Colo*; CON; Fer; Hep; Ign; KALI-BI; KALI-C; Lach; *Lyc*; Mag-m; Merc; Nat-c; NAT-M; NIT-AC; NUX-V; Petr; *Pho*; Pod; *Pul*; Rum; SEP; SIL; SUL; Ver-a; Vio-t; Zin.

AMEL: *Anac*; Bov; Cham; Chel; Con; Flu-ac; Grap; Hep; IGN; IOD; Kali-bi; Kalm; Lach; NAT-C; Nat-m; PHO; Plb; Psor; Radm; Rhod; Sep; Spo; Val; *Zin*.

A little
- AGG: Bry; Carb-an; *Chin*; Con; *Kali-c*; LYC; Nat-p; *Nux-V*; Petr; *Pho*; Pul; *Sul*.
- AMEL: Lob; Spo.

Breakfast agg and amel: See BREAKFAST.

Fatigue AGG: Ars; Bar-c; Carb-an; Kali-c; Lyc; *Nat-m*; Pho-ac; Zin.

Frequently
- Agg: Aeth.
- Amel: Flu-ac; Sul.
- Wants to, but least food oppresses+: Kali-c.

EATING
Hastily agg: Sil.
Long after AGG: Aeth; Anac; Carb-v; Fer; *Kali-bi*; *Kre*; Nat-m; PHO; PUL; Sul; Zin.
Night, at AGG: See DINNER.
Seldom and much: Ars.
Sleepy, feels while+: Kali-c.
Too much, overeating AGG: Aeth; *Ant-c*; Ant-t; Bry; Calc; *Carb-v*; *Lyc*; Nat-p; Nux-m; NUX-V; *Pul*; Sul.
Until satisfied AMEL: Ars; *Iod*; Pho.

EBULITIONS: See WAVES.

ECHYMOSIS, petechiae, purpura, etc: ARN; Ars; Bry; Crot-h; Ham; Kre; LACH; Led; Mur-ac; *Pho*; Pho-ac; Pyro; Rhus-t; Sec; Solid; *Sul-ac*; Tarn; Terb.

Advancing: Terb.
Blow, slight, from: Agar; Arn.
Old age: Sars.
Urticaria, with: Lob.

ECLAMPSIA: *Bell*; Cham; *Cic*; Cup; Hell; *Hyo*; Ign; Passif+; *Stram*; *Stry*; Thyr+; Ver-a; *Ver-v*.

Delivery, immediately after: Amy-n; Ant-t.
Labour pains, ceasing, from: Op.

ECSTASY: See DREAMINESS

ECTROPION (eyelids turned up): Ap; Arg-m; Arg-n; Grap; Psor; Spig.

ECZEMA: Alu; *Ars*; Ars-io; Bell; BOV; Calc; Calc-s; *Carb-v*; Cic;

ECZEMA

Clem; Crot-t; DUL; GRAP; *Hep*; *Kre*; *Lyc*; *Merc*; *Mez*; *Old*; *Petr*; *Pho*; Psor; Radm; *Rhus-t*; Solid; Stap; *Sul*; Sul-io.

Beard, of: Ars-io.
Crusts thick, with: Stap.
Digestive affections, with: Lyc.
Dry, children, in: Calc-s; Dul; Frax; Tarn; Vio-t.
Finger, toe of, with loss of nail: Bor.
Foul: Lapp; Vinc.
Hair margins, at: Hyds.
Itching, without: Cic.
Liver affections, with: Lyc.
Menstrual affections, with: Mang.
Moist: Kre; Lapp; Sul-io; Vinc.
 • **Foul:** Lapp.
Neurotic: Anac; Zin.
Recurrent: Como.
Scurfy: Kre.
Sun, exposure, from: Mur-ac.
Suppressed, head of, agg: Mez.
Urine
 • **Affections, with:** Lyc.
 • **Suppressed agg:** Solid.
Washing agg: Ars-io.

EDGE, on, as if: Rut; Val.

EFFECTS
Compensatory: Pru-sp.
Single: See SINGLE, parts.

EFFUSION, deposit: Abro; Ap; Bels; *Bry*; Canth: Hell; Kali-n; Ran-b; Sul; Sul-io.
Bloody: Carb-ac.

EGG
Albumin dried on, as if: Alu; Ol-an; Sul-ac.
Rotten odour of: Arn; Ascl; Cham; Psor; Stap; Sul.

EGOISM: See POMPOUS.

ELBOWS: Caus; Kali-c; Rhus-t; Sep; Sul.
Ankylosis: Sil.
Axilla, to: Ars.
Bandaged, as if: Caus.
Bend of: Kali-c.
 • **Eruptions yellow, scaly:** Cup.
 • **Straightening agg:** *Caus*; Hep; Pul.
 • **Warts:** Calc-f.
Bubbling, in: Rhe.
Carrying weight agg: Cham.
Cracking: Kalm.
Crusts thick, on: Sep.
Drawing: Ars.
Eruptions: Syph.
Hand, to: Cinb.
Herpes: Pho; Sep; Stap; Thu.
Itching: Nat-c; Syph.
Knitting agg: Mag-c.
Numb: Nat-s; Pul.
Painful, in heart disease: Arn.
Paralysis: Rhus-t.
Shiny: Ant-c.
Shoulder, to: Ther.
Sprain: Fer-p.
Stiff: Bry; Lyc.
Swelling: Bry; Merc.
Tendons, inflamed: Ant-c.
Tip, of: Hep.
 • **Touch agg:** Grap.

ELECTRIC
Shock AGG: Pho.

Sparks sensation: Agar; Arg-m; Calc; *Calc-p*; Lyc; Nat-m; SEC; Sele.

ELECTRICITY AMEL: Sil.

ELEPHANTIASIS: Ars; Hydroc; Grap; Iod; Lyc; Sil.

ELEVATING LIMBS AMEL
(See also HANGING, limbs agg): Calc; CARB-V; Pul; Ran-sc; *Sep*; *Vip*.

ELONGATED, as if: Alu; Hypr; Kali-c; Lac-c; *Pho*; Stram; Tab.

EMACIATION, atrophy:
Abro; Arg-n; ARS; Ars-io; *Bar-c*; Bism; Bor+; CALC; Calc-io; CALC-P; Caus; *Chin*; *Fer*; *Grap*; Hell; IOD; Led; LYC; Med; NAT-M; NIT-AC; *Nux-v*; Op; *Pho*; PLB; Sanic; Sars; Sele; *Sil*; Stan; Stram; Stro; SUL; Syph; Thu; Thyr; *Tub*.

Affected part: See Partial.

Appetite, with: Abro; Ars; Calc; Cina; *Iod*; Lyc; Nat-m; Petr; Psor; Sul; Thyr; Tub.

Ascending: Abro; Arg-n.

Cough, with: Amb.

Descending: Lyc; Nat-m; Sanic; Sars.

Flesh fell off from bones, as if: Tarn.

Glands
- Of: Con; Iod.
- Enlarged, with: Iod.

Grief, after: Petr; Pho-ac.

Infantile marasmus: *Abro*; Ars; Ars-io; *Aur*; Bor+; CALC;

EMACIATION, infantile ..
Calc-hyp; Calc-p; *Chin*; Iod; Kre+; *Lyc*; *Mag-c*; Nat-m; Plb; Sanic; Sil; SUL; Syph; Ther; Tub.

Insanity, with: Nat-m; Sil.

Loss of vital fluid, from: *Chin*; Lyc; *Sele*.

Neuralgia, after: Plb.

Painful: Caps; Plb.

Partial, affected parts of, etc: Bry; Calc; Grap; Led; *Mez*; Pho; *Plb*; *Pul*; Sec; *Sele*; Sul.

Pining boys: *Aur*; *Lyc*; Nat-m; Pho-ac; *Tub*.

Progressive, acute diseases, in: Arn+; Guai+; Ver-a.

Rapid: Ars; Calc-hyp; Chlor; Fer; Thu; Thyr.

Senile: Amb; Bar-c; Chin; Flu-ac; Iod; Lyc; Op; Sec; Sele.

Sensation, of: Naj.

Upper parts: Calc; Plb.

Upwards: Abro; Arg-n.

Well-nourished persons, of, suddenly: Bar-c; Grap; Samb.

EMBARASSMENT AGG: Amb; Gel; Ign; Kali-br; Op; *Sul*.

EMBRACES: Agar; Plat.
Everybody, even objects+: Ver-a.

EMBOLISM: Kali-m.

EMISSION: See SEMINAL EMISSION.

EMOTIONAL: *Aco*; Ant-c; ARS; *Aur*; Bell; *Cham*; Cina; Cof; Colo; Croc; Gel; Hyo; IGN; Lach; *Lyc*; *Nat-m*; Nit-ac; NUX-V; Pall; Pho; Pho-ac;

EMOTIONAL ..
  Plat; Psor; PUL; Stap; Stram; Sul; Sumb; Ver-a.

EMOTIONS
  AGG: See Mental excitement AGG.
  Dull: Anac.
  Lively AGG: Pall.
  Long-lasting, effects of: Petr.
  Mental excitement AGG: ACO; Amb; Amy-n; Anac; *Arg-n*; Aur; Bell; *Bry*; Caus; Cham; Cof; COLO; Con; Fer; *Gel*; Hyo; IGN; Kali-c; Kob; *Lach*; *Nat-m*; NUX-V; *Op*; *Pho*; PHO-AC; Phyt; Plat; Psor; PUL; Sep; Sil; Stan; STAP; *Stram*; Tub; Ver-a.
  Sexual AGG: Plat.
  Slight AGG: Psor.

EMPHYSEMA: See CHEST.

EMPTY, hollow, sinking: *Chin*; *Cocl*; Dig; Hyds; IGN; Kali-c; Murx; Nux-v; Old; PHO; Pod; SEP; *Stan*; *Sul*; Tell; Ver-a.
  Body, as if whole: Aur; Kali-c.
  Eating, after: Grat.
  Organs: Tab.

EMPROSTHOTONOS: Canth; Ip.

EMPYEMA: See CHEST.

EMPYOCELE: Kali-s; Sil; Sul.

ENAMEL, thin: Flu-ac; Sil.

ENERVATED: See DELICATE.

ENLARGED, swelled, as if: Aco; Alu; ARAN; ARG-N; Bap; *Bell*; Bov; Cocl; Coll; Gel; *Glo*; Guai; *Ign*; Lach; Merc; Merc-i-f; Nux-v; Op; Paeon; Par; Pul; *Ran-b*; *Rhus-t*; Sanic; Spig.

ENTROPION (eyelids turned down): Bor; Grap; Nat-m; Psor; Pul; Sil; Tell.

ENURESIS: See URINATION, involuntary and BED, wetting.

ENVY: See JEALOUSY.

EPIGASTRUM: ARS; *Calc*; Chel; Cocl; Colo; *Ign*; Ip; KALI-C; *Lach*; Lob; Lyc; *Nat-m*; NUX-V; Pho; *Pul*; Sep; Sul; Tab.
  Above: Nat-m; PHO; Pul.
  Aching: See PAIN.
  Anxiety at: *Ars*; Lyc; Nux-v; Pul.
  Axilla, to: Kali-n.
  Back, to+: Sabi.
  Burning: Ars; Med; Nux-v; Sep; Sil; Terb; Ver-a.
  • Hot coal, as if from: Ver-a.
  Chill, from: Arn.
  Cold: Cam; Hep; Kre.
  Cough, from: Bry; Nit-ac; Pho; Pho-ac.
  Empty, sinking, faint: Ant-t; Apoc; Dig; Glo; Hyd-ac; Ign; Kali-c; Latro; Lob; *Sep*; Strop; *Sul*; Tab.
  • Eating agg: Myr.
  • Meeting a friend, when: Cimi.
  • Nausea, with: Lac-c.
  • Urination, after: Apoc.
  • Vertigo, with: Adon.
  • Walking fast, amel: Myr.
  Everything affects: Sul.
  Lump
  • Above, as if: Nat-c; Nat-m; Pho; Pul.
  • In: *Agar*; Arn; Chel; Con; Cup; *Lach*; Sep.

EPIGASTRIUM

Pain
- Aching: Ars; Nux-v; Sil; Ver-a; Vip.
- Cramp, pinching: Lach; Laur; Merc; Sil; *Ver-a*; Vip.
  - down bowels: Arn.
  - taking breath away: Cocl.
- Cutting: Pul.
- Heavy, suffocating: Rum.
- Stitching: Arn; Bry; *Nit-ac*; Rhus-t; *Sep*; Sul.

Pressure, sense of: Cup; Lyc; Nat-m; Nux-v; *Pho*; *Pul*; Ver-a.

Radiating from: Arg-n.

Red spots on: Nat-m.

Scapula or vertebra, to +: Bad.

Sensitive, sore: Bry; Calc; Carb-v; Chel; Chin; Hyo; Kali-c; *Lach*; Lyc; Nat-m; Nux-v; Pho; *Ver-a*.
- Spot: Pho.

Shock felt in: Dig.

Stoppage in: Guai.

Sweat: Kali-n.

Swelled: *Calc*; Manc; Nat-m; Nux-v.

Talking agg: Nat-c.

Tense: Sang.

Throat to, upward: Aco; Ars; Calc; Carb-v; Fer; Kali-bi; *Kali-c*; Lyc; Nat-m; Nux-v; Pho.
- Worm, crawling: Zin.

Throbbing, pulsation: Ars; Asaf; Bry; Chin; Kali-c; Lach; *Nat-m*; Nux-v; Old; Pul; Rhus-t; Sep.
- Distension like a fist, with: Cic.

EPIGASTRIUM, throbbing
- Visible, perceptible: Asaf.

Tickling, in: Pul.

Torn loose, as if: Berb.

Transfixed pain: Latro.

Tremor: Sul-io.

Tumour: Hyds.

Wriggling in: Chel.

EPILEPSY (See CONVULSIONS):
Agar; Arg-m; Arg-n; *Ars*; Art-v; Bell; *Buf*; *Calc*; CAUS; Cic; Cina; CUP; Glo; Hyd-ac; Hyo; *Lach*; Oenan; Op; PLB; *Sil*; *Sul*; Visc; Zin-p; Zin-val.

Aura, without +: Art-v.

Chronic, with marked aura: Plb.

Coition, during: Buf.

Consciousness, with: Hell; Nux-m; Pho +.

Contradiction, from: Ast-r.

Drunkards: Ran-b.

Glow rise from feet to head +: Visc.

Haemoptysis, ending in: Dros.

Heart, diseases, with: Calc-ar.

Injury, after: Con; Cup; Nat-s; Oenan.
- Blows to head, from: Art-v; Meli.

Jealousy, from +: Lach.

Knee, aura begins +: Cup.

Masturbation, after: Buf; Lach; Stram.

Menses
- Absent, with: Pul.
- During: Buf.

EPILEPSY, menses
- After: Syph.

Minor: Art-v; Bell; Caus; Pho; Zin-cy.
- Injury to head, from: Nat-s.

Opisthotonus, with+: Stan.

Prepuce, adherent, removed from: Raph.

Priapism, with: Oenan.

Puberty, at: Caul; Caus.

Rage, then: Arg-m.

Sexual: Bar-m; Buf; Calc; Stan; Visc.

Shuddering, with: Mos.

Sleep, during+: Lach.

Status epilepticus: Abs; Aco; Buf; Hell; Oenan.

Stools, during: Nux-v.

Thumbs, clenching+: Stan.

Tooth extraction, after: Buf.

Tumour in brain, from: Plb.

Vertigo, before+: Hyo.

EPISTAXIS (See HAEMORRHAGE): Arn; *Fer-p*; HAM; Nit-ac; *Pho*; Vip.

After, agg: Pho.

AMEL: Bro; Elap; Meli+; Psor; Rhus-t; Tarn.

Bed, in, morning: Alo; Caps.

Blow or fall, from: Acet-ac.

Children (fat)+: Calc.

Coryza, with: Senec; Sil.

Coughing, from: Bell; *Dros*; Lach; Led; Merc; Nat-m; Nux-v; PHO.
- Night, at: Nat-m.
- Whooping cough in: Arn; Dros; Ip; Led; Merc.

EPISTAXIS

Drunkards+: Sec.

Easy: Con.

Eating, after: Am-c.

Face, washing agg: Amb; Am-c; Arn; Bry; Kali-c.

Fainting, with: Croc; Lach.

Feet, washing agg: Carb-v.

Fever, during: Rhus-t.

Frequent+: Meli.

Goose skin, with: Cam.

Habitual, young persons, in: Card-m.

Hands, washing agg: Am-c.

Hawking, after: Rhus-t.

Headache
- During: Aco; Agar.
- After: Ant-c; Sep.

Heat, with: Thu.

Hemiplegia, in: Ham.

Hot weather: *Croc*.

Infants, in: Sil.

Jarring, from: Carb-v; Sep.

Lying, on right side: Sul.

Menses
- Absent, with: Ap; Bry; Carb-an; Cham; Dul; Fer; *Lach*; Lyc; Pho; *Pul*; Senec; Sil.
- Agg: Amb; Grap; Lach; Nat-s; Pul; Sep.
- Profuse, with: Aco; Meli.

Morning
- Early: Bov.
- Rising, on: Chin.

Night: Carb-v; Nat-m; Nit-ac; Rhus-t; Sul.

EPISTAXIS, night
- Right nostril, from: Kali-chl; Ver-a.

Nose blowing, on: Arg-m.
Nursing child, when: Vip.
Old people, in: Agar; Carb-v; Ham; Sec.
Operations, after: Bur-p.
Overheated, being, agg: Thu.
Ozoena, in: Sang.
Persistent: Led.
Piles
- Suppressed, from: Nux-v.
- With: Sep.

Pregnancy, during: Sep.
Profuse+: Merc-cy; Meli.
- But, ceases soon+: Cact.

Prostration, with+: Sec.
Puberty, at: Abro; Kali-c; Pho.
Salivation, with: Hyo.
Singing, after: Hep.
Sleep, during: Bov; Merc; Nux-v; Ver-a.
Sneezing, when: Bov; Con.
Spasms, with: Caus; *Mos*.
Stools
- Agg: Pho; Rhus-t.
- Straining at, when: Cof.

Stooping, on: Nat-m; Rhus-t.
Sweat, with: Bry; Caus; Con; Nux-v; Op; Pho; Tarx; Thu.
Touch, slight to nose, on: Cic; Sep.
Typhoid fever, in: Arn; Bap; Crot-h; Lach.
Vertigo, with: Bell; Carb-an; Lach; Sul; Vip.
Vicarious: Bry.

EPISTAXIS
Vomiting
- With: Ox-ac; Sars.
- After: Ars.

Waking on: Am-c.
Weeping, when: Nit-ac.
Young
- Girls: Croc.
- Women: Abro; *Pho*; Sec.

EPITHELIOMA: See CANCER.
EPULIS: Calc; *Thu*.
ERECTION (of penis): *Canth*; Grap; Merc; Nat-c; Nat-m; *Nux-v*; *Pho*; Pic-ac; Plat; Pul; Thu.

Child, in a: Lach; Merc; Tub.
Coition, after: Sep.
Coughing, when: Cann; Canth.
Dysuria, after: Radm.
Emission, after: *Pho-ac*.
Excessive, strong, violent: Canth; FLU-AC; *Pho*; *Pic-ac*; Plat; Sabi+.
- Lascivious thoughts, during: *Pic-ac*.

Frequent, during day+: Chel.
Incomplete, deficient, failing: Agn; *Arg-n*; *Bar-c*; Calad; Calc-s; Chin; CON; Grap; *Lyc*; Med; *Nux-v*; Pho; Sele; Sep; *Sul*; Sul-io; Tab.
- Coition, during: Grap; Lyc; Sul.

Lasts all night+: Dios.
Pain in abdomen, with: Zin.
Painful (priapism, chordee): *Arg-n*; *Cann*; *Canth*; *Caps*: Grap; Merc; Merc-c; Nux-v; Oenan; Pho; Pic-ac; *Pul*; Sabal;

ERECTION, painful ..
Stap; *Terb.*
- Coition, during: Hep.
- Cutting in, with: Arg-n.
- Dreams, in+: Cam.
- Emission, after: Grat; Kali-c.
- Epilepsy, during: Oenan.
- Sleep, in: Merc-c.
- Urethra, burning in, with: Calc-p.

Presistent: Am-c.
Riding in carriage, when: Bar-c; Calc-p.
Shivering and sexual desire with: Bar-c.
Sleep, during: Flu-ac; Nat-c; Op.
Slow, delayed: *Bar-c*; Calc; Sele.
Standing agg+: Sul-ac.
Stools, during: Ign; Thu.
Toothache, with: Daph.
Urination
- Copious, after: Lith.
- Urging, with: Mos.

ERETHISM false: Merc; Mur-ac; Pho.
EROTIC: See AMOROUS.
Ability, without: Lach.
ERRATIC: See CHANGING MOODS.
Effects (motion): Ign; Lac-c; Med; Mos; Tarn; Ver-v.
ERRORS IN DIET agg: All-s; Calc-ar; Cep; Dios; Flu-ac; Grap; Nat-c; Sul-ac.
ERUCTATIONS: Amb; ARG-N; Arn; Asaf; *Asar*; *Bell*; BRY; CARB-V; Chin; *Cocl*; *Con*; Cup;

ERUCTATIONS ..
Guai; Iod; Iris; Kali-bi; Kali-c; LYC; Mag-c; Med; *Merc*; *Nat-m*; NUX-V; Pho; Psor; Pul; Rhus-t; *Saba*; *Sep*; *Sul*; Tarn; *Ver-a.*

AGG: Bry; Carb-an; Carb-v; CHAM; *Chin*; Cocl; Jal; Lach; Nux-v; Pho; Rhus-t; Sul.

AMEL: Ant-t; *Arg-n*; CARB-V; *Grap*; *Ign*; Kali-bi; KALI-C; *Lach*; LYC; *Nux-v*; Pul; Sang.

Abortive, incomplete: Ars; Chin; Con; *Grap*; Lyc; Med; Nat-m.

Acrid, hot: Ap; Carb-v; Con+; Fag; Gymn; Kali-bi; Lac-c; Lyc; Merc; Nat-m; Pod+.
- Eating agg: Nat-m.
- Foul air: Naj.
- Smoking agg: Lac-ac.

Apples, tasting like: Agar.
Ball moving up and down during, as if: Bar-c.
Barley water, tasting like: Naj.
Bitter: Arn; Chin; Nat-s; Nux-v; Pho; Pul; Sep; Tarx+.
- Hysteria, in: Tarn.
- Milk, after: Chin.

Bloody: Sep.
Bugs, odour of: Phel.
Cold: Cist.
Colic, with: Hyo.
Continuous: Chel; Con.
Convulsion
- Before: Lach.
- After: Kali-c.

Coughing, when, after: *Amb*;

ERUCTATIONS, coughing ..
Arn; Carb-v; Chin; Kali-bi; Lob; Sang; Sul-ac; Ver-a.
Difficult: *Arg-n*; Calc-p; Cocl; Con; Grap; Nux-v.
Drinking water, after: Ap+; Hypr.
Eggs, like bad: Agar; Ant-t; *Arn*; Cham; Mag-m; Plant; Psor; Sul; Val.
Empty: Bry; Calc; *Carb-v*; *Con*; Grap; Iod+; Pho; Sep; *Sul*.
Epilepsy, before+: Lach.
Faintness, causing: Arg-n.
Fecal: Plb.
Fever, in: Lach; Ran-b.
Foamy, frothy: Kre; Sep; Ver-a.
Food, of: See REGURGITATION.
Forcible, oesophagus would split, as if: Coca.
Gall stones, with: Dios; Lyc.
Garlicky: *Asaf*; Mag-m.
 • Spasms, after: Mag-m.
Greasy: Alu; Asaf; Caus; Iris; *Mag-c*; Thu; Val.
Headache, with: Calc; Cimi; Mag-m.
Hiccough
 • Alternating, with: Agar.
 • Like: Cyc.
Hot: See Acrid.
Incomplete: See Abortive.
Ingesta, tasting of: ANT-C; Ap+; Bism; *Bry*; Carb-an; Caus; Chin; Fer; Nat-m; *Pul*.
 • Drinking water agg: *Ap*.
Long-continued: Glo.

ERUCTATIONS
Loud, noisy: ARG-N; ASAF; *Chin*; Kali-bi; Petr; Pho; *Plat*; Thu; Vib.
 • Violent and+: Coca.
Lying amel: Aeth; Rhus-t.
Meat, from: Rum.
Menses, at: Lach.
Musk, tasting of: Caus.
Nauseous, foul: Arn; *Asaf*; Bism; Carb-v; Grap; Pul; Sul.
Onions, like: Mag-m.
Painful: Bry; Carb-an; *Cham*; Par.
Pressing
 • Painful part, on: Bor.
 • Stomach, on: Sul.
Pungent+: Petr.
Putrid: Acet-ac; Arn; Bism; Kre; Plb; Psor; Val.
Radish, tasting like: Osm.
Rancid: *Asaf*; Carb-v; Chin; Lyc; Merc+; Sep; Tell; Thu.
Relief, without: Carb-v; *Chin*; Lyc.
Salty: Carb-an; Kali-c; Nux-v; Sul-ac.
Shivering, with: Dul.
Sleep amel: Chel; Chin.
Smoking, after: Sele.
Sour: CALC; Carb-v; *Chin*; Grap; Gymn; Ign; Kali-bi; LYC; *Mag-c*; Nat-c; *Nat-m*; NAT-P; NUX-V; Pho; Psor; *Pul*; Rob; Sep; *Sul*; Sul-ac.
 • Bitter: Iris; Nux-v.
 • Cabbage, after: *Mag-c*.
 • Eating, after: *Nat-m*.

ERUCTATIONS, sour
- Hot: Fag, Gymn; Pod.
- Intermittent fever, in: Lyc.
- Milk, after: Chin; Sul.
- Sugar, after: Caus.
- Vertigo, during: Sars.
- Vomiting, sour, after: Caus.

Stale: Flu-ac.

Suppressed: *Am-c*; Calc; Con.
- Followed by pain, in stomach: Con.

Swallowing difficult, with: Ox-ac.

Sweetish: Dul; Plb; Sul-ac.
- Menses, before: Nat-m.
- Pregnancy, during: Nat-m; Zin.

Tea, tasting like: Lycps.

Tough, mucus, of: Sep.

Urinous: Agn; Ol-an.

Violent: *Mos.*

Vomiting, with: Cimi.

Water, tasting of: Naj.

ERUPTIONS (tendency to): *Aco*; ARS; Ars-io; Bar-c; Bell; CALC; Calc-s; *Caus*; *Clem*; *Dul*; *Grap*; Kali-c; Kali-s; *Lach*; LYC; MERC; *Mez*; *Nat-m*; *Nit-ac*; Petr; Pho; Psor; *Pul*; RHUS-T; SEP; SIL; SUL.

Acne: Ast-r; Bar-c; Bell; Carb-v; Cyc; Grap; *Hep*; Kali-br; *Merc*; Nux-v; Sele; Sep; Sul; Sul-io.
- Black: Ars; Ast-r.
- Cheese agg: Nux-v.
- Cosmetics+: Bov.
- Emaciation, with: Abro.
- Face, disfiguring: Cop.
- Hard: Ars-io.

ERUPTIONS, acne
- Masturbation, from: Crot-h; Pho-ac.
- Menses
  - before agg: Grap; Mag-m; Psor; Sep.
  - after agg: Med.
  - delayed: Crot-h.
  - scanty, with: Sang.
- Nose, on: Ars.
- Obstinate: Lapp.
- Pustular: Berb; Sul-io.
  - body, all over: Calc-hyp.
  - menses, during: Kali-br.
- Rosacea: Psor; Radm; Rhus-t+.
- Scars, remaining, after: Carb-an; Cop; Kali-br.
- Sore: Arn.
- Summer agg: Bov.
- Women, young: Cyc.

Acuminate, conical: Ant-c; Ant-t; *Ars*; Hyds; Pul; *Sil.*

Alternating with
- Dysentery: Rhus-t.
- Joints: Stap.
- Other complaints: Ant-c; Ars; Calad; Grap; Hep; Stap; Sul.

Black-tipped: Carb-v.

Bleeding: Am-m; Merc; Sul.

Blue: Ant-t; Hyd-ac.

Chalky, white: Mez.

Circular: See HERPETIC.

Clustered: Agar; *Calc*; Crot-t; Nat-m; Rhus-t.

Cold bathing agg: Thu.

Confluent: Ant-t; Bell; Caps; Cic; Pho-ac; Rhus-t.

ERUPTIONS

Coppery: Ars; *Carb-an*; Kre; Merc-d+; Rhus-t; Sars+.
Cosmetic agg: Bov.
Covered parts, on: Led; Thu.
Delayed: Ant-t; Ars; *Bry*; Stram.
Dry: Ars; Ars-io; Aur; *Bar-c*; *Calc*; Calc-s; *Carb-v*; *Hep*; Led; MERC; Mez; Pho; *Sep*; Sil; SUL; *Ver-a*.
Eczema: See ECZEMA.
Erythematous: Ars; Merc; Sul.
Favus: Ars; Sul.
Fine: Carb-v; Nat-m; Rhus-t.
Fish, after: Ars; Sep.
Flat: *Bell*; Lach; Pho-ac; Sep.
Freckles: *Ant-t*; *Calc*; Kali-c; *Lyc*; Nat-c; Nit-ac; *Pho*; *Pul*; Sep; *Sul*.
• Sun, from: Mur-ac.
Granular: Agar; Ars; Carb-v; Hep.
• Honey-coloured: Ant-c.
Hair, in apex of: Kali-bi.
Heated, when: Bov; Carb-v; Con; *Nat-m*; Psor; Pul.
Herpetic (ringworm): Aco; ARS; Bacil; Bell; Bov; Calc; Calc-s; Clem; Con; *Dul*; Grap; Hep; Lyc; Manc; *Merc*; NAT-M; Petr; Phyt+; Ran-b; RHUS-T; *Sep*; Sil; *Sul*; Tell; Vario.
• Body, all over: Psor; Ran-b.
Horny: Ant-c; Ars; Bor; Grap; Ran-b; Sil; Sul.
Impetigo: *Ant-t*; Ars; *Aru-t*; Calc; Grap; Rhus-t; *Sul*; Tarn; Vio-t+.
Indented: Bov; Thu; Vario.

ERUPTIONS

Intertrigo: Cham; Lyc; *Merc*; *Sul*.
• Dentition, during: Caus.
Itching, without: Cic; Cup-ac.
Itch-like, scabies: Ars; *Carb-v*; *Caus*; Hep; Lyc; MERC; Psor; *Sele*; *Sep*; SUL.
Leave a stain
• Blue: Abro; Ant-t.
• Brown: Berb.
• Purple: Abro.
• Red: Aru-t.
Lichen: Aco; Agar; Bry; *Cic*; Cocl; *Dul*; *Lyc*; Mur-ac; Nat-m; *Sul*.
• Fiery: Cic; Lyc; Rhus-t.
Menses, before, agg: See SKIN.
Mentagra: Calc; Grap; Sep.
Miliary: Aco; Ars; Bry; Cof; *Dul*; *Ip*; Merc; Phyt; *Sul*.
Moist: *Calc*; Caus: *Cic*; *Clem*; *Grap*; Kre; *Lyc*; MERC; Pho-ac; *Rhus-t*; *Sep*; *Sul*.
Newborn: Dul.
Nodular: Ap; Calc; Caus; Dul; Lach; Mez; Kali-io; *Nat-s*; Rhus-t; Sil.
Obstinate: Mang; Sul-io.
Painful: Arn; BELL: Hep; Lach; Lyc; Merc; Nux-v; Pho; *Pho-ac*; Sil; Sul.
Painless: Amb; Cocl; Con; *Lyc*; Old; Sec; Sul.
Papules: *Aco*; *Bry*; *Dul*; Kali-io; *Merc*; *Sul*.
Parts, covered, on: Led.
Patches, in (See MOTTLED): Ail; Ap; Sec.

ERUPTIONS

Pearly: Nat-m.
Pedunculated: Thu.
Pemphigus: Ars; *Aru-t*; Canth; *Dul*; *Hep*; Lach; Manc; Ran-b; Ran-sc+; *Rhus-t.*
Petechiae, with: Ail; Mur-ac.
Pimples: *Ant-c*; Ars; *Caus*; Merc; Nat-m; *Nit-ac*; Pho; Pho-ac; Pul; Rhus-t; *Sep*; Sul; *Zin.*
- Liquor, excessive use of, from+: Nux-v.
- Red, small, with scanty menses: Con.
- Small, body all over: Mag-s.
- White, with red areola: Bor.

Psoriasis: *Ars-io*; Berb-aq; Bor; *Clem*; *Dul*; *Grap*; Kali-m+; Mang; Merc; *Pho*; Phyt; Psor; Radm; *Ran-b*; *Sep*; *Sul*; Thyr; Tub+.
- Itching, without: Cup-ac.
- Scales, shining+: Iris.

Pustulating: *Ant-c*; *Ant-t*; *Ars*; Cham; *Cic*; Clem; Dul; Grap; Lyc; *Merc*; Nat-c; Nit-ac; Petr; *Pul*; *Rhus-t*; Sep; Sil; Stap; *Sul*; Thu; Thyr; Vario.
- Apices
  - black: Anthx; Kali-bi; Lach.
  - brown: Ver-a.
  - bloody: Carb-ac.
  - foul: Vario.
  - sunken+: Thu.

Receding: Ant-t; Ars; Bry; Cam; Caus; Cup; Lyc; Op; Sul; *Zin.*
Repelled+: Plb.
Ringworm: See Herpetic.
Roseola: Aco; Bry; *Kali-io*; Pul; Sars.

ERUPTIONS, roseola
- Syphilitic: *Kali-io*; Pho.

Rubella: Aco; *Bell*; Bry; Pul.
Rupia: *Ars*; Cham; Grap; *Merc*; Petr; Sep; *Sul.*
Scabby, crusty (See CRUSTS): Calc; *Con*; Grap; Hep; *Lyc*; Merc; *Rhus-t*; Sars; Sil; *Sul.*
- Bloody: Merc; *Sul.*

Scaly: Calc; *Clem*; Pho; Sul.
Scarlatinous: Ail; Am-c; *Ap*; BELL; Lach; Lyc; Merc; Nit-ac; Rhus-t; Stram; *Sul.*
- Maligna: *Ail*; Am-c; Carb-ac; *Lach.*

Scars from, unsightly: Carb-an; Cop; Kali-br.
Serpigenous: Ars; Sul.
- Symmetrical+: Thyr.

Skin, under: Hypr.
Soap, application of agg: Nat-c.
Sparse: Ail; Mur-ac.
Spring agg: Nat-s; Psor: Sang; Sars; Sep.
Stab wound, after: Sep.
Sticky: Lapp.
Summer agg: Kali-bi.
Suppressed, undeveloped: Ail; Ap+; Ars; Asaf+; BRY; *Cup*; Dul; Ip; Petr; Pho-ac; Psor; *Stram*; SUL; *Zin.*
- Childhood, in: Kali-c.,

Syphiltic: Ars-io; Kali-io; Merc; Merc-c; Merc-i-f; Merc-i-r; Nit-ac; Syph.
Tettery: Alu; *Ars*; Bov; Calc; Cham; Con; *Dul*; *Grap*; Lyc; *Merc*; *Mez*; *Nat-m*; Petr; Pho; *Rhus-t*; Sep; Sil; *Sul*; Vib.

ERUPTIONS

Touch agg: Ap; Chin; Coc-c; Cof; Hep; Lach; Mang; Plb; Thu.
Trade: Bor.
Urticarious: See URITICARIA.
Vesicles, blisters: ARS; ARU-T; CANTH; *Caus*; Clem; CROT-T; *Dul*; Euphr; *Grap*; *Lach*; Manc; Med; *Merc*; NAT-M; Nat-s; Nit-ac; *Pho*; RAN-B; RHUS-T; *Sep*; *Sul*; Urt.
- Abscess over: Rhus-t.
- Air, in: Asaf.
- Bloody: Carb-ac; Sec.
- Blue: Anthx; Ran-b.
- Dark: Ail; Anthx.
- Discharges, from: Tell.
- Large: Buf; Manc+.
- Yellow: Anac; Euphor; Nat-s; Ran-sc.

Winter
- Agg: Alu; Ars; *Petr*; *Psor*; Saba; Tub.
- Amel: Kali-bi; Sars.

Yellow: Cup.
Zoster: Ars; Crot-t; Grap; Lach; Merc; Mez; Pru-sp; *Ran-b*; *Rhus-t*; *Vario*.
- After effects+: Kali-m.
- Gastric disturbances, with: Iris.
- Pain
  - before: Stap.
  - after+: Zin.

ERYSIPELAS: Aco; AP; Arn; *Bell*; Canth; Crot-h; Euphor; *Grap*; *Lach*; *Merc*; Pul; *Rhus-t*; Sec; Sul.
Brain affections, with: Ver-v.

ERYSIPELAS

Bullosum: Euphor.
Gangrenous: Ars; Carb-v; Lach; Sec.
Menses, during: Grap.
Navel about, after injury: Ap.
Newborn babies: Bell; Cam.
Receding: Lyc.
Recurring: Ap; Fer-p; *Grap*; Hyds; Nat-m; RHUS-T; *Sul*.
Senile: Am-c; Carb-an.
Swelling, great: Ap; *Bell*; Merc; Rhus-t.
Traumatic: Calend; Psor.
Urticaria, with: Canc-fl.
Vesicular: Canth; Euphor; Rhus-t.
- Turning dark: Canth; Ran-b.

Wandering, creeping: *Grap*; Hyds; Rhus-t; Sul; Syph.

ERYTHEMA: See Under ERUPTIONS.
ESCAPE, impluse, to: *Bell*; Bry; Cup; *Hyo*; Mez; Nux-v; Op; Stram.
Hide, and: Meli.

EUSTACHIAN TUBES: Bar-m; Fag; *Fer-p*; *Kali-m*; Merc-d; Nux-v; Petr; Sil.
Right: Hyds.
Left: Sang.
Catarrh: Asar; Calc; Kali-s; Merc-d+; Petr; Pul.
Hypertropy: Ars-io.
Inflammation: Calc; Kali-s; Pul; Sil.
Itching: Nux-v; Petr; Senec; Sil.
Obstructed: Kali-m; Merc-d; Petr.

EUSTACHIAN TUBES
Open, with a pop: Merc-i-r.
Stricture: Lach.

EXACTING: See CRITICAL.

EXAGGERATES her symptoms: Asaf; Cham; Plb.

EXALTATION: See CHEERFUL.

EXANTHEMATA, in general: Aco; Ap; *Bell*; *Bry*; Cof; Euphr; *Merc*; Pho; *Pul*; Rhus-t; Sul.
Blue: Hyd-ac.
Checked+: Hell.
Diarrhoea, during: Ant-t.
Non-appearance+: Stram.
Undeveloped: Saba.

EXCESSIVE use: See OVERUSE.

EXCITABLE: See ANGER.

EXCITEMENT mental, nervous: ACO; *Bell*; COF; Gel; Hyo; Ign+; Lach; Mar-v; NUX-V; Op; Pyro; *Stram*; Val; *Ver-a*; Zin; *Zin-val*.
Pleasurable amel: Kali-p; Pall.

EXCORIATION: See DISCHARGES, acrid.

EXCRESCENCES: See FUNGUS GROWTH.

EXCRETIONS: See DISCHARGES.

EXERTION
Mental
- AGG: Agar; Anac; Arg-m; *Arg-n*; *Aur*; CALC; Calc-p; *Ign*; Kali-p; *Lach*; *Lyc*; *Nat-c*; *Nat-m*; Nat-p+; NUX-V; Pho; Pho-ac; Pic-ac; Pul; Rhus-t; Sele; *Sep*; *Sil*; Stap; Sul.
- AMEL: Fer; Gel; Helo; Nat-c.

EXERTION
Physical
- AGG: Alu; ARN; ARS; Ars-io; *Berb*; BRY; CALC; Calc-s; Carb-an; COCL; *Con*; *Dig*; *Fer*; Gel; Iod; Laur; Lycps; Nat-c; *Nat-m*; *Nat-s*; *Nit-ac*; Pic-ac; RHUS-T; Sele; Sep; Spig; Spo; Stan; *Stap*; Strop; *Sul*; Tub; *Ver-a*.
- AMEL: Adon; Aesc; Bur-p; Flu-ac; Hep; *Ign*; Kal-br; *Lil-t*; RHUS-T; SEP.
- Mental symptoms AMEL: Calc; *Iod*.
- Slight AGG: Sul-io; Thyr.
- Violent AGG: Lapp; Mill; Symp.

Will, of amel: Phyt.

EXHALATION
AGG: Ant-t; Arg-m; Ars; Caus; CHLOR; Colch; Dros; Med; Meph; *Pul*; *Samb*; Vio-o.
AMEL: ACO; Agar; Bry; Rhus-t; Sabi.
Forcible: Chin; Gel; Ox-ac.
Hot (See BREATH, hot): Kali-bi.

EXHAUSTION: See WEAKNESS.

EXHILARATION: See CHEERFUL.

EXOSTOSIS: See BONES.

EXOPHTHALMIC GOITRE: See GOITRE.
Choking: Meph.
Trembling, with: Meph.

EXPECTORATION (See DISCHARGES)
AGG: Coc-c; Dig; *Led*; *Nux-v*.

EXPECTORATION

AMEL: *Ant-t*; *Ap*; Aral; *Coc-c*; Grind; Hypr; Kali-bi; Kali-n; Sep; *Stan*; Sul-io; *Zin*.

Astringent: Chio.

Balls, of: Agar; Arg-n; Coc-c; Sang; Sil; *Stan*.
- Bitter, green: Med.
- Feels like a round, and rushed into mouth: Syph.
- Round, flying from mouth: Kali-c.

Bitter: Cham; Pul.

Bleeding from mouth, with: Dros.

Blood, pure, after cough+: Am-c.

Bloody (See HAEMORRHAGE): Bry; Chel; Laur; Mag-c; Stan; Sul-ac.
- Chest, burning in, with: Psor.
- Chronic: Sul-ac.
- Erection, violent, after: Nat-m.
- Fall, after: Fer-p; Mill.
- Lactation, during: Fer.
- Lumpy: Sele.
- Menses
  - agg: Pho; *Zin*.
  - before: Zin.
  - suppressed or instead of: Carb-v; Dig; Led; Lyc; *Nux-v*; Pho.
- Plugs: Sang.
- Water: *Gel*.

Bluish: Amb; Kali-bi; Pho.

Casts: See Membranous.

Cold (cool): Cor-r; Pho.

Corrosive: Iod; Kali-c; Sil; Thu+.

EXPECTORATION

Creamy: Amb.

Curdy, cheesy: Kali-c; Thu.

Difficult: *Ant-t*; *Caus*; Ip; Just; Kali-bi; Mag-c; Pul; Sang; Scil+; Seneg.
- Cough, loose, with: Hep.

Drinking amel: Am-c.

Easy: Agar; *Arg-m*; Dul; Nat-s; Pho; Scil; *Stan*; Tub.
- By day: Euphr; Mang; Pho.

Epistaxis, with: Dros.

Flies from mouth: Arg-n; *Bad*; *Chel*; Kali-c; *Kali-m*; Mang; Mez.

Foamy, frothy: *Ars*; *Ip*; Kali-io; Kali-p; Pho; Rum.

Foul taste: Asaf; Lach; Pul.

Granular: Bad; Calc; Chin; Kali-bi; Pho; Sil.
- Offensive: Sil.
- Sneezing, when: Mez.

Grayish (See GRAY): Amb; Arg-m; Lyc; Stan.

Greasy: Caus.

Greenish (See GREEN): Benz-ac; Par; Psor; Sul-io.

Hard: Nat-c.
- Calcareous: Sars.

Heavy: Scil.

Hot: Aral.

Loose: See COUGH, expectoration, with.

Lumpy: Calc-s; Kob; Lyc; Sil.

Lying amel: Cist; Thu.

Membranous, casts: Brom; Iod; Kali-bi; Merc-c; *Spo*.

Milky: Ars; Kali-chl; Sul.

EXPECTORATION, milky
- Odour: Spo.

Morning and evening: Scil.
Mouthful: *Euphr*; Pho; Rum.
Musty: Bor.
Offensive: Ars; Ars-io; Bor; Calc; Guai; Lyc; Meph; Nat-c; Phel; Sang; Sil; Stan.
- Bed bug, like: Phel.

Orange-coloured: *Kali-c*; Pul.
Profuse, copious: Am-c; Ars; Cact; Calc; Calc-s; Coc-c; Euphr; Hep; Lyc; Mag-c; Pho; Pul; Rum; Sep; Sil; Stan; Tub+.
- Glairy: Cist.
- Nasal discharge, with: Sabal.
- Old age: Alum; Bar-c.

Purulent: Bro; Bry; Carb-v; *Chin*; *Con*; Dros; Fer; *Kali-c*; Led; Lyc; Nat-c; Nit-ac; Pho-ac; Plb; Pul; RHUS-T; Samb; Sang; *Sep*; *Stan*; Sul.
Retching, with: Carb-v.
Rusty: *Bry*; *Lyc*; Sang+; Scil.
Sago, like: Sil; Stan.
- Yellow: Calc-f.

Salty: Aral; Ars; Lyc; Mag-c; Nat-c; Pho; Pul; Sep.
Slips back again: CAUS; CON; *Kali-s*; Sang; Seneg; Zin-chr.
Smeary: Nit-ac; Phel; Thu.
Sour: Kali-c+; Kali-n.
Spitting, with: Zin-chr.
Sticky, tough, viscid: Coc-c; *Hep*; KALI-BI; Sang; *Stan*; Sul-io; Zin-chr.
Swallow, must (See Slips back): Caus; Con; Kali-s; *Lach*.

EXPECTORATION
Sweet: Ap+; Calc; Lycps; Scil; Zin-chr.
- Frothy: Kob.

Syrub, like: Carb-an.
Thick: Arg-n; Bro; Hep; Hyds; Kali-bi; Kali-s; Sil; Tub.
Vomiting, with: Dig.
Warm: See Hot.
Weak, too, to cough out: Caps.
Yellow: Hep; Sil; Stan; Sul-io; Tub.
- Green: Ars-io; Lyc.

EXPIRATION: See EXHALATION.
EXPLOSIONS: See BLOWS and SHATTERED.
EXPRESS herself, cannot: Pul.
EXPRESSION: See FACE.
EXTENSION: See STRETCHING.
EXTREME goes, to: Bell; Caus; Con; Val.
EXTREMITIES: See ARMS and LEGS.
EXUDATION: See EFFUSION.
Continuous: Merc.
Fibrinous: Iod; Kali-chl; Kali-m; Merc-d.
Hard: Kali-m; Nit-ac.

EYES: Aco; *Agar*; Ap; *Arg-n*; *Ars*; BELL; CALC; Caus; Euphr; *Gel*; Grap; *Lyc*; MERC; NAT-M; Nux-v; Pho; PUL; *Rhus-t*; *Rut*; Sep; *Spig*; SUL; Ver-a; Zin.
Right: Am-c; *Bell*; Calc; Cann; *Colo*; Euphr; *Lyc*; Nat-m; Nit-ac; Petr; Pho; Plat; Rhus-t; Seneg; Sil.

EYES, right
- Closed, in hemiplegia: Ap.
- Protruding, looks larger than left: Arn.

Left: Ap; Ars; Asar; Bry; Chel; Chin; Hep; Laur; Mez; Nux-v; Plb; Scil; *Spig*; *Spo*; Stan; Sul; Tarx; Thu.
- Drawn, inwards+: Cyc.
- Pain, periodical, over: Mur-ac.
- Smaller, than right: Arn; Flu-ac; Scil.
- Vertex, to: Vio-o.

Alternating between: Aco; Agar; *Ars*; Bell; *Chin*; Cup; *Lyc*; Pul; *Ran-b*; Seneg; Sil.

Abdomen, with: Arg-n.

Above, something, as if cannot look up: Carb-an.

Air
- Cold
  - blowing on, as if: See Wind.
  - streaming out, as if: Thu.
- Hot, streaming out, as if: Dios.

Alternating with
- Abdomen: Euphr.
- Limbs: Kre.

Around: Asaf; *Cinb*; Hep; Ign; Kali-bi; Merc.
- Bluish: Ant-t; Ars; Bism+; *Chin*; Ip; Merc-i-f; Old; Rhus-t; Sec; Stap; Thu; Ver-a.
- Crawling: Cist.
- Dark circles under: Fer; Sep; Thu.
- Eruptions: Ant-c; Ap; Ars; Bar-c; Caus; Hep; Merc; Sil; Sul.

EYES, around, eruptions
- pimples, hard: Guai.
- Numb: Asaf.
- Red: Ap; Bor; Chin-ar; *Elap*; Lapp; MALAN; Pul; Rum; Sil.
- Swelling: Ap; Kali-c; Kali-io; Rhus-t.
- Yellow: Coll; Mag-c; Nit-ac; Nux-v; Spig.

Ascending into
- Right: Sang.
- Left: Spig.

Backwards (drawing etc): Ast-r; Bry; *Crot-t*; Grap; Grind; Hep; *Lach*; Old; *Par*; Pho; Pru-sp; Pul; Radm; *Rhus-t*; Seneg; Sil; Spig.

Ball round, or stick, in, as if+: Dios.

Behind: Bad; Bry; Chel; *Cimi*; Gel; *Lach*; Lith; Manc; Merc; Pod; Pul; RHUS-T; Sep; Ther.

Bending head backwards amel: Seneg.

Big, as if: Arg-n; Chel; Chlo-hyd; Cimi; Como; Glo; *Guai*; Lyc+; Meli; Mez+; Par; Pho+; Pho-ac; Seneg: Spig.

Bleeding: Both; Crot-h; Lach; Nux-v; Pho.
- Blowing nose, on: Nit-ac.

Blinking amel: See Winking.

Bloodshot: Aco; *Arn*; Cact; Chlo-hyd; Ham; Led; *Nux-v*; Phys; Thu.
- Water from, in new born: Cham.

Blowing nose amel: Aur.

Boils over, left: Nat-m.

EYES

Brilliant+: Ap.

Burning, heat: ARS; BELL; Bro; Bry; *Cham*; *Chin*; Cimi; Grap; *Kali-c*; Kali-p; Lil-t; *Lyc*; Mag-p; Merc-c; Pho; Rum; *Rut*; *Sul*; Zin.
- Closing, on: Echi; Manc.
- Cold iron thrust, as if from: Til.
- Dry: Aru-t; Croc.
- Fever, in: Sep.
- Fiery: Cedr; Clem.
- Hot, painful: Naj.
- Hot vapour coming out, as if: *Cham*; Clem; Dios.
- Indoors: Rum.
- Moving, eyes, on: Stic.
- Red+: Stro.
- Sand, as if, from: *Caus*; Nat-m.
- Sneezing, with: Como.
- Weeping, as from: Croc.

Bursting: Pho; Pru-sp; Sul.

Closing
- AGG: Arn; Bry; Carb-an; Chel; Con; LACH; *Sep*; Stro; THER.
- AMEL: Con; Gel; Kali-c; Sil; Tab; Zin.
- Difficult: Caus; *Nux-v*; *Par*; Pho; Sil.
- Frivolously on being questioned: Sep
- Heart affection, in: Spo.
- Light, penetrating the brain+: Kali-c.
- Must: Croc.
- Sees vision, on: Bell.
- Sitting, on: Mur-ac.
- Tightly, for relief+: Meli.

EYES, closing
- Walking in open air, when: Calad.

Coition agg: Kali-c; Nat-m; Pho; Sep.

Cold
- Application
  - agg: Ars; Clem; *Merc*; Thu.
  - Amel: Ap; *Arg-n*; Asar; Bry; Nux-v; Pho; *Pul*; Syph.
- Iron pressed through, as if: Til.
- Water, as if, in: Scil.

Coldness: Alu; Berb; *Calc*; Croc; Flu-ac; Mez; Plat.
- Icy: Seneg.
- Pain, with: Mez.

Cold taking agg: Dul; Merc; Pul; Rhus-t.

Combing hair agg: Nux-v.

Cotton piece in, as if: Radm.

Coughing agg: Seneg.

Covered, as if: Pul.

Cramp: Vio-o.

Crawling, in: Nat-s.

Crossed, as if: Bell; Calc; *Con*; Kali-bi; Nat-m; Op; Pod; *Pul*; Zin.

Crushing: *Bry*; *Pru-sp*.

Dark amel: Con; Lil-t.

Dermoid: Nit-ac.

Distorted: Hyd-ac.
- Spasms, during: Sil.

Drawn
- Back: See Backward.
- Downwards+: Aeth.
- Together, as if: Lach; Lyc; MERC; *Nat-m*; Op; Sul; Zin.

EYES

Dry: *Aco*; Alu; Ars; *Bell*; Glo; Ign; Lith; *Lyc*; Mez; NUX-M; Op; *Pul*; Stap; SUL; Ver-a; Zin.
- Lachrymation, with+: Stap.
- Using them, as if from: Lith.

Dull: Ant-t; Cep; Nux-v; Op; Stan+.

Ears, and: Vio-o.

Exertion, physical amel: Aur.

Falling out, as if: Bro; Carb-an; Colo; Guai; *Ign*; Hell; Lyc; *Pul*; *Sep*; Tril.

Fixed+: Hyd-cy; Merc-cy.
- Staring+: Cup.

Forced out, as if: Ham.

Foreign body
- As of a: Ap; Calc-p; Dios; Flu-ac.
- Between, lids and: Berb.

Formication: Nat-s.

Foundry work agg: Merc.

Glassy+: Pho-ac.

Glaucoma: Aco; Aur+; Bell; Berb; Bry+; *Colo*; Gel; Osm; *Pho*; Plb; Phys; Spig.
- Injury, after: Phys.
- Iridescent vision+: Osm.

Green: Canth; Cup-ac.

Haemorrhage, intraocular: Ham; Sul-ac.

Hair, before+: Euphr; Plant.

Hand, covering with amel: Aur; Thu.

Heat
- Agg: *Ap*; Arg-n; Cof; *Merc*; Pul; Zin.

EYES, heat
- Fire of
  - agg: *Ant-c*; Arg-n; Merc; Pho.
  - amel: Flu-ac.
- Steaming out: Dios.

Heavy, as if: Ars-io.

Hiccough, vomiting agg: Ap; Arn; Asar; Bry; Chin; Lyc; Nux-v; Pul; Sep; Sil; Ver-a.

Injected: Aco; *Ap*; Arg-n; *Arn*; *Bell*; Cep; Glo; Led; *Merc*; Nat-m; *Nux-v*.

Injuries: Arn; Erig; Euphr; Ham; Led; Stap; *Symp*.

Into, pains: Stap.

Itching: Calc; *Pul*; *Sul*.

Jerk, stare and: Cic.

Kidneys, and: Vio-o.

Lachrymation amel: Pru-sp.

Large, as if: See Big, as if.

Light
- Agg: Bar-c; *Bell*; Calc; Chin; Con; Nat-s; Rhus-t.
- Amel: Am-m.
- Artificial agg: Ars; Pic-ac.

Liver symptoms, with: *Corn*.

Looking
- Down
  - agg: Nat-m.
  - amel: Bar-c.
- Fire, at agg: Ap; Merc; Nat-s.
- Intently amel: Petr.
- Pieces of paper at agg: Calc-s.
- Red objects at agg: See Sun.
- Sun at, or anything white or red agg: *Ap*; *Lyc*.
- Up agg: Ars; Carb-v; Chel.
- White object at, agg: See Sun.

EYES

Looks down before him: Stan; Ver-a.
Loose, as if: Carb-an.
Menses, at agg: Croc; Naj; Nit-ac.
Moon light amel: Aur.
Motion of: Agar; Caus; Bell; Cham; Cup; Hyo; Mag-p; Stram.
- Constant: Kali-io.
- Directions, in all: Kali-br.
- One, other motionless: Apoc; Phyt.
- Oscillations: Agar; Benz-n; Cocl; *Cup*; Elap; Gel; *Zin*.
  - as if: Pho; Phys.
  - eyes
    closed with: Cocl; Stic.
    closing quickly on: Aeth; Cup.
- Sleep, in: Aeth; Ap.

Needles, as if in: Cimi; Rhod; Spig.
- Red hot: Rhod.

Neuralgia, operations, after: Mez.
Numb around: *Asaf.*
Nystagmus: See Motion.
Opening, amel: See Closing agg.
Open, half open, etc: Bap; *Bell*; Colch+; *Cup*; Hell; Hyd-ac; LYC; *Op*; *Pho*; POD; Samb; Stram; Thu.
- One: *Ant-t*; Chin; Ign; Ver-a.
- Rapid succession, in: Myg.

Opening difficult (See EYE-LIDS, closed tightly): Ars; Caus; Gel; *Nux-m*; Rhus-t.

EYES, opening difficult
- Faceache, with: Chel.
- Headache during: Nat-m; Tarn.
- Melancholy, in: *Arg-n.*
- Menses, during: Cimi.
- Sneezing, after: *Grap.*
- Swallowing amel: Terb.

Operations, after: Alum; Asaf; Mez; Stap; Zin.
Ovaries, with: Onos.
Over: Arn; *Ars*; *Bell*; Bism; Bry; Calc; *Carb-v*; Cedr; Chel; *Chin-s*; *Gel*; Iris; Kali-bi; *Lach*; *Lil-t*; Lyc; Naj; *Nat-m*; *Nux-v*; *Pho*; *Pul*; Sang; Sil; *Spig*; Thyr; Zin.
- Right: Bell; Cedr; Chel; Lyc; Nat-m; Pul; *Sang*; Senec; *Sep*; Syph.
- Left: Ars; Bry; Fer; Kali-c; Nux-m; Sele; Sep; *Spig*.
  - pain periodically: Mur-ac.
  - veins distended: Dig.
  - warm flowing: Nit-ac.

Paralysis, post-diphtheritic: Phys.
Pink: Euphr.
Pressed
- Apart: Asar; Pru-sp.
- Forward: *Bry*; Kali-m; Merc-c; Nux-v; Pru-sp; Sang; *Spig*.
  - throat, pressing, on: Lach.
- Outward: Cedr; Glo; Gymn; Lach; Nat-m.

Pressing amel: Asaf; Caus; Chel; Pic-ac.
Protruding: Aco; Ars+; BELL; Bro; Chlor; Cocl+; Fer-io; Glo; *Guai*; HYO; IOD; Jab; Laur; Lycps; Nat-m; Stram.

EYES

EYES, protruding
- As if: Med; *Par*; Spo.
- Brilliant, and +: Aeth.
- Convulsions, during: Dros.
- Cough, during: Caps; Dros.
- Injury, from: Led.
- Mania, during: Cam.
- Measles, during: Dros.
- Right more than left: *Como*.
- Trembling, with: Meph.
- Tumour behind eyeball, from: Thu.

Puckered, as if: Ars.
Puffy: Kali-io.
Pulsating, throbbing: Bell.
- Night: Asaf; Merc.

Quivering: Sul.
Radiating pain: Mez; Spig.
Raw: Arg-n; Kali-io; Lyc.
Reading and writing agg: Chin+; Phyt.
Red: Asar; Bell; Merc; Merc-i-r; Radm; Rhus-t; Spig; Thu.
- Bluish: Plb.
- Bulging +: Ap.
- Lower: Glo.
- Prostate, enlargement, with: Sabal; Solid.
- Reading, sewing agg: *Arg-n*; *Nat-m*; Radm; Rut.
- Sexual excess, after: Stap.
- Styes, with: Sep.
- Vision, yellow, with: Alo.
- Vomiting agg: See Hiccough.

Reflex symptoms: Kali-p.
Restless: Chin-s; Stram; Ver-a.
Rubbing amel: Caus; Cina; Croc; *Pul*; Ran-b.

EYES
Rubs: Cep; Gamb; Gymn; Ign; Sanic; Scil; Seneg.
- Brain affections, in: Scil.
- Measles, in: Scil.

Sand in, as if: Ars; Calc; Caus; Chin; Flu-ac; Nat-m; Sul.
- Headache, during: Lac-d.
- Night: *Zin*.
- Right: *Sep*.

Seeing, sight, cinema, etc. agg: Arn.
Sewing agg: Mang.
Skin overhanging, as if: Ol-an.
Sleep, afternoon, amel: Am-c.
Small, as if: Lach.
- Left than right: Arn; Flu-ac; Scil.

Smart: Manc; Radm; Ran-b.
- Lids, closing, on: Manc.

Smoke in, as if +: Croc.
Sneezing amel: Lil-t.
Snow, exposure to, agg: Aco; Cic.
Sore, bruised, aching: Arn; Bap; *Bry*; Chio; *Cimi*; Como; EUP-P; *Gel*; Mag-p; Merc; Onos; Pho; Pul; *Phyt*; Rhus-t; Sang; Spig; Tub+.
Sparkling: *Bell*; *Cam*; Stram; Strop.
Sprained, as if: Lil-t.
Squint: *Alu*; BELL; Calc; Cic; Con; Cup; *Cyc*; HYO; Nat-m; Spig; Stram; Zin.
- Brain diseases
  - during: Stram.
  - after: Kali-p.
- Convergent: *Cic*; *Cyc*.

EYES

EYES, squint
- Convulsions
  - during: Stram.
  - after: Cyc.
- Day, on alternate: Chin-s.
- Dentition, during: Alu.
- Diarrhoea, with: Stram.
- Divergent: Agar; Colo; Con; Hyo; Jab; *Nat-m*.
- Double: Alu.
- Meningitis, with: Tub.
- Menstrual irregularities, with: Cyc.
- Night terrors, after: Kali-br.
- Operations, after: Jab.
- Sensation of: Calc.
- Terror, fear, from: Stram.

Staring: Ant-t+; *Bell*; *Cic*; Cup+; Glo; *Hell*; HYO; *Ign*; Iod; Laur; Lyc; Merc; Naj+; *Op*; Sec; *Stram*; Ver-v.
- Everything at, as if: Med.
- Eyes wide open+: Scil.
- Frightended, as if+: Zin.
- Headache, during: *Bell*; *Glo*; *Stram*.
- Person, at, but does not understand what he speaks: Merc-c.
- Thoughtless+: Guai.
- Unconscious, when: Caus.
- Vacantly, in space: Bov.

Stiff: *Kalm*; Nat-m; Onos.

Stitching: Pru-sp; Spig.
- Coughing agg: Seneg.

Stools agg: Nat-c.

Strain agg: See Reading agg.

Sunken: *Abro*; Ant-c; Ant-t; *Ars*; Cam; *Chin*; Cina; Cup+; Fer;

EYES, sunken ..
Glo; Iris+; Merc-cy+; *Pho-ac*; Sec; Spig; Stan; Stap; Sul; Ver-a.
- Menses, during: Cedr.

Sunlight, bright, complaints from+: Clem.

Sunrise to sunset agg: Kalm; Nat-m.

Swallowing agg: Arg-n; Tarn.

Sweat
- On: Mag-c.
- Under: Con.

Swelled, as if: Como; *Guai*; Mez; *Nat-m*; Par; Pru-sp; Rhus-t; Rum; Seneg; SPIG; Spo.

Swelling
- Between, and brows: *Kali-c*.
- Morning: Rum.
- One, of, in coma: Terb.
- Under: Ap; Arn; Ars; Med; Merc; Merc-i-f; Pho.
  - right: Merc-i-f; Polyg.

Swimming in cold water, as if: Scil.

Tension: Rut.
- Decreased: Nat-m.

Thinking of it agg: Lach; Spig.

Tingling: Clem; Pic-ac; *Phyt.*

Tongue, protruding agg: Syph.

Touch agg: Aur; Bry; Hep; Pho.

Turned
- Down: Aeth; *Hyo*.
- Left, to: Dig; Pho.
- Outward+: Pho.
- Up: Buf; Cam; Cup; Glo; Hell; Mos; Op.
  - fever, in: Hell.

EYES

Turning agg: Sang; Sil; Spig; Tub+.
Twisting, revolving as if: Pho; Phys; Pop-c+.
Upward, from: Berb; Grap; Lach.
Urination amel: Gel; Ign; Kalm.
Veil falling over, as if: Con.
Veins, distended, on: Dig.
Vertex, to: Bur-p; Lach; Vio-o.
Vomiting agg: See Hiccough agg.
Water, warm, flowing over: Nit-ac.
Watery: Tell; Thu.
Weight on, as if+: Carb-v.
Wild look: Bell; Lil-t; Lyss; Nux-v; Sec; Ver-v.
Wind blowing on, as if: Cham; Flu-ac; Lach; Mez; Pul; Sep; Syph; Thu.
 • Cold: Croc; Syph.
Wine agg: Gel; Zin.
Winking: Bell; Croc; Euphr; Flu-ac; Merc-d; Mez; Spig.
 • Amel: Bell; Croc; Euphr; Old.
 • Absent: Caus.
 • Convulsions during: Kali-bi.
 • Inclination to: Mez+; Spig.
 • Must+: Flu-ac.
 • Painful: Kali-io.
 • Rapidly: *Ast-r*; Merc-d.
 • Reading, while: Calc; Croc.
 • Writing, after: Hep.
Wipe, must: Calc; Croc; Euphr; Nat-c; Nat-m+; Pul; Seneg.
Wiping amel: *Calc*; Cina; Cyc; Euphr; *Nat-c.*

EYES

Writing agg: Calc-f; Nat-m; Phyt.
Yawning agg: Agar; Saba.
Yellow: Chin; Crot-h; Lach; *Nux-v*; Plb; Sep; Spig.
 • Lower part: Nux-v.
 • Spots: Agar; Pho-ac.
EYE BROWS: See BROWS.
EYE GUM, sticky: Euphr; Kali-bi.
EYE LASHES
Dandruff: Sanic.
Falling: Ars; Med; Petr; Rhus-t.
Ingrown: See ENTROPION.
Long, curved: Pho.
Stiff, points towards nose: Nit-ac.
EYE LIDS: Aco; Agar; Ap; Bell; Calc; *Caus*; Hep; Merc; Rhus-t; *Sep*; Spig; *Sul*.
Edges: See TARSI.
Inner surface: *Arg-n*; Ars; Rhust-t.
Upper: *Caus*; GEL; Kalm; *Sep*; Spig.
 • Foreign body between eyeball and: Berb; Coc-c; Fer-p.
 • Hard: Med.
 • Swelled: *Kali-c*; Sep.
  - between brows, and *Kali-c.*
Lower: Calc; Pho-ac; Rut; Seneg.
 • Contraction: Colch.
 • Swelled: Ap; Arn; Ars; Merc-i-f; Pho.
Agglutinated, suppuration: Arg-n; Asaf; Calc; *Caus*; Cham; Euphr; Glo; Grap; Guai; Kre; *Lyc*; NUX-V; Pho; PUL; RHUS-T; *Sep*; Sul.

EYE LIDS

EYE LIDS, agglutinated
- Menses, during: Calc.
- Sneezing, with: Gamb.

Bleeding: *Hep*; Nat-m; Nux-v. Sul.

Blue: Dig; Kali-c.

Burning: Colo; Ran-b+; Stic.
- Closing, on: Manc.
- Fiery: Phyt.

Chemosis: Ap; Arg-n; Kali-io; Lyc; Rhus-t.

Closed, shut: *Colo*; Mur-ac; Nux-m; Rhus-t.
- Headache, with: Nat-m.
- Sleepiness, with: Vio-o.
- Tightly, spasms: *Ars*; Bell; Cham; Colo; Croc; Cup; Euphr; HYO; Ip; Kali-c; *Merc*; *Nat-m*; Sil; Stram.

Cold: Kali-c

Crusty: Bor.

Cyst, on: Fer-p.

Dry: Rhus-t; Ver-a.

Eczema: Kre.

Epithelioma: Sep.

Everted: See ECTROPION.

Eye ball, stick to: Asaf; Sanic.
- Sneezing, when: Gamb.

Granular: Ap; Arg-n; Ars; Bor; Grap; Kali-bi; Lyc; Merc-i-r; Nat-s+.

Gummy: Bor; Psor.

Heavy, falling, drooping, paralysis: Alu; *Caus*; Cham; Chlo-hyd; Cocl; Con; GEL; KALI-P; Manc; Naj; Nit-ac; Nux-v; Rhus-t; *Sep*; Spig; Syph; Thu; Ver-a.
- Right: Caus.

EYE LIDS, heavy
- Left: Bar-c; Buf; Colo; Kali-p; Thu.
- Bending head backward amel: Seneg.
- Coal gas from: Sec.
- Leucorrhoea, with: Caul.
- Lying Agg: Nat-m.
- Sore, and: Manc.
- Weekly: Stan.

Half open, as if: Bell.

Inflamed: Aco; Ars; Bell; *Lyc*; *Pul*; *Stap*; Sul.
- Gonorrhoeal: Aco; Pul; Sul; Thu.

Inverted: See ENTROPION.

Itching+: Arg-n; Gamb; Tell.

Jerking+: Cocl.

Motion of AGG: Colo.

Narrowing, space between: Agar.

Nodes: Grap; Stap.

Oedema: Ap; Ars+.

Pricking: Spig.

Puffy: Fer.

Quivering, constant+: Caus; Kre.

Red: Aco; Lyc; Myr.

Retracted: Iod.

Rubs: Gamb; Ign.

Spasms, of: Ars.
- Lower+: Rut.

Sticks
- In, as if: Med.
- Eye balls, to+: Asaf; Sanic.

Stiff: *Ap*; *Kalm*; Nat-m; Onos; Rat; RHUS-T.

Styes: Calc-f; Con; *Grap*; Kre;

EYE LIDS, stye ..
  Lyc; PUL; Sep; Sil; *Stap*; *Sul*; Zin.
  • Crop of: Lapp.
  • Recurrent: Ap.
Tense: Phys.
Thick: Alu; Arg-m; Arg-n; Bar-c; Merc; Tell.
Twitch: AGAR; Bell; Calc; Cic; Colo; Ol-an; *Phys*; Plat; Rhe; Sul.
  • Asthma, during: Cup.
  • Closed, when: Polyg.
  • Cold air, in: Dul.
  • Constant: Kre.
  • Convulsions, during: Kali-bi.
  • Lower: Iod; Kali-io; Rut.
  • Lying, when: Polyg.
  • Opening, on: Kali-bi.
  • Painful: Colo.
  • Rapid succession, in: Myg; Rat.
  • Reading, when: Berb.
  • Vertigo, with: Chin-s.
Ulcer on: Ars+; Lyc.
Warts on: Caus; Thu.
FACE: Aco; Ant-c; Ap; Ars; *Bell*; Bry; Caus; Cham; Chin; Fer; Hyo; Lyc; Mag-p; *Merc*; *Nux-v*; *Rhus-t*; Stram; *Sul*; Ver-a.
Right: Ap; *Bell*; Cact; Calc; Canth; Chel; *Kalm*; Lyc; Nat-c; Nux-v; *Sang*; Zin.
  • Left, to: Grap.
Left: Aco; *Colo*; Con; *Lach*; Rhus-t; Sep; *Spig*; Stap.
Albumin, covered with, as if: Alu; Petr; Pho-ac.
  • Dried on, as if: Mag-c; Sul-ac.

FACE
Alternating sides: Chin; Lyc; Pho.
Angioma: Abro.
Besotted, stupefied: Arn; *Bap*; Bry; Crot-h; Gel; Hyo; Op; Stram.
Black pores, in+: Sabi.
Blemishes, clearing for: Berb-aq; Cimi; Sars.
Bluish: Aco; Ant-t; ARS; Asaf; Bap; *Bell*; Cam; Carb-v; Con; CUP; Dig; Hyo; *Ip*; Kali-m; LACH; *Op*; Samb; VER-A; VER-V; Zin.
  • Chill during: Nux-v; Stram.
  • Cough, whooping, with: Dros; Ip; Samb.
  • Laughing, when: Cann.
  • Menses, before: Pul.
  • Pregnancy, during: Pho.
  • Red, evening, in: Phel.
Blushing: See RED.
Boils: Bro.
  • Small, menses, at: Med.
Brown: See Earthy.
Changing colour: Aco; Bell; Fer; IGN; *Pho*; *Plat*; Sep; Stram.
Chewing
  • Agg: Pul; Stap.
  • Amel: Cup.
Childish+: *Anac*.
Chloasme: Caul; Kali-p; Sep.
Cobweb, on: Alu; Bar-c+; Bor; Bro; Calad; Grap; Ran-sc; Sumb.
Cold: Abro; Ant-t; *Ars*; Cam; *Caps*; CARB-V; Cina; Cocl+; Colch; Hell; Lyc; Plat; VER-A.

FACE, cold
- Children, fleshy, in: Iod.
- Drops of water were spurting out, as if: Berb.
- One side, with severe pain in other: Dros; Polyg.
- Water
  - holding, in mouth amel: Clem.
  - running about, which amel: Bism.
- Wind amel: Arg-n.

Congested: Aco; Amy-n; Aur; *Bell*; Glo; Hyo; Nux-v; Op; Pul; *Stram*.

Coughing agg: Kali-bi; Samb.

Cramp: Colo; Mez; *Plat*; *Verb*.

Crawling: See Flies.

Desires to wash with cold water: Ap; Asar; Flu-ac.
- Thereby amel: Asar; Calc-s; Pho.

Death-like, pinched, collapsed: See Hippocratic.

Dirty: See Earthy.

Distorted: Ars; BELL; Cam+; Cocl; *Colo*; Hyd-ac; *Hyo*; Ign; Ip; Lyc; Nux-v; *Op*; Sec; STRAM; Tell; Ver-a.
- Pain, by+: Cham.
- Speaking, when: Ign.
- Waking, on: Crot-h.

Down on, in hysteria: Nat-m; Psor.

Drawn: Aeth; Ant-c; Ars; Bell; Lyc; Op; Sec; Stram; Tab; Ver-a.
- To a point: Bism; Bro; Kali-n.
- To root of nose: Bro; Par.

FACE
Dusky, dark, sooty: Alu; Ant-t; *Bap*; Colch; Crot-h; Gel; Hell; Iod; Mur-ac; Op; *Pho*; Psor; Stram; Tub.

Earthy, dirty brown: Anthx; Ars; Calc-p; *Chin*; *Fer*; Iod; Lyc; Merc; Nat-m; Nux-v; Op; Psor; Sul; Terb+; Thu.
- Yellow: Lycps.

Eating
- Agg: Mez; Pho.
- Amel: Kalm; Rhod.

Egg, white of, on: See Albumin.

Elongated, as if: Stram.

Emaciated, thin: Acet-ac+; Alu; Ars; Calc; Carb-v; Fer; Iod; Nat-m; Sele; Stap; Tab+; Tarn.
- Neuralgia, after: Plb.

Embarrassed+: Amb.

Epithelioma+: Kali-s.

Eruptions: *Ant-c*; Calc; Caus; Dul; Kali-br; Kali-c; *Kre*; *Led*; Merc; Mez; Nat-m; Petr; Psor; Pul; *Rhut-t*; *Sep*; Sul.
- Burning: Am-m.
- Coryza, with: Mez.
- Eczematous: Ars; Bor; Calc; Cic; Grap; Hypr; Kre; Merc; Mez; *Rhus-t*; Sars; Vio-t.
- Fine: Aur.
- Menses, at: Am-c; Grap; Sars.
- Nodular: Chel.
- Pimples: Carb-an; *Carb-v*; Nat-c.
  - red: Led.

Expression changed: Aco; Ap; Arg-n; *Ars*; Bell; Cam; *Gel*; Hyo; Lyc; Mang; *Op*; Pho; Pho-ac; Sec; STRAM; Ver-a.

FACE

Expressionless: Anac+; Gel+; Kali-br; Lycps.
Flies or spiders, crawling on, as if: Calad; Coc-c+; Gymn; Laur.
Foolish look+: Abs.
Formication: Crot-t; Gymn; Nux-v; *Plat*; *Sec*.
- Prickling, and: Ap.

Freckles: See under ERUPTIONS.
Frightened look: *Aco*; Cup; Spo; Stram; Ver-a.
Frowning: Cham; Hell; Hyo; *Lyc*; Sep; Sul; *Stram*; Ver-a.
Fuzzy: Caus; Psor.
Glistens, shining, waxy: Ap; Ars; Med; Sele; Thu.
Green: Carb-v; Chel.
Grimaces: See GRIMACES.
Haggard look+: Ant-c; Ars; Cam.
Hair on, as if: Sumb.
Hand, passes contantly over: Nux-v.
Hectic spots: Aco; *Ars*; Calc; Chin; Fer; Iod; Kali-c; Kre; *Lyc*; *Pho*; Pho-ac; Pul; *Sang*; Sil; Stan; *Sul*; Tub.
Heat: BELL; Bry; CALC; Cham; Cina; Fer; Grap; Hep; *Nux-v*; Pul; Stram; Tub.
- Affected side: Tub.
- Eating, after: Petr.
- Feet cold, with: Samb.
- Hands cold, with: Arn; Dros+; Stram.
- Headache, with: Chin-s.

FACE, heat

- One side, other cold: Cham; Dros; Ip.
- Palpitation, with: Mag-m.
- Rises, into: Kali-bi; Sang.
- Sitting, while: Val.

Hippocratic, death-like, pinched: Aeth; Ant-t; ARS; Cam+; Carb-v; Chin; Sec; Tab; VER-A.
Idiotic+: Agar.
Injuries: Symp.
Itching: Calc; Caus; Rhus-t.
Jerks, talking, while: Sep.
Mask-like, immobile: Lycps; Mang.
Miserable+: Zin.
Mouth opening, agg: Cocl.
Noise agg: Spig.
Numb: Aco; Asaf; Caus; Cham; Gel; Kalm; Mez; PLAT; Sep; *Verb*.
- Affected side: Caus; Nux-v; Plat.
- Right: Chel; Gel; PLAT.

Old look: *Alu*; *Arg-n*; Bar-c; *Calc*; *Con*; Guai+; Lyc; OP; Sanic; Sars; Sep+; Sul; Syph; Tub.
- Few weeks old infant: Op.
- Wrinkled+: Pulex.

Pain, neuralgia, prosopalgia
- Aching: Aco; *Ars*; Aur; Bell; *Bry*; Calc; Cam+; *Caus*; Cedr; *Chin*; COLO; Gel; Kalm; MAG-P; *Mez*; Nat-m; *Nux-v*; *Pho*; Plat; Pru-sp; *Rhus-t*; Sep; SPIG; *Stan*; *Stap*; Stram; *Verb*.

FACE, pain
- Alternating with pain in
  - coeliac region: Colo.
  - stomach: Bism.
- Boring: Aur; Hep; Mag-c; Mez; Plat.
- Chewing agg: Alo+; Hell; Kali-chl; Pul+; Stap+.
- Chilliness, with: Colo; Rhus-t.
- Cold washing
  - agg: Fer; Mag-c.
  - amel: Caus.
  - body becoming agg: Mag-p.
  - water, holding in mouth, amel: Clem.
- Coming and going÷: Spig.
- Cramp: Colo; Mez; *Plat*; *Verb*.
- Eating amel: Kalm.
- Eye
  - open, cannot: Chel.
  - symptoms, with: Colo.
- Heated, when agg: Fer.
- Kneeling and pressing the head firmly against ground amel: Sang.
- Lachrymation, with+: Plant; Pul.
- Linear: Caps; Cep.
- Lips, from+: Stap.
- Lying agg: Fer.
- Menses scanty, with: Caus; Lob; Mez.
- Mouth, opening agg: Mag-p.
- Nasal discharge, with: Spig.
- Noise agg: Spig.
- Paralysis, with: Caus; Cur; Gel; *Nat-m*.
- Pregnancy, in: Ign; Mag-c; Sep.

FACE, pain
- Radiating: Sang; Spig.
  - fingers, to: Cocl.
- Tea agg: Spig.
- Teeth
  - carious, or extraction, after: Hekla.
  - chattering, with: Sul-ac.
- Temples, to+: Plant.
- Urination frequent, with: Calc.
- Yawning+: Alo.

Pale
- Cachectic+: Sil.
- Cough, during: Cina.
- Deathly+: Crot-h; Sul-ac.
- Exertion, from: Spo.
- Hot, and: Cimi; Cina; Croc; Hyo; Op.
- Linea nasalis: *Aeth*; Ant-t; Carb-ac; *Cina*; Ip; Merc-cy; *Pho*; *Stram*; Tarn.
- Menses
  - absent, with: Lob.
  - during: Ign.
- Migraine, with: Amy-n; Ars.
- Red and, alternately: *Aco*; Cam+; Caps+; *Fer*; Fer-p; Glo; *Lac-c*; Op; Stram; Stro+; Zin+.
- Rising, on: Aco; Ver-v.
- Sickly+: Pho-ac.
  - waxy+: Mag-c.
- Sudden: Cimi.
- Wilted: Nat-c.
- Yellow+: Kali-bi.

Paralysis: *Cadm*; *Caus*; Grap; Kali-io; Merc; Seneg; Syph.
- Chewing difficult, with: Syph.
- Distortion of muscle, with: Grap.

FACE, paralysis
- Eyes
  - close, cannot: Cadm.
  - closed, with: Ap.
- Goitre, suppression, from: Iod.
- Mouth, opening agg: Caus.
- Neuraigia, after: Kali-m.
- Swallowing difficult: Cadm.
- Talking difficult: Cadm; Syph.
- Twitching of
  - muscle, with: Kali-m.
  - eyelids with: Syph.

Peaked: Stap.
Pinched: See HIPPOCRATIC.
Puffy, bloated: Acet-ac; *Aco*; AP; Apoc; *Ars*; *Bry*; *Calc*; Crot-h; *Lach*; Laur; Lyc; Manc+; Merc; Merc-d; Pho; Psor; Samb; Stram; Tarn; Ver-v.
- Lying agg: Apoc.
- Pale: *Ap*; *Ars*; *Calc*; Grap; Hell; Lyc.
  - coughing, when: Samb.
- Red: *Aco*; Arn; Chin; Fer; Lach; Op; Stram.

Red (See CHEEKS and EYES around): Aco; *Bell*; *Caps*; Hyo; Nux-v; Op; Stram; Stro; Tarn.
- One side: *Aco*; *Arn*; Bar-c; Bell; CHAM; Chel; *Ign*; Lac-c; Merc; Mos; Nux-v; *Pho*; Pul; Ran-b; Spig; Sul.
  - other pale: Cham; Ip.
  - right: *Ars*; *Calc*; Lachn; Merc; Mos; Nat-c; Sang; Sul-ac; Tab.
  - left: Acet-ac; Agar; Am-c; Ap; Bor; Cham; *Lyc*; *Nat-m*; PHO; *Rhus-t*; Stram; *Sul*; Thu; Ver-a.

FACE, red
- Alternating: Chel; Lach; Nat-p; *Pho.*
- Asthma, in: Caps.
- Blotches: Iod; Kre; Oenan.
- Circumscribed: Chin; Fer; Lyc; Pho; Sul; Tub.
- Cold, but: Asaf; Caps; Fer; Mos.
- Coma, in: Chin.
- Convulsions, during: Glo; Op.
- Cough agg: Bell; Sang; Tub.
- Eating, after: Caps; Lyc; Nux-v; Sul.
- Fiery: Amy-n; *Meli*; Saba+; Tarn.
- Flushes, blushing: Amy-n; Coco; Strop; Tell.
- Glowing: Mur-ac.
- Headache, during: Bell; Glo; Meli.
- Hot, and: Bell; Chin; Hell; Stram+.
- Loss of vital fluids, from: Chin.
- Old men+: Fer.
- Spots: Am-c; Bell; Elap; Pho; Saba; Strop; Sul.
- Stool, during: Caus.
- Toothache with: Bell; Cham.
- Unconsciousness, during: Glo; *Mur-ac.*
- Vertigo, during: Kalm.
- Walking, when+: Pho.
- Yellow spots: Kre.

Reddish yellow: *Chel*; Gel; Lach; NUX-V.
Rubs while coughing, with
- Fist (children): Caus; Pul; *Scil.*
- Hand: Nux-v.

FACE

Ruddy, florid: Arn; Fer.
Sallow+: Ant-t; Arg-m.
- Sunken+: Chel.

Shaving agg: Aur-m; Carb-an.
Sickly: Ant-t; Arg-n+; Ars; *Chin*; Cina; Lach; Lyc; *Nit-ac*; *Nux-v*; Stap+: Sul-ac.
- Cough, during: Cina.

Skin tight, as if: Cann.
Spiderlets, red+: Med.
Spotted, blotched: Aco; Aeth+; Ars; Carb-an; *Kali-bi*; Lach; Manc; *Rhus-t*; Sil; Sul.
Stupid look: Bar-c; Cann; Hell; Kre.
Suffering: Ars; Cact; Kali-c; Lyss; Mang; Sil; Sul.
Sunken: Ant-t; Arg-n+; ARS; Berb, *Cam*; Carb-v; CHIN; Dig; Hyds; Ign; Kali-m; Mang; Op; Par; *Rhus-t*; Sec; *Ver-a*.
Sunrise to sunset agg: Kalm; Spig; Stan; Verb.
Swallowing agg: Kali-n; Pho; Stap.
Sweat on (See SWEAT, partial): Bell; Cam; Cina; Ign; Merc; Lyc; Op; Spo; Val.
- Cold: Ant-t; ARS; Cam; Carb-v; *Cina*; *Merc-c*; Spo; Tab; VER-A.
- diarrhoea, in: Apoc.
- Convulsions, during: Buf; Cocl.
- Drinking agg: Cham.
- Eating agg: *Cham*; Ign; *Nat-m*; Sul.
- Hot: Cham.

FACE, sweat
- One side, on: Nux-v; Pul.
- Spots on, while eating: Ign.

Swollen, turgid: Ail+; Am-m; *Ap*; ARS; BELL; *Bry*; Cham; Kali-c; Lac-d; *Lyc*; Lycps; *Manc*; Merc; *Nux-v*; Oenan; Op; Pho; Rhus-t; Stram; Tarn; *Ver-v*.
- Dark, and+: Ail.
- Morning: Kali-chl.
- One side: *Arn*; *Bell*; *Bry*; *Cham*; *Merc*; *Merc-c*; Sep; Spig.
  - right: Arn; Merc-i-f; Polyg; Sang.
- Stiff: Rhus-t.

Talking
- Agg: Bry; Kali-chl; Mez; Pul; Sep; Tell.
- Amel: Kali-p.

Tension: Pul; Verb; Vio-o.
Terrified look: ACO; Ap+; Spo; Tarn; Ver-a.
Thinking of it agg: Aur.
Tired: Hell.
Tongue, protruding agg: Hyo; Syph.
Tough agg: Lapp.
Twitching, trembling: *Agar*; Ars; BELL; Cham; Gel; Ign; Laur; LYC; Myg; Oenan; *Op*; Plb; Rhe; Sele; Senec; STRAM; Tell; Thu.
- Asthma, before: Bov.
- Coughing, while: *Ant-t*; Kali-m.
- Eating, when: Kali-m.
- Sleep, in: Rhe.
- Speaking, when: Kali-m.

FACE, twitching
- Spreads, all over body+: Sec.
- Tongue, protruding, when: Hyo.
- Vision, misty, with: Mill.

Ulcer, cancerous: *Con.*
Veins, distended: Chin; Dig.
- Spider-like+: Thu.

Walking amel: Mag-c; Rhus-t.
Warts on: Dul; Sep+.
Wash, desire to, in cold water: See Desire to wash.
Waxy+: Acet-ac; Sil.
Wild look+: Anac; Sec; Val.
Wind, cold, blowing on, as if: Colo; Mez.
Wrinkled (See FOREHEAD): Abro; Alu; Calc; *Lyc*; Syph.
Yellow: *Ars*; Bry; Card-m; *Chel*; *Chin*; Fer; Kre; Lach; *Lyc*; Merc; Nat-s; *Nit-ac*; NUX-V; *Plb*; Pod; SEP.
- Hair, at the edge of: Caul; Kali-p; Med.
- Red: See Reddish yellow.
- spots: Kre.
- Spots: Nat-c.

FAG, enervation: See DELICATE.
FAILURE, feels himself a: Naj; Sul.
FAINT, fainting (See also UNCONSCIOUS): ACO; ARS; *Asaf*; BRY; Cam; *Carb-v*; CHAM; Caus; CHIN; Cof; Croc; *Crot-h*; *Dig*; Glo; Hep; IGN; Iod; LACH; *Mos*; NUX-M; NUX-V; Op; Plb; Pod; *Pul*; SEP; Stram; Strop; SUL; Sumb; Tab; Thyr; Val; VER-A.

FAINT
Accompaniment, as a: Lach.
Afterpains, after every: Nux-v.
Arms extending above head, on: Lac-d; Spo.
Ascending stairs: Anac.
Bath, hot agg: Lach.
Blindness, after: Nux-m.
Blood, at the sight of: Nux-m.
Cause, without: Asaf.
Chill, during: *Sep.*
Close, crowded room, in: Asaf; Plb; *Pul.*
Coition
- During, in women: Murx; Orig; *Plat.*
- After: *Agar*; Dig; Nat-p; Sep.

Die, as if would: Vinc.
Dinner, during, after: Mag-m; Nux-v.
Disturbed, when: Asaf.
Easy+: Ign; Mos.
Eating, while+: Mos.
Emission, after: *Asaf*; Pho-ac.
Emotions, on: *Ver-a.*
Exertion, on: *Sep.*
- Slight: Ver-a.

Fever, during: Arn; Nat-m; Pho; *Sep.*
Frequent: *Ars*; Pho; *Sul.*
- Sweat, profuse, with: Hyds.

Gastric origin: Ol-an.
Haemorrhage, with: Ver-a.
Heat, then coldness, with: *Sep.*
Heated, when: Ip; Tab.
Hour, at a certain: Lyc.
Injuries, slight: Ver-a.

FAINT

Looking
- Steadily at any object: Sumb.
- Up: Tab.

Medicine, taking, on: Asaf.

Menses
- During: Lach; Laur; Mag-c; Mos; *Nux-m*; Nux-v; Sep; Tril.
  - coldness, with: Laur.
- Pain, from: Kali-s; *Lap-alb*.
- Start, at+: Merc.
- Suppressed from: Nux-m.

Music, from: Sumb.

Nursing child, when: Vip.

Odours, from: Colch.

Pain, from: Asaf; *Cham*; Cocl; *Hep*; Mos; *Nux-m*; Nux-v; Ran-sc; Stro; Val.

Palpitation, during: Lach; Nux-m.

Prolonged: Hyd-ac; Laur.

Reading, when+: Merc-i-f.

Rising, on: *Bry*; *Cadm*; Merc-i-f; Phyt; *Ver-v*; Vib.

Room
- Entering: Plb.
- Hot: Ip; Lil-t; Pul; Sep.

Sitting up, on: Vib.

Standing, on: *Alu*; Lil-t; Nux-m.

Stool, at: Con; *Nux-m*; Nux-v; Ox-ac; Pod; Spig; Sul; Ver-a.

Stooping, on: Elap; Sumb.

Sudden: Ip; Pho; Ran-b; Sep.

Summer: Ip.

Sweat, with: Dig; Hyds.
- Cold: Lach.

Thinking after: Calad.

FAINT

Trifles, from: Sep; Sumb.

Vertigo, with: Berb.

Vomiting, from: Cocl; Nux-v; Ver-a.

Waking, on: *Carb-v*.

Walking in open air: Seneg.

Washing clothes, on: Ther.

Wound, from slight: Ver-a.

Writing, after: Calad.

FALLING: Bro; Caus; Coll; Con; Kre; Laur; Nat-c; Pho-ac; Rat.

As if: BELL; Thu.

Backward, as if: Bry; Chin; Led; Rhus-t.

Down, as if: Laur.

Easily: Calc.

Forward, as if: Alu; Dig; Elap; Mang; Nat-m; *Nux-v*; Rhus-t.

Ground to, suddenly when walking or standing: Mag-c.
- Cries, and+: Hyo.
- Rolls about and: Cic.
- Through, as if: Benz.
- Unconscious: Cocl.
  - screams, and: Buf.

Height from, as if: Caus; Gel; Mos.
- Sleep in+: Caps.

Inward, wall as if, before epilepsy: Carb-v.

Out, as if: *Bell*; Cocl; Laur; *Lil-t*; Nux-v; Pod; Sep.

Rising and falling: See DIRECTIONS Up and Down.
- As if: Bar-c; Lach.

Sideways, as if: Calc; Cocl; Nux-v.

FALLING

Street, in: Chin-s.

Without any cause or from least obstacle: Nat-c.

FALTERING: See HESITATES.

FALLOPIAN TUBES

Inflammation of (salpingitis): Ars; Coll; Lach; Merc; *Pul*; Sep; Stap.

Cutting along: Polyg.

Serum or pus, escapes from uterus: Sil.

FANATICISM: Thu

FANCIES: See PERCEPTIONS Changed.

FANNED, as if: See AIR, blowing, on part.

FANNING

AGG: Mez.

AMEL: Ant-t; Ap; Arg-n; Bap; CARB-V; *Chin*; Chlo-hyd; Crot-h; Fer; Kali-n; Lach; Med; Sec; Xanth.

FANTASY: See IMAGINATIONS.

FAR OFF feeling: Med; Syph.

FASTIDIOUS: *Ars*; Grap; Nux-v.

FASTING

AGG: *Calc*; *Croc*; Dios; *Flu-ac*; IOD; Kre; Lach; *Laur*; *Nat-c*; *Pho*; Plat; Plb; Ran-b; Sep; Stap; Sul; Tab; Val.

AMEL: *Cham*; *Con*; Kali-s; Nat-m.

As if: Ars; Bry; Chin; Cocl; Ign; Pul; Ver-a.

- **Meals, after:** Lyc.

FATIGUE

AGG: Act-sp+; Berb; Cof; Epip; Helo; Nux-v; Pho-ac.

FATIGUE

Scientific labour, from AGG: Grap.

FATS: See FOOD & DRINKS

FATTY: See GREASY.

Degeneration: *Ars*; Aur; Cup; Kali-c; *Lyc*; Mang+; Merc; Pho; Vanad.

FAUCES

Itching: Phyt; Rhus-t.

Numb+: Arg-m.

Sensitive: Coc-c.

FAULT FINDING: Ars; Helo; Sul; Ver-a.

FAVUS: See under ERUPTIONS.

FEAR, anxiety, fright: Abro+; ACO; *Arg-n*; ARS; *Bell*; Bor; Bry; CALC; Calc-p; *Carb-v*; Cist; Cocl; Cof+; *Dig*; Gel; Grap; Hyo; IGN; *Lyc*; Lyss; Med; Merc-c; Mos; Murx; Nat-c; Nat-m; Nit-ac; *Nux-v*; *Op*; PHO; Psor; *Pul*; Rat; Rhus-t; Samb; *Sec*; Spo; Stram; Sul; Ther; Tub; *Ver-a*.

Alone, of being+: Ant-t; Con; Naj.

- **Lest, he injures himself:** Ars; Merc; Nat-s.
- **Darkness, in:** Kali-br; Radm; Val.

Animals, dogs etc: *Bell*; Buf; *Chin*; Tub.

Appearing in public, (stage fright etc): Anac; Arg-n; *Gel*.

Approach, of: *Arn*; Bar-c; Caus; Cup; Ign+; *Lyc*; Petr; Pho; Plb; Sep; Tarn; Ther+.

Arrest, of: Ars; Meli; Plb; Tab; Zin.

FEAR

Ascending steps, on: Nit-ac.
Assassins: Plb.
Bad news: Ast-r.
Bed or coach, of: Alum; Cann; Cedr.
Bed wetting: Alu.
Bitten by beast, being: Hyo.
Brilliant, shining objects, mirrors, etc: Canth; Lach; Lyss; Stram.
Cause, without: Plb; Zin-val.
Children, about one's: Rhus-t.
Closed carriage, riding in: Cimi; Succi.
Coition, at the thought of, in women: Kre.
Corners, to walk past certain: Arg-n; Kali-br.
  • Something, creeping out of+: Pho.
Crossing streets: Aco; Hyd-ac; Plat.
Crowd: Aco; Arg-n; Aur; Fer-p; Gel; Nat-m; Pul.
Cruelties, hearing: Calc.
Dark: Arg-n; Cam; *Cann*; Carb-an; Kali-br; Sanic; STRAM; *Val.*
  • Eyes, Closing on: Carb-an.
Death, of: ACO; Arn; ARS; Cact+; *Calc*; Cimi; *Gel*; Hyd-ac; Kali-c; Kali-n+; Lac-c; Mos; Nit-ac; *Pho*; Plat.
  • Starvation, from: Ars.
Desire, to escape from: Merc.
Disease, of: Arn; Calad; *Calc*; Kali-c; Lac-c; Lil-t; Nux-v; Pho; Sele.

• Cholera: Lach; Nit-ac.
• Contagious: Bor.
• Incurable, being: Cact; Lil-t.
• Lungs, of: Aral.
• Pneumonia: Chel.
• Small-pox: Vario.
• Syphilis: Hyo.
• Tuberculosis: Calc.

Door
• Bell, ringing: Lyc.
• Opening, on: Cic; Con; Lyc.

Downward motion: See Falling.
Emission, after: Carb-an; Petr.
Endure, cannot: Lyss.
Every thing, of: Calc; Hyd-ac; Lyc+.
Evil, of+: Kali-m.
Examination, of: Aeth; Anac; Gel; Pic-ac.
Exertion
• Amel: Tarn.
• Slight of: Sul-io.
Eyes, closing on: *Carb-v*; Mag-m.
Fall upon him, high walls and buildings: Arg-n; Arn.
Falling
• Downward motion of: Bor; Gel; Hypr; Lac-c; Sanic; Sil; Zin.
• Forwards: Alu.
• Height, from: Hyo.
• Houses, of: Hyd-ac.
• Stairs, down: Lac-c.
  - up, and: Onos.
Fever, during: Aco; Amb; Ars; Bar-c; Ip; Sep.

FEAR

Financial loss, of: Ars; Calc-f; Stap.
Friends, of: Cedr.
Fright, of, remains: Op.
Future, misfortune, evil forebodings: ACO; ARS; Ast-r; CALC; Caus; Cham; Chin-s; Cimi; Dig; Grap; Grat+; Kali-c; Kali-m; Lil-t; Merc; Nat-m; *Nux-v*; Pho; Plat; PSOR; PUL; Thu; *Ver-a*.
- Imaginary: Kali-c; Laur.
- Sense, of: Merc.
- Twilight agg: Caus.

Ghosts: Carb-v; Kali-c; Pho; Pul+; Ran-b+; *Stram*.
Glistening objects: See Brilliant.
Green stripes, seeing on: Thu.
Health
- Of others, about: Cocl.
- One's own: Arg-m; Kali-p+.

Heart will stop+: Lach.
Hurt, being: *Arn*; Chin; Hep; Kali-c; Rut; Spig.
Husband will never return, something will happen to him: Plat.
Imaginary things: *Bell*; Hyd-ac; Laur; Pho.
Impulse of his own: Alu.
Insanity, of: Alu; *Calc*; *Cann*; Chlor; *Cimi*; Kali-br; Lil-t; Lyss+; Manc; Med; *Pul*; Sumb.
Knives, of: Alu; Ars; Chin; Hyo; Lyss; Nux-v.
Lightning: Sil.

FEAR

Long lasting: *Aco*; Hyo; Op; Petr.
Lying down of
- Heart will stop: Lach.
- One will die: Mos.

Maniacal: Sec.
Mirrors, of: See Brilliant.
Murdered
- Of being: Cimi; Op; Pho; Plb; Stram; Tab.
- Somebody: Ars.

Narrow or shut places: *Arg-n*; Cimi; Lac-d; Stram; Succi; Val.
Never, get well+: All-s.
Night at, cannot lie in bed: Rhus-t; Syph.
Noise: Bor; Cocl; Mos; Ther.
- Door, at: Aur; Lyc.
- Least: Aur.
- Street, in: Bar-c; *Caus*.

Observed, her condition being: CALC; Chel.
Open
- Air, of: Cyc.
- Space: See AGORAPHOBIA.

Ordeals: Arn; *Arg-n*; *Gel*; Kali-br; Lyss; Strop.
Pain
- Becomes unbearable: Cep.
- From+: Sars.

Paralysis, of: *Anac*; Arn; Bap; Syph.
People, of: See ANTHROPOPHOBIA.
- Yet if alone AGG: Ars; Clem; Con; Kali-br; Lyc; Sep; Stram; Tarn.
- menses during: Con.

FEAR

Physician: Iod; Thu; Ver-a.
Places, buildings: Arg-n; Calc; Kali-p; Visc.
Pointed things, needles, pins: Ap; Ars; Bov; Merc; Plat; *Sil*; *Spig*.
Poison: All-s+; Anac; Ap; Bell; Glo; *Hyo*; Lach; Kali-br; Rhus-t; Ver-v.
Poverty: Bry; Calc; Calc-f; Nux-v; Psor; Sep.
Pursuit: Hyo.
Rain: Elap; Naj.
Rats: Cimi.
Riding carriage, in: Bor; Lach; Psor; Sep.
Robbers: Ars; Ign; Nat-m.
Say something wrong, lest he should: Lil-t; Med.
Self control, losing: Arg-n; Gel; Stap.
Shadows: Calc.
- His own: Calad; Lyc; Stap.

Sharp things (See Pointed things): Alu; Ars; Merc; Plat.
Shut places: See Narrow.
Sleep
- Falling to: Calad; Lach; Sabal.
- Loss of, from: Cocl; *Nit-ac*.

Society: Cup; Cup-ac; Sele; Til.
- Position, his own in: Ver-a.

Stool, after: Calc; Caus; Kali-c; Nit-ac.
Strangers: *Bar-c*; Buf; Carb-v; Caus; Cup; Thu.
Sudden, wakes from sleep: Arn.

FEAR

Talking, loudly: Meli.
Telephone: Visc.
Thunderstorm, lightning: Bor+; Lyc; Nat-c; Nit-ac; *Pho*; Rhod.
Touch of (See Approach): ANT-C; *Arn*; CHAM; Cina; Con; Cup; Ign; Kali-c; Lyc; Tarn.
- Others passing, by: Aco.
- Sore parts: Tell

Trembling and chattering of teeth, with: Elap.
Tremulous: Mag-c.
Trifles, over: Aco+; Ign+; Sep; Thu.
Tunnel: Stram.
Twilight agg: Caus.
Undertaking any new thing: Arg-n; Ars; Lyc; Sil.
Vehicles, approaching of: Hyd-ac.
Waking, on: Ant-t; Arn; Ars; Cina; Lach; Psor; Spo; Tub.
Walk
- Rapid, must; Tarn.
- Slowly must, otherwise something will happen: Cup.

Water (See WATER): Hyo; Lyss; Stram.
Women: Pul.

FEARLESSNESS: See BOLDNESS.

FEATHER: See DUST.

FEATHER BED AGG: Cocl; Colo; *Mang*; Merc; Psor; Sul.

FEEBLE: See WEAK.

FEELS
Good and bad by turns: Alu; Psor.
Not normal, but cannot tell why+: Bro.
Too hot: See HEAT agg.
FEET: Arn; Ars; Bell; Bry; Caus; Kali-c; Lyc; *Pul*; Sep; Sil; Zin-ch.
Arches: Rut; Sil.
Bed, out of: Ars; Cham; Sang; Sec; *Sul*.
Blotchy: Led.
Bones: Chin; Cup; Hypr; *Led*; Mez; *Rut*; Stap.
- Broken, as if: Zin.
Border, of: Grap; Kali-bi; Led; Lith; Zin.
Braces, stretching, amel: Ign; Med; Pul.
Broken, as if: Hep; Zin.
Bunions: Grap; Lyc; Paeon; *Sil*.
Burning: Cham; Med; Pho-ac; *Pul*; Sec; *Sul*.
- Hands cold, with: Sep.
- Menses during, at night: Nat-p.
Clubby: Nux-v.
Cold
- Agg: Bar-c; Con; Lach; *Nux-v*; *Pul*; Sil.
- As if, though warm: Sul.
- Water in, as if: Gel; Sanic; *Sep*.
- Wet agg: See Wetting agg.
Coldness (See COLDNESS, partial): Kali-chl; Raph.
- Bed in: Am-c; Calc; Grap; Psor; Rhod; Senec; *Sep*; Sil.

FEET, coldness, bed in
- right: Lyc; Raph.
- left: Ars; Tub.
- icy: Bell.
- Chorea, in: Laur.
- Colic, with: Colo.
- Constant+: Old.
- Day time, burn at night: Nat-p.
- Fever, during: Arn; Lach; Stram; Sul.
- Headache, during: Gel; Meli; Sep; Vario.
- Hot days, summer in: Asar.
- Icy: Cam; Carb-v; Elap; Lach; Pho; Samb; Sep; Sil; Ver-a.
- menses during: Nat-p.
- Menses, with: Nux-m.
- One of: Chel; Con.
- right: Bar-c; *Lyc*; Pul; Sabi.
- left: Carb-v; Psor; *Sul*; Tub.
- other, hot: *Lyc*; Pul.
- Pregnancy, duing: *Lyc*; *Ver-a*.
- Smokers: Sec.
- Soles, burning: Cup.
- Urination, during: Dig.
- Walking, while only: Anac; Chin; Plb.

Cramp: Bell; Caus; Cup; Frax; Lac-c; Rum; Sanic; Sec; Val; Ver-v.
- Pregnancy during: Calc; Frax.
Crawling: See Formication.
Crippled: Ant-c.
Damp: CALC.
Desquamation: Manc.
Dorsum, of: Calc; *Caus*; Hep; Led; *Pul*; Spig; Tarx.

FEET

FEET, dorsum
- Cramp: Anac; Lach; Ver-v.
- Itching: Caus; Led.
- Stitches, in: Berb.
- Sweat: Iod.
- Swelled: Bry; Pul; Thu.

Dry: *Sul.*
Emaciation: Caus.
Enlarged, as if: *Ap*; Colo.
Fanned, wants: Med.
Fidgety: Kali-p; Tarn; Zin.
Flat: Calc-p.
Floating, as if: Spig.
Formication: Agar; Hypr; Sec.
Frost bitten, as if: Kali-p.
Furry: Hypr.
Galled: Cep.
Glued to floor, as if+: Pho.
Hanging down agg: See HANGING down limbs agg.
Hard floor agg: Rut.
Head to, glowing sensation: Visc.
Heavy: *Alu*; *Ars*; Cyc; Ign; Mag-c; NAT-M; Pho; Pic-ac; *Pul*; *Rhod*; *Rut*; Sep; SUL.
- Walking amel: *Mag-c*; Nat-m; Sul.
- Weight, hanging, as if: Rhod; Rut.

Held to earth, by magnet, as if: Led; Pho.
Higher than head, as if: *Spig.*
Hot: See Burning.
- Cold and alternately: Gel; Polyg.
- Water in AMEL: Buf.

Instep: Sang.

FEET
Inversion: Cic; Nux-v; Sec.
Itching: Led; Pic-ac; Sep; Strop; Sul.
Knee, to: Cedr.
Motion
- Amel: Ars; *Rhus-t*; *Zin.*
- Spasmodic of left foot: Cina.

Numb: Ap; Arg-n; ARS; *Cocl*; Con; Form; Grap; Lyc; NUX-V; Pho; Pho-ac; Pic-ac; *Plat*; Sep.
- Right: Alu; Am-c; Ant-c; Ars; Cam; Kali-bi; Mang; Rhus-t; Sep.
- Left: Grap; Kali-c; Med; Nat-m; Pho; Psor; Thu.
- Legs crossing, on: Laur.
- Sitting, when: Ant-t; Helo.

Offensive, sweat without: Grap; Sil.
Painful
- Menses during: Am-m; Ars; Mag-c.
- Sciatica, with: Mag-p.
- Standing, from: Scil.

Paralysis: Caus; Plb; Vip; Zin.
- As if: Cham.

Pressing to floor AMEL: Cup-ar; Ign; Med; Zin-io.
Pricking: Kali-p.
Restless: Ars; Rhus-t; ZIN.
Shop girls, of: Scil.
Spasms: Bism; Ver-a.
Stamps: Ant-c; Stram; Ver-a.
Stiff in A.M.: Led.
Stretching
- Amel: See Braces.
- Spasmodic: Cina.

FEET

Sweat: *Bar-c*; *Calc*; Calc-s; Carb-v; Cocl; Colo; Grap; *Iod*; *Lyc*; Mag-m; Merc; Psor; *Pul*; SEP; *Sil*; *Sul*; *Thu*; Zin.
- Acrid: Flu-ac; *Grap*; Manc; Sep; Sil; Thu.
- Burning, with: Calc; Lyc; Sul.
- Cold: Aur; *Bar-c*; *Calc*; Calc-s; Carb-v; Kali-m; Lach; Lyc; Mur-ac; Pul; Sec; Stap; Tarn; Ver-a.
  - bed in, morning: Merc.
- Destroys shoes: Grap; Hep; Naj; Sanic; Sec; Sil.
- Foul, offensive: Aur; *Bar-c*; Calc-s; Grap; *Kali-c*; *Lach*; Lyc; *Nit-ac*; Ol-an; Psor; *Pul*; Sec; Sep; SIL; Tell; *Thu*.
  - menses, after: Sep; Sil.
- Injuries of spine, after: *Nit-ac*.
- Sour, between toes: Kob.
- Sticky, hose stiff: Am-c; Calc; Kali-c; Lyc; Manc; Sanic.
- Stubborn: Psor.
- Suppressed: *Bar-c*; Ol-an; Pho; Sep; *Sil*; *Zin*.
- Swelling, with: Lyc.
- Toes, sore with: Grap; Zin.
- Walking agg: Carb-v.
- Warm: Led.
- Wilting the skin: Ant-c.

Swelling, oedema etc: *Ap*; *Ars*; Caus; Chel; Grap; Led; *Lyc*; *Med*; Merc-c; Pul; Pru-sp; Samb; Sil.
- Right: Bov; Lac-c; Lach; Lyc; Sars; Sec; Spig; Spo; Stro; Sul.

FEET, swelling
- Left: *Ap*; Colo; Como; Kali-c; Kre; Lyc; Sang; Sil; Tell.
- Cold: Ap; Calc.
- Diarrhoea
  - with: Acet-ac.
  - after or amel by: Med.
- Hands of, with: Fer.
- Hot: Ars; *Bry*; Lyc.
- Menses, during: Ap; Grap; Lyc; Pul.
- One foot, only: Kali-c.
- Paralysis, with: Cocl.
- Sensation of: *Ap*.
- Soles, painful, with: Saba.
- Sprain, after: *Bov*.

Swing in half circle, while walking: Cic.

Tingling: Cocl.

Touch agg: Ars; Calc; Chin; Kali-c; Sep; Sul.

Touch, do not, ground, as if+: Calc-ar.

Trembling: Aur; Bar-c; Merc; Ox-ac; Pul.
- Menses, during: Hyo.

Turn
- Inwards: Cic.
- Under: See ANKLES, weak.

Ulcer, on: Sil

Uncover, must: Cham; Flu-ac; Med; Pul; *Sul*.

Veins, distended: Sul-ac.

Vesicles: Nat-c.

Weakness: Ars; Mag-c; Ox-ac; Sil.
- Sitting agg: Card-m.

Weight, hanging: See Heavy.

FEET

Wetting of AGG: Cep; Cham; Cup; *Dul*; Merc; Nat-c; Nat-m; *Pho*; PUL; Rhus-t; *Sep*; SIL.

Winter agg: Caus.

Wood, as if were: Plb.

FEIGNING sick: See MALINGERING.

FELON: See FINGERS.

FEMALES

Affections in general: Aco; Ap; *Bell*; Calc; Caps; Cham; Chin; Cimi; Cocl; Con; Croc; Helo; *Lach*; Mag-m; Mos; PUL; Sabal; SABI; SEP; Val; Vib.

Afterpains: See AFTERPAINS.

Coition
- Agg: Ap; *Arg-n*; Fer; Fer-p; Hep; Kre; Lyc; Lyss; Nat-m; Pul; Sep; Sul; Tarn; Thu.
- After agg: Ap; Plat; Stap.
- Aversion to: Agn; Bor; Caus; Grap; *Nat-m*; *Sep*.
  - menses after: Caus; Pho.
  - orgasms painful, from: Nat-m.
- Enjoyment absent: Berb; Caus; Kali-br; Sep.
- First agg: Stap.
- Haemorrhage, after: *Arg-n*; Arn; Hyds; *Kre*; Nit-ac; Sep; Tarn.

Conception, easy: Bor; Merc; Nat-m.
- Promotes: Canth; Nat-c+.

Desire, sexual
- Diminished: Agn; *Caus*; *Grap*; Helo; Ign; *Nat-m*; Onos; Sabal; Sep.

FEMALE, desire
- Increased: AGN; *Calc*; Calc-p; Cam; *Canth*; Con; Flu-ac; Grat; HYO; Lach; *Murx*; *Nux-v*; *Orig*; *Pho*; PLAT; Pul; Stram; Tarn; *Ver-a*.
  - contact, least, from: Lac-c; Murx.
  - dysmenorrhoea, with: Cann.
  - menses
    before: Ars; Calc-p; Pho; Stan; Stram; Ver-a.
    during: Ars; Canth; Hyo; Lach; *Lyc*; Plat; *Pul*.
    after: Ars; Kali-p.
    suppressed, from: Ant-c.
  - musk keep busy to repress it: Lil-t.
  - nursing, while: Calc-p; Pho.
  - old women in: Mos.
  - parturition, after: Chin; Ver-a; Zin.
  - pregnancy, during: Pho.
  - scratching, distant parts from: Stan.
  - sterile, women, in: Cann.
  - worms, from: Saba.
- Perverted: Sabal.
- Supressed, ill effects from (See SEXUAL DESIRE, male): *Con*; Sabal.
- Violent, insatiable, nymphomania: AGN; Ast-r; Calc; Grat; *Hyo*; Lach; Murx; Orig; *Plat*; Stan; Stram; Sumb; *Ver-a*; Zin.
  - love, disppointment from: Ver-a.
  - lying in women: Ver-a; Zin.
  - masturbation, driving her to: Orig; Plat+; Zin.

FEMALE, desire, violent
- unsatisfied sexual desire from: Ver-a.
- virgins, in: Con; *Plat.*
- widows, in: *Ap*; *Orig.*

Frigidity+: Ign.

Orgasm
- Delayed, wanting: Berb; Bro.
- Easy: Stan.

Sexual excitement easy: Bur-p; Lac-c; Manc; Orig; Sumb; Zin.
- Frigidity: Ign.

Sterility: Agn; Aur; Bor; Merc; Nat-c; *Nat-m*; Pho; Sep.
- Acid vaginal secretion from: Nat-p.
- Atrophy of mammae and ovary, from: Iod.
- Excessive sexual desire from: Kali-br; Orig; Pho; Plat.
- Menses, copious, from: Calc; Merc; Mill; Nat-m; Sul.
- Non retention of semen, from: Nat-c.
- Ovarian atony, from: Eup-pur.
- Sycotic: Med.
- Uterine torpor, from+: *Goss.*
- Weakness, from: Merc; Sil.

To complete full term in delicate and sheer nervous women: Rat.

Women
- Pregnant, late in life: Bell.
- Who deliver, still born children: Cimi.

FEMALE ORGANS

In general: Amb; Ap; BELL; *Calc*; Cham; *Cimi*; Con; Grap; Kali-c; Kre; *Lach*; *Lil-t*; Lyc;

FEMALE ORGANS ..
Nat-m; *Nux-m*; Nux-v; Onos; Pho; *Plat*; PUL; *Sabi*; *Sec*; Senec; SEP; *Sul*; *Thu*; Til; Tril; Ust; *Vib*; Visc.

Backward, pains: Bell; Lil-t; Sep.

Burning: Ars; Berb; *Canth*; Carb-an; *Kre*; Nit-ac; Sec; Sul.

Cold: Plat.

Consciousness of, internal: Vib.

Crossing legs amel: Lil-t; Sep.

Dryness: Berb; Lyc; *Nat-m*; SEP.

Gangrene: Sec.

Hard: Con; *Kre*; Merc.

Heart, to: Naj; Xanth.

Heavy: Lob; Plat.
- Menses, during: Plat; Sep.

Itching: Amb; Am-c; CALAD; *Calc*; *Carb-v*; *Con*; Kre; Merc; NAT-M; Nit-ac; Petr; Plat; Rhus-t; SEP; Sil; *Sul*; TARN.
- Burning: Am-c; Calc.
- Coition
  - agg: Nit-ac.
  - desire for+: Sabi.
- Cold water amel: Calad.
- Desire strong to embrace+: Alu.
- Intolerable: Agar; *Amb*; Calc.
- Lying amel: Berb.
- Menses
  - after agg: Nit-ac; Tarn.
  - from: Sul; Tarn.
- Pregnancy, during: Calad; Flu-ac; Helo; Merc; Sabi; *Sep.*
- Urine, contact of agg: *Merc.*
- Voluptuous: *Orig*; *Plat.*
- Walking agg: *Nit-ac*; Thu.

FEMALE,

Labour like, bearing down pains: Agar; Alo; BELL; *Caul*; CHAM; GEL; *Lil-t*; Murx; Nat-m; NUX-V; Plat; PUL; *Sabi*; *Sec*; SEP; Stan; Vib.
- Colds agg: Hyo.
- Fear of death with: Cof.
- Menopause, after: Agar.
- Noise agg: Cimi.
- Riding in carriage agg: Asaf.
- Rubbing amel: Pall.
- Standing
  - agg: Dict.
  - amel: Bell.

Lying
- Agg: Amb; Fer; Kre; Murx; *Pul*.
- Back on, amel: Onos.
- Doubled up amel: Cact; Cimi; Nux-v.

Moist, as if: Petr.

Pressure on
- Back amel: Mag-m.
- Vulva amel: Lil-t; Murx; Sanic; Sep.

Sitting agg: Sul.

Sore, sensitive, painful: Ap; Bell; Canth; Cof; *Con*; *Kre*; *Lach*; Lil-t; Mur-ac+; *Plat*; Stap; Sul; Thu.
- Redness of, with+: Til.

Stool agg: Amb; Pod; Stan.

Swelled: Ap; Ars; Bell; Canth; *Kre*; *Nit-ac*; Nux-v; *Pul*; Rhus-t.

Thighs, to: Cham; Stap; Xanth.

Tingling, voluptuous: *Orig*; *Plat*.

Upward, going: Alu; Cact; Calc-p; Coc-c; Elap; Lach; Lil-t; Nit-ac; Pul; Sabi; *Sep*.

FEMALE, upward going
- Right: Alu; *Ap*; Croc; Lach; Lyc; Murx.
- Left: *Bro*; Caul; Cimi; Kali-c; Lac-c; LACH; LIL-T; NAJ; Sul.
- mammae, to: Murx.

FEROCIOUS: See DELIRIUM, maniacal.

FESTERING, as if: Buf.

FESTINATION: Alu; Mang; Syph; Tarn.

FEVER: ACO; Ant-t; *Ap*; Arn; ARS; BELL; BRY; *Canth*; Caps; *Carb-v*; *Caus*; Cham; Chin; Chin-s; Con; Fer-p; *Gel*; Ign; Ip; Kali-s; Lach; LYC; Med; *Merc*; Merc-c; Mez; *Nat-m*; NUX-V; Op; PHO; Pic-ac; PUL; RHUS-T; Sang; *Sul*; Tarx; Ver-a.

Adynamic+: Ail; Bap; Mur-ac.

After AGG: *Ars*; Bell; *Chin*; Hep; Nux-v.

Alternating with chill: See CHILL.

Anticipating: Nux-v.

Before AGG: Arn; *Ars*; Calc; *Carb-v*; *Chin*; Cina; Ip; *Pul*; Rhus-t; Spig; Sul.

Black water: *Ars*; Crot-h; Lyc.

Catarrhal: See Coryza.

Chill absent: Ap; Ars; Bell; Bry; Cham; Gel; Rhus-t.

Coition, after: Grap; Nux-v.

Continued: See BLOOD, sepsis, TYPHOID etc.

Conversation, from: Sep.

Cough
- Agg: Arn; Ars; Chin; Ign; Mur-ac; Nat-m; Thu.

FEVER, cough
- Whooping, with: Dros.

Covers, warmth
- Agg: *Ap*; Chin; *Ign*; Mur-ac; Nat-m; Op; *Pul*.
- Amel: Bell; Nux-v; Pul; Pyro; Rhus-t; Stram; Stro; Tub.

Dentition, during: Aco; Calc; *Cham*; Nux-v; Sil; Sul.

Drinks, warm agg: Sumb.

Dry, burning: ACO; *Ap*; *Ars*; Carb-v; Dul; Gel; *Mur-ac*; Nux-v; Op; Pho; *Pul*; Sec; Tub.
- Night, at: Samb.

During AGG: *Ars*; Bry; Calc; Cham; *Chin*; Ip; Kali-c; Lyc; *Nat-m*; Nux-v; Op; *Pul*; Rhus-t; *Sep*; Sul.

Dysenteric: Bap; Fer-p; Nux-v.

Eating
- Agg: Pho; Tub.
- Amel: Anac; Chin.

Emotion, from: Caps.

External: *Aco*; Ars; *Bell*; Bry; *Canth*; Cham; *Ign*; Pul; Rhus-t; Sil; Stram.

Fanned desire to be, in place of thirst: *Carb-v*.

Feet, cold with: Tarn.

Fright, from: Cheno.

Gastric: Ant-c; Ant-t; Ars; *Bap*; Bry; Fer-p; Ip; Pul.

Hands, cold with: Thu.

Hectic: Ars; Ars-io; Bap; Caps; Chin-ar; Fer-p; Iod; Pho; Sang; Sep; Sil; Tub.

High, hyperpyrexia: *Aco*; Bap; Chin-ar; Iod; Mur-ac; Pho; *Pyro*; Sul; Ver-v.

FEVER, high
- Erratic, rise of: Pul.
- Evening in, below normal in morning: Ver-v.

Home sickness, from: Caps.

Insidious: Ars; Chin; Sec; Sul; Tub.

Intermittent, ague: Aran; ARS; Calc; Calc-ar+; Caps; Cedr; *Eup-p*; Fer; Ign; *Ip*; Kali-s; Lyc; *Nat-m*; Nat-s; Nit-ac; *Nux-v*; Pho-ac; Psor; Pul; Pyro; Sul; Tarn; Tub; *Ver-a*.

Internal: *Aco*; Arn; *Ars*; *Bell*; Bry; Laur; Mag-c; Merc; *Nux-v*; Pho; Pho-ac; Rhus-t; Sul; *Ver-a*.
- External
  - coldness with: *Aco*; Ars; Cam; Mos; Sul-io; Ver-a.
  - cold parts, with: *Aco*; Ant-t; Ap; Arn; *Ars*; Bell; Calc; *Cam*; Carb-v; Cham; Cina; Cof; Dig; Dros; Hyo; Ign; Ip; Kali-c; Mez; *Mos*; Nit-ac; Nux-v; Pho-ac; Plat; Rhus-t; Sul; *Ver-a*.

Intolerance of both cold and warmth: Cocl; Cor-r.

Menses, with: Calc; Grap; Pho; *Pyro*; Rhod; *Sep*.

Mental exertion agg: Old; Spo.

Milk fever: *Aco*; *Bry*; *Calc*; Cham.
- Delirium with+: Aco.

Motion
- Agg: Cam; *Chin*; Sep.
- Amel: Caps; Lyc; Pho; Pul.

Night agg: *Ars*; Bap; Bell; Bry; Calc; Cham; Grap; *Hep*; Iod; Lach; Merc; Petr; Pho; *Pul*; *Sil*; Sul; Urt.

FEVER, night agg
- Periodically: Flu-ac.

Noise, from: Bry.

One sided: Alu; Bry; Cham; Dig; Lyc; Mos; Nux-v; Par; Pul.
- Right: Alu; Bry+; Cham+; Pho.
- Left: Lyc; Rhus-t; Stan.
- Lain on: Mag-m.

Oscillating: Chel; Chin-ar; Echi; *Pyro*; Sul-ac; Ver-v; *Zin*.

Pain, from: Carb-v; Cham.
- Abdomen, in: Sec.

Painful: Bry; Canth; Rhus-t.

Painless: Pho; Pho-ac.

Paroxysms, irregular: Ars; Nux-v; Psor; Pul; Sep.

Puerperal: See PUERPERAL sepsis.

Pulsations, with: Urt.

Relapsing: *Calc*; *Fer*; *Psor*; *Sul*; Tub.

Remittent: Aco; Ars; Bell; Bry; Cham; *Gel*; Merc.
- Bilious: Merc-d.
- Infantile: Ip.

Septic: See BLOOD SEPSIS.

Shivering, with: Arn; Caus; Gel; Kali-io; Nux-v; Sul.

Sleep
- Agg: *Calad*; Mez; Op; *Samb*.
- Amel: *Calad*; Pho; Sep.

Stupid form: Bap; Carb-v; Hell; Hyo; Mur-ac; Op; Pho-ac.

Subnormal, persistent: Cact; Chin-s; Kali-p; Nat-sal.

Suppression, from: Cham; Merc.

Sweat
- Absent: Ars; Bell; Bry; Cact; Gel; Nux-m; Scil.

FEVER, sweat
- Amel: Ars; Lyc; Rhus-t.
- Thighs on, with: Spo.
  - cold: Caps.
- With, continues, after: Calc; Chin; Hell; Merc; Op; Pho; Pho-ac; Pul; Pyro; Stram; Sul; Tub; Ver-v.

Then sweat, then chilliness: Calad; Kali-bi.

Thirst, without: Cham; Cina; Ign; *Pul*.

Traumatic: Cof.

Vertigo, with: Urt.

Weakness disproportionate+: Sul-ac.

Yellow: Ars; Cadm; Canth; Carb-v; Crot-h; *Nux-v*.

FIBROID (See GROWTHS, new): CALC; Calc-f; Calc-s; Con; Grap; Kali-br+; *Pho*; *Sil*; Thyr+; Tril; Ust.

Bleeding: Bur-p; Calc; Hyds; Led; Nit-ac; Pho; Sul-ac; Tril; Vinc.

Burning: Lap-alb.

Cramps, with+: Bur-p.

Hard, stony: Merc-i-r.

FIBROID TISSUE, ligaments: *Bry*; *Calc*; Calc-f; Colch; FLU-AC; *Grap*; GUAI; *Kali-m*; *Lyc*; Phyt; Rhod; RHUS-T; Rut; Sabi; *Sec*; *Sil*; Stap.

FICKLE: See PERSEVERE, cannot.

FIDGETY: Ap; Bor; Cimi; *Grap*; Kali-br; Meny; Pod; Sep; Sil; Sumb; Tarn; Vib.

Women, urinary troubles, with: Meny.

FIGWARTS: See FUNGUS GROWTH.

FILM: See VALVE.

FINANCIAL LOSS AGG: Arn; Ars; Aur.

FINE PAIN: See PAIN, stitching, NEELES, HAIR sensation, THREAD sensation.

FINGERS: Am-m; Lyc; Ran-b; Rhus-t; Sil; Sul; Thu.

Along: Fago.

Alternating, with gastric symptoms: Kali-bi.

Around: Calc-p; Kali-bi; Lith.
- Ulceration: Grap; Pul; Sil.

Atrophy: Sil.

Backward, bent: Sec.

Between: Grap; Nit-ac; Sele.

Bites: Med; Plb.

Blue: Agar; *Carb-v*; Sec.

Bones
- Devloped imperfectly: Stap.
- Pain, pressing, in: Vio-o.

Burning: Kali-c; Mag-c; Mur-ac.
- Between, on touching water: Laur.

Children, put in mouth: Calc; Cham; *Ip*.

Clenched: Aeth+; Arg-n; Sec.

Closed: Cup; Merc; Plb.
- Motion, constant, with: Colch.

Clubbing: Laur.

Cold: Abro; Agar; Chel; Grap; Kali-c; Tarx; Thu.

Contracted
- Hysterical: Zin.
- Sprain, from: Cann.

Convulsions, spasms: Agar; Chel; Cup; Sec.

FINGERS

Cracks: Calc; Nat-m; Petr; Sanic; Sars.
- Nails, around: Nat-m.

Cramps: Arn; Chel; Merc; Sec; Ver-a.
- Contraction, with: Cyc.
- Cutting with shears: Con.
- Dysmenorrhoea, alternating with: Dros.
- Periodical: Pho.
- Picking small objects: Stan.
- Single, in: Tab.
- Washing Agg: Tab.
- Writing, while: See Working with; Writing Agg.

Crooked: See Deformed.

Crossed: Carb-v; Grap.

Deformed: Kali-c; Lyc.
- Sprain, from: Cann.

Desquamation: Am-m; Elap.

Drawn together: Pho.

Eczema, with loss of nails: Bor.

Electric current flowing through, on touching any thing, as if: Alu.

Emaciated: Sil.

Extend, cannot: See Straighten, cannot.

Felon, runround, panaritium: Am-c; Anthx; *Ap*; Ars; Dios; *Flu-ac*; Hep; *Lach*; *Merc*; NAT-S; Nit-ac; Psor; *Sil*; Sul; Syph; TARN-C; THU.
- Chronic tendency: Dios; Hep; Sil.
- Cold water amel: Ap; Flu-ac; Led; *Nat-s*; *Pul*.
- Deep: Calc; Merc-c; *Sil*; Sul.

FINGERS

FINGERS, felon
- Injury, from: Led.
- Parturition, after: Cep.

Flexed
- Constant motion, but+: Colch.
- Spasmodically: Rhod.

Formication: Lyc; Sec; Thu.
- Extending on lower limbs: Thal.

Fuzzy, smokers, of: Sec.
Grasping amel: Lith.
Growth stunted: Stap.
Hair, back on, as if: Flu-ac.
Heavy: Plb; Strop.
Hypertropy: Am-m.
Itching: Anac; Psor; Sul; Urt.
Jerking: Caus; *Cic*; *Cina*; Cyc; Rhe; Stan; Sul.
- Sleep during: Sul-ac.
- Writing, when: Sul-ac.

Joints: Ant-c; Calc; Calc-f; *Caul*; Caus; Lyc; Nat-m; Sep; Spig; Sul.
- Closing agg: Caul; Nat-m.
- Dark, dirty: Pic-ac.
- Dilocation, easy: Hep.
- Distorted: Colch.
- Nodes, on: Stap.
- Swollen: Nit-ac.
- Ulcers, on: Bor; Mez; Sep.

Knitting amel: Lyc.
Lame: Calc; Kali-m; Sep.
Lift, cannot: Cur.
Mashed: Hypr.
Middle: Calc; Nat-m; Syph.
Mobility, affected: Calc.
Motions, of: Kali-br; Mos.
- Flexed, with: Colch.

Nails: See NAILS.

FINGERS

Nodes: Abro; Benz-ac; Berb; Calc; Caul; Kali-m; Led.
Numb: Abro; Aran; Bar-c; *Calc*; Dig; Grap; LYC; Merc; Nat-m; PHO; Plat; *Rhus-t*; Sec; Sil; Sul; Thu; Thyr.
- Extending to other parts: Thal.
- Left, then right leg: Thyr.
- Night, on waking: Nat-m; Thu.
- Ring and little: Arg-n.

Pale: Kre.
Paralysis, of: Mez.
Peeling of: See Desquamation.
Picks, plays with: Aru-t; Calc; Con; Hyo; Kali-br; Lach; Tarn; Ther.
Prickling: Abro.
Red: Mur-ac.
Rough, everything feels: Par.
Sensitive: Berb; Lac-c; Led; Sec.
Sides: Sars.
Single: Tab.
Skin, tight: Mag-p.
Spread apart: Glo; Lac-c; Lyc; Med; *Sec*.
Stiff: Kali-c; Led; Lyc; Rhus-t.
- Book, while holding: Lyc.
- Grasping anything when: Carb-an; Dros.
- Paralytic: Lil-t.
- Scissors, cutting with, while: Con.

Straighten, cannot: Ars; Cam; Colo; Cup-ar.
Sweat, on: Lyc.
Swelled: Mur-ac.
- As if: Kali-n.

FINGERS

Tense: Crot-h; Mag-p; Pho; Pul.
Thumbs, as if were: *Pho.*
Tingling: Aco; Ars; Cact; Nat-m; Ran-b; Sil.
Tips: Am-m; *Calc-p*; Kali-c; Lach; Mar-v; Pho; Sec; Thu.
- Brown: Tub.
- Burn: Canth; Mar-v; Med; Nat-m.
- Bursting: Caus.
- Cold: Chel; Lac-c; *Tarx.*
  - dry: Ant-t.
  - icy: Ant-t; Lac-d+.
- Cracked: Am-m; Bar-c; Bell; Grap; Med; Merc; Nat-m; *Petr*; Ran-b; *Sars*; Sil.
- Dead: Mag-m.
- Dry, as if made of paper: Ant-t; Sil.
- Formication: Am-m; Mag-s; Nat-m; Sec.
- Fuzzy: Tab.
- Heavy: Plb; Strop.
- Knobby: Laur.
- Numb: Arg-m; Arg-n; Kali-p; Lach; Nat-m; *Pho*; Spo; Stap; Sul.
  - chill, with: Stan.
- Painful: Calc; Cist; Kali-c; Lac-c; Sil; Sul.
- Peeling: See Desquamation.
- Prickling, grasping when: Rhus-t.
- Red: Aco.
- Sensitive: Berb; Calc-p; Cist; Lac-c; Nat-c; Sars; *Sul*; Tarn.
- Sweat, on: Carb-an; Carb-v; Pho; Sep; Sul.
- Tearing, fine: Stap.

FINGERS, tips
- Tingling: Am-m; Kali-c.
- Ulcers: Ars; Pho; Psor; Sars.
- Vesicles: Nat-c.
- Warts, on: Caus.

Touching one another unbearable: Lac-c; *Lach*; Sec.
Twitching: Cic; Lyc.
- Cough, with: Osm.
- Sleep, during: Lyc; Rhe.

Using agg: See Working with.
Water soaked: Sec.
Weak: Calc; Carb-v; Kali-m; Sep.
Working with, grasping, sewing, playing instrument etc, AGG: Agar; Bov; *Calc*; CAUS; *Cham*; *Cimi*; Cocl; *Cyc*; *Dros*; Gel; KALI-C; Mag-p; NAT-M; Pho; Pic-ac; Plat; Sep; *Sil*; *Stan*; *Val*; ZIN.
Writing
- Agg: Anac; Arg-m; Arn; Caus; Cyc; Dros; Kali-c; Mag-p; Pic-ac; Stan; Sul-ac.
- Amel: Fer; Nat-c; Zin-ar.

Yellow spots, on: Saba.
FIRELIKE: See BURNING, fiery.
FISHY odour, taste etc: Calc; Grap; Med; Ol-an; Sanic; Sep; Tell; Thu.
FISSURE: See CRACKS.
FISTULA: *Berb*; Bry; CALC; Calc-f; Calc-p; Carb-v; CAUS; Con; *Flu-ac*; Hep; Kali-c; LYC; Nat-s; Nit-ac; Petr; *Pho*; *Pul*; SIL; Stram; SUL.
Chest symptoms and: Berb; Calc-p; Sil.
Closing, after: Kali-c.
Recto vaginal: Thu.

FITFUL: See CHANGING MOODS.

FIT OF PASSION, ill effects+: Mag-c; Nat-m; Plat.

FIXED IDEAS: See IDEAS.

FLABBY FEELING: See RELAXATION.

FLATULENCE: Alo; *Amb*; ARG-N; Arn; Ars; *Asaf*; Calc; Carb-an; CARB-V; CHAM; CHIN; *Cocl*; Colch; GRAP; Hyds; *Ign*; *Kali-c*; LYC; Mag-c; Nat-s; *Nit-ac*; Nux-m; NUX-V; Old; Op; *Pho*; Pic-ac; *Pul*; *Sil*; SUL; Tarn; Terb; Val; Ver-a; Vib.

Abdomen
- Upper in: Carb-v; Pul.
- Lower, in: Aco; Lyc; Nat-m; Nux-m; Sil; Sul; Zin; Zin-val.
- Right side: Bism; CALC; Grap; Lil-t; *Nat-s*; Ox-ac; *Pho*; Thu.
- Left side: Am-m; *Aur*; *Carb-v*; CON; Crot-t; Dios; Euphor; Lyc; Nat-m; Pho-ac+; Seneg; Stap; SUL.

Air hunger, with+: Kali-io.

Back, felt in: Rhod.

Bath, after: Calc-s.

Croaking: Arg-m; Colo; Lyc; Saba.

Discharge, of: *Carb-v*; Chin; Grap; Kali-c; *Old*.

Dysmenorrhoea with: Vib.

Fermenting, as if: Chin; Lyc; Rhus-t.

Food, all turns to gas: Carb-v; Kali-c; Nux-m; Nux-v.

FLATULENCE

Generation of: Carb-v; Kali-c; Mar-v.

Here and there: See Wandering.

Hysterical: Asaf; Ign; Pul; Raph; Val+.

Menses, with: Kali-p; Nux-m; Vib.

Noisy, rumbling, growling, borborygmy: Agar; Anac; Ant-c; CARB-V; *Caus*; *Chin*; *Hell*; Hep; LYC; Nat-m; NAT-S; NUX-V; *Pho*; *Pho-ac*; *Pul*; Sep; *Sil*; *Sul*; Ver-a.
- Annoying, in women: Rum.
- Empty, feeling with: Sars.
- Lying, on left side: Colo.
- Sleep, during: Agn; Cup.
- Stools
  - before: Mag-c.
  - after: Petr.

Numbness, with: Med.

Obstructed, retained: Ant-t; Arg-n; Calc+; Carb-v; Cham; *Chin*; COCL; Colch; Grap; IGN; LYC; Mos+; Nat-c; Nat-s+; *Nit-ac*; Nux-v; Plb; *Pul*; RAPH; Sil; STAP; Tarn; Ver-a.
- Left Side: *Aur*.
- Stools
  - before: Lyc.
  - after: Lyc; Pic-ac.

Painful, wind colic: Carb-v; *Cham*; Chin; Coll; Lyc; Mag-p; Nat-s; *Nux-v*; Ox-ac; Pul; Rhod; Step; Ver-a; Zin-val.
- Hot drinks amel: Pho.

Post operative: Chin; Raph.

Pressing
- Bladder, on: *Carb-v*; Ign; Kali-c.

FLATULENCE, pressing
- Out+: Lyc.
- Rectum, on: Calc; Ign; Nat-s.
- Upward: Arg-n; Asaf; Carb-v; Grap; Thu.

Pushing: Nat-s.
- Upward: Asaf.

Rectum, in: Hep; Nux-v; Sep.
Rolling: Thyr.
Sour food, from: Pho-ac.
Squeaking: Kali-io.
Vegetables, from: Caps.
Wandering: *Carb-v*; Chin; LYC; Nat-m; Pul; Sil.

FLATUS
Back, felt in: Rhod.
Cold: Con.
Coughing, on: Sang.
Hot: Agar; *Alo*; Carb-v; Mar-v; Stap; Zin.
Involuntary: Pho.
Moist: Ant-c; Carb-v.
Offensive, foul: Alo; Arn; *Ars*; *Asaf*; Bry; CARB-V; Caus; *Cocl*; Lach; Nat-m; Nat-s; Nit-ac; *Pul*; *Sil*; Spig; *Sul*; Zin.
- Eggs, like spoiled: Arn; Stap; Sul.
- Garlicky: Agar; Pho-ac.
- Urine, like: Agn.
- Writing, after: Ant-t.

Passing
- AGG: Chin; Cocl; Flu-ac.
- AMEL: CARB-V; Colo; *Lyc*; Nat-s; *Nux-v*; Pul; Sang; Scop; Stap; Sul.
- Difficult: Op; Ox-ac.
- Up and down AMEL: *Arg-n*; Grap; Kali-c; SANG; Ver-a.

FLATUS
- Upward, not down+: Asaf.
- Walking when: Myr.

Profuse, inodorous+: Agar.
Sour: Calc; Mag-c; Nat-c; Rhe.

FLEETING PAINS: See PAIN.
FLESHY: See GROWTHS NEW and FUNGUS GROWTHS.
FLEXURES: See SKIN, folds.
FLOATING, flying as if: Aco; Arg-n; Asar; Calc-ar; Cann; Cocl; Cof; Hyo; Hypr; LAC-C; Lach; Nat-m; Nux-m; Op; *Pho-ac*; Phys; Spig; Stic; Stram; Thu; Val; Zin-io.

Lying on left side agg: Zin-io.

FLOWING: See TRICKLING as of water.
FLUCTUATION: See WAVES.
FLUIDITY: See DISCHARGES, increased.
FLUSHES: See WAVES.
FLUTTERING: See VIBRATIONS.
FLYNG to pieces: See SHATTERED.
FOAMY, frothy: See DISCHARGES, foamy.
FOETID: See OFFENSIVE.

FOETUS
Expels, dead+: Canth.
Lying crosswise, as if: Arn.
Maldisposition: Pul.
Movement, as if: Nat-c; Tarn.
- Causes nausea and vomiting: Arn.
- Disturb sleep: Con.
- Intolerable: Sep.
- Lively: Lyc; Op.

FOETUS, movementcj
- Painful: Con; Croc; *Sil.*
- Somersault, like: Lyc.
- Violent: Croc; Lyc; Op; Psor; Sil; Thu.
  - vomiting, with: Psor.

FOGS: See CLOUDY WEATHER.

FOLDS: See SKIN.

FONTANALLES: See Under CHILDREN.

FOOD AND DRINKS

Acid: See Sour.

Alcoholic
- Agg: *Ars*; Asar; Bar-c; Calc; *Carb-v*; Chin+; Cimi; Hyo; *Kali-bi*; *Lach*; NUX-V; *Op*; Pho; Pul; *Ran-b*; Sele; *Stram*; Sul; *Sul-ac*; Terb+; Zin.
- Amel: *Aco*; Agar; Canth; *Con*; *Gel*; Lach; Op; Sele; Sul-ac.

All Disagee: Arg-n+; Carb-an; *Carb-v*; Fer; Lach; Mos; Nat-c; Syph.

Apples
- Agg: Ars-io; Bell; Bor.
- Amel: Guai.
- Sour Agg: Merc-c.

Artifical AGG: Alu; Calc; Mag-c; Sul.

Bacon amel: Ran-b; Ran-sc.

Baked agg: Carb-v; Pul.

Beans agg: See Legumes.

Beer
- Agg: Bap; Card-m; *Kali-bi*; Led; Nux-v; Rhus-t.
- Amel: Nat-p; Ver-a.

Berries agg: Ip.

Bitter agg: Nat-p.

FOOD

Brandy
- Agg: Nux-v; Op; Sul.
- Amel: Old.

Bread
- Agg: *Bry*; Hyds; Lyc; Nat-m; *Nux-v*; *Pul*; Sul.
- Amel: Caus; Nat-c.
- Butter, and agg: Acet-ac+; Chin; Nit-ac; *Pul*; Sep.

Buckwheat agg: Ip; *Pul*; Ver-a.

Butter
- Agg: Carb-an; *Carb-v*; Nat-m; *Pul.*
- Tastes too sweet: Ran-b.

Buttermilk agg: Bry; Pul.

Cabbage agg: *Bry*; Carb-v; Kali-c; *Lyc*; Mag-c; *Petr*; Rob.

Cakes
- Agg: Ant-c; Ip; Pul.
- Hot Agg: Kali-c; Pul.

Carrot agg: Calc; Lyc.

Cereal agg: See Farinaceous.

Cheese, old agg: Ars; Bry; Ptel; Rhus-t.

Cherries agg: Merc-c.

Chilli (green or red) agg: Pho.

Chocolate agg: Bry; Calad; *Kali-bi*; Lyc; *Ox-ac*; Pul.

Coffee
- Agg: Ars; Canth; Caus; *Cham*; Colo; IGN; Merc; NUX-V; Ox-ac+; Pul.
- Amel: Arg-m; Cham; Colo; Fago; *Ign.*
- Odour of, agg: Flu-ac; Lach; *Nat-m*; Osm; *Sul-ac*; Tub.

Cold
- Agg: ARS; Bell; Calc; *Canth*;

FOOD, cold, agg ..
  Caps; Cham; Chel; Chin; Dul; Fer; *Hep*; Kali-io; Kali-m; Kre; Lach; LYC; Manc; Merc-i-r; NUX-V; *Rhus-t*; Saba; Samb; Sep; *Sil*; Stap; Ver-a.
  • Amel: *Ap*; Arg-n; *Bell*; *Bism*; *Bry*; Cann; CAUS; Cup; Ign; Kali-m; LACH; Merc-i-f; *Pho*; Phyt; *Pul*; Radm; Sang; Sele; Sep.
  • Drinks, in hot weather agg: Bry; Kali-c; Nat-c; Ver-a.

Condiments, spices
  • Agg: *Nux-v*; Pho; Sele.
  • Amel: Hep; Nux-m.

Cucumber agg: Ars; Cep; Pul; Ver-a.

Dainty agg: Pul.

Dry
  • Agg: *Calc*; Lyc; Nat-c; Pul.
  • Too, seems, while eating: Calad; Chin; Fer; Ign; Kali-io; Ox-ac; Raph.

Eggs agg: Calc; Colch; Fer; Led; *Pul*; Sul.

Farinaceous
  • Agg: Bry; Caus; *Lyc*; Nat-c; NAT-M; NAT-S; Pul.
  • Children in amel: Nat-c.

Fat, oils
  • Agg: Ant-c; Ars; Calc; CARB-V; *Chin*; CYC; *Fer*; *Grap*; Kali-m; Lyc; Nat-p; PUL; Rob; Sep; Tarx.
  • Amel: Nux-v.

Fish
  • Agg: Ars; Carb-an; Carb-v; Kali-c; Nat-s; *Plb*; *Pul*; Urt.
  • Amel: Lac-c.

FOOD, fish
  • Fried agg: Kali-c.
  • Herring agg: Fer-p.
  • Pickled agg: Calad.
  • Salmon agg: Flu-ac.
  • Shell agg: Carb-v; *Lyc*; *Urt*.
  • Spoiled agg: Ars; Carb-an; Carb-v; Pul.

Flatulent agg: Bry; Chin; *Lyc*; *Petr*.

Frozen: See Ice.

Fruits
  • Agg: *Ars*; *Bry*; Caus; Chin; Colo; Elap; Glo; Ip; Nat-c; Nat-s; *Pul*; Rum; Sep; VER-A.
  • Amel: Lach.
  • Banana agg: Rum.
  • Canned agg: Pod.
  • Grapes agg: Ox-ac.
  • Guava agg: Sep.
  • Juicy agg: Ant-c; Calc; Iod; Pul; Sul.
  • Oranges agg: Pho-ac.
  • Peach agg: Cep; Flu-ac; Glo; Psor.
  • Pears agg: Bor; Bry; *Ver-a*.
  • Plantains agg: Rum.
  • Plums and prunes agg: Rhe.
  • Sour
    - agg: Ant-c; Ip; Lach; Ox-ac; Pho-ac; Pod; Psor.
    - amel: Lach; Naj.
  • Unripe agg: Ip; Rhe; Rob; Sul-ac.

Garlic, odour of agg: Saba.

Honey: Nat-c; Pho.

Hot
  • Agg: Bry; Chlo-hyd; Nat-s; *Pul*; *Sep*.

FOOD

FOOD, hot
- Amel+: Chel.
- Drinks amel: Ail; Ars; Lyc; Nux-v; Sul-ac.

Ice, frozen things
- Agg: Arg-n; *Ars*; Calc-p; Carb-v; Dul; Ip; Kali-bi; *Pul*; Rob.
- Amel: Xanth.

Ice water agg: Dig.

Indigestible
- Agg: *Iod*; Ip; Rut.
- Amel: Ign.

Legumes, beans, peas agg (See Flatulent): *Bry*; Calc; *Lyc*; Petr.

Lemonade
- Agg: Phyt; *Sele*.
- Amel: Bell; Cyc; Phyt.

Lemons
- Amel: Bell; Stram.
- Peel agg: Ip.

Liquids agg: ARS; *Chin*; *Cocl*; Colo; Crot-t; *Fer*; Ign; *Lach*; *Nat-m*; PHO; *Rhus-t*; *Sil*; Ver-a.

Malt liquor+: Kali-bi.

Maple sugar agg: Calc-s.

Meat, mutton
- Agg: Arg-n; *Ars*; Caus; Carb-v; Chin; *Colch*; *Fer*; Kali-bi; Lept; Lyss; Merc; Ptel; *Pul*.
- Amel: Ver-a.
- Fresh agg: *Caus*; Chin.
- Spoiled, agg: See PTOMAINE POISONING.

Melons agg: Ars; *Flu-ac*; Zing.

Milk
- Agg: Aco; AETH; Amb; Bry; CALC; Calc-s; *Chin*; Con; Lac-d; Lyc; Mag-c; Mag-m; Merc; Nat-c; *Nit-ac*; Nux-m;

FOOD, milk, agg ..
Ol-j; Pho; *Pul*; Sep; Sul.
- Amel: Aco; Ars; Chel; Cina; Fer; Iod; Merc; Mez; *Nux-v*; Pho-ac; Scil; Stap; Ver-a.
- Boiled agg: Nux-m; Sep.
- Cold
  - agg: Kali-io; Spo.
  - amel: Iod.
- Sour agg: Pod.
- Sweet amel: Ars.
- Warm
  - agg: Amb.
  - amel: Chel; Crot-t; Grap.

Mixed agg: Ant-c; Ip; *Pul*.

Nuts agg: See Fats.

Odour of cooking agg: Ars; Cocl; *Colch*; Dig; Ip; Merc-i-f; Sep; Stan.

Onions
- Agg: Bro; *Lyc*; Nux-v; *Pul*; Thu.
- Amel: Cep.

Oysters agg: Alo; Bro; Carb-v; *Lyc*; Pul; Sul-ac.
- Amel: Lach.

Pastry: Ant-c; Ip; Kali-chl; Lyc; Pho; *Pul*.

Pepper
- Agg: Ars; *Cina*; Nat-c; Sep; Sil.
- Cayenne agg: Pho.

Pork agg: Ant-c; CARB-V; *Cyc*; *Grap*; Ham; Ip; PUL; Sep.

Potatoes
- Agg: *Alu*; Colo; Mag-c; Nat-s; Pul; Sep; Ver-a.
- Amel: Acet-ac.

Poultry agg: Carb-v.

Pudding agg: Ptel.

FOOD

Raisins agg: Ip.
Raw agg: Pul; *Rut*; Ver-a.
Rich agg: Ars; Bry; *Carb-v*; Ip; Kali-m; Nat-s; Nit-ac; PUL; Sep.
Salads agg: Ars; Bry; *Calc*; Carb-v; Ip; Lach; Lyc.
Salt
- Agg: Alu; Ars; Carb-v; Dros; Mag-m; NAT-M; *Pho*; Sele.
- Amel: Mag-c; Nat-m.

Sausage agg: Acet-ac; *Ars*; Bell; Bry; Pul.
Seasoned highly, amel: Nux-m.
Sight or smell agg: Ars+; Colch; Nux-v; Pho; Sul.
Soup agg: Alu; Kali-c.
Sour
- Agg: *Ant-c*; Ant-t; Arg-n; Ars; Carb-v; Dros; Flu-ac; Merc-c; Nat-m; Nat-p; Pho-ac; Pod; *Pul*; Sep; Sul.
- Amel: Arg-n; Ign; Lach; Ptel; Pul; Sang.
- Becomes: Lapp.
- Odour agg: Dros.

Sourkraut agg: Bry; Lyc; Petr; Pul.
Spices: See CONDIMENTS.
Spoiled agg: See PTOMAINE POISONING.
Starchy agg: Colo; Mag-c; Nat-c.
Stawberries agg: Ant-c; Bur-p; Ox-ac; Sep.
Sugarcane juice agg: Ars.
Sweet potato agg: Calc-ar.
Sweets
- Agg: Ant-c; *Arg-n*; Ars; Cham; Cina; Grap; *Ign*; Ip; Lyc;

FOOD, sweets, agg ..
Med; Merc; Nat-p; Ox-ac+; Sang; Sele; Sul; Zin.
- Amel: Bell.

Tamarind water agg: Sele.
Tea
- Agg: Ars; Calad; Chin; Cocl; Dios; *Fer*; Pul; *Sele*; Strop; THU.
- Amel: Alo; Dig; Fer; Glo; Kali-bi.

Thought of agg: Carb-v; Grap; Nat-m; *Pul*; Sep.
Tobacco agg: See TOBACCO.
Tomota agg: Lith; Pho.
Turnips agg: Calc-ar; Bry; Lyc; Pul; Rob.
Uncooked: See Raw.
Unripe agg: Rhe.
Veal agg: Calc; Caus; *Ip*; *Kali-n*; Sep; Zin.
Vegetables (green) agg: Alu; Ars; Bry; Caps; Hell; Hyds; Lept; Lyc; Nat-c; *Nat-s*; Ver-a.
- Decayed: Carb-an.
- Potatoes except+: Acet-ac.

Vinegar
- Agg: *Ant-c*; *Ars*; Sul.
- Amel: Asar; Hell; Pul.

Warm
- Agg: *Bry*; *Lach*; *Pho*; Phyt; *Pul.*
- Amel: *Ars*; Lyc; *Nux-v*; Rhus-t.

Water
- Agg: Ars; Chin-ar.
- Drinking too much agg: Grat.

Wine agg: LED; Nux-v; Ox-ac+; Rhod; Zin.

FOOLISH: See CHILDISH.
Happiness and pride: Sul.

FORCED

Apart: See SEPARATED as if.
Out as if: See PAIN, pressing.
Through narrow opening, as if: BAR-C; Bell; Buf; Carb-ac; Coc-c; Cocl; Dig; Glo; *Lach*; Op; *Plb*; Pul; Sul; *Tab*; Thu; Val.
• Fluids, as if: Coc-c.

FORCEPS DELIVERY after:
Bur-p; Hypr.

FORE ARM : See under ARMS.

FOREBODINGS: See FEAR of future.

FOREHEAD: *Aco*; *Am-c*; Arn; Ars; BELL; *Bry*; Chin; Ign; Lach; Lyc; *Merc*; *Nat-m*; NUX-V; *Pho*; Phyt; Pru-sp; *Pul*; Sep; Sil; *Spig*; *Sul*; Thu.

Aching: Merc-i-f.
Adhesions of skin: Sabi.
Alternating sides: *Iris*; Lil-t; Pho; Saba.
Ascending, into: Lach; Zin.
Ball, lump, knot: Ant-t; Carb-ac; Caus; Kali-c; Stap.
• Hot: Carb-ac.
Band, constriction: *Cact*; Gel; Merc; *Sul*.
Block, solid, as of a: Kali-bi; Kre.
Blood boils: Led.
Board, pressed against+: Dul; Rhus-t.
Brown yellow: Kali-p; Sep.
• At the edge of hair: Caul; Kali-p; Med; Nat-m.
Bubbles: Form.
Centre: Crot-h.
Cold: Cimi.

FOREHEAD, cold
• Spot on: Arn.
Crackling: Aco.
Crawling, as of a worm: Alu.
Deep, pigmented patches, in liver complaints+: Van.
Eyes, close must+: Pod.
Flattened, or pressed flat, as if: Cor-r; Ver-a.
Formication: Colch; Zin.
Frowning: Lyc; Ver-a.
Fullness: Carb-s; Cinb.
Heat, burning: Ap; Bell; Kali-io; Nux-v; Pho.
Heavy: Ant-c+; Rut; Stap.
Hollow: Caus.
Loose: Sul-ac.
Menses amel: Cep.
Nasal discharges amel: Cep; Kali-bi; *Lach*; Zin.
Navel, with: Lept.
Nodes: Caus.
Nose, to: Lach; Phys.
Numb: Mur-ac; *Plat*.
Occiput, to: Caus; Tub.
• Right: Pru-sp.
• Left: Senec.
Oily, greasy: Hyds; Psor.
Pimples, disappear in open air: Hep.
Presses against something: Nux-v.
Pricking: Mur-ac; Vio-o.
Projecting: Apoc.
Pulsation: Bell; Glo; Iris; Lac-d; Pul.
• Right: Ant-t; Bell; Ign.
• Left: Aco.

FOREHEAD

Rub, inclination, to: Glo; Ver-a.
Skin, drawn in folds, as if: Grap.
Sweat
- Cold: Ant-t; *Carb-v*; Chio; Cina; Dros; Ip; Op; Stap; *Ver-a.*
- Drinking
  - agg: Cup; Ip.
  - amel: Ver-a.
- Epistaxis, with: Croc.
- Sudden: Val.
- Vomiting, with: Chio.

Swelled: Ap; Hell; *Nux-v*; Rhus-t.
Tongue, protruding agg: Syph.
Upper: Colo.
Veins: Abro; Calad; Cam; Chin; Cub; Sul.
Vertigo felt in: See VERTIGO.
Warts, on: Cast-eq.
Water, as of: Plat.
Waving, shaking, as if: Bell; Merc; Sep.
Weight in, as if: Rut.
Wrinkled: Hell; Hyo; LYC; Rhe; Sep; *Stram*; Ver-a.
- Brain symptoms, with: Grat; Hell; *Stram.*
- Chest symptoms, with: Lyc.
- Headache, during: Caus; Grat; Stram; Ver-a.

FOREIGN BODIES: Aco; Anac; Calc-f; Hep; Lob; Sil.

FORGETFUL: See MEMORY, bad.

FORGETS

Errand: Bar-c; Manc; Med.
Events, recent: Abs; Ail; Grap; Rhus-t.

FORGETS

Everything+: Gymn; Merc.
- When busy: Ant-c.

Name
- His own: Med.
- Objects, of: Lith.
- Persons, of: Chlor; Guai.

Sentence, cannot finish: Med.
Suddenly+: Anac.
Time and place: Merc.
What
- He wishes to do next: Manc; Mill.
- She wanted to say: Hypr; Iod.

Words, in mouth: Anac; Arn; Bar-c; Cann; Med; Pho-ac; Rhod.
- Hunts, for: Thu.

Words, whole, while writing+: Rhod.

FORGOTTEN

Something constantly, as if he had: Caus; *Iod*; Mill.
Things come to mind in sleep: Calad; Sele.

FORMICATION, crawling (See also skin): Aco; *Agar*; Arn; Bar-c; Bor; Calc; Carb-an; Colch; Lyc; Merc; *Nux-v*; Oenan; Op; Osm; *Pho*; Pic-ac; *Plat*; *Rhus-t*; Saba; Sang; SEC; Sep; Spig; Stram; Stro; *Sul*; Tell; Vario; *Zin.*

Affected part: Colo.
Angina, during: Dig.
Anxiety, with: Cist.
Bad news, after: Calc-p.
Body, all over: Ail; Aran; Cist; Dig; Mag-m; Med; Zin-p.

FORMICATION
Cold: Frax; Lac-c.
- Body around: Helod.
- Menses, before: Ant-t.

Dyspnoea, with: Cist.
Here and there: Op.
Internal: Med.
Knocking against anything agg: Spig.
Pain
- With: Hypr.
- After: Sec.

Paralysed part: Cadm; Pho.
Root of hairs, at: Pho-ac.
Rubbing amel: Sec.
Skin, under: Cadm; *Sec*; Zin.
Sweat, with: Rhod.

FORSAKEN, lonely: Arg-n; *Aur*; Bar-c; Calc; MENY; Plat; *Psor*; *Pul*.

FRACTURES: See BONES, brittle.

FRAGILE: See BRITTLE and BONES, brittle.

FRAIL as if body were: Sars; Thu.

FRANTIC: See BESIDES HIMSELF.

FRECKLES: See Under ERUPTION.

FRETFUL: See ANGER.

FRICTION AGG: Con; Sep; Tell.

FRIGHT
Complaints, from (See fear, emotions agg): Aco; Anac; Ap+; Caus+; Cup; Hyo; Hypr; Ign; Lyc; Nat-m; Nux-m; *Op*; Pho; Pho-ac; Pul; Sil; Stram; Ver-a; Vib; Zin.

FRIGHT
Animals, from: Stram.
Cause, without: Plb.
Sudden, pleasant surprise from+: Cof.
Tendency to take: Sul-ac.

FRIGHTENDED
Easily: Aco; Arg-n; *Arn*; Ars; Bar-c; Bor; Cact; Carb-an; Carb-v; *Cocl*; Grap; IGN; Kali-c; Kali-p; *Lyc*; Nat-c; *Nat-m*; Petr; *Pho*; Saba; *Stram*; Ther; Zin.
Emissions, after: Alo.
Noise, every: Bor.
Suffocative attacks, follow+: Samb.
Trifles, at: Ant-t+; Kali-c; Kali-s; Lach; Lyc; Nit-ac; Pho.

FROST
Air AGG: *Agar*; *Calc*; Caus; CON; Lyc; Nux-v; *Pho-ac*; *Pul*; Rhus-t; SEP; *Sil*; *Sul*; Syph.
Bite: See CHILBLAINS.

FROTHY: See DISCHARGES, Foamy.

FULLNESS: See CONGESTION.

FUMES: See VAPOUR.

FUNGUS GROWTH, excrescences, warts, condylomata, proud flesh, haematodes etc:
Ant-c; Ars; Aur; Bar-c; *Calc*; *Carb-an*; Caus; Clem; *Dul*; Lach; *Lyc*; *Merc*; Merc-c; Med; Nat-c; *Nat-s*; NIT-AC; Petr; *Pho*; *Pho-ac*; Phyt+; Ran-b; Rhus-t; *Sabi*; Sang; *Sil*; *Stap*; Sul; *Thu*.

Bleeding: Nit-ac; Pho.

FUNGUS GROWTH
Burning: Sabi.
Fleshy: Calc; Stap; Thu.
Foul: Sabi.
Granular: Calc; Nit-ac; Stap; Thu.
Itching: Sabi.
Pedunculated: Lyc; *Nit-ac*; *Sabi*; Stap+; Thu.
Ragged: Nat-c; Pho-ac; Rhus-t; Thu.
Spongy: Calc; Lyc; Nit-ac; Stap; Thu.
Summer disappear, winter reappear+: Psor.

FURIBUND: See DELIRIUM, maniacal.
FURRY: See COATED.
FURY, rage: See DELIRIUM, maniacal.
FUSSY: Ap; Calc-p; Samb; Sele; Zin.
GAGGING: See RETCHING.

GAIT
Body trembles while walking: Lac-ac.
Bent: See Stooped.
Dragging: Lach; Lathy; *Myg*; Naj; Nux-v; Pho; Rhus-t; Tab.
Feet, swing at each step: Cic.
Festination: See FESTINATION.
Heels do not touch ground when walking: Lathy.
Knees knock against each other: Arg-n; Caus; Colch; Con; Glo; Lathy; Zin.
Legs
 • Apart: Pho.
 • Involuntarily thrown forward when walking: Merc.

Limping: Caus; Colo; Dul; Kali-c; Rhus-t; Tab.
 • Involuntary: Bell.
Missing steps when going down stairs: Stram.
Reeling: Agar; Alu; Cocl; Lol-t; Pho.
Shuffling: Ol-an; Op; Sec; Stap+; Tab; Vip.
Slapping: Mang.
Slovenly: Sil.
Slow, sluggish: Gel; Pho; Pho-ac; Tab.
Spastic: Lathy; Zin.
Staggering: Alu; Buf+; Calc; Helod; Lil-t; Mur-ac; Nat-c; Onos; Pic-ac; Pul; Ver-v.
 • Coition, after: Bov.
 • Places one foot over the other: Mar-v.
 • Unobseved, when: Arg-n.
 • Walking in dark or closed eyes when: Alu; Ap; Arg-n; Gel; Iodof; Stram; Zin.
Stairs ascending agg: Tab.
Stepping
 • Backwards: Mang; Oxytr; Stram.
 • Down form high step agg: Phyt.
 • High: Agar; Bell; Carb-v; Merc; Nat-m; Onos; Rhus-t.
 • Left, towards: Lach.
 • Puts down heel hard: Helod.
Stooped, bent: Am-m; *Arg-n*; *Carb-v*; Cocl; Colo; Con; Gel; Lathy; Mang; Nat-m; *Pho*; *Sul*; Terb; Ver-a.

GAIT

Stumbling: Agar; Arg-n; Bar-c; Caus; Con; Hyo; Ip; Nat-c; Nux-v; Pho; Pho-ac; Rut; Zin.
- Against everything+: Ip.
- Ascending and descending when: Phys.
- Easily: Agar; Pho; Pho-ac; Rut.

Tottering: Op; Pho; Rhod; Ver-a; Zin.
- Drunkards: Ran-b.

Unsteady: *Agar*; Arg-n; Ast-r; Bar-c; Caus; Cocl; Con; Kali-br; Lol-t; Nat-c; Ol-an+; Sec; Stan; *Sul*; Tab; Tarn-c.
- Sciatica, in: Kali-cy.

Waddling: See Legs apart.

GALL BLADDER

Burning: *Lept*; Myr.

Anger, after agg: Stap.

Bursting: Bap; Lept; Myr.

Clawing: Lyc; Med; Nat-s.

Duct: Hyds.
- Obstruction, duodenum at: Canc-fl.

Eating amel: Mag-m.

Fullness: Myr.

Gripping: Sep.

Inflammation: Lach; Pho.

Septic: Bry; Buf; *Lach*; Pho.

Sore: *Bap*; Lept; Myr.

Stomach, to+: Berb.

Stones: Bell; Berb; *Bry*; *Calc*; Card-m; *Chel*; Chio; Euon; Lach; *Lept*; Lyc; Mag-p; MERC; Merc-d; Myr; Nat-s; Nux-v; *Pho*; Pod; Sang; Sul; Tarx+; Ver-a.

Stooping agg: Sep.

GANGLIA (bursae):
Am-c; Ap; *Arn*; Benz-ac; Carb-v; *Nat-m*; Pho; RUT; Sil; *Stic*; Sul.

GANGRENE:
Anthx; ARS; Bell; Canth; CARB-V; Chin; Cist; Crot-h; Kre; LACH; Mur-ac; Plb; *Sec*; *Sil*; Solid; Sul-ac; Tarn-c; Vip.

Burns or scalds from: Anthx; Ars; Caus; Sec.

Cold: Ars; Lach; Sec; Sil.

Diabetic: Con; Lach; Solid.

Dry: Ant-c; Sec.

Hot: Aco; Ars; Bell; Sabi; Sec.

Leeches, application from: Sec.

Moist: Carb-v; *Chin*; Hell; Pho.

Mustard, application from: Calc-p; Sec.

Senile: Carb-v; Cep; Euphor; Pho-ac; SEC; Sul-ac.

Threatened, with blue parts: Ars; Asaf; Aur; Con; Hep; *Lach*; Merc; Sil; Ver-a.

Traumatic: Arn; Lach; Sec; Sul-ac.

GARGLING AGG: Carb-v.

GARLICKY, odour of discharges, taste, etc:
Art-v; Asaf; Cup-ar; Kali-p; Lach; Osm; Petr; *Tell*.

GASTRIC FEVER: See FEVER.

GASTRITIS:
Aco; Ars; Bry; Merc-c; Nux-v; Pho; Ver-v.

Alcoholic: Arg-n.

Enteritis with: See VOMITING, purging with.

GATHERED together: See CONSTRICTION.

GAY: See CHEERFUL.

GELATINOUS: See DISCHARGES.

GENITALS (in general, both sexes): Agn; Arn; Berb; Calad; Cof; Erig; Gel; Hyo; Merc; Nat-p+; Nit-ac; *Pul*; Rhus-t; Sabal; Sele; *Sep*; Sul.

Right: Ap; Calc; Caus; *Clem*; Hep; *Lyc*; Merc; Nux-v; Pall; Spo; Sul-ac; Ver-a.

Left: *Lach*; Naj; *Pul*; Rhod; *Thu*.

Alternating between: Cimi; Colo; Lac-c; Lycps; Ol-an; Onos; Rhod.

Burning, heat: Cof; Tarn; Tub.
• Eating Agg: Tub.

Cold: Berb; Calad+; Sabal.

Crawling: Calc-p; Plat.

Dry: Tarn.

Eruptions: Petr; Radm; *Rhus-t*.

Flabby+: Bar-c.

Flowing, everything towards (male): Colo.

Fumbles, grasps: Aco; Bell; Buf; Canth; *Hyo*; Merc; Sep; *Stram*; Zin.
• Constantly: Stram.
• Coughing when: Zin.

Inflammed: *Merc*.

Itching: Cof; Plat; Radm; Sabi; Tarx.
• Burning: Nat-m; Urt.

Motion agg: Sabi.

Numbness: Bar-c.
• Ascending: Form.

Offensive: Psor; Sars; Sul; *Thu*.
• Briny, coition, after: Sanic.

Pulsating, coition, after: Nat-c.

Raw: Merc+; Tarn.

GENITALS

Sensitive: Cof; Plat; *Stap*; Tarn; Zin.

Sitting agg: Sul.

Sweat, moisture, on: Dios; Sars; Sele; *Sep*; Thu.
• Coughing agg: Thu.

Swelled: *Rhus-t*; Tarn.

Thighs, down: Cham; Chel; Cimi; Kali-c; Ox-ac; Rhus-t; Sep; Ust.

Tickling: Alu; Plat.

Upward: Murx.

Varicose: Zin.

Weakness, after stool: Calc-p.

GENTLE: See TIMID.

GESTURES, makes: Bell; Cocl; Hyo; Mos; Nux-m; Stram; Tarn.

Ridiculous: Cic; Hyo; Nux-m.

GHOSTS: See FEAR.

GIDDY: See VERTIGO.

GIRDLE

Pains: See under PAIN.

Sensation: Stan.
• Yawning, with: Stan.

GIRLS: See PUBERTY.

Pampered+: Mos.

GLABELLA

Aching, fulness, and: Kali-bi.

Nodes+: Caus.

Puffy: Flu-ac; Kali-c; Sele; Sil.

GLANDS (in general): Ap; Ars; Aru-t; Aur; BAR-C; *Bell*; Bro; Bry; CALC; Carb-an; Chin; *Clem*; Cist; Con; Hep; Iod; Kali-m; *Lach*; *Lyc*; MERC; Nit-ac; *Pho*; *Phyt*; PUL; Rhod; Rhus-t; SIL; Spo; Stap; Sul; Tab; Tub.

GLANDS

Bead like, knotted: Aeth; Aur; Bar-io; Bar-m; Berb; Calc-io; Nit-ac; Sul-io; Tub.

Burning: Ars; Pul.

Cervical: Am-m; Bar-c; *Calc*; Canc-fl; Cist; Grap; Kali-c; Lap-alb; Lyc; *Merc*; Merc-i-f; Rhus-t; *Sil*; *Sul*; Vio-t.
- Malignant: Cist.
- Milk crusts, with: Canc-fl+; Vio-t.
- Neck, moving agg: Ign.

Constriction: Calc; Ign; Iod; Plat; Pul.

Ductless: Spo.

Emaciated: Con; Iod.

Enlarged, swelled: Bell; Calc; Carb-an; Cist; Dul; Iod; Kali-m; *Merc*; Phyt; *Rhus-t*; Sil; Sul; *Sul-io*; Syph; Tub.
- Atrophy, or+: Kali-io.
- Body, all over: Med.
- Emaciation, with: Ther.
- Fever, during, over body: Bell; Kali-c; Sep.
- Many: Tub.
- Menses, during: Kali-c; Lac-c.
- Painful: Merc-i-r; Stap.

Flaccid: Cham; Con; Iod.

Formication: Con; Spo.

Hard: Alum; Bad; Bar-m; Bro; Calc; Calc-f; Carb-an; Clem; Con; Iod; *Phyt*; Sele; Sil; Spo; Sul.

Hot and throb, all over+: Asaf.

Inflamed: Aco; Bell; Bry; Calc; Merc; Pho; Sul.

Inguinal: See GROINS.

GLANDS

Itching: Anac; Caus; *Con*; Kali-c; Pho; Sil; Spo.

Mesenteric: Calc; Iod.

Pulsation: Con; Merc.

Sore, bruised: Con.

Stitches: Bell; Ign; *Merc*; Nit-ac; Pul; Thu.

Submental: Led; Sil; Stap.
- Hard: Anthx.
- Head, moving agg: Calend.
- Swallowing agg: Chin.

Tearing: *Chin*; Merc; Pul; Thu.

Tension, in: Pho.

Ulcerative pain: Pho; Sil.

Uterine haemorrhage, with: Carb-an.

GLANS (penis): Merc; Nit-ac; Rhus-t; Thu.

Aching, steady: Chel: Osm.

Burning, when urinating: Anac.

Cold: Berb.

Cracks: Ars.

Crushed: Rhod.

Dry: Calad.

Flaccid: Mag-m; Nat-c.

Inflammation: Cinb; Kali-chl.

Into: Par-b.

Itching: Chel; Mez; Sul.

Numb: Berb.

Pimples, small, red: Cinb.

Pulsation: Coc-c; Pru-sp.

Rag like+: Calad.

Sore, on slight rubbing: Cyc; Nat-c.

Swelled: Merc.

GLANS

Tumour
- Soft: Bell.
- Yellow, behind: Lyc.

Urinating agg: Ox-ac; Pru-sp.
Urine, reaches and then returns: Pru-sp.
Warts, on: Ant-t.

GLAUCOMA: See Under EYE.
GLEET: See URETHRA, discharge gleety.
GLISTENING, shining: Aco; AP; *Aur*; *Bell*; *Bry*; Calc-f; Carb-ac; Caus; Cist; Euphr; Glo; *Kali-bi*; LAC-C; Lach; Mang; Nat-m; *Pho*; Rhus-t; Sabi; Sil; Syph; *Terb*.

Objects AGG: Bell; Canth; Hyo; Lyss; Mur-ac; Stram.

GLOBUS: See BALL, hysteria.
GLOOMY: See SAD.
GLOSSITIS: See INFLAMMATION, and TONGUE.
GLOTTIS spasms of (laryngismus stridulus): *Bell*; Calc; Calc-p; *Gel*; IGN; *Mos*.

Alternating, with constriction of fingers and legs: Asaf.

GLUEY: See DISCHARGES, gluey.
GLUTTONY: Ab-c; All-s; Ant-c; Bry; Chin.
GNAWING: See PAIN, gnawing.
GODLESS, want of religious feeling: See IRRELIGIOUS.
GOITRE: Ars-io; Bro; Calc; Flu-ac; Hep; *Ign*; *Iod*; Iris; Nat-m; *Spo*; Strop; Thyr; Vip; Zin-io.

Right side: Hep.

GOITRE

Left side: Chel.
Air, passing through, as if, on breathing: Spo.
Cardiac
- Pain, with: Spo.
- Symptoms, with: Cact.

Choking, from: Grap; Merc-i-f; Spo.
Diarrhoea, with: Cist.
Exophthalmic: *Bell*; Buf; Fer-p; *Iod*; Jab; Lycps; *Nat-m*; Strop.
- Grief, from: Amy-n; Chlo-hyd.
- Trembling, with: Meph.

Hard: Buf; Iod; Nat-c; Spo.
Heart action, rapid with: Buf.
Lumpy: Grap.
Menses
- Agg: Calc-io; Cimi; Iod.
- Suppressed, from: Fer; Fer-io.

Nodulated: Grap; Phyt.
Pain, into head, with: Hep.
Palpitation, with: Pho.
Pinched, as if: Nat-ar.
Pregnancy, during: Calc-io; Hyds.
Pressing, inward: Zin-io.
Puberty, during: Calc-io; Hyds.
Small, causing agg: Bar-c; Bro; Caus; Crot-h; Grap; Lach; Pho.
Suffocation, with: See Choking.
Touch, pressure agg: Kali-io.
Toxic: Bell; Cact; Crot-h; Lycps.
Vascular: Ap.

GONORRHOEA: *Arg-n*; Calc; CANN; Canth; Dig; Fer-p; Kali-chl; *Med*; *Merc*; Nat-s; Nit-ac; Petros; *Pul*; *Sep*; *Sul*; THU.

GONORRHOEA
Chronic+: Kali-io.
Thick, green discharge+: Kali-io.
Haematuria, with: Mez.
Ill effects: See SYCOSIS.
Suppressed: Agn; Clem; *Nat-m*; Med; PUL; *Sars*; Thu.

GOOSE SKIN: Buf; Hell; Nux-v; Par; Ver-a.
Drinking, after: Cadm.
Hands, hot with: Cadm.
Heartburn, with: Cadm.
Nose bleed, with: Cam.

GOSSIPING: Hyo.

GOUT: *Colch*; Colo; Kali-io; Led; Lyc; Nux-m; Radm; Ran-sc; Sul; *Urt*.
Acute: Colch; Sabi; Urt.
Diarrhoea, after: Ant-c; Benz-ac; Colch; Merc-d; Nat-s.
Joints, small of: Ran-sc.
Metastasis, from: Abro; Ant-c.
Rheumatic: Rhod.

GRACILE: Pho.

GRANULAR APPEARANCE: *Carb-v*; *Grap*; *Hep*; Nat-m; Pho-ac.

GRANULATION
Poor: Carb-v; Hep; Kre; Nit-ac; Sil.
Warty: Arg-n.

GRAPES like: See GROWTH.

GRASPED and RELAXED: See OPENING AND SHUTTING.

GRASPING
AGG: See Fingers, working with.
AMEL: Anac; Cimi; Lith; Spig.

GRASPING
Cold objects AGG: *Hep*; Merc; *Nat-m*; Pho; Sil; Thu; *Zin*.
Involuntarily: Sul.
Smooth objects agg: Plb.
Tightly
 • AGG: Rhus-t.
 • AMEL: Mez; Nux-v+.

GRAY, dirty (discharges, discolouration etc): Arg-m; *Ars*; Berb; Calc; Caus; *Chel*; Cup; Dig; Diph; Fer-p; KALI-C; Kali-m; Lach; *Lyc*; *Merc*; Merc-cy; Ox-ac; PHO; Pho-ac; Sil; Sul.

GREASY, oily, fatty (skin, discharges etc): *Bry*; CAUS; Flu-ac; Iod; Iris; Kali-p; MAG-C; Malan; *Merc*; *Nat-m*; Ol-an; Pho; Psor; Pul; Sele; *Thu*; Val.

GREEDY: See AVARICIOUS.
Eating in: Nat-c; Zin.

GREEN, greenish (skin discharges etc): Aco; Ap+; ARS; Carb-v; Cham; Con; Ip; Kali-bi; Kali-io; Lyc; Mag-c; Med; MERC; *Nat-s*; Par+; Pho; PUL; Rhus-t; Sec; *Sep*; Stan; *Sul*; Sul-ac; *Ver-a*.
Spots: Arn; Buf; *Con*; Lach.
Turns: Arg-n; Bor; Calc-f; Nat-s; Psor; Rhe; Sanic.
Yellow: *Merc*; Pul.

GRIEF, sorrow: Am-m; Ars; Aur; *Caus*; Cocl; Colch+; Colo+; Con; Cyc; Grap+; IGN; Lach; Lyc; Naj; Nat-m; Petr; *Pho-ac*; *Pul*; Samb+; *Stap*; Zin.
Boisterous: Nat-m.
Brooding: Ign.

GRIEF
Cannot cry: Am-m; Gel; *Nat-m*.
Financial loss, from: Arn; Aur.
Imaginary, broods over: Cyc; Ign.
Paralytic state of body and mind, from: Phys.
Prolonged: Nat-m; Pho-ac.
Silent: *Ign*; *Nat-m*; Pho-ac; Pul.
Trifles, over: Bar-c.
GRIMACES: Agar; Cup; *Hyo*; Plat; Stram.
GRINDING: See PAIN, boring.
GRIPING: See PAIN, cramping.
GRISTLY: Nit-ac; Sil.
GRIT want of+: *Sil.*
GRITTY feeling: Con.
GROANING: See MOANING.
Every little thing from: Bar-c.
GROINS: Alo; Am-m; Cocl; Gran; Guai.
Right: Calc; Cham; Kali-c; Lach; *Lyc*; Nux-v; Pul; Rhod; Rhus-t; Sul-ac; Thu.
 • Swelling painful, on extending leg: Ars-io.
Left: Euphor; Mag-c; Naj; *Zin*.
Afterpains, felt in: Caul; Cimi.
Alternating between: Colo; Phys.
Body, as of a: Carb-an; Plant.
Clothes, feel uncomfortable: Hyds.
Coition agg: Ther.
Cord like swelling, to knee: Buf.
Coughing agg: Bor.
Creeping cold, menses before: Ant-t.

GROINS
Cutting: Thu.
Dragging: Calend.
Eruption, moist, menses before: Sars.
External ring: Ars; Merc.
Internal ring: Am-m; Aur; Lyc; *Nux-v*; Sul-ac.
 • Coughing agg: Nat-m.
Glands: Calc; *Hep*; *Merc*; Nit-ac; Oci-c; *Thu*.
 • Indurated and visible+: Tub.
 • Swollen: Calc; Clem; *Hep*; Lach; *Merc*; Nit-ac; *Sul*.
  - colds agg: Merc.
  - pain
     in legs, with: Calc-ar.
     jerking, with: Clem.
Hollow: Con; Nux-v; Pall.
Jerking, penis, to: Zin.
Knees, to: Pod.
Lumps, hard, painful: Pul.
Operations, after: Naj.
Pressing in, both, to sexual organs+: Alu.
Rash, menses, before: *Ap*; Ars.
Sore, menses, before: Ant-t; Bry.
Sprained, as if: Hyds.
Stitches, menses, during: Bor.
Swelling
 • As if: Am-m.
 • Fall, after: Aur.
 • Painful, extending to legs+: Ars-io.
Tense, sprained: Am-m; Nat-m.
GROPING in dark, as if: Croc; Hyo; Op; Plb.

GROUND gives way: Arg-n; Con; Kali-br; Sul; Visc.

Or stairs came up to meet him: Bell; Calc; Cann; Pic-ac; Sil.

GROWING PAINS: Calc; Calc-p; Guai; Mang; Pho-ac.

GROWLING: See HOWLING.

GROWTH

Affected, disorders of: Bar-c; Calc; Calc-p; Pho; Pho-ac; Sil; *Thyr*.

Rapid: Guai; Pho.

GROWTHS NEW, tumours, etc. (See CANCER and CYSTS): *Ant-c*; Ars; Bell; Bels; Calc; Carb-an; Carb-v; Caus; Clem; Con; Grap; *Lyc*; Med; *Nit-ac*; Ran-b; Sil; *Stap*; Sul; Thu.

Angioma: Abro; Lyc; Sul.

Burns after: Calc.

Dispersing, for: Croc.

Encephaloma+: Croc.

Erectile: *Lyc*; Nit.ac; Pho.
 • Menses, before agg: Lyc.

Fleshy: Merc; Nit-ac; *Stap*; Thu.

Fungus: See FUNGUS GROWTH.

Grapes like: Alo; Calc; Dios.

Horny: Ant-c; Ran-b; Sil; *Sul*.

Lipoma (See CYSTS): Aur; Croc; Lap-alb; Pho; Phyt.

Lymphangioma: Vip.

Lymphoid: Radm; Sec.

Neuroma: Calend: Cep.

Pain severe: Stram.

Rapid: Iod; Pho.

Sensitive, convulsions from least touch: Stap.

GRUMBLING: Alu; Aur; Sang; Thyr; Val.

His value is not understood by others: Calc-s.

GUILT, sense of: Alu; Arn; *Ars*; *Aur*; Chel; *Cocl*; Con; Croc; Cyc; Dig; Hyo; Kali-br; Kalm; Kob; *Med*; Psor; VER-A.

Trifles, about: Sil.

GULLET: See OESOPHAGUS.

GUMMATA: Carb-an.

GUMMY: See DISCHARGES, Gluey.

GUMS: Bor; Carb-v; Kali-c; Kre; Merc; Nux-v; Stap.

Lower: Sars.

Upper: Calc; Rut.

Inner: Pho; *Stap*.

Alternating sides: Aeth.

Abscess: Bell; Calc-f; Echi; Hep; Merc; *Sil*.
 • Recurrent: Caus.

Black wedges on: Bism.

Bleeding: Amb+; Am-c; Bar-c; Bov; Cist; Kre; *Merc*; Nat-m; Nit-ac; Pho-ac; Psor; Stap.
 • Easily: Ant-c+; Caus+; Lach+; Sul-ac.
 • Pressing with finger large quantity oozes: Bap; Grap.
 • Sour: Grap.
 • Sucking them: Bov; Carb-v.
 • Touch, on: Lyc; Merc; Pho.

Blue: *Kre*.
 • Line along margin: Plb.

Boring: Calc; Merc.

Burn like fire: Nat-s.

Clenches: Lyc; *Phyt*; Pod.

GUMS

Edge, at: Am-c; Calc; Flu-ac; Mez; Syph; Thu.
Epulis: Nat-m; Thu.
Excoriated: Carb-v; Sep.
Excrescences: Nat-m; Stap.
- Hard: Plb.

Grasps, at: Sil.
Incisors, behind: Merc-cy; *Pho.*
Itching: Kali-c.
Nodes
- Painful: Pho-ac.
- White, small, on: Berb.

Painful: Ars; Kre; Merc; Stap.
Ragged: Merc.
Receding, detached, scorbutic: Ars; *Carb-v*; Caus+; Kali-chl; *Kali-p*; Kre; *Merc*; Mur-ac; Psor.
Sore, sensitive: Am-c; Ars; *Carb-v*; *Merc*.
- Chewing, while: *Carb-v*; Nit-ac.
- Cold and warmth agg: Nat-m.
- Eating, while: Clem; Pho.

Spongy: Kali-p; Kre; Lach; Merc; Merc-c; Mez; Psor; Sep; Thu.
Sucking agg: Bov; Nit-ac; Nux-m; Sil.
Suppuration, pyorrhoea: Calc; Carb-v; Cist; Hep; Kali-c; *Merc*; Merc-i-f; *Pho*; PUL; *Sil*; Stap.
Swelled: Merc; Nux-v; Sep; Stap; Sul.
- White: Nux-v.

Tubercles, on: Plb.
Vesicles: Sil.

GURGLING:
Agar; ALO; Berb; Cic; Cina; *Crot-t*; Cup; *Gamb*; Hyd-ac; Jat; Kali-c; Kre; *Laur*; Lil-t; *Lyc*; *Pod*; *Pul*; Scil; Sul; Thu.

GUSHING:
Ars; Bell; Berb; Bry; CROT-T; Elat; *Gamb*; Grat; Ip; *Jat*; Kali-bi; Mag-m; *Nat-c*; Nat-m; *Nat-s*; Pho; *Pod*; Sabi; Stan; *Thu*; Tril; *Ver-a*.

HABITS
Dirty: See DIRTY.
Intemperate agg: Arg-n.

HACKING, like a hatchet:
Am-c; Ars; Aur; Clem; Kali-n; Lyc; Pho-ac; Rut; Stap; Thu.

HAEMATEMESIS:
See VOMITING, blood and HAEMORRHAGE.

HAEMATOCELE:
Arn; Con; *Ham*; Rut.

HAEMATODES:
See FUNGUS GROWTH.

HAEMATOMA:
Calc-f; Merc; Sil.
Ear, on: Bell.

HAEMATURIA:
See URINE, bloody and HAEMORRHAGE.
Gonorrhoea with: Mez.
Menses, suppressed, from: Nux-v.

HAEMOPHILIA:
Arn; Ars; Carb-an.; Crot-h; Ham; Kre; Lach; Nat-s; *Pho*; Sil; Visc.
Suppuration, with: Hyds.

HAEMOPTYSIS (See HAEMORRHAGE):
Aco; Am-c; Ars; Bell; Bry; Chin; Fer; Hyo; Ip; Mill; Nit-ac; Pho; Plb; Pul; Rhus-t; Sabi; Sec; Sul; Sul-ac; Terb+.

Blood, black, watery: Elap.
Chest, heat in, with: Psor.
Convulsions
- With: Hyo.

HAEMOPTYSIS, convulsions
- After: Dros.

Drunkards: Ars; *Nux-v*.
Dyspnoea, with: Arn.
Exertion, violent, after: Urt.
Intermittent: Kre.
Masturbation, from: Fer.
Menses
- Before: Dig.
- Suppressed, with: Ars; Senec.

Palpitation, with: Mill.
Periodical+: Kre.
Repeated+: *Pho*.
Rheumatism, alternating with: Led.
Valvular heart disease, in: Cact+; Cratae; Lycps.

HAEMORRHAGE (bloody discharges): Acet-ac+; *Aco*; ARN; Ars; BELL; Bur-p; *Cact*; CALC; Canth; *Carb-v*; CHIN; Croc; *Crot-h*; FER; Ham; Hyds; Ip; *Kre*; Lach; Led; Lept; Lyc; Lycps; Mang; MERC; Merc-c; *Mill*; NIT-AC; *Nux-v*; PHO; PUL; Rhus-t; Sabi; *Sec*; *Sep*; Solid; Sul; *Sul-ac*; Terb; Tril; Urt; Ust; Vib; Vip.

Acrid: Kali-c; Sil.
Acute: *Aco*; *Bell*; Croc; Fer; Hyo; Mill; Pul.
Agg and amel from: See BLEEDING.
Altered blood of: Crot-h; Pul; Sec.
Bright: *Aco*; Arn; *Bell*; Carb-v; *Dul*; *Erig*; Fer; *Hyo*; *Ip*; Led; Meli; Mill; Nit-ac; Pho; Plb; *Sabi*; Sul; Tril.

HAEMORRHAGE, bright
- Clots, dark with: Fer; Sabi; Sang; Ust.
  - gelatinous, with: Laur.
- Frothy: Led.

Clotted (See DISCHARGES, lumpy): Arn; Bell; Bur-p; Canth; Chin; Fer; Hyo; Ip; Nux-v; Pul; Sabi; Sul.
- Rapidly: Ip.

Clots, mixed with: Sabi; Ust.
Dark: Aco; Bur-p; Canth; Carb-v; Cham; Chin; Croc; Crot-h; Elap; Ham; Helo; Kre; Lach; Nux-m; Nux-v; Pul; Sec; Sep; Sul-ac; Ust.
- Thin: Am-c; Sul-ac; Ust.

Easy: Kali-chl.
Effects, chronic: Stic; Stro.
Face flushed, with: Amy-n.
Frothy: Led.
Gushing: Aco; *Bell*; Cham; Erig; Ham; Ip; Lac-c; Pul; Sabi; Sec; Tril.
- Intermittently: Psor; Sul.

Heart symptoms, with: Cratae; Lycps.
Hot: *Bell*; Sabi.
Leech bite, form+: Alum.
Lifting agg: Petr.
Mind tranquil, with+: Ham.
Offensive: Bell; Bry; Carb-v; Helo; Sabi.
Orifices of the body, from: Bothr; Crot-h; Ip; Pho.
Passive, oozing: Bov; Buf; Carb-v; *Chin*; Crot-h; Fer-p; Ham; Kre; Pho-ac; Sec; Terb; *Ust*.

HAEMORRHAGE, passive
- Mucous, mixed with: Caps.
- Wounds, closed, edges from: Mill.

Post-partum+: Mill.
Riding in carriage agg: Petr.
Scratching agg: Psor.
Slight, causing great agg: See under BLEEDING.
Sticky, stringy: Croc; Merc; Naj; Ust.
Thick: Agar; Bov; Croc; Cup; *Nux-m*; Plat.
Thin, watery: Carb-v; Crot-h; Grap; Laur; Nit-ac; Rhus-t; Sabi; Sec; Sul-ac.
- Clot
  - mixed, with: Arn; Bell; Caus; Pul; Sabi.
  - won't: Lach; Pho.

Violent: Mur-ac.
Weakness, undue: Alu; Bry; Carb-an; Ham; Hyds.

HAEMORRHOIDS: See PILES.

HAIR (Condition)
Affections of: Bell; Bor; Calc; Carb-an; Carb-v; Con; *Grap*; *Hep*; *Kali-c*; *Lyc*; Merc; *Nat-m*; *Nit-ac*; *Sul*; Ust.
Blond: Bro; *Calc*; Caps; Cocl; Hyo; *Pul*; Sele; Seneg; Sil.
Body, all over: Med; Thu; Thyr.
Bristling, erect: Aco; *Bar-c*; Cham; Canth; Chel; Glo; *Laur*; Meny; Mur-ac; Sul-io; *Ver-a*; Zin.
Brittle+: Grap; Zin.
Chin and upper lip, on (women): Ol-j.

HAIR
Cold: Sul.
Dark: Aco; Cina; Iod; Nit-ac; *Nux-v*; Pho; Pho-ac; Plat; Sep.
Dry: Alu; Kali-c; Psor; Sul; *Thu*.
- Oily, becomes: Lyss.

Falling: Alu; *Ars*; Ars-s-fl; Aur; *Calc*; Carb-v; Flu-ac; GRAP; Hell; *Hep*; *Kali-c*; Kali-s; Lach; *Lyc*; Nat-m; Nit-ac; PHO; Sep; Sil; Stap; SUL; Thal; Thu; Thyr; *Ust*.
- Beard, of: Grap; Kali-c; Plb; Sele.
- Bregma, from: Ars; Nat-m; Pho.
- Children, in: Nat-m.
- Climaxis, at: Sep.
- Colour changes, after: Kali-io.
- Combing, when: Canth.
- Fevers, after: Flu-ac.
- Genitals, from: Sele.
- Gray hair, replaced by: Vinc.
- Grief, from: Pho-ac.
- Handfuls, bunches, in: Carb-v; Mez; *Pho*; Syph; Thal.
- Headache, after: Ant-c; Hep; Nit-ac; Sep; Sil.
- Illness, severe after: Carb-v; Manc; Thal.
- Injury from: Hypr.
- Itching of head, with+: Ant-c.
- Lactation, during: Nat-m.
- Nails, with: Hell; *Ust*.
- Occiput, from: Carb-v; Chel; Merc; Petr; Stap.
- Parturition, after: Carb-v; Lyc; Sul.
- Pregnancy, during: Lach.
- Pubis, from: Nat-m; Nit-ac; Zin.

HAIR, falling
- Rapidly: Thal.
- Sides, from: Grap; Pho; Stap.
- Spots, in: Alu; Flu-ac; Grap; Hep; Lyc; *Nat-m*; Pho.
- Sweat, offensive from: SUL.
- Temples, from: See HEAD, bald.

Gray, early: *Ars*; *Lyc*; *Nat-m*; *Pho-ac*; Sil.

Letting down, AMEL: Bell; Cina; Fer; Kali-m; Kali-n+; Kali-p; Pho.

Margins, edge at: Hyds; Kali-p; Med; Nat-m; Old; Petr; Sep; *Sul*; Tell.
- Brown, stripe: Kali-p.
- Moisture: Diph.
- Yellow: Med.

Matted: Ant-c; Grap; Lyc; Ust; Vinc; Vio-t.
- Secretion, sticky, from: Ust.

Offensive, foul: Vinc.

Oily, greasy: Bry; Merc; Pho-ac.

Painful, touch to, etc: Ap; *Ars*; Bry; *Chin*; Hep; *Nux-v*; Sele; *Ver-a*; Zin.
- Root, at: Colo.
- Vertex, on: Zin.

Pulled, as if: ACO; Aeth; *Arg-n*; Kali-n; Lach; Mag-c; Mag-m; *Pho*; Sele.

Pulls her: See DESIRE, to pull her hair.

Sensation, of: Arg-n; Ars; Kali-bi; Pul; Sil; Sul.

Soppy, wet: *Rhe*.

Split: Thu; ZIN.

Standing, as if: Mur-ac; Rhod; Spo; Sul-io.

HAIR
Stiff: Sele.

Tangled, tousy: Bor; Flu-ac; *Lyc*; Med; Mez; Nat-m; *Pho-ac*; Psor; Sul.

Thick: Ant-c; Grap; Lyc; Ust; Vio-t.

HAIR (Modality)
Combing or brushing
- AGG: Bry; *Chin*; Carb-ac; Form; Glo; Ign; Mez; Sele; Sil.
- AMEL: Form; Tarn.
- Back agg: Pul; Rhus-t.
- Electric crackling, when: Sanic.

Cut AGG: *Bell*; Glo; Led; Pho; Sep.

Touching AGG: Ap; *Ars*; Bell; *Chin*; Fer; Lach; Nux-v; Pul; SELE; Sep; Ver-a; Zin.

HALLUCINATIONS: See PERCEPTIONS CHANGED and IMAGINATIONS.

HAMMERING: See PAIN, hammering and HEAD.

HAMSTRINGS, short, tense: Am-m+; Bry; Dios; Guai+; Nat-m.

Left: Sul.

HAND
Laying on part amel: Carb-an; Croc; *Cup*; Meny; Pho.

Moving, body on, as if: Carb-v.

HANDS: *Calc*; Caul; Lyc; Nux-v; Pho; *Sul*.

Back of: Kre; Nat-c; Rhus-t; Sep.
- Brown: Iod.
- Cramp: Mag-c; Ver-a.

HANDS, back
- Eruptions: Kre; Mez; Mur-ac; Nat-c; Petr; Pul.
- Spiders, were crawling: Visc.
- Sweat, cold: Bothr; *Chio*; Zin-s.
- Swollen, as if: Iod.
- Warts: Nit-ac.
- Wrinkled: Pho-ac.

Behind him AGG: Ign; Sanic.

Bites, sleep, during: Elap.

Burning heat: Agar; Asar; Carb-v; *Lach*; Med; Mur-ac; *Petr*; Pho; Sang; Sep; Spig; *Stan*; *Sul.*
- Body, spreads to, from: Chel.
- Chill, with: Kali-c.
- Cold
  - agg: Caps.
  - feet, with: Sep.
  - weather in: Rhod.
- Fanning, desires: *Med.*
- Feet, and: Flu-ac.
- One: Mez.
- Then; cold: Cocl.

Callosities: Grap; Sul.
- Cracked: Cist.

Clammy: Sanic; Tarn; Sul.
- Feet, and : Sanic.

Clasps: Bell; Stram.
- Head over: Sec.

Cobweb sensation: Bor.

Cold (See COLDNESS of single parts): Bro.
- One: Chin; Dig; Ip; Lyc; *Pul*; Rhus-t; Sul.
  - other warm: Chin; Ip.
- Right: Gel.
  - then, left: Med.
- Left: Thyr.
- Coughing, when: Rum.

HANDS, cold
- Dead, as if+: Ox-ac.
- Diarrhoea, during: *Pho.*
- Face, dark red, with: Mur-ac.
- Feet, and: Kali-m; Sanic.
- Headache, during: Amb; Vario.
- Hot
  - feet, with: Calc; Sep.
  - weather, in: Asar.
- Icy: Cact+; Hyd-ac; Nux-m; Thyr; Ver-a.
  - emission, after: Merc.
  - fever, in: Thu.
  - headache, with: Vario.
- Room, warm, in: Sep.
- Smoker's: Sec.
- Sweat, during: Thu.
- Uncovering on: Mag-c.
- Water, in
  - AGG: Con; Lac-d; Mag-c; Mag-p; Pho; Tarn.
  - AMEL: Flu-ac; Gel; Jat.

Contraction, involuntary, as if grasping: Sul.

Cover, cannot: Mag-c.

Cracks (See also FINGERS): Alu; *Calc*; *Grap*; Hep; Nit-ac; *Petr*; Rhus-t; Sanic; *Sars*; Sep; Sil; Sul; Zin.

Cramps: Anthx; *Bell*; *Calc*; Lyc; Pyro; Sec; Val.
- Broom, cannot let go: Dros; Stan.
- Closing, on: Chin.
- Feet, and: Lyc; Lyss.
- Grasping
  - agg: Amb.
  - cold things agg: Nat-m.
- Sleep prevents+: Val.
- Writing, while: Nat-p.

HANDS

Crawling: Hypr.
Dry: Anac; Bar-c; *Lyc*; *Sul*.
Eczema: Berb; Cor-r; Grap; Nat-c; Sep; Zin.
- Dorsum+: Mur-ac.
- Trade: Bor.

Emaciation+: Sele.
Formication+: Hypr.
Heavy: Bell; Pho.
Hot: See Burning.
- Constant: Lyc.

Itching: Agar; Anac; Sul.
Jerking: Nat-c.
Lame: *Caus*; Cup; Kali-bi; Mez; Sil; Zin.
- Exertion or writing while: Mez; Sil.

Large too, as if: Cact+; Hyo.
Laying, affected part on: See HAND laying on.
Motion, automatic, towards mouth: Nux-v.
Numb: Ap; Calad; Carb-an; Cocl; Form; Kali-n; Lyc; Stro.
- Alternating: Echi.
- Chest affections, with: Carb-an.
- Cold, and: Lach; Ox-ac.
- Electric shock, as from, as if: Flu-ac.
- Grasping anything: Calc; Cham; Cocl.
- Heat, insensitive to: Plb.
- Left, formication, extending with up: Grap.
- Putting in pocket: Nat-m.
- Sewing when: Crot-h.
- Ulnar nerve, along: Cup-ac.

Offensive: Phys.
Open and shut: Stram.
Paralysis: Plb.
Pins and needles: Colch.
Pricking: Kali-p.
Puffy
- A.M. in: Just.
- Feet and: Naj.

Purple: Sep.
Restless, busy: Kali-br; Sul; Tarn; Ther; Thyr; Ver-v.
- Delirium, during: Ver-v.
- Feet, and: Stic.

Rubs: Bap.
Soft+: Cact.
Stiff, when
- Knitting: Kali-m.
- Writing: Kali-m.

Sweat, on: Agn; Ars; CALC; Naj; Nit-ac; Pho; Sep; Sil; *Sul*; Thu; Thyr; *Tub*.
- Cold: Canth; Nit-ac; Sep.
  - feet on, with: Cimi; Ip; Kali-bi; Tarn.
  - heat, during: Am-c; Fer-p; Nit-ac.
  - stools, during: Chio.
  - vomiting, with: Chio.
- Cough, with: Naj.
- Feet, and: Flu-ac; Naj; Nit-ac.
- Injuries to spine, from: Nit-ac.
- Opthalmia, during: Flu-ac; Sul.
- Palms, put together, when: Sanic.
- Profuse: Stic; Sul.

Swelled, as if: Coll; Kali-n; Stro; Terb.
- Ankles, and: Stan.
- Feet, and: Fer; Just.

HANDS, swelled
- Hanging down arms, when: Am-c.
- Left, heart disease, in: Cact.
- Opening and closing on: Mang.

Tremble: Glo; Lach; Lol-t; Mag-p; Ox-ac; Tarn; Zin.
- Carrying something to mouth: Merc; Plb; Sil.
- Concomitant, as a: Calc-p.
- Grasping, objects: Led; Merc; Plb.
- Menses, during: Hyo; Zin+.
- Moving, when: Led.
- Palpitation, with: Bov.
- Vomiting, with: Calc-p.
- Waking: Nat-s.
- Writing when
  - agg: Cimi; Merc; Nat-m; Nat-s; Plb; Sul; Zin+.
  - fast amel: Fer.
  - presence of others agg: Ign.

Ulnar nerve, along: Cup-ac.
Using: See FINGERS, working.
Veins, swelled: Am-c; Arn; Chin; Ham; Laur; Nux-v; Op; *Pho*; PUL; Thyr; Vip.
- Chill during: Chel.

Vesicles: Kre; Ver-v.
Wants
- Covered: Ign.
- Fanning: Med.

Warts, on: Dul; Nat-m+.
- Horny+: Ant-c.

Wash, tendency to: Coca; Lac-c; Psor; Syph.
- Dry, when: Pho.

Water, in AGG (See cold of single parts): Ign; Nat-m; *Pho.*

HANDS, water in
- Cold: See under COLD.

Weak: Bov; Caus; Kali-bi; Mez; Ox-ac; *Zin*.
- Drops things: Bov; Stan.
- Menses, during: Alum.
- Writing, while: Mez; Sil.
- Wens+: Pho-ac.

Withered, skin: Lyc.
Wooden sensation: Kali-n.
Wrings: Ars; Kali-br; Stram; Sul; Ther.
- Walks the floor, and: Buf.

Yellow, colic with: Sil.

HANGING

Affected parts agg and amel: See Hanging limbs agg and amel.

Down, loose, suspended as if: Alu; Aur; Bar-c; *Ign*; *Ip*; Kali-c; LACH; Lil-t; Med; Merc; PHO; Saba; Sep; Sul; Val.

Limbs
- AGG: Alu; Am-c; Bar-c; BELL; Calc; CARB-V; Con; Pul; Ran-sc; Sabi; Thu; Vip.
- AMEL: Aco; *Arn*; Asar; Berb; CON; *Lyc*; Mag-c; Mag-m; Mang; Mar-v; Merc; Pho; Rat; Rhus-t.

HAPPY, seeing others, agg: Hell; Helo.

HARD

Bed sensation: See BED.
Pain: See PAIN, aching.
Parts, feel soft: Merc; Nit-ac; Nux-m.

HARDNESS, induration: Alu; Ant-c; *Ars*; Bad; Bar-c; Bell; Bro; *Bry*; Calc; CALC-F;

HARDNESS ..
CARB-AN; Carb-v; Chin; Cist; *Clem*; CON; Flu-ac; Grap; Iod; KALI-M; Lach; *Lyc*; Mag-m; Merc; Merc-i-r; *Pho*; *Phyt*; Plb; *Rhus-t*; Sele; *Sep*; *Sil*; Spo; Stap; *Sul*; Tarn-c.

Injury after: Calc-f.

Pressure constant, from: Sep.

Stony: Calc-f; Carb-v; Kali-bi; Kali-m; Merc-i-r; Sul; Tarn-c.

HARSH: Kali-io.
HASTE: See HURRY.
HATEFUL: Led; Lyc; Nat-m; Nit-ac; Tarn.
HATRED: See MALICE.
Male, female, each other for: Sep.

Others, by as if: Lach.

HAUGHTY: See INSOLENT.
HAUTEUR: See PRIDE.
HAWKING (mucus): Arg-n; Caus; Con; Cor-r; Hep; KALI-BI; *Kali-c*; LACH; LYC; Mang+; Merc; *Nat-c*; *Nat-m*; Nux-v; PHO; Pul; Rhus-t; Rum; Sele; *Sep*.

AGG: Am-m; Arg-n; Coc-c; Nux-v; Sil.

AMEL: Kob; Lach.

Bitter: Arn; Ars; Cist; Menis; Nat-m.

Blood, bright red: Saba.

Brown, gluey: Ol-an.
- Effort, with: Bry.

Clear, morning, in: Sele.

Cold: Sinap.

Constantly: Mang; Spo.

Coppery: Cimi.

HAWKING
Drawn from posterior nares: Cinb; Cor-r; *Hep*; Hyds; Kali-bi; Mag-c; Nat-c; Nat-m; Nit-ac; Nux-v; Sele; Sep; Spig; Sul; Tell.
- Brown: Bry.
- Vomits, from: Sep.

Eating agg: Sil; Tub.

Glairy: Pall.

Green: Colch; Par; Syph.
- Comes involuntarily in mouth: Colch.

Lumps
- Cheesy, of: *Agar*; *Hep*; *Kali-bi*; KALI-M; Kali-p; *Mag-c*; Merc; Merc-i-f; PSOR; Sanic; Sep; *Sil*.
- Foul: Kali-m; Lach; Med; Petr; Sil.
- Solid: Calc; Lith; Mar-v; Merc; Merc-i-f; Sep.

Nausea
- From: Stan.
- With: Lil-t.

Salty: Calc; Nat-m; Tell.

Singing, before: Calc-p.

Sleep, during: Calc-p.

Sour: Tarx.

Sticky: Arg-n; Cinb; Coc-c; Hyds; KALI-BI; *Lach*; Mag-m; Phyt; Rum.

Sweetish: Aesc+; Mag-p.

Talking, while: Arg-m; Calc-p.

Tough: Aesc; Kali-c; Ol-an; Par; Rum.

Vomiting, with: Calc-p.

HAY
Asthma: See ASTHMA.

Fever: See CORYZA, annual.

HEAD

Affections in general: BELL; *Bry*; Calc; *Carb-v*; Chin; Gel; *Glo*; *Lach*; *Lyc*; *Nat-m*; *Nux-v*; Par; *Pho*; *Pul*; Sang; Sep; *Sil*; Spig; Sul; Tub.

One sided: Alu; Anac; Arg-n; *Ars*; Asaf; Calc; *Chin*; *Chin-s*; Cof; *Colo*; Con; IRIS; Kali-c; Kali-io; Nux-v; *Pho-ac*; Plat; PSOR; *Pul*; Saba; SANG; Sars; *Sep*; Spig; Sul-ac; Verb; Zin.
- Begins on one, goes to and agg. on other: Arg-n; Fer; Iris; Lac-c; LYC; Mang; Nat-m; Tub.
- Right: *Bell*; Cact; *Calc*; Carb-v; Chel; IGN; *Iris*; Kalm; Lyc; Nat-c; Plat; Plb; Pru-sp; Pul; Rhus-t; *Saba*; SANG; Sars; *Sil.*
  - cut off, as if: Lach.
- Left: Arn; Ars; Asaf; Bro; Chin-s; *Colo*; Ip; Kali-c; *Lach*; Lil-t; *Merc*; Mur-ac; Naj; Nit-ac; Nux-m; *Nux-v*; Onos; *Rhod*; Sele; *Sep*; SPIG; Sul.
  - growth retarded: Flu-ac.

Absent, as if: Asar; Calc-io; Nit-ac.

Aching: See Pain.

Active, when amel: Merc-i-f.

Alternating with
- Others: Alo; Alu; Ars; Cina; Gel; Glo; Ign; Psor; Strop.
- Back: Ign; Meli.
- Lumbago: Alo.
- Pelvis: Gel.
- Stomach: Ars; Bism; Ox-ac; Plb; Ver-a.

HEAD

Air
- Blowing on, as if: Petr.
- Cold amel: Seneg.
- Streaming through eyes: Thu.
- Wind, through: Aur; Cor-r; Ver-a.

Anger agg: Mez.

Arms over: Ars; Lac-c; *Pul.*

Ascending
- Agg: Bell; Bry; Calc; Sil; Spig.
- Into: Aco; BELL: Bry; *Calc*; Canth; Chel; Chin; Cimi; Gamb; Gel; Glo; Kalm; Mang; *Meny*; Merc; Nat-m; Pho; SANG; Sep; SIL; SPIG.
  - Right: Alo; *Bell*; Gel; Ign; Meny; Nat-m; Nux-v; Pho; SANG.
  - Left: Arg-n; Chel; Cimi; Colch; Lac-c; Lil-t; Par; Petr; Sabi; Sil; SPIG.
- Stairs agg: Ant-c.

Backward, extending: Arn; BELL; BISM; BRY; *Cimi*; *Glo*; Kali-bi; Lac-d; Lach; Lyc; Med; Mur-ac; Nat-m; *Nit-ac*; Par; Pru-sp; Rut; Sep; Syph; *Thu*; Tub; Ver-v; Verb; Zin.
- Pulled, as if: Syph.

Bald: Alum; Aur; Bar-c; Flu-ac; Grap; Lyc; Syph; Zin.
- Gonorrhoea, from+: Kali-s.
- Premature: Bar-c+; Sil.
- Soreness of scalp, with: Zin.
- Spots covered with
  - lock of white hair: Psor.
  - wooly hair: Vinc.

HEAD

Ball, lump, knot: Con.
- Striking in, while talking: Sars.
- Throat, rising from, to: Plb.

Band, constriction: Anac; Ant-t; Carb-ac; Carb-v; Caus; Coca; Cocl; Gel; Glo; Grap; *Merc*; Nit-ac; Ox-ac; Sars; Sul.
- Green tea and smoking amel+: Carb-ac.
- Hot: Aco; Chlo-hyd.
- Tight
  - around+: Xanth.
  - painful, removes the hat involuntarily, without amel: Sars.

Bandaging, binding amel: Ap; *Arg-n*; Glo; Lac-d; Mag-m; Pic-ac; *Pul*; Pyro; *Sil*.

Base, of: Cimi; Gel; Syph; Ver-v.

Bathing, washing
- Agg: Canth.
- Feet amel: Ascl.

Beats, the: Aco; Ap; Hyo; Mill; Syph; Tub.

Bed, early, in agg: Hell; Rhod.

Belongs to another, as if: Ther.

Bend, backwards
- Amel: Seneg; Thu.
- Must: Ant-t; Arn; *Cham*; Kali-n; Nat-c; Stram.
- Sneezing, when: Lyss.

Big with
- Big belly: Calc.
- Body wasted: Sil.
- Jaws small: Kali-io.

Blow, shock, thrusts etc. as of: *Ap*; Cann; Croc; *Glo*; Ign;

HEAD, blow ..
Naj; *Nat-m*; Nux-v; *Spig*; Sul-ac; Tarn.
- Biting, chewing, while: Am-c.
- Talking, when: Sars.

Blowing nose
- Agg: Amb.
- Amel: Chel.

Boiling water, side lain on as if: Mag-m.

Bores into pillow: See Drawn backwards.

Breathing deep agg: Anac; Cact; Rat.

Burning, heat: *Aco*; Ap; *Bell*; Bor; Bry; Cact; Calc; *Frax*; *Grap*; Lach; Merc; *Merc-i-r*; Nat-c; Oenan; Pho; *Pic-ac*; SUL.
- Mental exertion
  - amel: Cham.
  - from: Calc.
- Spot, in: Con.

Cap, hat
- Aversion to: Iod; Led; Lyc.
- On, as if: Berb; Eup-p; Phys; Pyro.

Carriage, riding in amel: Kali-n.

Catarrhal: Kali-bi; *Merc*; NUX-V.

Children, thin agg: Lyc.

Chronic: Arg-n; Ars; Calc; Nat-c; Nat-m; Psor; Sep; *Sil*; Zin.

Clothes, warm agg+: Aru-t.

Coffee, hot agg+: Aru-t.

Coition agg: Bov; Pho-ac; Sil.

Cold
- Application amel: Alo; *Ars*; Bry; Cyc; *Glo*; Pho; Sul.

HEAD

HEAD, cold
- Water
  - agg: Ant-c.
  - poured over, as if: Cup; Tarn.
- **Coldness:** Agar; *Bell*; *Calc*; Calc-p; Cann; Chel; Cup; Dul; Hypr; *Laur*; Lyc; Merc-c; Nat-m; Pho; Rhus-t; Sep; Sil; Stan; Stro; Tarn; VER-A; *Ver-v*.
  - Hand touch cold, as if: Hypr.
  - Hands and feet+: Vario.
  - Heated, from being: *Carb-v*.
  - Upper part: Val.
  - Warm room, in: Laur.
- **Commotion, painless in:** Caus.
- **Compression, cap, squeezing:** Agn; Arg-n; *Berb*; Bry; Cact; Glo; Ign; Lach; *Meny*; Merc; Onos; Pho-ac; Plat; *Pul*; *Stap*.
  - Vise like: Arg-n+; Nit-ac; Pul.
- **Congestion:** *Aco*; Amy-n; Ap; Ars; BELL; *Bry*; Calc; FER; *Gel*; GLO; Hyo; *Lach*; Meli; NUX-V; *Op*; Pho; *Pul*; *Psor*; Rhus-t; *Sang*; STRAM; Sul; VER-A.
  - Palpitation, with: Scop.
- **Constipation agg:** *Bry*; Colch; Nux-v; Op.
- **Conversation amel:** Dul; Eup-p; Lac-d+.
- **Cough**
  - Agg: Bell; BRY; *Caps*; Carb-v; Con; Fer; Iris; Kali-c; Lac-d; NAT-M; Nux-v; Pho; Psor; Scil; *Sul*; Vio-o.
  - Amel: Chel.
- **Cover, must:** Bro; *Rum*.
- **Crash, explosion, in:** Alo; Dig; Glo; Pho; Zin.
  - Sleep, falling to, on: Dig; Zin.

HEAD
- **Crawling, formication:** Aco; Arg-m; *Arg-n*; Colch; Cup; Hyo; Pho; *Plat*; *Pul*; *Rhus-t*; Sul.
- **Crowded room in, company etc. agg:** Lyc; Mag-c; *Plat*; *Plb*; Stap.
- **Crushed down, as if:** Dios.
- **Crushing in:** Bry; Nat-s+; Nit-ac; Syph.
- **Cut off, as if:** Lach.
- **Damp day agg:** Glo.
- **Dancing from, agg:** *Arg-n*.
- **Dark room**
  - Amel+: Nat-s.
  - Working in agg: Cedr.
- **Deep, in:** Aco; Arg-n; Bov; Calc; Dul; Lach; Nux-v; Pho; Sul; Tub.
- **Delicate literary persons+:** Arg-n.
- **Descending agg:** *Bell*; Fer; Rhus-t.
- **Diarrhoea**
  - Alternating with: Alo; Pod.
  - Amel: Pod.
  - With: Iris.
- **Diuresis, polyuria, with:** Aco; *Gel*; Glo; *Lac-d*; Ol-an; Phys; Sele; Sil; Vib.
- **Downward to nose, face, neck etc:** *Agar*; Ant-t; Bism; Calc; Calc-p; Cham; *Chin*; Dul; Guai; Hypr; Ign; Ip; *Lach*; *Led*; Mang+; *Med*; Meny; *Mez*; NUX-V; *Pho*; Pic-ac; Plat; *Pul*; Rhus-t; Sep; *Stap*; Stro; VERB; *Zin*.
- **Draft agg:** Bor; Chin; Hep; *Mag-m*; *Naj*; Nux-v; *Psor*; SIL.

HEAD

Drawn
- A point to, as if: Grap; Hypr; Lachn; Stro; Ther.
- Backward, bores into pillow, etc: Ap; Aru-t+; Bell; Cic; *Cimi*; Cup+; Hell; Med; Op; Pod; Syph; Tub; Ver-v; *Zin*.
- Shoulder, to: Agar.
- Side to, from enlarged glands: Cist.

Drinking
- Hot tea amel: Fer-p; Glo.
- Iced drinks
  - agg: Con; Dig.
  - amel: Alum.

Ear to ear+: Pall; Plant.

Ear, with: Fer-p; Merc; Pul; Sang.
- Jarring agg: Med.

Eating
- Amel: Cist; Elap; Lith; Lyc; Mag-c; Pho; Phyt; Psor; Rhod; Sang; Sil; Thu.
- Frequently amel: Sul.

Electric shocks
- Spasms before: Cep+; Hell; Mag-p.
- To all parts of body: Mag-p.

Emission agg: Ham.

Empty, hollow: Arg-m; *Cocl*; Cor-r+: Manc; Naj; Pho; Pul.
- Menses, during: Fer-p.
- Vertigo, with: Manc.
- Walking agg: Manc.

Enlarged, as if: Agar; *Arg-n*; Arn; Bapt+; *Bell*; Bov; Cor-r+; Gel; *Glo*; Hypr+; Lith; Mang+; Nat-c; Nux-m; *Nux-v*; Ran-b.
- Pain during: Cup.

HEAD, enlarged
- Pregnancy, during: *Arg-n*.
- Stools agg: Kob.

Epilepsy, after: Caus; Cup; Kali-br.
- Before, and: Cina.

Expanding and contracting: Calc; Glo; Lac-c.

Explosions: See Crash.

Eyes
- Extending into: Carb-v; *Chin*; Cimi; Ign; LACH; Lith; Mang; Nat-c; NIT-AC; PHO; Pho-ac; Pul; *Sil*; SPIG; *Sul*; Val; *Zin*.
- Closing
  - agg: Cep; Chin; Sil; Ther.
  - half amel: Alo.
- Motion of
  - agg: Bell; Bry; Nux-v.
  - lids agg: Colo.
- Out through, as if: Nat-c; Sil.
- Over head, to nape: Bur-p.
- Pressure on, amel: Nat-m.
- Straining of, exertion agg: Gel; Nat-m; *Onos*; Pho-ac; Rut.
- Symptoms, with: See Visual symptoms, with.

Fear, fright agg: Aco; Chin-ar; Cimi; Glo.

Feet
- And: Mag-m.
- Bathing amel: Ascl.

Fingers, tip to: Cam.

Fixing attention on, amel+: Pall.

Flatus passing amel: Aeth; Cic; Sang.

Food, going without agg: Ars; Cact; Cist; Lach; Lyc; Sang; Sil.

HEAD

Forward, extending: Aco; Alu; Arg-n; *Bell*; Canth; *Carb-v*; *Chin*; Cimi; *Con*; *Gel*; Laur; Lyc; Mur-ac; Pho-ac; *Rhus-t*; Saba; Verb.
- Right: Kali-c; SANG; *Sil*.
- Left: Chel; Sabi; SPIG; Thu.

Frowning
- Agg: Ars; Mang; Nat-m.
- Amel: Caus; Pho; Sul.

Fullness: Aco; Bry; *Glo*; Merc; Sul.

Fungus: Ap; Calc-p; Pho.

Gastric symptoms+: Tarx.

Hair
- Binding amel: Sul-io.
- Cut agg: *Bell*; Glo; Pho; Sep.
- Down amel: Bell; Cina; Fer; Kali-m; Kali-p; Pho.
- Dragged by, as if+: Alu.
- Washing amel: Bell.

Hammering: See Pain.

Hands, holding near amel: Carb-an; Glo; Petr; Sul-ac.

Hat on head agg: Nit-ac.

Heart symptoms, with: Cact; Crot-h; Dig; Glo; Kalm; Merc-i-f; Naj; Spig.
- Pain after: Merc-i-r.

Heated if, agg: *Aco*; Ant-c; Bell; *Bry*; Carb-v; *Glo*; Lyc; Nit-ac; *Ver-v*; Zin.

Heat of sun agg: See Sunlight.

Heavy: Ap; Carb-v; Chin; Gel; Lach; Lol-t+; Mang+; Mur-ac; Nat-m; Nux-v; Petr; Pic-ac; Sul.
- Pillow, on: Buf; Glo; Sang.

Hold, unable to (See Wobbling about): Ap; Cocl; Cup; *Gel*; Sanic; Ver-a.

Holds, while coughing: Bry; Nic; Nux-v.
- Groans, and: Cimi.

Hot
- Air, about: Ast-r; Flu-ac; Plant; Pul; Ver-a.
- Application amel: Arg-n; Aur; Bry; Gel; Kali-c; *Mag-p*; Pho; *Sil*.
- Cold limbs, with: Aco; *Arn*; BELL; Bry; Calc; Carb-v; *Chin*; Fer; Gel; Lach; Mur-ac; *Sul*.
- Spots, on: Con.
- Vapour, rising to top: Buf; Ol-an.
- Vertigo, after: Aeth.
- Weather agg: Nat-c.

Hysterical, young women+: Arg-n.

Injuries, to: *Arn*; Calc; *Cic*; Con; Glo; Hep; Hypr; Lach; *Nat-s*; Pul; Rhus-t; Sil; Sul-ac; Symp.
- Delirium, after: Bell; Hyo; Op; Stram; Ver-a.
- Distress in, after: Lac-d.
- Stupefaction, after: Arn; Cic; Con; Pul; Rhus-t.
- Tender, after: Nat-m.

Inward extending: Agar; Anac; Arn; Ars; Calc; Canth; Hep; *Ign*; Nit-ac; *Stan*; Thu.

Ironing clothes, agg: *Bry*; Pho; Sep.

Jarring+: Ther.
- Cars, in agg: Med.

HEAD

Jaw, into: Lach; Pho; Stro.
Jerks: *Bell*; Bry; Caus; Cic; PUL; Sep.
- Sexual excitement, with: Ver-v.
- Up, and drops it again: Stram.

Kneeling and pressing the head to floor, amel: Sang.
Knotted, up, as if: Cam.
Larger than body, as if: Nux-v.
Laughing agg: Nat-m; Zin.
Lean
- Hand, on: Iod.
- Side, to one: Cina.
- Something on, desires to or amel: Bell; Fer; Kali-c; *Merc*; Nux-v; Saba; Spig
- Table, on AMEL: Ign; Saba.

Left to, face and neck: Tarn.
Lift it up, desire to: Ther.
Loose, something, in, as if+: Kali-c.
Lying
- Agg: Ther.
- Amel: Con; *Nat-m*; Nux-v; Sang; Sele.
- Dark in agg: Onos.
- Occiput, on
  - agg: Bry; Cact; *Cocl*; Kali-p; Onos; PETR; Pho; *Sep*; Spig.
  - amel: Kali-p; Pho-ac.
- Right side, on agg: Pho.
- With head low
  - agg: Pul; Sang.
  - amel: *Bry*; Phys; Ver-v.

Lying, something, in+: Plant.
Male voice, hearing agg: Bar-c.

Meals, missing agg: See Food going without agg.
Menses
- Before and after agg: Glo; Kali-p; Lil-t.
- During agg: Croc; Glo; Kali-p; Lac-d.
- Instead, of: Croc; Glo; Lith.
- Profuse, after agg: Glo.
- Suppressed agg: Lith; Naj; Psor.

Mental exertion agg: *Anac*; Cimi; Glo; *Iris*; *Kali-br*; NAT-C; Nat-p; Pho-ac; *Pic-ac*; Pul; *Sep*; *Sil*; Zin.
Milk
- Agg: Bro; Lac-d.
- Amel: Bry; Ver-a.

Motions, of: Alu; *Bell*; Cam; Cic; Cina; *Cup*; Hyo; Ign; Sep; Spo; Stram; Ver-v.
- Agg: Tub.
- Convulsive, cannot talk or swallow: Nux-m.
- Eyes, agg: Nat-m.
- Nodding to and fro: *Agar*; Chin; Hyo; Hypr; Ign; Nat-m; Sep; Stram; Ver-v.
  - bending forward, when: Hyo.
- Rolling: See Rolling
- Swinging backwards and forwards, as if: Pall.
- Writing, while: Caus.

Music agg: Cof; Pho; Pho-ac.
Narcotics agg: Acet-ac; Cof.
Neck, to: Bry; Cimi; Cocl; Kali-c; Lach; Nux-m; Nux-v.
Noises, clang, reverberations etc. in: Ars; *Aur*; Calc-f; Chin; Cop; Iod; Kali-c; Kalm; Kre;

HEAD, noises ..
  Lyc; *Phel*; Pho; Plat; PUL; Sars; Sil; *Stap*; *Sul*; Zin.
- Seminal emission after: Carb-v.
- Sleep, falling to, on: Zin.
- Talking, when: Sars.

Nose
- Bleeding amel: Bry; Buf; Fer-p; Meli; Pic-ac; Psor+.
- Boring, in amel: Tarn.
- Discharge, from amel: Cep; Kali-bi; *Lach*; Zin.
- Into: Cimi; *Lach*; Mez.

Numb: Grap; *Kali-br*; Nit-ac; Petr; Plat.
- Side, one: Mez.

Odours, strong agg: Anac.

Opening and shutting, as if: Calc; Cann; Cimi; *Cocl*; Glo; Lac-c; Sep; Sul; Vib.

Opens, and cold air enters in, as if: Cimi.

Opera, seeing after: Cact.

Outward extending: Aco; Arn; *Asaf*; BELL; Bism; *Bry*; Canth; Cham; Chin; Con; Dul; Ign; Lach; Lyc; *Mez*; Nat-c; Rhus-t; Sep; Sil; Spig; Sul; Val.

Over lifting agg: Calc.

Over work+: Pul.

Pain
- Aching, dull, heavy: Aco; Agar; Alo; Am-c; Ars; Bell; Bism; Bry; Cact; Calc; *Carb-v*; *Chel*; Chin; *Gel*; Glo; Meny; NAT-M; *Nux-v*; *Petr*; Pho; Pho-ac; *Pul*; Rhus-t; Sep; Sil; *Sul*; Thu; Zin.
- Boring, digging: ARG-N; *Caus*; Colo; Hep; IGN; Sep; Spig.

HEAD, pain
- Bruised, crushed: Bry; Chin; *Ign*; Ip; Nit-ac; *Nux-v*; Syph.
- Bursting, distended: Aco; Arn; *Bell*; BRY; Chin; Fer; *Glo*; Lach; Meli; Merc; Nat-m; *Nux-v*; Spig.
- Coition, desire for, with: Sep.
- Coldness
  - with: Mos.
  - hands and feet: Vario.
- Crampy: Aco; Ign; Plat.
- Cutting sharp, shooting: Arn; *Bell*; Calc; Lach; Tub.
  - right: Spig.
  - left: Sep.
- Drawing: Carb-v; Cham; Chin.
- Eructation, with: Calc.
- Eye
  - inflammation with: Bad.
  - over, one: Pho.
- Hair, being pulled as if: *Chin*; Mag-m+; Sul.
- Hammering: Calc; *Fer*; Lach; Manc; Nat-m; Psor; Sul.
- Heart pain, after: Merc-i-f.
- Hunger, with: Kali-p.
- Lachrymation, with: Mez.
  - scalding+: Pul.
- Linear: Tell.
- Maddening, shrieks, with: Aco; Ap; Ars; *Bell*; *Cham*; Colo; Cup; Gel; *Meli*; Sep; *Stram*.
- Nail, clavus, plug: Cof; *Ign*; Nux-v; Thu.
  - coryza, with: Form.
- Persistent: FER; Lac-d; Terb.
  - for years+: Lac-d.
- Pressing, pressure: *Bry*; Chin; Ign; *Nux-v*; Saba; Stan; Sul.

HEAD, pain
- Screwed as if+: Kali-io.
- Shattered, as if: Aeth; *Arg-m*; Bar-c; *Bell*; *Bry*; Calc; *Chin*; Cimi; *Ign*; *Iris*; Merc; *Nux-v*; Pho; Rhus-t; Sil; Sul.
- Shooting: Kali-c; Tub.
- Sleep, felt during: Ther.
- Sore: *Chin*; Gel; Ip; Nux-v; Phyt.
- Spot, in a: Cann; Colch; *Ign*; Kali-bi; Kali-io.
- Squeezing: See Compression.
- Stitching, stinging: *Arn*; *Bry*; Caus; *Kali-c*; Nat-m; *Pul*; Sul.
  - sun, standing, in: Bar-c.
- Stools pressing at: Lyc; Rat.
- Stuperfying, stunning: *Bell*; Calc; Cocl; Flu-ac; Gel; Hell+; Hyo; *Nux-v*; Pho-ac; Spig; Stan; Stap; Verb.
- Sutures, along: *Calc-p*; *Flu-ac*.
- Tearing, rending: *Chin*; *Lyc*; *Merc*; Nux-v; Pul; Sul.
- Throbbing, pulsating: *Aco*; BELL; Bry; Cact; Calc; *Chin*; GLO; Jab; LACH; Laur; Led+; Lyc; Meli; Nat-m; Pyro; Sep; *Sil*; Stap; Sul; Ver-v.
  - cough, after: Lyc.
  - painless+: Pyro.
- Twinging: Bell; *Bry*; Chin; *Pul*; Sul.
  - vertigo, with+: Rhus-t.
- Waked, by: Aco; Ars; Chin; Kali-c; Lach; Nux-v; Sil; Sul.

Pressure
- Amel: Am-c; Ap; ARG-N; Bell; *Bry*; Cact; Fer; Lach; Mag-m; Mag-p; Meny; *Nat-m*; Nux-m; *Pul*; *Stan*; VER-A.
- Back, on amel: Sang.
- Eyes, on amel: Nat-m.
- Hand, of cold amel: Calc.
- Hard amel: Chin; Mag-p.
- Hat, of agg: Carb-v; Nit-ac.
- Nose, root at amel: Kali-bi.
- Vertex, on agg: *Chin*; Lach; Phys; Ther.

Pulled back, as if: Syph.

Pushed forward, as if: Fer-p.

Rain
- Agg: Phyt.
- Amel: Cham.

Reading amel: Ham; Ign.

Reclines: Carb-v.

Remove, desire to: Ther.

Retching amel: Asar.

Reverberation: See Noise.

Rolling, of: Agar; Ap; *Bell*; Cina; *Hell*; Hyo; *Lyc*; Merc; *Nux-m*; POD; Pyro; Tarn; Ver-v; *Zin*.
- Bending, forward, when: Hyo.
- Brain, concussion of from: Hyo.
- Business worry, from: Pod.
- Moaning, and: Merc; Pod.
- Side to side, from amel: *Agar*; Kali-io; Med; Pho-ac.
- Teeth, grinding with: Zin.

Room, crowded agg: See Crowded room Agg.

Rubbing
- Amel: Ars; Chin; Tarn; Thu.
- Soles, amel: Chel.

HEAD

Rubs
- Against something: Tarn.
- Hands, with: Ver-a.

Running agg: *Pul.*

School girls agg: Calc; *Calc-p*; Cimi; Mag-p; Nat-m; Pho-ac; Pul; Saba; Zin.
- Diarrhoea, with: Calc-p.

Scratching amel: Mang.

Seminal emission agg: Ham.

Seperated from body, as if: Alo; Alu; Ant-t; Cann; *Daph*; Nat-c; Nat-m; *Nux-m*; *Psor*; Ther.

Sewing agg: *Lac-c*; Petr.

Sexual desire, suppression from agg: Con; Pul.

Shaking
- Agg: Bell; Glo; Nux-m.
- Amel: Cina; Gel; Lach; Pho.
- Up and down amel: Chin.

Shakes, without cause+: Lyc.
- Involuntarily, slow, then rapid+: Lyc.

Shopping, exertion agg: Epip; Sep.

Sinking downwards, from: Arg-n.

Sitting
- Erect amel: Cic; Gel.
- Still amel: Nat-m.

Skull cap, sensation of: Carb-v; Cyc; Grap; Lach.

Sleep during
- Agg: Ther.
- Amel: Nat-m; Sang.

Smoking amel: Calc-p; Carb-ac; Lycps.

HEAD

Sneezing
- Agg: Carb-v; Kali-c; Nat-m; Nit-ac; *Pho*; Spig; *Sul.*
- Amel: Calc; Calc-p; Lil-t; Lyc; Mur-ac.

Soup, warm, amel: Kali-bi.

Sour things agg: Bell; Sele.

Speech
- Hearing agg: Bar-c; Lyss; Mag-m.
- Incoherent+: Stram.

Standing, (head) on, as if: Ars; Dios; Elap; Glo; Lach; Pho; Pho-ac; Thu.

Stiff: Caus.

Stool
- Agg: Manc; Ther.
- Amel: Aeth; Agar.
- Pressing at agg: Lyc; Mang.

Stooping
- Agg: Fer; Kali-c.
- Amel: Cina; Con; Hyo; Ign; Meny; Mez; Nat-s+.

Student's: Ars-io+; Aur; Cimi; Iris; Kali-p; Pic-ac+.

Sun
- Down amel: Gel; Lac-d; Sul-io.
- Light, Shine
  - agg: Ant-c; *Bell*; *Bry*; GLO; *Lach*; *Nat-c*; Nux-v; Pul; Val.
  - amel: Grap; Stro.
- Shade in amel: Bro.

Supports with hand, when rising or stooping: Stram.

Suppression
- From: Ant-t.

HEAD, suppression
- Sexual excitement+: Pul.

Sutures, along: *Calc-p*; Flu-ac.

Swashing of water, as if+: Hell.

Sweat, on: Am-m; Anac; CALC; CHAM; *Chin*; Guai; Kali-m; Mag-m; MERC; Mur-ac; Pho; *Pul*; Rhe; Sanic; SIL.
- Air open, when walking in: Chin.
- Cold: Hep.
- Musty: Ap.
- Palpitation, with: Calc.

Sweet things agg: Ant-c.

Swimming, in, as if+: Ab-c.

Talking
- Agg: *Aco*; Cact; *Chin*; Cof; Ign; Mez; NAT-M; *Sil*; SUL.
- Amel: Dul; Eup-p; Ham; Lac-d; Sil.
- Hearing, distant agg: Cact; Mur-ac.

Tea, green amel: Carb-ac.

Teeth, pressing together
- Agg: Am-c.
- Amel: Sul.
- With: Merc; Plant+.

Thick, as if: Ther.

Tightness: Nit-ac; *Nux-v*.

Tip, fingers of, to: Cam.

Tired, weary, as if: Pho; Psor.

Tobacco smoke amel+: Calc-p; Naj.

Tongue, protruding agg: Syph.

Touch agg: Aur; *Chin*; Hep; Lyc; Mez; Nit-ac; *Nux-v*.

Turning
- AGG: *Calc*; *Cic*; Kali-c; Pul; Spig; *Spo*.

HEAD, turning
- Quickly agg: Sang.
- Side to side agg: Cina.

Twisting
- In: Kali-c; Mur-ac; Til.
- To one side: Cic; Cup.

Uncovering agg: Ars; Aur; *Bell*; Calc-p; Colch; Con; *Hep*; Hyo; Kali-bi; Lach; Mag-c; Mag-p; Nux-m; Nux-v; *Psor*; *Rhus-t*; Samb; SIL; Stro.

Unsteady, as if: Sul.

Uraemic: See Urination, suppresion, from.

Urination
- Before, if call is not attended to agg: Flu-ac; Sep.
- During agg: Colo; Nux-v; *Tab*.
- After amel: Agar; Flu-ac; Gel; Ign; Meli; Sang; Sil.
- Frequent, and profuse amel+: Kalm.
- Frequent, and scanty then agg: Iod; Ol-an.
- Profuse
  - agg: Mos.
  - amel: GEL; *Ign*.
  - with: Aco; *Gel*; *Ign*; Lac-d; Mos; Ol-an; Sele; Sil.
- Suppression, from: Arn; *Glo*; Hypr; Sang.

Uterus, with: Cimi; Helo; Plat; Pul; Sep.

Variable intensity: Zin.

Vertigo, after agg: Calc; Rhus-t.

Vise, in as if+: Arg-n.

Visual or eye symptoms with: Bar-c; Bell; Bry; Cocl; Cyc; *Gel*; Hyo; Kali-c; Lach; Lil-t; Nat-c; Pul; Sang; Sep; Sil; Stram; Zin.

HEAD

Vomiting
- Agg: Phyt.
- Amel: Eup-p; Nat-s; Sang; Stan.
- With: Dig; Eup-p; Ip; Sang.

Waked, by pain: See under Pain.

Walking, motion
- Agg: Bell; Bry; Carb-v; Led; Mez; Nit-ac; Tub.
- Amel: Guai; Rhus-t.
- Jarring, of agg: Stan.

Walks
- Tip toe on: Crot-h.
- With head thrown backward: Arn.

Washer women's of agg: Bry; Pho.

Washing
- Agg: Canth; Tarn; Zin-chr.
- Cold water, with amel+: Ant-t.
- Feet with cold water amel: Nat-s.

Water were poured over: Cup.

Waving in, as if: Glo; Sep.
- Occiput to sinciput: Senec.

Weak persons+: Sabal.

Weekly agg: Calc; Epip.

Wild feeling+: Lil-t.
- Sleep, prevents+: Lil-t.

Wind through: See Air.

Winter agg: Bism.

Wobbling about: Abro; Aeth; Bell; *Calc-p*; Cham; Dig; Hyo.
- Falls backwards: Dig.
  - forwards, or: Colch.
- Whooping cough, in: Ver-a.

HEAD

Wrapping
- Agg: Iod; Led; *Lyc*; Pho; Pul.
- Amel: Cor-r; HEP; Led; *Nux-v*; Pho; *Rhus-t*; Rum; Sil.

Wrinkling forehead agg and amel: See Frowning.

Writing amel: Fer.

Yawning
- Agg: Kali-c.
- Amel: Mur-ac; Nat-m; Stap.

HEAD EXTERNAL (Scalp and skull): *Aco*; Ap; *Arn*; *Ars*; *Aur*; *Bar-c*; *Bell*; CALC; CALC-P; Caps; Chin; Clem; Hep; *Lyc*; *Merc*; Mez; *Nit-ac*; *Nux-v*; *Old*; Pho; *Pho-ac*; Rhod; RHUS-T; *Rut*; *Sil*; *Stap*; Sul; *Vio-t*.

Right: *Calc*; Canth; Con; Mez; Sil.

Left: Clem; Rut; Thu.

Front: Hep; Led; Pho-ac; Sul.
- Bregma: Ars; Merc.

Occiput: Carb-an; *Carb-v*; *Petr*; Sil.

Scalp
- Boils, on: Aur; Sanic.
- Contracted, as if: Carb-v.
- Crawling+: Arg-m.
- Creeping: Ran-b.
- Damp agg: Led.
- Drawn back and forth, as if: Nat-m.
- Eruptions, on: ARS; Bar-c; *Calc*; *Grap*; HEP; *Lyc*; Merc; Mez; OLD; *Petr*; RHUS-T; *Sul*; Vio-t.
  - ringworm: Dul.
- Fissure: Kali-io.

HEAD EXTERNAL, scalp
- Gathered, as if: Chin; Sele.
- Hard: Fer-p.
- Ice cold+: Calc.
- Itching: Anac+; Bar-c; Calc; Calc-s; GRAP; *Lyc*; Mez; NAT-M; *Old*; *Pho*; *Saba*; *Sep*; SUL.
  - damp weather+: Mag-c.
  - day and night: Old.
- Lice: Carb-ac; Merc; *Psor*; Stap+.
  - as if+: Led.
- Lumps, nodes: Caus; Daph; Grap; Sil.
  - headache, with: Sil.
  - sore: Hep; Kali-io.
  - under: Aur.
- Milk crusts: *Calc*; *Grap*; *Lyc*; *Old*+; Ol-j; Psor; Sep; *Sul*; Tub; Ust; Vio-t.
  - cervical glands swelling of, with: Canc-fl; Vio-t.
  - eroding: Stap.
  - foul: Calc; Stap; Sul.
  - suppressed agg: Vio-t.
- Numb: Plat.
  - one side: Mez.
- Oedema: Ap; Ars.
- Sensitive, painful: Ars; Bell; Bry; Chin; Hep; Kali-io; Merc; Merc-d; Nit-ac; Nux-v; Par; Sil; Spig; Tub.
  - hair combing, on: Kre; Nat-s.
- Shivering: Mos.
- Stiff: Rhus-t.
- Sweats: *Calc*; Cham; *Pul*; Rhe.
  - gushing+: Stry.
- Swelling, puffy
  - on: Nit-ac.
  - beneath: Sil.

HEAD EXTERNAL, scalp
- Tension: Alo; Asar+; Merc; Plat; Vio-o+.
- Tight+: Adon; Caus.
- Under: Rhod.
- Wounds, bleeding, from: Calend.

Sides: Zin.

Skull
- Lifted, as if: Lac-d.
- Must press+: Carb-an.
- Painful: Mez.
- Small, too, as if: Chel; Cof+; Glo; Grat.
- Tumours, painful: Kali-c.
  - perforating: Lach.

Temples: Nat-m.

Tubercles, all over+: Syph.

Vertex: Carb-v; Grap.
- Itching: Ver-a.

HEADSTRONG: See STUBBORN.

HEALING difficult (Wounds, ulcers, etc.): *Arn*; *Ars*; Bor; Calc; *Cham*; Con; Grap; *Hep*; Kali-bi; *Lach*; *Lyc*; Merc; Petr; Sil; *Sul*; Visc+.

HEARING

Acute, sensitive to noise: ACO; Aur; BELL; Caus; Cham; *Chin*; COF; Con; *Lach*; *Lyc*; Mur-ac; Nat-c; Nit-ac; *Nux-v*; *Op*; Sabal; Sep; *Sil*; Spig; Tab; THER; Zin.
- Distant sound: Calend; Nux-m.
- Dull, and alternately: Cic.
- Heat, during: Caps; Con.
- Menses, during: Hypr.
- Nausea, causing: Cocl; Ther.

HEARING

HEARING, acute
- Rumpling of paper, to: Bor; Nat-c; Nat-s.
- Scratching on linen and silk, to: ASAR.
- Voices and talking, to: Zin.
  - her own (autophoney): Bell.
  - her own seem too loud: Caus.

Bad, deafness, impaired: Aur; Bar-c; BELL; CALC; Carb-an; Carb-v; *Caus*; Chin; Chin-s; CIC; CON; Cup; Grap; *Hyo*; Kali-m; Led; LYC; Med; MERC-D; Nat-m; NIT-AC; Op; *Petr*; *Pho*; PHO-AC; PUL; *Sec*; Sep; SIL; SUL; Ver-v; Verb.
- Abdomen, coldness in, with: Amb.
- Adenoids, from: Stap.
- Adhesions in middle ear, from: Iod.
- Bending head backwards amel: Flu-ac.
- Blowing nose
  - agg: Sul.
  - amel: Mang; Merc; Sil.
- Cause, without: Syph.
- Cholera, after: Sec.
- Colds agg: Fer-p; Gel; Kali-m; Mag-c; Merc-d; Pho.
  - menses, during agg: Fer-p.
- Concussions, blows, after: *Arn*; Chin-s; Croc.
- Confusion of sounds: *Carb-an*.
- Convulsion, after: Sec.
- Cotton, stuffed with, as if from: Led.
- Coughing
  - agg: Chel.
  - amel: Sil.

HEARING, bad
- Direction of sound, cannot tell: Arg-n; Carb-an; Kali-bi.
- Discharges, suppressed from: Lob.
- Earache, recurring, from+: Nat-c.
- Eating agg+: Sul.
- Enlarged tonsils from: Hep; Kali-bi; Merc; Nit-ac; Stap.
- Eruptions, suppressed after: Lob; Mez.
- Eustachain tubes
  - hypertrophy, from: Ars-io.
  - occlusion, from+: Kali-m.
- Exanthemata, after+: Carb-v.
- Hear, can distant sound: Calend.
- Heated, from being: Merc.
- Human voice, to: Ars; Cheno; Pho; Sul.
  - except for: Ign.
- Indistinct: Bov.
- Infectious diseases, after: See Typhoid fever, after.
- Leaf or membrane before the ear, as if from: Ant-c; Verb.
  - shaking head and boring in ear amel: Sele.
- Measles, after: Nit-ac; Pul.
- Menses, at: Fer-p; Kre.
  - absent with: Nat-c.
- Misunderstanding of: Bov; Pho.
- Morning amel: Rhod.
- Moving quickly, on: Ver-v.
- Nervous: Aur; Jab; Syph.
- Night, at: Elap.
- Noise amel: Calend; Grap; Jab; Nit-ac.

HEARING, bad

- Old people, in: Bar-c; *Cic*; *Petr.*
- One, in, noises in other: Amb.
- Otalgia, after: Caps; Nat-c.
- Paralysis of auditory nerve from: Caus; Glo; Hyo; Kali-n; Kali-p; Sil.
- Periodically+: Spig.
- Pressure on ear amel: Pho.
- Quinine+: Calc.
- Riding in carriage amel: Calend; Grap; *Nit-ac*; Pul.
- Room, warm in amel: Pul.
- Rubbing amel: Pho.
- Scarlet fever, after: Carb-v; Lyc; Sul.
- Sexual excess, after: *Petr.*
- Snap, report amel: Sil.
- Sound seem far off: Lac-c.
- Speech, embarassed, with: Aur.
- Spinal fever, after: Sil; Sul.
- Stooping amel: Croc.
- Sudden: Elap; Gel; *Mag-c*; Plb; Sep; Sil.
  - plugs as from: Sep.
- Swallowing amel: Merc.
- Syphilis, hereditary, from: Lac-c.
- Tympanum, injury, from: Tell.
- Typhoid fever, after: Ap; Arg-n; Ars; Nit-ac; Pho-ac.
- Walking, motion (quick)
  - agg: Chin-s; Ver-v.
  - amel: Merc-i-r.
- Water
  - getting in ear, from: Verb.
  - working, in+: Calc.

HEARING, bad

- Wax, hardened from: Sele.
- Weather, damp agg: Mang.
- Wisdom tooth, cutting from+: Mag-c.
- Yawning amel: Sil.

Ear, not his own, with: Psor.
False, misunderstanding: Bov; Pho.
Foot steps, in next room: Nat-p.
Forehead, through, as if+: Sul.
Illusory sounds, noises: *Bell*; Cact; *Calc*; Cann; *Caus*; CHIN; *Chin-s*; Cimi; Grap; *Kali-io*; Lyc; Mang; Petr; Pho-ac; Psor; *Pul*; Radm; Sang; Spig; Spo; *Sul*; Thyr; Tub; Val.

- Blowing nose on: Bar-c; Carb-an; Mang; Pho-ac; Stan.
- Chewing, while: Bar-m; Calc; Grap; Iod; *Kali-s*; Meny; Nat-m; *Nit-ac*; Petr.
- Climaxis, at: Sang.
- Coition agg: Carb-v; Dig; Grap.
- Confused, voices: Benz-ac.
- Convulsions, after: Ars; Caus.
- Coughing, on: Kali-m.
- Crackling: Ars; Cof; Dig; Glo; *Phel.*
- Crashings, explosions: Alo; Ars; Bar-c; *Dig*; Glo; Grap; Kali-c; Mos; Nit-ac; Petr; *Phel*; Pho; *Rhus-t*; Saba; Sil; Zin.
- Deafness, with: Cimi.
- Door, beating at: Ant-c.
- Ear, passing hand over, agg: Mar-v.
- Echoes, reverberating: *Caus*; Colo; Lyc; *Pho*; Sep.

HEARING, illusory, echoes
- loud: Pho-ac.
- music+: Pho.
- words: Bell; Sars.
• Fever, during: *Ars*; Lach; *Nux-v*; *Tub*.
• Fluttering: Plat; Spig.
• Gurgling, bubbling: Lyc; Nat-c.
• Headache, during: *Chin*; Form; Naj; Pul; Sil.
• Hissing: Dig; Mar-v.
• Horn blowing: Kalm.
• Humming, buzzing: Arg-n; Calc; Cann; *Chin*; Chin-s; Kali-c; Lyc; Nux-v; Plat; PUL; Sep; *Sul*.
- vertigo, with+: Arg-n.
• Inspiring forcibly, when: Mar-v.
• Lying
- agg: Fer-p.
- amel: Bar-c; *Pho-ac*.
• Morning amel: Rhod.
• Music, as if: Cann; Merc.
• Nauseous taste, with: Naj.
• Pain, with: *Ars*; Lach.
• Pulsating: Bell: *Calc*; Cann; Fer-p; Nit-ac; *Pho*; Pul.
• Ringing: Bell; Cact; Calc; Calc-s; Cann; Carb-v; CHIN; Kali-c; Kali-io; Kali-s; Lyc; *Nux-v*; Petr; Plat; Psor; *Pul*; Sep; Sul.
- bell: Pyro.
- deafness with+: Arg-n.
- haemorrhage, during: Chin.
- headache, during: Chin.
- menses, before: Fer.
• Roaring, rumbling: *Aur*; Bar-c; *Bell*; Bor; Carb-v; *Caus*;

HEARING, illusory, roaring ..
Chin; Chin-s; *Grap*; Lyc; *Nux-v*; Pho-ac; *Pul*; Sil; Spig; *Stap*; *Sul*.
- music amel: Ign.
- pulse, synchronises with+: Kali-br.
• Rushing: Kali-c; Lyc; Nat-m; Nit-ac; *Pho*; *Petr*.
- water, as of: *Cham*; Cocl; Pul; Radm+; Ther.
• Singing: Chin: Kali-c.
• Sneezing agg: Bar-c; Bar-m.
• Stools
- during: Lyc.
- after: Calc-p.
• Stooping on: Croc.
• Swallowing, on: Bar-c; Benz-ac; Calc; Cic.
- empty: Thu.
• Swashing: Sul.
• Talking agg: Mar-v; Nat-c; Op; Spig.
• Ticking: Chin; Grap; Zin-val.
• Vertigo, during: Bell; *Chin-s*; Dig; Op; Pho; Psor.
• Voices of absent persons+: Cham.
• Water
- boiling, as if in: Cann+; Dig; Thu.
- falling from height+: Nat-p.
• Yawning agg: Mang.
Perversion of: Calc.
Sound, seem distant, while: Lac-c; Sabal.
Variable: Cheno.
HEARING talk agg: See TALK, hearing agg.

HEART: ACO; Ars; *Aur*; *Bell*; Bry; Buf; CACT; *Calc*; *Carb-v*; Chin; DIG; *Fer-p*; Glo; Iod; *Kali-c*; *Kalm*; *Lach*; Lith; *Lil-t*; Lob; LYCPS; *Naj*; *Nat-m*; PHO; Pru-sp; PUL; Scil; Sep; SPIG; Spo; Strop; SUL; Tab; Tarn; Thyr; Ver-a; Ver-v; Zin-io.

Aching: Lith; Spo; Strop; Tab; *Ver-v*.
- Dysmenorrhoea, with: Crot-h.
- Headache, with: Crot-h.

Alternating with
- Others: Benz-ac; Glo; Kalm; Nat-m; Nat-p; Strop; Visc.
- Abdomen: Merc-i-f.
- Aphonia+: Ox-ac.
- Piles: Coll.

Anger agg: Cup.

Angina: See ANGINA PECTORIS.

Anus, wiping agg: Ap.

Anxiety, anguish, with: ACO; Arn; Ars; *Aur*; Calc; Carb-v; Dig; Ign; Ip; *Pho*; Plat; *Pul*; Spig; Strop; Sul; Ther; Ver-a.
- Evil, something going to happen, as if: Meny.

Apex region: Ap; Lil-t; Sul.
- Base to: Med.
- Cutting: Zin-chr.
- Painful: Lil-t.

Arms, to: Alu; Bar-c; *Cact*; Carb-v; Dios; Glo; Kali-n; Kalm; Latro; Lyc; Pho; Spig; Stic.
- Right: Bor; Kre; Ox-ac; Pho; Plb; Phyt.
- Left: *Aco*; Ars; Cact; Cimi; *Dig*; *Kalm*; Lach; *Latro*; Lil-t; Pho; Pul; RHUS-T; SPIG; Strop; Tab; TARN; Thyr.

HEART, arms to, left
- shoulder, and: Fago; Scop; Thu.
- Mammae, from: Lith.

Ascending agg: Ars; Aur; Calc; Nit-ac.
- Descending, and : Lac-d.

Axillae, to: Kali-n; Latro; Thyr.

Backward (to left scapula): *Agar*; Alo; Cimi; *Kali-c*; *Kalm*; Lach; Laur; *Lil-t*; Mez; *Naj*; Rhus-t; Rum; SPIG; Sul; Tab; Ther; Thu.
- From: Cimi; Kali-c; Spig; Ther.

Ball, as of a: Lil-t.

Base
- To apex: Syph.
- Painful: Lob.

Beats
- Audible: Ars+; Ars-io; Bism; *Pul*; Saba; *Spig*; Sul.
- Back, heard in: Abs.
- Body over whole: Bell; Fer; *Glo*; *Kali-c*; Lach; Nat-m.
- Ceases
  - as if: *Aur*; Chin-ar; Cic; Cimi; *Conv*; DIG; Gel; Lob; Rum; Vib.
  - and starts suddenly: *Aur*; Conv.
  - then heavy throbbing: Rum.
  - trembles and throbs, inspiration amel: Arg-m; Arg-n.
- Ear, felt in: Glo; Pyro; Thyr.
- Face, felt in: Mur-ac.
- Hard: Spo; Zin.
  - occasional: Sep.
- Head, felt, in: Phys.
- Heavy: Lycps.

HEART, beats
- Neck, upto: Bad.
- One hard: Sep; Zin.
- Shaking the body: Ap; Arn; Mur-ac; Nat-m; Rhus-t.
- Strong: Rhod.
  - occasional: Hyd-ac.
- Throat, felt, in: Phys.
- Thumping: Aur; Iod; Rhod; Spo; Zin.
- Unsteady: Tab.
- Violent: Gel; Ver-v.
- Visible: Ars; Iber; Kalm; Lach; *Spig*; Sul; Ver-a.
- Water in, as if+: Sumb.

Bending double agg: Lith; Spig.
Big, seems, too: Lach; Sul.
Bladder (urinary), with: Lith.
Block, as of a: Stro.
Boiling, in region: Glo; Lachn.
Breath, holding agg: Cact.
Bubble starts from, and passes into arteries: Nat-p.
Bubbling, in region: Bell; Lach; Lachn; Lyc.
Burning: *Aco*; Ars; Aur; Bry; Calc; Cup; Hyo; Kalm; Op; *Pho*; Pul; Rhus-t; Sul; Syph; Ver-v.
- Ascends, impeding breathing: Croc.
- Fire, on, as if: Kali-c; Op; Tarn.

Bursting, distended: Glo; Pho; Zin.
Cavity, in place of+: Med.
Chocolate agg: Raph.
Church bell ringing agg: Lyss.
Clutched and released alternately: *Cact*; Iod; Lil-t.

HEART
Clutching: Thyr.
- Short breath, from: Thyr.

Coition after agg: Dig.
Cold: ACO; Ars; Bov; Carb-an; Grap; *Helod*; Kali-bi; Kali-chl; Kali-m; Lil-t; Nat-m; Petr; Rhus-t; Sul-io; *Ver-a*.
- Drops were falling on, as if: Cann.
- Horripilation, with: Carb-an.
- Icy, chill, during: Nat-m.

Compression, constriction, squeezed, grasped: Am-c; Arn; *Ars*; Ars-io; CACT; Colch; IOD; Lach; LIL-T; Radm; Spig.
- Cap like: Zin.
- Drinking water amel: Pho.
- Walk erect, cannot: Lil-t.

Congestion: Aco; Glo; Pho.
Coughing agg: Aur; Pho.
Crackling: Spig; Spo.
Cutting: Ars; Colch; Sul; Ver-a.
Debility, after influenza: Iber.
Dilatation: Adon; *Cact*; Chlo-hyd; Cratae; Dig; Grind; Naj; Spig; Tab.
- Shock, from: Tab.

Drawn down, as if: Thu.
Drinking agg: Con; Cup.
Drop down, as if: Hypr.
Dropsy (hydro-pericardium): Ars; Ascl; Colch; Dig; Lyc.
Ears, to: Thyr.
Empty, hollow, as if: Cocl; Grap; Med; Sul.
Endocarditis: Ars; Aur; Kalm; *Lach*; Naj; Spig; *Zin-io*.
- Septic: Naj.

HEART

Exertion agg: Cact; Dig; Lil-t; Nit-ac; Strop; Tab.
Eyes, with: Lith; Spig; Spo.
Falling down, as if: Laur.
Fatty degeneration: Adon+; Arn; Ars; Ars-io+; Aur; Aur-m; Cact; Kali-c; Pho; Phyt.
Floats: Bov; *Buf*; Kali-io; Sumb.
Fluttering, trembling: Ars; *Calc*; Chin; Cic; Cimi; Crot-h; DIG; Kalm; *Lil-t*; Naj; Nat-m; Nux-m; Nux-v; Rhus-t; SPIG; Strop; Tarn.
- Air, in as if: Buf.
- Body, all over: Phys.
- Excitement, least+: Amy-n.
- Head, felt in: Phys.
- Menses, after: Nat-p.
- Then blood rushes to head: Cinb.
- Throat, felt in: Phys.
- Vexation, after: Lith.

Foot sweat suppressed agg: Aur; Bar-c.
Foramen ovale, non-closure of: Calc-p.
Forceps delivery, after: Cact.
Formication, crawling: Canth; Kalm; Nux-v.
Fulness: Aur; Lach; Sul; Ver-v.
Goitre, during: Ars; Buf; *Crot-h*; Lach; Latro; Lycps; Pho; *Spo*; Thyr.
Gurgling: Psor.
Hands
- Over: Buf; Cup; Hyd-ac; Laur; Lil-t; Naj; Nat-m; Pul; Tarn.

HEART, hands

- Wetting in cold water agg: Tarn.

Hanging
- By the thread, as if: Aur; *Kali-c*; Lach; Lil-t; Nux-m.
- Rib, left, floating from: Kali-c.

Hard, as if: Nat-c.
Head
- Alternating, with: Amy-n; Glo; Nux-m; Strop; Tab.
- Congestion, with: Scop.
- Extending, to: Glo; Lachn; Lith; Med; Nux-m; Pho; Sep; Spig; Spo; Strop.
- Then: Merc-i-f.
- With: Lach; Naj.

Heat, ascending to: Croc.
- Yawning amel+: Croc.

Heavy: Aur; Lil-t; Pul; Spig; Tub.
Hollow: See Empty.
Hypertrophy: Aco; Aur; Bro; Cact; Iber+; Kali-c; Kalm; Lith; Lyc+; Naj; Pru-sp+; Spo; Thyr.
- Compensatory: Adon.
- Gymnastics, from: Bro; Rhus-t; Thyr.
- Palpitation, with: Bro.

Impeded: Rum.
Infectious diseases, after: Naj; Scop.
Influenza, after+: Adon.
Joints, alternating with: Nat-p.
Jumping: Aur; Merc-i-f; Tarn; Thyr.
Knocking at+: Pru-sp.
Large, feels+: Buf.
Leaning, backwards agg: Glo.

HEART

Lifted up or rising up, as if: Colo; Pod; Spo; Val.
- Throat, to: Caus; Glo; Phyt; Pod.

Lively: Strop.

Liver symptoms, with: Agar; Aur; Cact; Calc; Dig; Mag-m; Myr.

Loose, as if: Aur; Crot-h.
- Walking on: Aur.

Love sickness, from: Cact.

Lung affections, with: Pho.

Lying
- Agg: Aur; Spo; Thyr.
- Amel: Laur; Naj; Psor; *Spig*.
- Back on amel: Cact; Fago; Psor; Tell.
- Right side on agg: Alu; Arg-n; Bad; Cimi; Kali-n; Lach; Lil-t.
- Left side on agg: Crot-h.

Masturbation agg: Bar-c.

Menses, at agg: Lith.

Metastasis to: Aur; Kalm; Lach; Lyc.

Motion
- Agg: Con; Dig; Mag-m; Spig.
- Amel: Aur; Caus; Colch; Gel; Glo; Mag-m; *Rhus-t*.

Muscle exhaustion: Arn; Chin-ar; Zin-io.

Myocarditis+: Ars-io.

Narrow space, as if, in: Eup-p.

Neck and throat, to: Ars; Bad; Bell; Glo; Naj; Pho; Phys; Scop; Spig; Spo.
- Electric shock: Grap.

Needles, at: Cimi; Lyss; Manc.

HEART

Nephritis, after+: Adon.

Numb: Kalm.

Occiput to: Ars.

Oppressed: Ars; Aur; Cact; Ip; Lycps; Pul; Scop; Spig.
- Walking amel: Colch.

Palpitation: ACO; Agar; Amy-n; Arg-n; *Ars*; Ars-io; *Aur*; *Cact*; CALC; *Cham*; *Chin*; Colch; Con; CRATAE; *Dig*; *Glo*; IOD; Kali-bi; *Kali-c*; *Kalm*; Lach; *Lil-t*; LYC; MERC; Naj; Nat-c; NAT-M; Nat-p; *Nit-ac*; NUX-V; PHO; Pho-ac; PUL; *Rhus-t*; SEP; SPIG; *Spo*; Strop; SUL; Tab; *Thu*; *Thyr*; VER-A; Zin-io.
- Head
  - beating in, with: Nat-m.
  - congestion+: Scop.
- Anxious, nervous: ACO; ARS; *Aur*; Bro; Calc; Carb-v; Chin; *Cof*; CRATAE; *Dig*; Grap; Lach; *Mos*; Naj; *Nat-m*; Ol-an; *Pho*; *Pho-ac*; PUL; SPIG; Strop; Sul; Sumb; Thu; *Val*; *Ver-a*.
  - thunderstorm, after+: Nat-p.
- Aphonia, alternating, with: Ox-ac.
- Arm, left holds, during: Aur.
- Attacks of: Bar-c; Cann; Mang; Old; Pho.
- Attention is directed to anything, when: Nat-c.
- Audible, extending to limbs: Aesc.
- Back pain, with: Tub.
- Bathing
  - agg+: Bov.

HEART, palpitation, bathing
- cold amel: Iod.
- Body, through out+: Arg-n.
- Breath
  - holding agg: Cact.
  - offensive, with: Spig.
- Breathing deep
  - agg: Spig; Tub.
  - amel: Arg-m; Carb-v.
- Breathlessness, with: Strop.
- Chest
  - expanding on: Lach.
  - tightness, with: Chel.
- Chill
  - before: Chin.
  - during: Merc; Nat-m.
- Chronic: Strop.
- Climaxis, at: Sumb.
- Coition
  - during: Agar; Calc; Lyc; *Pho*; Pho-ac; Visc.
  - after: Dig; Sec; sep.
- Continuous: Calc; Carb-v; Cratae; Sul.
- Convulsions, before: Cup; Glo.
- Coryza, with: Anac.
- Coughing agg: Calc; Iber; Nat-m; Ol-j; Pul; Sul.
- Dinner, after: Pul.
- Disappointed love, from: Cact; Ign; *Nat-m*; Pho-ac.
- Drinking
  - after: *Con.*
  - cold water: Thu.
- Dyspnoea, with: Merc-i-f; Spo.
- Emissions, after: Asaf.
- Emotions
  - pleasurable+: Bad.
  - slight agg: Calc-ar; Lith.

HEART, palpitation
- Epigastrium, in: Med.
- Epistaxis, with: Grap.
- Eructation amel: Aur; Bar-c; Carb-v; Mos.
- Excitement, after: Arg-n; Pho.
- Exertion
  - amel: Mag-m.
  - slight agg: Ars; Calc; Calc-ar; Chin-s; Con; Dig; Lil-t; Rhus-t; Spig; Sumb; Thyr.
- Eyes, closing amel: Carb-an.
- Face
  - felt, in: Mur-ac.
  - pale, with: Amb.
  - red+: Agar.
- Faintness, with: Cocl; *Crot-h*; Hyd-ac; Lach; Laur; Lil-t; *Nux-m*; Pul; Ver-a.
- Fear, with: Nit-ac.
- Fever, in: Ars; Calc; Nit-ac; Pul.
- Fistula in ano, with: Cact.
- Foetus, first movement from: Sul.
- Fright
  - after: Dig.
  - as from: Nux-m.
- Goitre, with: Pho.
- Grief, from: Dig; Op.
- Growth fast, with+: Pho-ac.
- Haemoptysis, with: Mill.
- Hammering: Thyr.
- Hands
  - tremors, with+: Bov.
  - washing in cold water from: Tarn.
- Head
  - aching in, with: Bro; Calc-ar.

HEART, palpitation
- beating in, with+: Nat-m.
- congestion, with: Scop.
• Hot
- drinks amel: Nux-m.
- feeling, with: Ant-c.
• Hunger, from: Kali-c.
• Hymn tune in church, from: Carb-an.
• Hysterical: Sumb.
- nose bleeding with: Agn.
• Lachrymation, with: Am-c.
• Laughing, on: Iber.
• Limbs, trembling, with: Cof.
• Lying
- agg: Kali-n; Merc; Nux-v; Ox-ac; PUL; *Sul*; Thyr.
- back on
  agg: Ars; Merc-i-f.
  amel: Kalm; Lil-t.
- left side on
  agg: Bar-c; Bro; Cact; Nat-c+; Nat-m; *Pho*; *Psor*; Pul; Sep; Zin-io.
  amel: Ign; Mag-m.
- right side on
  agg: Alu; Arg-n; Bad; Kali-n; Kalm; Lil-t; Plat.
  amel: Lach; Nat-c; *Pho*; *Psor*; Tab.
• Maids, old, in: Bov.
• Masturbation agg: Fer.
• Menses
- before: Cact; Cup; *Spo*.
- with: Buf; Crot-h; Ign: Phys.
- amel: Eupi.
- suppressed from: Cyc.
• Mental exertion agg: Calc-ar; Cocl.

HEART, palpitation
• Metastasis, from: Abro; Aur; Cact; Colch; Dig; Iod; Kalm; Lach; Naj; *Pho*; Spig; Spo; Sul.
• Morning, waking, on: Kali-c; Nux-v.
• Motion, walking
- agg: Aur-m; Cact; Chin; Dig; Naj; Pho; Psor; Spig.
- amel: Arg-n; *Fer*; Gel; Lob; Mag-m; Nux-m; Rhus-t.
- every agg: Chin.
- quick agg: Cocl.
• Mouth, foul odour from, with: Spig.
• Music, when listening to: Amb; Kre; Stap.
• Nausea, with: Arg-n; Bro.
• Nervous: See Anxious.
• Noise from every strange: Nat-c; *Nat-m*.
• Occiput, to: Cimi; Sep.
• Pain changing locality when: Lach.
• Painful: Mag-m; Spo.
• Periodical: Chel.
• Pleasurable emotions, from: Bad; Cof.
• Preaching agg: Naj.
• Pregnancy during: Arg-m; Lil-t.
• Pressure with hand amel: Arg-n.
• Puberty agg: Aur.
• Pulsations, through the body with: Saba.
• Sadness, as from: Nux-m.
• Sexual excess, from: Sec.
• Sighing amel: *Arg-m*.

HEART, palpitation
- Sitting, when
  - agg: Asaf; Mag-m; Pho; Rhus-t; *Spig*.
  - amel: Cact; Lach.
- Sleep
  - in: Merc-c.
  - unable to: Cimi; *Ign*; Spig.
- Stiff, as if: Aur-m.
- Stool
  - during: Ant-t.
  - after agg: Agar; *Ars*; *Con*; Cratae; Grat.
  - loose, with: Ant-t.
- Stooping agg: Nat-c; Spig; Thyr.
- Stop, must: Aur.
- Sudden: Mos.
- Suffocative feeling, with: Calc-ar.
- Sun heat agg: Cof.
- Sweat
  - with: Jab; Spo; Tab; *Ver-a*.
  - cold, with: Am-c.
- Takes the breath, away: Chin.
- Talking
  - agg: *Naj*; Pul.
  - impossible: Naj.
- Thinking
  - of it agg: Alum; Sumb.
  - wrong of, on, agg: Iod.
- Throat, to: Nat-m; Spo.
- Thunderstorm, after+: Nat-p.
- Tobacco amel+: Agar.
- Tumultous+: Agar; Amy-n.
- Urination
  - affections, of, with: Laur.
  - profuse with: Cof.
  - scanty, with: Ap.

HEART, palpitation
- Uterus, soreness of, with: Conv.
- Vertigo, with: Adon; Aeth; Cact; Cocl; *Iber*; Spig.
  - and throat choking: Iber.
- Violent: Arg-n; Calc; *Cratae*; Dig; Glo; Iod; Kali-c; *Lycps*; Mur-ac; Nat-m; *Pul*; Sep.
- Visible: Bov; *Carb-v*; Glo; Kalm; Naj; Sep; *Spig*; Ver-a.
  - apex beat, through, clothing: Mag-p.
- Waking
  - on: Lach; Naj; Pho.
  - suddenly, on: Chin-s.
- Washing hands in cold water: See Hands Washing.
- Water in, as if: Bov; Sumb.
- Weakness with: Hyds.
- Women, looking at: Pul.
- Writing, when: Fer-p; Nat-c.
- Wrongs, real of imaginary, from+: Iod.

Plug at: Ran-sc.
Pressure of hands amel: See Hands over.
Purring: Glo; Iod; Pyro; *Spig*.
Radiating, from: Aco; Glo; *Kalm*; Spig.
Reflex from: Asaf; Naj.
Restless: Ars.
Revolving as if: Ant-t.
Rheumatism, after: Adon+; Aur; Benz-ac; Gel; Kalm; *Lach*; Spig.
Riding in carriage agg: Naj.
Right side, as if, on: Bor; Ox-ac; *Phyt*.

HEART

Rising
- As if: See Lifted.
- Seat from agg: Gel.

Rubbing amel: Lil-t.

Scapula, to, left: Agar; Kalm+; Naj+.
- Arm, and+: Kalm.

Senile+: Ars-io.

Shocks, at: Calc; Con; Lith; Nux-v.
- Coughing agg: Agar.
- Electric: Sep.
- Eructation agg: Agar.
- Noise, sudden agg: Agar.

Short breath: Strop; Thyr.

Shoulder and neck, to: Naj; Scop.
- Left, arm and: Fago.

Sitting
- Agg: Mag-m.
- Erect agg: Aco.

Smothered, as if: Stro; Thyr.

Sneezing agg: Agar; Bor; Dros; Merc.

Sore, bruised: AP; ARN; Bap; BAR-C; Cact; *Cimi*; Flu-ac; Lach; *Lith*; *Lycps*; *Nat-m*; Spig.
- Foot sweat suppressed agg: Aur; Bar-c.

Space too small, as if, in: Eup-p.

Spine, touching agg: Tarn.

Squeezed, as if: Iod.

Stagnated sensation: Lyc; Saba; Zin.

Stairs, going up and down agg: Lac-c.

Stooling agg: Con.

HEART

Stooping agg: *Lith*; Lil-t; Old.

Stops, as if: See Beats, ceasing as if.

Surging upward: See Lifted up.

Swelled, full, as if: Asaf; Cimi; Glo; *Lach*; Pyro; Sep; Sul.

Swaying by the thread, as if: Tub.

Symptoms
- Few, with: Naj.
- Vary, with: Lycps.

Tension: Radm.

Throb, one: Zin.

Tired, feeling: Crot-h; Kali-bi; Lil-t; Naj; Nux-v; Op; Pho; Pyro; Rhus-t; Strop; Ver-a; Zin-io.
- Lung troubles, chronic after: Ars-io.

Tobacco agg: Cact; Kalm+; Scop.

Toe, big, alternating, with: Nat-p.

Torn loose and swinging by thread, as if: Dig.

Tremors: See Fluttering.

Tumultous: Aco; Amy-n; Lycps.

Turns over, twists: Ap; Arn; Cact; Caus; Crot-h; *Lach*; Rhus-t; *Sep*; Tab; Tarn.

Twitching: Aesc; Arg-m; Cam.

Undulating, as if: Benz-ac; Spig.
- Warm: Rhod.

Unsteady: Tab.

Urinating amel: Lith; Nat-m.

Vacuum, beating in, as if: Nux-m.

Valves: *Bar-c*; Calc; Calc-f; *Kali-c*; Lach; Laur; Naj+; Pho; *Pul*; Spo; *Strop*; *Tarn*; Thyr+; Zin-io.

HEART, valve
- Aortic obstruction+: Kalm.
- Incompetent: Cact; Cratae; Kali-c; Spo.
- Mitral and tricuspid regurgitation: Apoc; Cact; Laur; Psor; Strop.

Walking amel: Colch.

Water, as if in: See Floats.

Weak: See Tired feeling.
- Entering cool room from a walk in hot sun: *Rhus-t.*

Whirling about, as if: Cact; Iod.

Wine agg: Glo.

HEARTBURN: Aesc+; Amb; Am-c; *Calc*; *Carb-v*; Cic; *Con*; *Croc*; Fer-p; Lyc; Mag-c; NUX-V; PUL; Sumb.

Dinner, after: Merc-i-r.

Fats agg: Nat-c.

Horripilation, with: Calend.

Milk, after: Amb.

Palpitation, with: Nat-m.

Sweets agg: Zin.

Water, burning: Ars.

HEAT (Modalities)

AGG (Feels too hot): Aco; Alo; *Ant-t*; Ap; *Arg-n*; *Bell*; *Bry*; *Carb-v*; Cham; Coc-c; Cyc; Dros; Euphor; *Flu-ac*; GEL; *Glo*; Guai; IOD; Kali-io; Kali-m; LACH; Led; *Lil-t*; Lyc; Med; Merc; Nat-c; NAT-M; *Nat-s*; Op; *Pul*; Rat; Sabi; *Sang*; *Sec*; *Sul.*

AMEL (Warmth of bed; external heat AMEL): *Ars*; *Bell*; *Bry*; Caus; *Cham*; Chin; Clem; Cocl; Dros; GRAP; HEP; Hyo; *Kali-bi*; KALI-C; Led; *Lyc*;

HEAT amel ..
Mag-c; *Mag-p*; MERC; Nat-c; *Nux-m*; NUX-V; Pho; RHUS-T; Rum; *Samb*; *Scil*; Sep; SIL; STRO; SUL; Zin.

Cold, and
- AGG: Ant-c; Calc; *Caus*; Cimi; Fer; *Flu-ac*; Grap; Hell; Kali-c; Lach; MERC; *Nat-m*; *Pho-ac*; Phys; Sep; Sil; Sul; Sul-ac; Syph.
- AMEL: Syph.
- Extreme AGG: Ant-c; Caus; Ip; Lach; Sul-ac; Syph.

Fire of amel: See Stove of amel.

Radiating
- AGG: Ant-c.
- AMEL: Mez.

Steam, of AGG: Kali-bi.

Stove, of AMEL: Ars; Bov; Hep; Ign; Lach; Rum; Tub.

HEAT (Conditions): See BURNING, FEVER.

Exhaustion: Aco; Helo; Nat-c; *Sele*; Ver-v; Zin-io.

Fever without: Cham; Grap; Ign; Lach.

Flushes, in: *Amy-n*; Buf; *Calc*; Carb-an; Caus; Cocl; Coll; *Flu-ac*; Glo; LACH; Lyc; Mang; Nat-s; Nit-ac; *Pho*; Psor; *Sang*; Sep; Stro; *Sul*; *Sul-ac*; Sumb; Thu; Thyr; TUB.
- Bone pain, with: Flu-ac.
- Cardiac pain, with: Spo.
- Chill, then: Thyr.
- Eating, after: Tub.
- Face, in: Caus; Sang; Stro.

HEAT, flushes
- Fixed, ideas, with: Pho.
- Head, to: Sang.
- Headache, with: Sang.
- Hot water, immersed in, as if: Pho.
- Menses, during: Nat-m.
- Motion amel: Sul-ac.
- Pain, with: Cam.
- Palpitation, with: *Kali-c.*
- Piles, with: Coll.
- Sleep, falling to, on: *Con*; Lach.
- Steam, being over, as if: Pulex.
- Stooping agg: Merc-c.
- Sudden: Mang; Sep.
- Sweat
  - with: Sep; *Tub.*
  - cold, then: Amy-n; Sul-ac; Thyr.
  - sticky: Kali-bi.
- Thinking of it agg: Spo.
- Throbbing, general, with: Sul.
- Tired, when: Helo.
- Trembling, then: Sep; Sul-ac.
- Upper parts, in: Sul-ac.
- Upwards: Glo; Sep.
- Waking, on: Lach.
- Warm
  - ingesta agg: Sul-ac.
  - water dashed over one, as if: Pul; Rhus-t.
  - water were poured over one, as if: *Ars*; *Psor*; Pul; Rhus-t; *Sep.*

Intolerable: Sabi.
Itching, with: Alu.
Lively impression, from: Pho.
Mental, exertion agg: Old.
Only, disagreeable: Val.

HEAT
Partial: *Aco*; *Ap*; ARS; *Bell*; Bor; Bry; Calc; *Canth*; Caps; Carb-v; Caus; Cham; Lyc; *Merc*; Mos; *Nux-v*; PHO; Pho-ac; *Pul*; *Rhus-t*; Sep; SUL; Ver-v.
- Affected part: Guai.
- External: Ars; Bell; Merc; Pho; Pho-ac; Sul.
- Internal: Aco; Bell; Bry; Canth; Laur; Merc-c; Pho; Sul.

Pungent, glowing: Cep; Rut; Tarn-c.
- Head to, from feet: Visc.

Shivers, with: Ars; Sec.
Side
- One of, other cold: Ap; Par.
- Lain on: Mag-m.

Spots, in: Tub.
Stooping, on: Merc-c.
Sweat hot, with: Glo.
Weakness, with: Spo.

HEATED by fire, sun, becoming heated
AGG: *Aco*; *Ant-c*; BELL; Bor; *Bry*; Carb-v; *Gel*; GLO; Iod; Ip; Kali-c; Kali-s; Lach; Lyss; Merc; *Nat-c*; Nat-m; Op; Pul; Samb; Sele; Sil; Ther; Ver-v; Zin.
AMEL: ARS; IGN.
Easily: Bro; Kali-n; Nit-ac.

HEAVINESS, LOAD: Aesc; Alet; Alo; Alu; Ap; Arg-n; Ars-io; Bell; Bism; Bry; *Calc*; Chel; *Con*; GEL; Helo; Ip; Lach; Lapp; Lil-t; Lith; Lyc; Meny; *Nat-m*; NUX-V; Par; Petr; PHO; Pho-ac; Pic-ac; PUL; Ran-b; *Rhus-t*; SEP; Scop; Sil; Spig; *Spo*; *Stan*; Stic; SUL.

HEAVINESS
Affected part on+: Elap.
Lightness, alternating, with: Nux-v.
Paralytic: Stan.
Whole body+: Am-c; Cast-eq.

HECTIC
Fever: See FEVER.
Spots: See FACE.

HEEDLESS+: Am-c.

HEELS: Am-m; Calc; Caus; Con; Fer; Grap; Ign; Led; Mang; Nat-c; Pul; Sabi; Sep.
Bone would push through, as if: Con.
Burning: Cyc; Grap; Ign.
- **Coal red hot applied to, as if:** Visc.
- **Near each other, when:** Ign.

Calf, to: Anac.
Cold: Merc; Sang; Sep.
- **Touching each other when:** Ign.

Contraction: Colch.
Corns: Pho.
Cutting: Mag-m.
Elevating amel: Phyt.
Formication: Grap; Sul.
Itching: Caus; Med; Pho; Pho-ac.
Kicks: Stic.
Numb: Alu; Ign; Lyc; Stram.
- **Sitting, while:** Con.
- **Stepping on:** Alu.

Os calcis painful: Aran; Cinb.
Painful: Am-m; *Mang*; Med; *Pul*; *Rhod*; Val.
- **Intermittent:** Sabi.
- **Lying back, on agg:** Fer.

HEELS, painful
- **Standing long, after:** Zing.
- **Walking amel:** Cyc; *Val.*

Piercing: Nat-s.
Pinched, by narrow shoes, as if: Chel; Ran-b.
Purple: Pul.
- **Red:** Petr.

Shooting: Con; Sabi.
Sitting agg: Cyc; *Val.*
Sore, bruised: *Cep*; Cimi; Kali-bi; Lac-c; *Led*; Polyg.
- **Burning:** Cyc.

Stand, cannot, on: Caus.
Sticking: Petr; *Val.*
Stone under: Aur; Berb; Bro; *Cann*; Hep; *Lyc*; *Rhus-t.*
Sweat, fishy on: Ol-an.
Tearing: Am-m.
Tension: Caus.
Throbbing: Nat-s.
Tingling: Nux-m.
Ulcer: Am-m; Aran; Ars; Cep.
Walking
- **Agg:** Zin.
- **Amel:** Cyc; *Val.*

Vesicles, on: Petr.

HELD, being amel: See HOLDING amel.

HEMICRANIA: See HEAD, One sided symptoms.
Climacteric: Croc.
Menses, instead of: Croc.

HEMIOPIA: See VISION, half.

HEMIPLEGIA (See also PARALYSIS): *Arn*; *Aur-m*; *Caus*; Cheno; COCL; Elap; LACH; *Nux-v*; *Old*; *Pho*; *Rhus-t*; Xanth.

HEMIPLEGIA

Right side: *Caus*; *Chel*; Elap; Merc-i-r; Nat-m; Plb.
- Aphasia with: Canth; Cheno.

Left side: Ap; Gel; *Lach*; *Nux-v*; Op; *Rhus-t*; Stro; Vip.

Anger, after: Stap.

Apoplexy, after: Arn; Bar-c; *Bell*; *Cocl*; Lach; Nux-v; Op; PHO; Stan; Zin.

Contraction of limbs, with: Cheno.

Convulsions of other side: Hell; Stram.

Diphtheria, after: Nux-v.

Hyperesthesia of other side with: Plb.

Masturbation, after: Stan.

Mental shock, after: Ap.

Numbness of other: Cocl.

Slowly advancing: Caus; Syph.

Spasms, after: Stan.

Sweat, with: Stan.

Twitching, with: Stram.

HERE AND THERE: See DIRECTIONS.

HERNIA: Am-m; Aur; Cham; Lyc; *Nux-v*; Sul; Sul-ac; Ver-a.

Femoral: Cub; Lyc; Nux-v.

Infantile: *Aur*; Calc; Cham; Lyc; Mag-m; Nit-ac; *Nux-v*; Sul-ac.
- Congenital: Thu.

Strangulated: Aco; Alu; Aur; Bell; Calc; Caps; Cham; Colo; Lach; Lyc; Nit-ac; Nux-v; Op; Plb; Sil; Sul; Sul-ac; Tab+; *Ver-a.*
- Tender: Sil.

Umbilical: Calc; Lach; Nux-m; Nux-v; Op; Plb.

HERPES: See ERUPTIONS.

HESITATES: Anac; Arg-n; Grap; Kali-br.

Trifles, at: Grap.

HICCOUGH: Am-m; Ars; Ars-io; Carb-an+; *Cic*; *Cyc*; *Hyo*; IGN; Iod; Lyc; Mag-p; *Mar-v*; Merc; Nat-c; Nat-m; Nux-m; NUX-V; *Pul*; Ran-b; Sec; Tab; Ver-v; Zin-val.

AGG: *Am-m*; Bry; Cyc; Hyo; Ign; Nux-v; Stro; Zin-val.

Alcoholic drinks, after or drunkards, in: *Ran-b*; Sul-ac.

Alternating with spasms of chest: Cic.

Asthma, before: Cup.

Back, pain, with: Mar-v.

Brain
- Affections, in: Arn; Cina.
- Concussion, from: Hyo.

Breath, short, with: Phys.

Chest pain, with: Stro.

Colic, with: Hyo.

Consumption, in: Lyc.

Convulsion
- With: *Cic*; *Hyo*; Ran-b.
- Before: Cup.

Convulsive: Gel; Mag-p; Ran-b.

Cough, after: Tab; Trifo.

Cramps, with: Cup-ar.

Day and night+: Mag-p.

Dinner, after and during: Mag-m.

Drinking, after: Ign.

Ear ache, with: Tarn.

HICCOUGH

Eating or nursing
- After: Hyo; Ign; Mar-v.
- Amel: Carb-an.

Eructations
- With: Cyc; Dios; Ign; Nux-v.
- Amel: Carb-an.
- Bitter: Ign.
- Empty: Ign.

Evening+: Gel.

Fever
- During: Mag-p.
- After: Ars; Lach.
- Same hour when fever ought to come: *Ars.*
- Typhoid, in: Pho.

Hawking agg: Calc-f.

Incessant+: Merc-cy.

Injury to head, from: Hyo.

Laughter agg: Calc.

Loud: Cic.

Nervous (hysterical): Gel; *Ign*; Mos; Nux-m; Zin-val.

Obstinate+: Stram.

Peritonitis, in: Hyo; Lyc.

Persistent: Kali-br; Laur; Merc-cy; Sul-ac; Zin-val.

Pregnancy, during: Cyc; Op.

Retching, vomiting with: Mag-p; Merc; Nux-v.

Sleep
- During: Ign; Merc-c.
- Amel+: Phys.

Smoking agg: Arg-m; Calend; Ign; Pul; Sele.

Thirst, with: Nic.

Unconscious when: Cup.

HICCOUGH

Violent: Nat-m; Nicc; Stram; Ver-v.
- Painful: Rat; Ver-v.
- Sleep, in+: Merc-c.
- Thirst, with+: Nic.

Vomiting
- Before: Cup; Jat.
- With: Bell; Bry; Lach; Rut.
- After: Jat; Ver-v.

Yawning, with: Cocl; Cyc.
- Stretching and with: Amy-n; Mag-c.

HIDE

Desire to: *Bell*; Hell; Pul; Stram.

Children, behind furniture: Bar-c.

Run away, and: Meli.

HIGH

Living+: Dig.

Places (See ASCENDING) agg: *Arg-n*; *Aur*; Coca; Gel; Pul; Stap; *Sul.*

Hills AMEL: Syph.

HIP JOINT: Bry; *Caus*; Led; Merc; Pho-ac; Rhus-t; Stram; Thu.

Buttocks, with: Card-m.

Cracking, in: Cam; Cocl; Croc.

Cramps: Led.

Dislocation spontaneous: Colo; Rhus-t; Thu.

Leg, too long, as if, with: Kre.

Motion
- Agg: Ant-t.
- Amel: Am-m; Calc-f; Iris.

Rising agg: Nat-s.

Stooping agg: Card-m.

HIP JOINT
Tuberculosis (morbus coxarious): Calc; Calc-p; Card-m; Chin; Colo; Hep; Kali-c; Kali-s; Led; Pho-ac; Pul; Rhus-t; Sil; Stram; Tub.
- Right: *Led.*
- Left: Stram.

HIPS (Region): Arn; Caus; Euphor; Lyc; Phyt; Rhus-t; Rut; Sep; Sul.

Alternating, between: Euony.

Above: *Caus.*

Aching, loss of power of legs with: Stap.

Bruised: Mag-m; Rut.

Bubbling: Led.

Burning: Mag-m.

Change of weather agg: Phyt.

Coition, after agg: Mag-m.

Contracted (drawn together): Colo; Polyg.

Coughing agg: *Caus*; Val.

Cramp: Colo; Led.

Dragged down, from: Visc.

Drawn together: See Contracted.

Forced apart, disjointed as if: Agar; Calc-p; Con; Sep; Sul; Tril.

Hollow: Pall.

Motion
- Agg: Ant-t.
- Amel: Am-m; Calc-f; Iris.

Pain, violent: Stram.

Pregnancy
- In: Calc-p.
- After: *Hypr.*

HIPS
Rising agg: Nat-s; Sep.

Sitting down agg: Nat-s.

Sore: Visc.

To hip: Arn; Cimi; Colo; Lac-c; Lil-t; Onos; Thu; Ust.

Up, back: Pho.

Urination agg: Berb.

Weak: Calc-p; Rut; Sep; Thu; Tril.
- Coition preventing: Cep.
- Sudden: Kob.
- Walking agg: Kob.

Wrenched: Iris.

HIVES: See URTICARIA.

HOARSENESS: See VOICE.

HODGKIN'S DISEASE: Ars; Ars-io; Bar-io; Iod; Pho; Syph.

HOLDING
Or being held AMEL: Ars; *Bry*; Carb-an; Diph; Dros; Eup-p; *Gel*; Glo; *Lach*; Lil-t; Murx; Nat-s; Nux-m; Nux-v; Rhus-t; Sang; *Sep*; Sil; Stram; Sul; Sul-ac.

Anything agg: Caus.

Attendant, to: Ant-t.

HOLE, blowing through: See AIR; blowing through.

HOLLOW: See EMPTY.

HOMESICK: *Bry*; CAPS; Carb-an; Eup-pur; Hyo; IGN; Merc; Op; *Pho-ac*; Sil.

Ailments, from: Clem.

HONOUR wounded: See PRIDE, wounded.

HOOK WORM DISEASE: Carb-tetra; Cheno; Thymol.

HOPEFUL: Sul; Tub.
  Despair, alternating with: Aco; Kali-c.
  Lung disease, in: Aur.
HOPELESS: See DESPAIR.
HORNY: See GROWTH and ERUPTIONS.
HORRIPILATION: See GOOSE SKIN.
HORROR: *Calc*; Cic; Plat; Zin.
  Solitude and work+: Cadm.
HORSE BACK: See RIDING on horse back.
HOT
  Application AMEL: Anac; *Ars*; Calc-f; *Hep*; Kali-c; Mag-p; Nux-v; Radm; *Rhus-t*; *Sil*; Syph.
  Ball: See BALL.
  Bath
    • **AGG:** Ap; Bels; Op.
    • **AMEL:** See BATHING, Hot.
  Days, weather agg: See SUMMER agg.
  Days and cold nights agg: See COLD nights with hot days agg.
  Drinks amel: See Drinks hot, under FOOD AND DRINKS.
  Iron, wires, needles etc. as if: Agar; Alu; Ap; *Ars*; Bar-c; Lith; Mag-c; Naj; Nit-ac; Ol-an; Rhus-t; Spig; Vesp.
  Water
    • **As if, in:** Pho.
    • **Breast to abdomen:** Sang.
    • **Flowing through part, as if:** Sumb.
    • **Pain during:** Terb.
    • **Poured on part, as if:** Ver-v.

HOUR exact agg: See PERIODICITY.
HOUSE in
  AGG: Bry; Lyc; Mag-m; *Pul*; Rhus-t; Til.
  AMEL: Agar; Cyc; Ign.
HOWLING: Aco; Arn; *Bell*; Cham; Cic; Ver-a.
  Anger, with: Arn.
HUMERUS
  Aching, right: Bry; Gel; Phyt.
  Broken, as if: Bov; *Cocl*; Pul.
    • **Middle:** Merc-i-r.
  Cramp, left: Val.
  Crushing: Stan.
  Electric shock: Val.
  Night, only agg: Dros.
  Writing agg: Ars-io.
HUMID (warm, damp) weather
  AGG: Alo; Ars; Bap; *Bro*; Bry; Carb-s; *Carb-v*; *Gel*; Iod; *Ip*; Kali-bi; LACH; Lyss; Nat-m; *Nat-s*; Old+; Op+; Pul; Rhus-t; Sil; *Ver-a*.
  AMEL: Sil.
HUMMING, buzzing, whizzing, purring: Caus; Kali-m; Kre; Mos; Nux-m; Old; Op; Pul; Spig; Sul.
HUNGER: See APPETITE.
  AGG: *Grap*; Iod; *Kali-c*; *Sil*; Spig; *Sul*.
HURRY, impatience: Aco+; Alu; Ap; *Arg-n*; ARS; BELL; Calc-p+; Cham; HEP; Hyo; IGN; Ip; Kali-s; Lach; *Lil-t*; Lycps; Med; *M-rc*; Mos; Nat-m; Nit-ac; NUX-V; Rhe; Sep; *Stram*; Sul; *Sul-ac*; Tarn; Thu; Val+; Ver-a.

HURRY
Cannot do things fast enough: *Sul-ac.*
Complaints, from: Arn.
Drinking, in: Anac; Bry; Hep.
- **Unconsciousness, during:** Hell.

Eating, while: Caus; Hep; Lyc; Plat; Sul-ac.
- **Can not eat fast enough:** Zin.

Every body must: Tarn.
Execution slow, with: Alu.
Menses, during: Ign.
Movements, in: Arg-n; Stram; Sul-ac; Tarn.
Time, for the appointed to arrive: *Arg-n.*
To do several things at once: *Lil-t.*
Trifle things, in: Med; Sul; Sul-ac.
Walking, while: Arg-n; Sul-ac; Tarn.
Writing, when: Sul-ac.

HURT
Fears being: *Arn*; Chin; Hep; Kali-c; Rut; Spig.
Feelings, others, of: Chin.
Little, pains terribly: Colch.

HYDRARTHROSIS: See JOINTS, water in.

HYDROCELE: Ap; Calc; Grap; Iod; Pul; *Rhod*; Sele+; SIL; Sul+.
Left side: Dig; *Rhod.*
Boys, of: Abro+; Pul; Rhod; Sil; Sul-io.
- **Birth, from:** Rhod.

Children+: Aur; Calc.
Gonorrhoeal orchitis, after: Pho.

HYDROCELE
Injury, from: Samb.
Multilocular: Ap.
Overlifting, from: Rhus-t.
Suppressed eruptions from: Hell.

HYDROCEPHALUS: *Ap*; Apoc; *Calc*; Calc-p; Iodof; Hell; Lyc+; Merc; *Sil*; Sul; Tub; *Zin*.
Convulsions, with+: Sul.
Diarrhoea, after (infants): Zin.
Vision, loss of, with: Apoc.

HYDROGENOID: Dul; Nat-m; Nat-s; Thu.

HYDRO-PERICARDIUM: See Dropsy, under HEART.

HYDROPHOBIA: *Bell*; Canth; Cup; *Hyo*; Lyss; Pho; Saba; *Stram.*
Prophylactic: *Bell*; Hyo; *Lyss*; Stram.

HYDRO-THORAX: See under CHEST.

HYGROMA: See GANGLION.

HYPERCHLORHYDRIA: See STOMACH, sour.
Hypochlorhydria, alternating, with: Chin-ar.

HYPERMETROPIA: See VISION, far sight.

HYPERPYREXIA: See FEVER, high.

HYPERTENSION: See BLOOD PRESSURE, high.

HYPERTROPHY: *Ant-c*; Ars; Calc; *Clem*; *Dul*; *Grap*; Ran-b; Rhus-t; Sep; *Sil*; Sul.
Exertion, excessive, from: Thyr.
One sided: Lyc.

HYPOCHONDRIAE: Aco; Chin; Lyc; Merc; Nat-s; Ran-b; Stap.
  Left: See SPLEEN.
  Right: See LIVER.
  Ache: Scil; Sil.
  • Leucorrhoea amel: Phyt.
  Anxiety, felt in: Arn; Nux-v.
  Around: Ran-b.
  Ball: Bro; Cup.
  Band, about: Aco; Card-m; Dros; Ign; Nux-v.
  Bruised, sore: Bry; *Chin*; *Eup-p*; *Ran-b*; Visc.
  Constriction: Cact; Lyc.
  Coughing agg: Dros; *Eup-p*; Kali-c; Nat-s.
  Full: Sep.
  Hard: Iod.
  Heavy: *Coc-c*; Zin.
  Holds: Dros.
  Sticking: Sil.
  Tension: Aco; Lyc.

HYPOCHONDRIASIS: Ars; Asaf+; AUR; Card-m+; Con; Grat+; Ign; *Nat-c*; Nat-m; NUX-V; Plat; PUL; *Sep*; Stan; Stap+; *Sul*; Val.
  Sexual: Mos.

HYPOCRISY: Pho.

HYPOGASTRIUM: *Bell*; Bry; Carb-v; Lyc; *Merc*; Ran-b; Scil; *Sep*.
  Aching, painful: Ars; Plat; Pul; *Sep*; Sul; Ver-a.
  • Coition, after agg: Cep.
  • Heavy: Vib.
  • Menses, during: Calc; Sec.
  Backwards
  • Right: Caus; Pho; *Sep*; Ust.

HYPOGASTRIUM, backward
  • Left: Aco; Carb-v.
  Bearing down: Bell; Dict; Lil-t; Lyc; Nux-v; Plat; Pul; *Sep*; *Sul*.
  Board, across: Nux-m.
  Clawing: Bell.
  Coldness: Plb.
  Constriction: Bell; Chel; Hyo.
  Cramps: Vib.
  Cutting: Bell; Hyo; Pul; Thu.
  • Menses, during: *Kali-c*; Lil-t.
  Distension: *Kali-c*; Phys.
  Empty: Kali-s; Sec.
  • Flatus passing amel: Kali-s.
  Flatulence: Zin; Zin-val.
  Fulness: Aesc; Bell.
  Heavy: Med; Pho-ac; Sec; Sep; Sul; Tarn.
  • Menses, amel: Vib.
  Legs, down: Con.
  Sore: Calc; Lach; Phys; Terb; Ver-a.
  • Standing agg: Phys.
  Tension: Sep.
  Trembling: Calc-p; *Lil-t*.
  Weak: Am-c; Apoc; Calc; Chio; Pho; Plb; Sul; Ver-a.
  • Stools, before: Merc-i-f.

HYPOSTASIS: Am-c; Rhus-t; Sep.

HYSTERIA: ASAF; AUR; Caus; Cham; *Cocl*; CON; Gel; Grat+; IGN; Kali-p; Lach; *Mag-m*; Mos; Nat-m; Nit-ac; NUX-M; NUX-V; *Plat*; *Pul*; Sep; *Sul*; Sumb; TARN; Ther; VAL; Ver-a.
  Climaxis, at: Pho-ac; Ther.
  Coition, agg: Lac-c.

HYSTERIA

Faints: Cocl; Ign.
Fright, after: Saba.
Globus: Aco; Con; *Mag-m*; Mos; Plb; Senec; Val; Zin.
- Eructation amel: Mag-m.
- Warm: Val.

Haemorrhage, after: Stic.
Lascivious: Plat; Tarn.
Looked at, when: Plb.
Menses
- Before: Hyo; Mos; Plat.
- First day, of: Raph.

Morning agg, sighing amel: Tarn.
Music amel: *Tarn*.
Puberty, at: Ther.
Sexual
- Excess, after: Pho-ac.
- Orgasm, at the height of: Lac-c.

Suppression of discharges, after: *Asaf*; Lach.
Twitchings, menses
- Before: Cup; Kali-c; Nat-m; Pho; Pho-ac; Plat; Pul; Sep; Sul.
- During: Aco; Bry; Calc; Caus; Cham; Chin; Cocl; Cof; Cup; Form; Hyo; Ign; Ip; Lyc; Mag-m; Merc; Nat-m; Nux-v; Pul; Sul.
- After: Chin; Cup; Pul.

Violent+: Aur.
Watched, only when: Plb.
ICHTHYOSIS: *Ars-io*; Pho; Syph; Thyr.
ICE factory complaints+: Dul.
ICY COLD: See COLDNESS, icy.

IDEAS: See IMAGINATIONS.

Compelling: *Lach*; Nit-ac.
Erroneous: Saba; Val.
Fixed: Anac; Ars+; Chin; Hell; Nat-m; Saba; Stan; Sul; Thu.
Many: Med.
- But uncertain in execution: Med.

Murdering her family, of: Jab; Kali-br.
Persistent: Med.
Strange: Arg-n.
Vanish: Anac; *Nux-m*; Ol-an; Ver-a.
Wander: Dul; Pho; Thu.

IDIOCY: See CHILDISH.
IDLENESS agg: See BUSY when amel.
ILEOCAECAL region: See APPENDICITIS.
ILEUS: See ABDOMEN, paralysis of intestine.

ILIAC

Down thigh: Berb.
Urinating agg: Berb.

ILL or sick feeling: Aco; Ant-t; Bap; Chel; Cimi; Lach; Lob; Nux-v; Petr; *Pod*; Psor; Pul; Sang; Stro; Tab; Tarx.
All over, in pelvic complaints+: Vib.
Does not know why: Bro.
Pain, from: Stro.
Queer, menses, before: Bro.

ILLUSIONS: See IMAGINATIONS.
IMAGINARY DISEASE: Arg-n; Mos; Saba; Ver-a.
Broods over: Cyc; Lil-t; Naj.

IMAGINATIONS, illusions, fancies, delusions: Aco; Amb; Anac; *Arg-n*; Ars; *Bar-c*; BELL; Calc; *Cann*; COCL; HYO; *Ign*; Kali-br; Lac-c; Lach; Merc; Mos; Nux-m; *Op*; Petr; Pho; *Pho-ac*; Plat; Pyro; SABA; STRAM; SUL; Thu; Val; Ver-a.

Animals, objects are: Hyo.

Behing him, somebody: See BEHIND.
- **Walking:** Calc.

Dead, he is: Lach.

Deceived, being: Dros; Rut.

Depressive: Amb; Kali-br.

Done something wrong: Cina.

Eat, cannot: Myr.

Front of him, someone: Con.

Furniture, to be persons: Nat-p.

He is not himself: Syph.

Heavy being+: Alu.

Horrid: Lac-c.

House, full of thieves+: Ars.

Husband, neglecting her: Stram.

Insults, of: Stap.

Larger, of being+: Alu.

Limbs, talking together: Bap.

Nose, wears, somebody else's: Lac-c.

Numb, being: Alu.

Odour, smell of: See under SMELL.

Pass, cannot a certain point: Kali-br.

Rich, as if, he is: Pho; *Plat*; Pyro; *Sul*; Ver-a.

Smooth, being: Alu.

IMAGINATIONS

Snakes, around: Hyo; Lac-c; Tub.

Starve, he must: Kali-m.

Strange surroundings: *Cic*; Hyo; Plat; Tub.

Stepping hard somebody, as if: Alo.

Super human control, under: *Anac*; *Lach*; Op; Plat; Thu.

Touch, sensory: Anac; Canth; Op; *Rhus-t*; Stram; *Thu*.

Voices, of: Aco; Anac; Ast-r; Cham; Chlor-hyd; Coca; *Elap*; Med; Nit-ac; Stram.
- **Unpleasant, about himself:** Coca.

Walks on knees, as if: Bar-c.

Wife is faithless: Stram.

World is on fire: Ver-a.

IMBECILITY: See CHILDISH.

IMITATES: Cup; Lach; Nux-m.

IMMOBILE: Lycps; Mang; Stro.

Side, one: Stro.

IMMORAL: See MORAL PERVERSIONS.

IMPATIENCE: See HURRY.

IMPETIGO CONTAGIOSA: See under ERUPTIONS.

IMPOTENCY (See ERECTION, incomplete): Calad; Iod; Kob+.

Diabetes, with: Coca; Mos; Pho-ac.

Fright, during coition, from: Sinap.

Gonorrhoea, after: Calad.

Imaginary: Stry-p.

Melancholy, with+: Kali-br.

IMPOTENCY

Nightly emissions, with+: Uran-n.
Onanism, after: Arg-n; Grap+.
Psychical: Onos.
Sexual excess, after: Arn; Grap+.

IMPUDENT CHILD+: Grap.

IMPULSES

Contradictory: *Anac.*
Fears, his own: Alu.
Horrid: Alu; Ars; Caus; Hep; Iod; Lach; Merc.
• Busy when amel: Iod.
To do strange things: Cact.
To tough things: See under TOUCH.

IMPULSIVE: Arg-n; Croc; Cup; IGN; Med; PUL; Tarn.

INACTIVE, lethargic, apathetic, lies down: Ail; Alu; Ant-t; Ap; *Arn*; Ars; Bels+; Bism; Calad; *Calc*; Carb-v; Caus; Chel; *Chin*; Con; Cup; Fer; *Gel*; Grap; *Hell*; Kali-c; Lach; Mar-v+; *Mur-ac*; NUX-V; Old; OP; PHO; PHO-AC; Pic-ac; Psor; Radm; Rut; Sang; Sele; SEP; Sil; *Stram*; *Sul*; Sul-ac; Tarn; Thyr; *Zin*.

Activity, alternating, with: Alo; Aur.
Coition, after: *Calc.*
Conversation, from: Sil.
Eating, after: Lach; Lyc; *Pho-ac*; Sele.
Stool, after every: Arn.
Stormy weather, in: Sang; Tub.

INATTENTION AGG: Gel; *Hell.*

INCITING OTHERS: Hyo.

INCOHERENCE: See CONFUSION.

INCONSTANCY: IGN.

INCONTINENCE stool, urine, sexual, etc: *Alo*; Arg-n+; *Arn*; Ars; BELL; CAUS; Chin; Con; Dios; *Gel*; *Hyo*; Mur-ac; Nat-m; *Pho*; PHO-AC; *Pod*; *Pul*; Sele; Sep; Stap; *Sul*; Uran-n+.

Fright, from: Op.

INCOORDINATION: See COORDINATION disturbed.

INCREASES AND DECREASES: See DIRECTIONS.

INDIFFERENCE: Ap; Arn; Ars; *Bap*; Berb+; CALC; *Carb-v*; *Chin*; Clem; CON; Gel; HELL; *Ign*; Lil-t; Mez; *Nat-c*; *Nat-m*; Nat-p; Onos; *Op*; PHO; PHO-AC; PLAT; PUL; SEP; Stap; Sul; Tab.

Complain does not: Hyo; *Op*; *Stram.*
Everything, to: Carb-v; Merc+; Mez; Nat-p; Pho-ac.
• Done for her: Lil-t.
Household matters, to: Cimi.
Loved ones, to relations: Flu-ac; *Hell*; Nat-p; *Pho*; *Sep.*
• Her own children: Lyc; *Pho*; *Sep.*
Opposite sex: Thu.
Pain, to: Op.
Pleasure, to: Fer-p; Hell; Nat-m; Op; Sul.
Society, when in: *Arg-n*; Kali-c.
Stoic: Ail; Op.
Sullen+: Ver-a.

INDIFFERENCE

Surroundings, about: Pic-ac+; Rum.

Welfare of others, to: SUL.

INDIGESTION (See DIGESTION affected): Aeth; *Ant-c.*

Coition, after: Dig; Pho.

Hurriedly eating and drinking from: Anac; Cof; *Old.*

Sprain, from: Rut.

INDIGNATION: Ars; Calc-p; Colo; *Stap.*

Pregnant, while: Nat-m.

INDOLENT, sluggish: Alu+; Bor; *Caps*; Carb-v; Chel; Chin; *Grap*; Kali-bi; Lach; *Merc*; Nat-m; Nit-ac; Nux-v; Pho; Psor; Sabi+; Sep; Sil; SUL.

Suddenly: Calc.

INDURATION: See HARDNESS.

INDUSTRIOUS: Aur; Tarn.

INFANTS: See CHILDREN.

INFERIORITY: See COWARDLY, ANTHROPOPHOBIA and COMPANY agg.

INFILTRATION: Calc; Carb-an; Grap; Iod; Kali-io+; Kali-m; Rhus-t; Sul; Sul-io.

Stubborn+: Kali-m.

INFLAMMATION: *Aco*; Ap; *Ars*; BELL; BRY; Calc; Cann; *Canth*; Cham; Echi; Fer-p; GEL; Hep; HYO; *Iod*; Kali-c; Lach; MERC; NUX-V; *Pho*; Plb; PUL; RHUS-T; Sec; Sep; SIL; *Stap*; Sul; Terb; *Ver-v.*

INFLUENZA: Ars-io; Bap; Bry; Cam; Caus; *Eup-p*; Fer-p; *Gel*; Merc; *Nux-v*; *Rhus-t*; Saba.

INFLUENZA

Gastric: Bap.

Pain remaining, after: Lycps.

Weakness, remaining after: Abro; Con; Kali-p; Nat-sal+.

INGUINAL GLANDS: See under GROINS.

INHALATION: See INSPIRATION.

INJURIES

In general, shocks, wounds, bruises etc: *Arn*; Bels; *Calend*; Cic; *Con*; Echi; Glo; Ham; Hep; Hypr; Kali-io; *Lach*; Led; Lith; Nat-s; Nit-ac; *Pul*; *Rhus-t*; *Rut*; Stap; Stro; *Sul-ac*; Symp.

Bites of poisonous animals, from (rats, snakes, cats, dogs etc.): Anthx; *Ap*; Arn; *Ars*; Cedr+; Cist; *Echi*; Hypr; *Lach*; LED; Mos; Pyro; Seneg+; Sul-ac.

- Bees+: Tab.
- Boots, tight form: Paeon.
- Bruised, sore spot, from: Lith.
- Insects+: Cedr.
- Mosquitoes: Calad; Tab+.
- Leeches: Alum.
- Snakes+: Cedr; Plant.

Bones, to: Arn; Calc; Iod; *Petr*; Pho; Pho-ac; Pul; RUT; Stap; Symp.

Bruises, contusions: Arn; Con; Ham; Hypr; Rhus-t; Rut; Symp.

- Trifles, from every: Terb.

Cold become: Led.

Constitutional effects: ARN; Carb-v; Con; Glo; Iod; Lach; *Led*; *Nat-s*; Nit-ac; Pho; Stap; *Stro.*

INJURIES

Crushed: Arn; Con; Hypr; Rut; Stap.
Deep: Bels.
Dissecting: Ap; *Ars*; *Lach*.
Falls+: Stap; Stic; Sul; Tell.
Fester: *Anthx*; *Ap*; *Ars*; Echi; Led; Pyro.
Gaping (wounds): Hypr.
Glands, to: Bels; *Con*.
Head, to: See HEAD.
Height, falling from: Mill.
Incisions, cuts, stabs: Arn; Lach; *Pho*; Pul; *Stap*; Sul-ac.
Lacerated: Calend; Ham; Hypr; Stap.
Little, pains terribly: Colch.
Mental effects: Cic; *Glo*; Hypr; Mag-c; *Nat-s*.
Muscles, to: Rhus-t.
Nerves, to: Bels; Cep; *Hypr*; Pho; Pho-ac; Xanth.
Old: Cep; Symp.
- Pains, in: Cep; Kali-io; Sil; Symp.

Pains, returning: Glo; Kali-io; Nat-m; *Nat-s*; *Nit-ac*; Nux-v.
Pelvic organs, of: Bels.
Punctured, shot gun etc: Ap; Arn; *Hypr*; Lach; *Led*; *Nit-ac*; Plant+; Sul-ac.
- Perineum, to: Symp.
- Soles and palms to: *Hypr*; *Led*.

Reopening of old: Carb-v; Crot-h; Flu-ac; Lach; Nat-m; *Op*; *Pho*; *Sil*.
Salt, sprinkled, on as if: Sars.
Slight agg: Val; Ver-a.

INJURIES

Slow to heal (See HEALING difficult): Carb-v; *Hep*; Kre; Lach; Nit-ac; Petr; *Sil*; Sul.
Splinters, from: Cic; Hypr.
Tendons, to: Anac.
Twitching: Led.

INQUISITIVE: Agar; Aur; Lach; Laur.

INSANITY, mania, craziness: Amb; Ars; BELL; CUP; *Hyo*; Kali-br; Kali-chl; Lyc; Med; *Merc*; *Nux-v*; *Op*; STRAM; Syph; *Tarn*; VER-A; Vip.
Apoplexy, after: Hell.
Brutal: Abs.
Busy: AP; Kali-br.
Crazy things, does all sorts of: Gel+; Stram.
Depressive narcosis, alternating with: Ap; *Hyo*.
Erotic: *Ap*; *Bar-m*; Buf; Canth; HYO; *Orig*; Pho; *Plat*; Stram; *Tarn*; Ver-a; Zin.
- Menses, before: Dul; Stan.

Females, of: *Aco*; Ap; *Bell*; Cimi; *Orig*; Plat; *Pul*; Stram; Ver-a.
- Self accusation, from: Hell.
- Stupor, alternating with: Ap.

Haemorrage, after: Chin; Cup; Sep.
Head, washing in cold water amel: Saba.
Loquacious: Par.
Malignant: Cup.
Masturbation, after: Buf; *Cocl*; *Hyo*; Op.
Menses
- Before: Cimi.

INSANITY, menses
- Profuse, with: Sep.
- Suppressed, with: Ap; Ign; *Pul.*

Neuralgia, disappearance of, after: Cimi; *Nat-m.*

Overstudy, mental labour, from: Kali-p; Lach; Pho.

Periodical: Con; Nat-s; Plat.

Puerperal: Aur; Bell; Cam; Cimi; Cup; Hyo; Lyc; Plat; Pul; Sec+; Stram; Thu+; Ver-a; Ver-v.
- Modesty, lost+: Sec.

Quarrelsome: Hyo.

Religious: Anac+; Cam+; Lach+; Nat-c; Stram; Ver-a+.

Sexual excess, from: *Ap.*

Strength increased: Agar; Bell; Stram; *Tarn.*

Suicidal: Ars; Naj.

Suppressed, eruptions, after: Caus; Sul; Zin.

Sweat, cold, with: Stram.

Syphilitic: Syph.

Taciturn, alternating with+: Ver-a.

Urine, passes on the floor: Plb.

Wedding preparations of: Hyo.

INSECT
Bites: See INJURIES, bites.

Crawling: See CRAWLING and FORMICATION.

INSECURITY, sense of: Ail; Alo.

INSENSIBLE: See UNCONSCIOUSNESS and NUMBNESS.

INSOLENT, rude, haughty: Lil-t; Lyc; Lyss; Med; Pall; Par; PLAT, Sul; VER-A.

INSOMNIA: See SLEEPLESSNESS.

INSPIRATION
AGG: Crot-h; Ip; Kali-n; Lob; Mez; Nux-m; Spo; Sumb.

AMEL: *Colch*; Cup; *Ign*; Lach; *Spig*; Stan; Verb.

Cold
- Air amel: Sele.
- Expiration, hot: Sul.

Did not reach the pit of stomach: Pru-sp.

Nose, through, expiration through mouth, while lying on back: Chlor-hyd.

Short, jerking+: Ox-ac.

Slow, expiration quick: Stram.

INSTEP ulcer: Lyc.

INSULTS, on the look out for+: Caps.

INSUSCEPTIBILITY: See NUMBNESS.

INTELLECT: ACO; Anac; Aur; Bap; BAR-C; BELL; Cann; Cocl; HELL; HYO; Ign; LACH; Laur; LYC; Merc; Nat-c; Nux-v; OP; PHO; PHO-AC; *Plat*; *Pul*; *Rhus-t*; SEP; STRAM; *Sul*; VER-A.

INTEMPERANCE AGG: Stram.

INTERCOSTAL REGION: Aesc; Amy-n; Bry; Cimi; Mez; Ran-b; Sil; Verb.

Neuralgia: See PLEURODYNIA.

Plug sensation: Caus; Cocl; Lyc; Ran-sc; Ver-a.

INTERMITTENCY: ARS; Calc; Chin; Ip; Lach; Nat-m; Nit-ac; *Nux-v*; Pho-ac; *Pul*; Sec; Sul.

INTERMITTENT FEVER: See under FEVER.

INTERNAL AFFECTIONS: Calc; Canth; Nux-v; Pho.

INTERTRIGO: See under ERUPTIONS.

INTESTINES

Breaking, as if, bending on: Adon.

Bitten off, as if+: Pall.

Burning: Manc.

Cancer: Rut.

Cold
- As if: Plant.
- Balls running through, as if: Buf.
- Water flowing through, to anus: Mill.
  - menses, during: Kali-c.

Colds agg: Dul.

Contents, fluid as if were: Polyg.

Cord, bound and loosened, as if: Chio.

Eating, something in, as if+: Kali-bi.

Falling out, as if+: Kali-br.

Falls to side lain on: Merc.

Hanging down, as if: Agn; *Ign*; Psor; *Stap*.
- Bed turning in, when: Bar-c; Merc; Merc-c.

Inactive: Aeth; Phys.

Inflammation, high fever with: Ver-a.

Intussusception: Ars; Cup+; Op; Plb; Ver-a.

Knotted: Asaf; Elap; Saba; Sul; Ust; Ver-a.

Liquid, flows from stomach, to: Mill.

INTESTINES

Loose, shaking, and: Mang.
- Walking, while: Mang.

Marble, dropped down at stool as if: Nat-p.

Neuralgia: Cup-ar.

Obstructed, as if: *Op*.

Paraysis of: See under ABDOMEN.

Running, alive, in: Cyc.

Shivering, in: Arg-n.

Sore: Manc.

Stricture: Con.

Weak: Merc.

Worm, writhing along in, as if: Calad.

INTOXICATION: *Caps*; *Gel*; Lach; NUX-V; Op; Ran-b.

Easy: Bov; Con; Zin.

Feeling of+: Naj.

INTROSPECTION, introverted: *Cocl*; *Ign*; Mur-ac; Ol-an; *Pul*.

INTUSSUSCEPTION: See under INTESTINES.

IRIS: Bell; Merc; *Merc-c*; Nit-ac; Sul.

Haemorrhage after iridectomy: Led.

Inflammation: Arn; Merc-c; Rhus-t.
- Adhesions, with: Calc; Clem; Merc-c; Nit-ac; Sul; Terb.
- Hypopion, with: Hep; Merc; Sil.
- Prostate gland, with: Sabal.
- Syphilitic+: Stap.

Jagged: Sil; Stap; Thu.

Paralysis, of: *Ars*; Par.

Prolapse, cataract operation after: Alum; Stap.

IRREGULAR: See COORDINATION, disturbed.

IRRELIGIOUS: Anac; Colo; Croc; Laur; Kali-br.

IRRESOLUTE, vacillating, wavering: Anac; *Ars*; Asaf; Bar-c; Cocl+; *Grap*; Hell; *Ign*; Lach; Lyc; *Nux-m*; *Onos*; Op; Petr; Pho; PUL; Sul-ac+.

IRRITABLE: See ANGER.

  Children: Abro; Cham; Cina; Kali-p; Lac-c; Mag-c; Rhe.
  • Towards: Kali-io.

  Coition
  • Agg: Petr.
  • Amel: Tarn.

  Day time, only: Lyc; Med.

  Day and night: Cham; Lac-c; Op; Psor; Stram.

  Headache, during: Syph.

  Night, only: Ant-t; *Jal*; Lac-c; Nux-v; Psor; Rhe.

  Questioned, when: Arn; Cham; *Nux-v*; Pho-ac.

  Sends the doctor home, says he is not sick: ARN; CHAM.

  Sexual appetite, loss of, from: Sabal.

  Stools, before: Bor.

  Takes, everything amiss: See BAD, parts.

  Touched when: Ant-c; Tarn.

ISOLATED effects: Agar; Gel; Ver-a; Zin.

ITCH: See ERUPTIONS, itch like.

  Baker's, barber's: Ant-t; Cic; Grap; Lith; Mag-p; Phyt; Rhus-t; Scop+; Sul-io; Tell.

ITCHING: Aco; *Agar*; Amb; *Ant-c*; *Ap*; Ars; Bov; Bry; *Calc*; Carb-v; CAUS; Chel; Cist; Con; Fago; Grap; *Lyc*; Mag-c; *Merc*; Mez; Nat-m; *Nit-ac*; Nux-v; Ol-an; Op; Pho; Psor; *Pul*; Radm; *Rhus-t*; Sabi; Sep; *Sil*; Spo; *Stap*; *Sul*; Sul-io; Tarn; Thu; Urt.

Affected part, over: Agar.

Air
• Agg: Ars; Hep; Old; Petr; Rum.
• Amel: Stro.

Bathing
• After: Bov; Calc; Clem; Mag-c.
• Amel: Clem.

Bed in, agg: Kali-ar; Led; Pic-ac; *Psor*; Sil; *Sul*.

Biting: Agar; Led; Ol-an; *Old*; Pul; *Stap*; Urt.

Body all over+: Pall.

Burning: AGAR; AP; Ars; Bry; *Caus*; Grap; *Lach*; Lyc; *Petr*; Pul; *Rhus-t*; *Sil*; SUL; Thu.
• Hairy parts, of: Rhus-t.
• Mosquito bites, after+: Calad.
• Painful part, in: Alu.

Cold
• Agg: Clem; Thu; Tub.
• Amel: Berb; Calad; Fago; Grap; Mez.

Corrosive+: Vinc.

Crawling: Agar; Colch; Lyc; Plat; Plb; Pul; Rhus-t; Sep; Spig; Stap; Sul; Tarn; Tell.

Desquamation, with: Clem.

Diabetes, in: Mang.

Eating amel: Chel.

Erosive: Rut.

ITCHING

Eruption, without: Alu; Ars; Cist; Cup; Dol; Mez; Thyr.
- Night agg: Thyr.

Heat of stove amel: Clem; Rum; Tub.

Here and there+: Am-c.

Hot bath amel: Syph.

Internal (tickling): Amb; Ap; Caus; Coc-c; *Cham*; Cist; *Con*; Fer; Hyo; IOD; Ip; Kali-bi; Kali-c; *Lach*; Nat-m; NUX-V; PHO; Rhus-t; *Rum*; Sang; Sep; Stan; Sumb; Sul.
- Intolerable: Coc-c.

Intolerable+: Kali-ar.

Jaundice, in: Dol; Hep; Myr; Pic-ac; Ran-b; Thyr.

Meat agg: Rum; Rut.

Menses
- During: Kali-c.
- Amel: Cyc.

Mosquito bite, after: Calad.

Nausea, with: Lob.

Nervous: Arg-m.

Old people, in (pruritus senilis): Alu; Ars; Dul; Fago; Merc; Mez; Old; Sul; Urt.

Pain, alternating with: Stro.

Painful: Bar-c; Sil; Sul.

Pleasurable: Sul.

Pregnancy, in: Sabi; Tab.

Prickling, with: Lob.

Rubbing
- Changes place: Tub.
- Slowly, amel: Crot-t; Dios; Med.

Scratching
- Agg: Ars; Crot-t; Mez.

ITCHING, scratching
- Bumps form, after: *Dul*; Lach; *Mez*; *Rhus-t*; Ver-a.
- Changes, places: Mez; Stap.
- Eruptions, follow: Am-c; Old.
- Moisture, follows: Grap; Old; Radm; Rhus-t; Sele.

Scratch must: Agar; Arg-m; Cof; Psor; Stap.
- Until it bleeds: Alu; Arg-m; *Ars*; Cof; Psor.
- Until it is raw: Grap; Petr.

Soreness, with: Med.

Spots, in: Con; *Led*; *Sep*; *Sil*; *Sul-ac*; Zin.

Sweat agg: MANG; *Merc*; Rhod.

Thinking of it agg: Med.

Uncovering, undressing agg: Dros; Kali-ar+; Nat-s; Nit-ac; Nux-v; Old; Pall; Rhus-t; *Rum*; Stap; Tell; Tub.

Vomits, not relieved until he: Ip.

Warm on becoming: Aeth; Alu; Lyc; Merc; Psor; Sul; Urt.
- Bed, in+: Kob.

Wiping with hand amel: Dros.

JADED RAKES: *Agn*.

JARRING, shaking, stepping hard, riding (See SENSITIVE)

AGG: Alo; Anac; ARN; BELL; Berb; Bry; *Chin*; Cic; *Cocl*; Cof; Con; GLO; Hep; Kali-io; Lac-c; Lach; Led; *Nit-ac*; Nux-v; RHUS-T; Sang; SEP; SIL; Spig; Ther.

AMEL: Ars; Caps; Gel; *Nit-ac*.

Sudden agg: Vib.

JAUNDICE (See YELLOWNESS): Aesc+; Canc-fl; Card-m; Chio;

JAUNDICE ..
Iod; Lept; Mag-m; Myr; Nat-p; Pic-ac+: Tarx.
Abdomen, itching, with: Cham.
Anger, after: Nat-s; Nux-v.
Brain affection, in: Pho.
Chronic: Aur; Chel: *Con*; Iod; *Pho*.
- Relapsing: Sul.

Cider, from: Chio.
Concomitant, as a: Pho.
Diarrhoea
- During+: Dig.
- After: Chin.

Fever, with: Card-m; Vip.
Fright, from: Aco.
Fruits, unripe, from: Rhe.
Gall stones, with: Pod.
Haematogenous: Pho.
Headache, with: Sep.
Loss of vital fluids, from: Chin.
Lung symptoms, with: Card-m; Chel; Hyds.
Masturbation, after: Chin.
Menses, arrested, with: Chio.
Nervous excitement, from: Pho.
Newborn, infants: Aco; Bov; Chin; Elat; Myr; Nat-s.
- Stool, bilious, with: Elat.

Obstinate+: Choles.
Over eating, or rich food from: Carb-v.
Pregnancy, in: Aur; Pho.
Sexual excess, after: Chin.
Summer, every: Chio.
Urinary symptoms, with: Carb-v; Cham; Chin; Ign; Lyc; Nux-v; Plb.

JAWS
Upper: Am-c; Carb-v; Chin; Kre; *Pho*; Zin.
- Projects: Hep.
- Swelling: Nit-ac.
- Throbbing: *Pho*.

Lower: *Bell*; Caus; Cham; Cocl; Lach; Laur; Nat-c; Plb; Stap; Zin.
- Cold: Plat.
- Drawn backward, as if: Bell.
- Exostosis: Ang; *Calc-f*; Hep.
- Hard swelling: Anthx.
- Immovale, A.M. in: Ther.
- Motion
  - chewing+: Cup.
  - loud: Plb.
  - sleep in: Calc.
- Mouth opening agg: Hep.
- Necrosis: Merc-c; Pho+.
- Nodes, painful: Grap.
- Sore: Aur.
- Spasms: Tab.
- Swelling: Kali-c; Lach; Pho.
  - beneath right: Ol-an.
- Temples, to: Mang.
- Tension: Caus.
- Thickened: Hecla.
- Throbbing: Lach; Nat-m.
  - biting agg: Nat-m.
- Toothache, with: Sil.
- Twitching, trembling: Alu; Ant-t; Cadm; Carb-v; Cocl; Gel; Ol-an; *Pho*.
  - speak, on attempting to: Cocl.
  - yawning while: Old.
- Weak
  - eating, after: Bar-c.
  - feeling: Kalm.

JAWS
Ache: Merc; Phyt.
- Bending head back agg+: Sars.
- Sleep in, from clenching: Merc-i-f.

Angles, of: Ign; Merc; Phyt; Sang.
- Behind: Chel; Colch; Sang.
- Right: Radm.

Bones: Pho; Sil.
- Caries: Cist; Pho; Sil.

Boring: Plat.

Closure, spasmodic+: Dios.

Cracking, chewing, while: Lac-c; Nit-ac; Rhus-t.
- Mouth, opening wide, on: Saba.

Cramp: Kali-c+; Plat+; Tab; Ver-a.
- Chewing, on: Ver-a.

Dislocation, easy: Ign; Petr; *Rhus-t*; Stap.

Drop: See MOUTH, open.

Keeps closed: Kob.

Locked, clenched (lock-jaw): BELL; Cam; Cann; Cham; *Cic*; *Cup*; Hyd-ac; Hyo+; *Hypr*; Ign; Merc; Merc-i-f; NUX-V; Op; Phyt; Plat+; Sec; Tab; Ver-a.
- Emotional: Ign.
- Grinding of teeth with: Canth; Cic.
- Morning: Ther.
- Newborn, in: Amb; Cam.
- Sunstroke, from: Glo.

Painful: Caus.

Paralysed, as if: Nux-m.

Periosteoitis (lower): Calc-f.

Snap, shut: Bell; Cic; *Ign*; Lyss; Merc; Nux-v; Plat; Rhus-t.

JAWS
Stiff: Ap.
- Tired, and: Cham; Merc-i-f.

Wagging: See CHEWING, motion.

JEALOUSY: Ap; Hyo; Ign+; *Lach*; Lil-t; Pul; Stap.

Happy, seeing others: Hell.

Insane: Lach.

Irrational: Cocain.

JELLY, body were made of: Eupi.

JERKING pain: See under PAIN.

JERKS (See CONVULSIONS): *Bell*; Bor; Calc; Caus; Cic; Colch; Hyo; Hypr; Lyc; Meny; Merc; Nux-v; Plat; *Pul*; Rat; Sep; Spig; Stan; Sul; Sul-ac; Tab; Tarn; *Val*; *Zin*; Zin-io.

Convulsions, before: Ars; Bar-m; Laur; Ver-v.

Lightning like, head to foot: Hyd-ac.

Motion amel: Merc; Ther.

Night, at: Zin.

Pain, during: Colo; Ign; Lyc; Meny.

Painful: Rhod.

Paralyzed, part in: Sec.

Run, through whole body: Ign.

Side
- Lain on: Cimi.
- Not lain on: Onos.

Sleep, on falling to: *Ars*; cup; Ign; *Kali-c*.

Spinal origin: Thu.

Together: Ther.

JESTS, joking: *Caps*; Cocl; Cof; *Hyo*; Kali-io+; Lach; Op; Tarn.

JOINTS

Affections in general: Arn; Bell; *Benz-ac*; *Bry*; *Calc*; Caus; *Cham*; Cimi; COLCH; Dros; Dul; Grap; Guai; Kali-bi; Kalm; Led; Lith; Lyc; *Mang+*; MERC; Nat-m; Nux-v; Phyt; *Pul*; Radm; *Rhus-t*; Rut; *Sabi*; Sep; *Sil*; Stap; Stro; SUL.

Ankylosis, spurious, with: Kali-io.

Arthralgia: Arg-m; Symp.

Broken, as if: Par.

Colds agg: Calc-p; Rum.

Constriction in: Anac; Aur; Grap; Nat-m; Nit-ac.

Cracking in: Benz-ac; Cam+; Cann; Caps; Caus; Fer; Kali-bi; Led; *Nit-ac*; PETR; *Rhus-t*; Rut; *Sul*; Thu.
- Walking in open air agg: Rut.

Cramps: Calc; Pho-ac; Plat; Sul.

Crusts, on: Sep.

Deep, in: Cimi; Radm.

Deformed: See ARTHRITIS DEFORMANS.

Digging: Colch.

Dislocation spontaneous: See DISLOCATION, easy.

Dryness: Canth; Lyc; *Nux-v*; Pul.

Eruptions on: *Ars-io*; Bor; Clem; Dul; *Grap*; Kre; Merc; Pho; Psor; *Ran-b*; SEP; Sul; Thyr.

Fatigue+: Stap.

Give way, suddenly+: Pho.

Glistening: Mang.

Gritty feeling: Con.

Infiltrated: Mang.

Loose: Bov; Chel; Med; Pho-ac; Psor; Thu.

Nodes, hard, around: Form.

Oedema, about: Thu.

Oil, lacking in, as if: Gnap; Lil-t.

Peg, as of a: Buf.

Power, loss of: Med.

Quaking: Colch.

Red spots, on: Bell; Stic.

Rice bodies, in: Calc-f.

Rubbing, in: Con.

Skin, alternating, with: Stap.

Small: Act-sp; Benz-ac; *Caul*; Colch; Kali-bi; *Led*; Lith; Nat-p; Ran-sc; Rhod; Sabi; Sal-ac; Stic; Thu.
- Blisters on: Nat-c.
- Ulcers, on: Sep.

Sore, bruised: Arg-m; Aur; Lapp; Pul; Sul.

Sores, blisters: Ars; Bor; Lapp; Mez; Nat-c; Psor; *Sep*.

Sprained, easily: Pho; Rhus-t.

Stiff, little pain with: Pho.

Stitches, in: *Ap*; Colch; *Hell*; Kali-c; Mang; *Merc*; *Rhus-t*; Sil; Tarx; *Thu*.

Stretches, bends, or cracks: Caus.

Suppurating: Calc-hyp; Merc; Pho; Psor; Sil.
- Skin around: Mang.

Swelling
- Fatigue, slight agg: Act-sp.
- Oedematous, after fractures: Bov.
- Pale (white swelling): Ant-c; *Ars*; Colo; *Iod*; Kre; Merc;

JOINTS, swelling, pale ..
Pul; Rhus-t; *Sil*; Sul.
- Shining red+: Aco.

Synovitis: Ant-t; Ap; Bry; Calc-f; Iod; *Pul*; *Sil*; Sul.
- Chronic: Calc-f; Sil.

Thickened: Spo.

Tearing, very severe pain: *Arn*; *Chin*; Fer; *Guai*; *Hell*; *Hep*; Merc; Old; *Pul*; RHUS-T; Stro.

Tension, in: *Bry*; *Caus*; Led; Lyc; Nat-m; Pul; Seneg; Sep; *Sul*.

Tuberculosis, of: Ap; Calc; Calc-p; *Kali-c*; Kali-io; Pho-ac; Pul; Sil.

Ulcerated: Colo; Hep; Pho-ac; Sep; Sil.

Water in (hydrarthosis): Ap; Bry; Kali-io; Ran-b; *Sul*.

Weak: Aco; Arn; Bor; Bov; Calc; Kali-c; Lyc; Mang; Merc; Pho; Psor; Rhus-t; Sep; Sul.
- Dislocation, after: Rhe.
- Exertion agg: Pho.
- Pregnancy, during: Murx.
- Spasms, after: Rhe.

JOURNEY long, ill effects+: Cof.

JOYLESS+: Card-m.

JOYOUS (See CHEERFUL): Aco; Caus; *Cof*; Croc; Op.

Headache, during: Ther.

Misfortune, others, from: Ars.

JUMP
Animals, bed on, as if: Con.

Bed out of: Abs; Aeth; Bell; Cam; Chin; Hyo; Op; Stram.
- Crawls on floor, and: Acet-ac.

Bridge, crossing, when: Arg-n.

Dream, in: Calc-f.

Epilepsy, after: Arg-m.

JUMP
Everything seems to: Ther.

Height, from: Arg-n; *Aur*.

Runs and, recklessly: Saba.

Suddenly, pain, as from: Cina.

Tendency, to: Agar; *Aur*; Croc; Stram; Tarn.

Window, from: Aeth; Arg-m; *Aur*; Cam; Gel; Glo.

JUMPING AGG: Spig.

KELOID: *Flu-ac*; *Grap*; Nit-ac; Sabi; Sil.

KERATITIS: See CORNEA, inflammation.

KICKING: Bell; Lyc; Stram.
- Sleep, in: Bell; Sul.

KIDNEYS: *Ap*; *Ars*; *Berb*; CANTH; Helo; Kali-c; Merc-c; Polyg; Rhus-t; Samb; Scil; Scop; Solid; Stro; Terb.

Right: Berb; Coc-c; Lyc; Nux-v; Oci-c; *Sars*.

Left: Chin; Colo; Merc; Par-b; *Zin*.

Abscess (perinephritic): Ars; *Canth*; Chin; Hep; Lyc; Pul; Sil; Sul-io.

Ache: Helo; Phyt; Sep; Solid.

Bladder, to: Arg-n+; Nit-ac; Op+.

Bleeding: Merc-c.

Blowing nose, agg: Calc-p.

Breathing deeply agg: Arg-n; Benz-ac.

Bubbling: Berb; Med.

Burning: Nat-m; Nux-v; Pho; Pho-ac; Phyt; Sabi+; Sep; Terb.

Colic: Berb; Canth; Colch; Colo; Oci-c; Par-b; Polyg; Sars; Tab; Terb.

KIDNEYS, colic
- Glans, pressing amel: Canth.
- Haematuria, with: Oci-c.
- Urination, profuse, amel: Med.

Congested: Aco; Ars; Canth; Kali-bi; Scop; Solid; Terb.
Contracted: Dig; Nit-ac; Plb.
Dancing agg: Alu.
Distended: Helo; Solid.
Ear and eye symptoms, with: Vio-o.
Epigastrium to (left): Thu.
Floating, reflex symptoms, from: Bell; Ign; Stry-ar; Zin.
Fluttering: Brach; Chim.
Function, defective: Solid.
Heavy: Helo; Kali-bi.
Inactive: Benz-ac; Helo; Solid.
Inflammation (nephritis): Aco; Ap; Arn; Bell; Benz-ac; Cann; CANTH; Fer; Hep; *Kali-chl*; Lyc; Med; Merc-c; Nit-ac; Oci-c; Pul; Rhus-t; Samb; Solid; Stro; *Sul*; *Terb*; Thu.
- Bronchitis, with: Terb.
- Cardiac and hepatic affection, with: Aur; Calc-ar.
- Cold, exposure, from: Kali-c.
- Exanthema, after: Hep; Terb+.
- Frequency, of: Gel; Kali-p.
- Influenza, during: Eucal.
- Injury, from: Kali-c.
- Palpitation, with: Kali-ar.
- Pregnancy, during: Helo; Merc-c.
- Rheumatism, with: Radm; Terb.
- Scarlatinal: Ars; Canth; Hell; Hep; Terb.

KIDNEYS, inflammation
- Slow: Merc-c.
- Suppurative: Ars; *Canth*; Hep; Lyc; Merc; Polyg; Pul; Sil; Sul-io.
- Toxemic: Crot-h.
- Vomiting, with: Hell.

Laughing agg: Cann.
Lifting agg: Calc-p.
Lying on back, with knees drawn up amel: Colch.
Motion
- Agg: *Berb*; *Canth*; Chel; Kali-io.
- Amel: Thu.

Numb, region of: *Berb*.
Pressure
- Agg: Berb; Canth; Colch; Solid.
- Over: Thu.

Sneezing agg: Aeth; Bell.
Sore: Berb; Cadm; Grap; *Phyt*; Pul; Senec; Solid; Visc.
Standing amel: Berb.
Stretching legs agg: Colch.
Testicles, to: Dios; Op+.
Thighs, to: *Berb*; Ip.
Throbbing, pulsation: Berb; Sabi+.
Urination, after amel: *Lyc*; Med.

KILL
Desire to (See IMPULSES, horrid): Hyo; Iod.
Herself suddenly: Iod; Meli; Nat-s.
Threatens, to: Hep; Meli; Tarn.

KINDNESS agg: See SYMPATHY agg.

KISSES

KISSES everyone: Croc; Pho; Ver-a.

KLEPTOMANIA: Abs; Art-v; Cur; Nux-v; Tarn.

KNEADING bread or making similar motions agg: Sanic.

KNEELING

AGG: Cocl; Mag-c; Sep.

AMEL: Aesc; Euphor.

Difficult: Tarn.

Praying, and: Ars; Stram.

KNEES: Ap; Aur; Benz-ac; Caus; Chel; Chin; *Gel*; Kali-c; Led; Nat-m; Nux-v; Petr; Pul; Rhus-t; *Sep*; Sul.

Air, hot, through: Lach.

Ascending
- Agg: Alu+; Bad; Carb-v; Plb.
- And descending agg: Bad; Kali-c; Rut; Ver-a.

Bandaged: Anac+; Aur; Sil.

Bend suddenly, when standing: Arn; Cup.

Burning
- Below: Nat-s.
- In: Chel.

Catch, in: Nat-m.

Cold: Agn; Ars; Carb-v; Lach; Pho; Sep; Sil.
- Bed in: Pho.

Clutched by bird's claws, as if: Cann.

Contracted: Caus; Guai; Nat-m.

Cracking: Caus; Cocl; Con+; Sul.

Cramp: Calc; Colo; Terb; Zin.

Descending agg: Arg-m; Ver-a.

Drawn up involuntarily, while walking: Cup; Ign.

Effusion: Ap; Iod; *Rhus-t*; *Sul.*

KNEES

Elbow position amel: See LYING, hands and knees on amel.

Eruptions, on: Led.

Gnawing: Ran-sc.

Heaviness: Nux-v.

Hot, nose cold+: Ign.

House maid's: Nat-m.

Itching: Sul.
- Pain, with: Mang.

Jerking: Pul.

Jerks
- Absent: Cur; Oxyt; Sec; Sulfo.
- Increased: Lathy.

Kneeling
- Agg: Bar-c.
- Rising form agg: Spig.

Knock: Arg-n; Caus; Colch; Con; Glo.

Large, as if: Merc.

Neuralgia, pressure amel: Tarx.

Numb: Colo; Merc-i-f; Nat-p; Plat.
- Scrotum, extending, to: Bar-c.
- Sitting amel: Bar-c.

Paralysed+: Anac.

Restless: Anac; Lyc; Rhus-t; Thu.

Shocks, through: Pul; Val.
- Falling, asleep, on: Agar; Arg-m.

Spread apart: Lyc; Plat.

Sprained, as if: Elap.

Tension: Caus; Nat-m.

Throbbing: Kali-c.

Totter
- Ascending, on: Canth.
- Bend and, while walking: Bry.

KNEES

Tremble: Anac; Chin; Lil-t; Stan; Zin.
- Ascending stairs: Canth.
- Descending stairs: Sil.
- Standing, when+: Old.

Tubercular: Calc; Iod; Lyc; Sul.

Twitching, in: Chin.

Walking agg: *Chel*; Led.

Weak: Aur; *Cocl*; Con; Cyc; GEL; Mur-ac; Nat-m; Nat-s; Plb; *Sep*; Stap; Sul-ac.
- Ascending stairs: *Con*; Kali-c; Rut.
- Descending stairs: Gel; Kali-c; Rut.
- Emission, after: Dios.
- Kneeling, when: Tarn.
- Knock together, as if they would: Agar; Cocl; Colch; *Nux-v*.
- Lumbar ache, with: Kob.
- Nausea, with: Bor.
- Standing, when: Old.
- Walking, while: Cocl; Colo.

KNIFE, sight of AGG: Alu; Plat.

KNOT: See BALL.

KYPHOSIS: See SPINE, curvature of.

LABIAE: See VULVA.

LABOUR PAINS (See FEMALE ORGANS, labour like pains): Caul; Cimi; Gel; Kali-c; Kali-p; Pul.

Back, in: *Gel*; Petr.
- Downward: Nux-v.

Ceasing, weak: *Bell*; Cimi; Gel; *Kali-c*; Kali-p; Nat-m; *Op*; PUL; SEC.
- Shivering, nervous with: Cimi.

LABOUR PAINS

Easing: Caul; Cimi; Vib.

Eructations, with: Bor.

Excessive, laborious, violent: *Cham*; Pul; Sec; *Sep*.

False: Bell; Calc; Caul; *Pul*.

Fainting, causing: Cimi; *Nux-v*; Pul.

Inefficient: Caul; Cof; *Kali-c*; Nux-v; *Pul*.

Irregular+: *Caul*.

Spasms, with: Caul; Caus; *Cham*; Gel; HYO; Ign; *Pul*.

Upwards, going: Calc; Cham; Gel; Lach.

LACERATIONS: Calend; Stap.

LACHRYMAL

Duct: Ap; Fago; Hep; Merc-d; *Petr*; Plb; Sil; Stap.
- Obstructed: Merc-d.
- Pain, along: Fago.
- Stricture: Arg-m; Hep; Nat-m; Sil.

Fistula: Calc; Flu-ac; Nit-ac+; Petr; Phyt; *Pul*; Sil.
- Discharging on pressure: Nat-m; Pul; Sil; Stan.
- Eruptions on face, with: Lach.

Glands: Bro; Saba.

Inflammation: Iod.

LACHRYMATION: Ars; *Bell*; *Calc*; Caus; CEP; Colch; EUPHR; Flu-ac; Ip; Kali-p; Kre; *Merc*; *Nat-m*; Nit-ac; OP; *Pho*; PUL; *Rhus-t*; RUT; Saba; Sil; STAP; Stram; SUL; Thu.

Affected side agg: Lach; Nat-m; Nux-v; Pul; Spig.

LACHRYMATION

Air
- Cold, from: Dig; Sanic.
- Open agg: Saba.

AMEL: Phyt; Pru-sp.

Bending, head backward amel: Seneg.

Biting: Como.

Brain affections in: Dig; Kali-io; Zin.

Breathing deep, on: Grap.

Chill, with: Saba.

Cold: See Tears.
- Applications, from: Sanic.

Colds, during: Carb-v; Cep; Euphr; Sang; Tell; Verb.

Cough, with: Cep; Chel; Cup; Euphr; Grap; Nat-m; Pul; Saba; Scil.
- Whooping: Caps; Grap; Nat-m.

Dreams, during: Plant.

Eating agg: Ol-an; Zin.

Eyes
- Closed, with: Spo.
- Closing, on: Berb.
- Opening, on: Kali-bi.
  - forcibly: Ap; Con; Ip; Merc-c; Rhus-t.
- Using+: Stro.

Fever, during: Pul; Stram+.

Fire, looking, at: Mag-m; Merc.

Gushing: Am-c; Ip; Rhus-t.

Headache, during: Ap; Ign; Mez; Plat; Pul.

Heart symptoms, with: Am-c; Spo.

Hot, scalding: See Tears.

Larynx, tickling in, from: Chel.

Laughing, on: Nat-m.

LACHRYMATION

Light, bright, from: Dig.

Looking
- Broad day light when: Mag-m.
- Intently agg: Chel.

Lying agg: Euphr.

Menses, during: Calc; Phyt; Zin.

Morning, early agg: Calc; *Pul*; *Sul*.

Music, hearing: Grap.

Night agg: Ap; Nit-ac; *Zin*.

Pains
- Agg: Chel; Cinb; Lach; Mez; Nat-m; Plant; Pul; Ran-b; Saba.
- Throat, in: Sep.

Reading, while: Am-c; Croc; Old; Seneg; Stro; Sul-ac.

Room, in agg: Dig.

Sneezing, with: Just; Nat-m; Saba.

Spasms, alternating, with: Alu.
- Lids, lower of, after: Rut.

Sun, in agg: Bry.
- Looking, at: Stap.

Swallowing on: Arg-n.

Tears
- Acrid: Ars; Caus; Colch; Euphr; Led; Merc-c; Sul.
- Bloody, newborn, in: Cham.
- Brine, like: Bell.
- Burning, hot: Ap; Ars; Cadm; Cedr; Chin; Euphr; Grap; Phyt; Plb; Pul; Rhus-t; Sul; Verb.
  - sun, looking at: Sang; Stap.
- Cold: Lach.
- Easy, sheds+: Castr.
- Itching: Ars; Senec.

LACHRYMATION, tears
- Oily: Sul.
- Sticky: Plat.
- Suppressed: Sec.
- Thick: Tarn.
- Varnish mark, leave: Euphr; Grap; Nat-m; Petr; *Rhus-t*; Thu.

Throat, tickling in, with: Chel; Cocl.

Wind, in: Euphr; Pho; Pul.

Writing, while: *Calc*; Ol-an.

Yawning when: Ign; Nux-v; Saba; Stap.

LACK OF
Vital heat: See COLD agg.
Power: See CONTROL, lack of.

LACTATION
Affections of: Bell; Cham; Merc; *Pul*; Sep; Sil.

Milk
- Absent, scant: Agn; Alfalfa; BRY; *Calc*; Caus; DUL; LAC-C; *Lac-d*; LACT-V; *Lecith*; PUL; Stic; Urt; *Zin*.
  - night watching from: Caus.
  - parturition, after+: Urt.
- Altered: Bell; Merc.
- Bad, spoiled: Aeth; Bor; *Calc*; *Cham*; Merc; Sil.
- Bitter: Rhe.
- Bloody: Buf; *Cham*; *Phyt*.
- Blue, thin: Lach.
- Child refuses mother's: Bor; Calc; *Calc-p*; Cina; Merc; Rhe; Sil; Stan.
- Flowing: Calc.
  - as if: Dict; Kre; Nux-v; Pul.
- Increased: *Bell*; *Bry*; Calc; Phyt; *Pul*; *Sabi*.

LACTATION, milk, increased
- menses, before: Con.
- Painless gathering from not nursing+: Nux-v.
- Sour+: Acet-ac.
- Suppressed agg: Agar; Hyo; Mill.
- Thick: Bor; Kali-bi.
- Weaning, after: Con; *Lac-c*; Pul.
- Yellow: Rhe.

LAIN ON, parts AGG (See PRESSURE, agg and DIRECTIONS, side lain on): Cimi; Grap; Mos; Nat-m; Phys; Tell.

LAMENTING: See COMPLAINING.

LANCINATING: See PAIN, shooting.

LARYNX: Aco; *Arg-m+*; *Bell*; Bro; *Caus*; Cep; Dros; Hep; *Iod*; Kali-bi; LACH; Mang; Nux-v; PHO; *Pul*; Rum; Sele; *Spo*; Stan; Sul.

Right: Agar; Kali-n; Pul; Stan; Stic.

Left: Caus; *Crot-h*; *Hep*; *Lach*; Rhus-t; *Sul-ac*; Thu; Til.

Air, hot, from trachea: Rhus-t.

Bending backward
- Agg: Bell; *Lach*; Rum.
- Amel: Hep.

Blowing nose agg: Caus.

Burning, heat: Ars; Iod; Nit-ac; Rum; Sang; Seneg; Spo.
- Coughing, when: Gel+; Spo.
- Hoarseness, with: Am-m.

Closed, nearly, as if: Calc-f.
- Salivation with: Tarx.

LARYNX

Cold
- As if, on breathing: *Bro*; Cist; Rhus-t.
- Inspiration, hot expiration: Sul.
- Shaving amel: Bro.

Constriction, spasm: Aco; BELL; Cup; Ign; Iod; *Mang*; Meph; Mos; Pho; Samb; Stram; Ver-a.
- Auditory canal scratching, from: Sil; Sul; Tarn.
- Singing agg: Agar.
- Sleep
  - during: Lach; Nux-v; Spo.
  - falling to, on: Kali-c; Lach.
- Swallowing
  - on: Dig.
- Talking, while: Dros; Mang.
- Walking, amel: *Dros*.

Coughing
- Agg: Arg-m; Aru-t; Bell; Bro; Caus; Cep; Kre; Nux-v; Pho; Pul; Sul.
- Amel: Asar.

Crawling: Con; Kali-c; Nat-m.
Crumb, as if, in: Lach.
Cutting: Arg-m; Manc; Merc-c; *Merc-cy*; Nit-ac; Vinc.
- Coughing, on: *Cep*; Stap.

Downwards: Cham; Glo; Ip; Ver-a.

Drawn
- Backwards, with a thread, as if: Calc-ar.
- In: Ap.

Dry: Bell; Con; Lach; Seneg; Spo; Sul; Thyr.
- Singers in: Sang.
- Spot: con.

Ear to left: Zinc-chr.

LARYNX

Fissures in: Buf.
Flapping sensation: Lach.
Foreign substance, sensation: *Bell*; Kali-c; Sang.
- Fever, during: Ip.

Food drops into: Kali-c; Lach; Meph; Nat-m.
Full, singers, in: Sang.
Furry: Pho.
Grasps the: Aco; Ant-t; Aru-t; Asaf; Cep; Dros; Iod; Naj; Pho; Spo.
- Drinking, when: Aco.

Hair, in: Naj; Sil.
Hanging, in: Lach; Pho; Spo.
Leaflet, trachea over, as if: Ant-t.
Lifting agg: Sil.
Movement, up and down: Lyc; Op; Stram; *Sul-io*.
- Cough, with: Lach.

Mucous, in: Lyc; Pho; Seneg; Stan.
Numb: Kali-br.
Oedema, glotidis: Ap; Kali-io.
Painful, tender: Syph.
Paralysis: Caus; Lach.
Plug, wedge, valve etc: Lach; Pho; Spo.
- Trachea, closing, as if: Mang.

Polypus: Berb.
Pressure, on: Chel.
Rattling, in: Ant-t; Bro; Hep; Ip.
Rough, raw: Carb-v; Caus; Mang; NUX-V; PHO; Pul; Rhus-t; Spo; Stan; Sul.
- Talking, from: Arg-m; Tarn.

Singers of: Aru-t; Fer-p.

LARYNX

Skin in, as if: Pho.
Smoke inhaled, as if: Bar-c.
Streak: Caus; Ol-an.
Swallowing agg: Spo.
Talking, singing
- Agg: Cep; Pho; Spo.
- Amel: Rhus-t; Sele.

Tearing: Caps.
- Coughing on: Cep.
- Swallowing on: Ign.

Thickened: Led.
Tickling, in: Aco; Ap; Bro; Caps; Cham; Con; Ign; Kali-bi; Lach; Lyc; Nat-m; Nux-v; Op; Pho; Psor; *Pul*; Rhus-t; RUM; *Sang*; Sep; Sil; Stan.
Touch agg: Aco; Bell; LACH; *Pho*; *Spo*; Syph+.
Trachea, narrow, as if: Cist.
Tuberculosis of: Carb-v; Dros; Mang; Sele+; Spo; Stan.
- Cough and hoarseness, with: Stan.

Turning neck agg: Lach; Spo.
Upwards: Stan.
Vapour, as of a: Ars.
Vocal Cords
- Nodes, on: Sele.
- Oedema of: Lach.
- Paresis, of: Kali-p; Lach; Ox-ac; Seneg.
- Polypus, on: Thu.
- Spasms of: Ip.

Weak: Alu; Bar-c; *Caus*; Gel; Plb; Sul.

LASCIVIOUS: See AMOROUS.
Impotent, but: Sele.

LASCIVIOUS
Insanity: Hyo.
Ogling, women on the street: Calad; Flu-ac.
Prostate, enlarged, with: Dig.

LASSITUDE: See INACTIVE.

LAUGHING
AGG: Aco; *Arg-m*; *Ars*; Aur; Bell; BOR; Cann; Carb-v; Chin; *Cof*; Dros; Kali-c; Mang; PHO; Plb; STAN; Sul; Syph; Tell.
Aloud agg: Calc-f.
Excessive agg: Cof.

LAUGHS: Bell; Cann; Cic; Cof; Croc; Ign; *Hyo*; Nux-m; *Stram*.
Angry, or+: Lach.
Asthma, with: Bov.
Averse, to: Alu; Amb.
Cause, without: Syph.
Chorea, in: Caus.
Continuous: Cann.
Convulsions
- Before, during, after: Caus.
- Paroxysms, between: Alu; Plat.

Cries, and by turns: Asaf; Bov; Cof; Croc; Ign; Mos; *Nux-m*; Samb.
- Sleep, during+: Caus.

Eating, after: Pul.
Everything, at: Nux-m.
Foolish: *Hyo*.
Immoderately: Cann+; Fer.
Involuntarily: Croc; Ign; Mang; Pho.
- Pressure on spine, on: Agar.
- Speaking, when: Aur.
- Tears, with: Pho.
- Yawning, after: Agar.

LAUGHS
Loudly: Bell.
Menses, before: Hyo; Nux-m.
Nervous: Mos; Tarn.
Night, at: Stram.
Peculiar, to herself: Thyr.
Reprimands, at: Grap.
Screams, then: Tarn.
Serious matters, over: Anac; Cann+; Ign+; Nat-m; Pho; Plat.
Sexual excitement, with: Stram.
Sleep, during: Alu; Caus; Hyo; Lyc; Stram.
Spasmodic: Aur; Cup; Ign; Mos.
- Asthma, with: Bov.
- Epilepsy, after: Cup.

Tittering: Buf.
Trifles, over+: Cann.
Uncontrollable: Cann+; Caps+; Mos.
Weeps, and, by turns: Caps+; Ign; Sumb.
Wrong time, at: Plat.

LAUNDRY WORK AGG: Sep.
LAX: See RELAXATION.
LAYING HANDS on part amel: See HAND, laying on parts amel.
LAZINESS (See INACTIVE and INDOLENT): Ars; Caps; Chel; Chin; Lach; Nat-c; Nat-m; Nux-v; Sep; *Sul.*
LEAD agg: See DRUGS, abuse of.
LEAF, valve, skin, as of a: Alu; Ant-t; *Bar-c*; Fer; Iod; Kali-c; Kali-io; Lach; Mang; *Pho*; Saba; *Spo*; Thu.

LEANING
Against a support
- AGG: Cimi; Hell; Nit-ac; *Samb*; Ther.
- AMEL: *Carb-v*; FER; Gymn; Kali-c; Kali-p; Nat-c; Nat-m; Pho-ac; *Sep.*

Head, sideways: Cina.

LEAN people: See THINNESS.
LEARNS
Easily: Cam; Cof; Lach; Pho; Plat.
Poorly, with difficulty: Agn; *Anac*; *Ars*; *Bar-c*; Calc; Calc-p; Carb-v; Caus; Con; Nat-m; Old; *Pho*; Pho-ac.

LECHEROUS, lewd (See LASCIVIOUS): Flu-ac; Pic-ac.
Old men: Dig.

LECTOPHOBIA: See FEAR, bed.
LEECHES application of AGG: Sec.
LEGS (Lower limbs): Alu; *Ars*; Bell; *Calc*; CAUS; Grap; Kali-c; Lach; Led; LYC; *Mang*; Merc; Nit-ac; Nux-v; PUL; RHUS-T; Sep; SIL; SUL; Val; Zin.

Right: Ars; Bell; Bry; Colo; Grap; Lach; Nux-v; Pho; Pul; Rhod; *Sars*; Sec; Sep.
- Motion involuntary: Cocl.

Left: Amb; Asaf; Calc; Cina; Con; Fer; Hep; Lyc; Nit-ac; Rhus-t; Sil; Stram; Sul.
- To right: Mag-c.
- Trembling: Cic.

Alternating between: Aco; Alo; Ars; BRY; Calc-p; Cham; Cic; Colo; Cup; Dios; Grap; *Kali-bi*; Kali-c; Kali-n; Lach; Lil-t; Mag-p; *Nat-m*; Nat-s; *Pul*; *Rhus-t*; Sep;

LEGS, alternating between ..
Sil; *Sul.*

Aching: Ars-io; *Eup-p*; Gel; Guai; Helo; Lil-t; Med; Nit-ac; Pic-ac; *Phyt*; Polyg; Rhus-t; Sul-ac; Sul-io; Vario.
- Menses, before: Caul.
- Night, at: Med.
- Pregnancy, during: Ham.

Alternating with arms: See ARMS.

Band, about: Chin.

Bathing, cool amel: Aur; *Led*; Syph.

Bed, warmth of agg: Merc; Syph; Ver-a.

Belong, to him, not: See Not his own.

Below knees: Am-c; Calc; Lyc; Phyt; Pul; Sep; Sil; Stap; Sul-io.
- Burning: Nat-s.
- Jerking: Dig.

Blood rushes, to: Arg-m; Aur; Meph; Phel; Spo; Sul; Thyr.

Blotchy: Led.

Blue: Nux-v; Ox-ac; Vip.
- Menses, during: Amb.

Bones: Merc; Pho; Pul; Rut; Sil; Stap.

Bruised, as if: Caus; *Eup-p*; Gel; Rhus-t; Rut.

Burning: Ars; Crot-h; Nat-s; Pho-ac; Pic-ac.

Clammy: Lil-t.

Coition agg: Calc; Nat-m.

Cold: Calad; Carb-v; Dig; Lac-c; Tab.
- Chorea, in: Laur.
- Clammy: Laur.

LEGS, cold
- Day during, burn at night: Lathy.
- Icy: Calc; Jat.
- night, in bed: Lil-t.
- Pains: Syph.

Cramp: Cham; COLO; CUP; Kali-m; Med; Stro; *Sul*; Vip.
- Extending agg: Calc.
- Pressing foot on floor amel: Cup-ar; Zin-io.

Crosses: Gel; Lil-t; Murx; Rhod; *Sep*; Thu.

Crossing
- Agg: *Rhus-t.*
- Amel: Ant-t; Lil-t; Murx; Rhod; Sep; Thu.
- Impossible: Lathy.

Descending agg: Arg-m.

Down to feet, pain: Alu; Caps; Lyc; Pul; Rhus-t.
- Burning: Pho-ac.

Drawn up: Arg-n.

Dropsy: Ant-t; Eup-p; Samb.

Elevating amel (See ELEVATING LIMBS amel): Bar-c; Grap; Ham; Sep.

Elongated, as if: Colo; Kali-c; Kre; Rhus-t; Sul.

Emaciation: Abro; Nux-v; Rhus-t; Sele+.

Eructation amel: *Pul.*

Fever, in agg: Pyro; *Rhus-t*; Tub.

Flexes when changing position: Hell.

Floating: Aco; Pho-ac; Spig; Zin-io.

Formication: Calc; Nux-v; *Sec*; Sep.

LEGS

Fulness, bursting: Ham; Vip.
- Fever, during: Chin-s.

Hanging out of bed amel: Ver-a.

Heat, flushes, of: Kob.

Heavy: Alu; Calc; Gel; Kali-c; Med; Nat-c; Pho; Pic-ac; Pul; Rhus-t; Rut; Sul.
- Ascending agg: Med; *Nat-m*; Pho.
- Exertion agg: *Gel*; Pic-ac.
- Feet glued to the floor: Pho.
- Lead like, while walking: Med.
- Painful: Bov.
- Sitting while: Alu.

Hot wind or wire darting through, as if: Dig.

Immobile: Ox-ac.

Inverted: Cic; Merc; Nux-v; Petr; *Psor*; Sec.

Itching: Agar; Calc; Caus; Mez; Rhus-t; Sil; Sul.

Jerking up: Lach; *Lyc*; Myg.
- Lying down, on: Meny.
- Pain, with: Lyc.

Lift cannot, when lying down: Lathy.

Long, too, as if when standing: Kre.

Many, as if: Pyro.

Not his own, as if: Agar; Bap; Coll; Op.

Numb: Calc; Cup-ar; *Grap*; Kali-c; Onos; Ox-ac; Plant; Plb; Pul; Rhus-t; Tarn; Thyr.
- Right: Cedr; Eup-p; *Kali-c*; Nux-m; Zin.
  - arm, left: Tarn.

LEGS, numb
- Crossing on: Agar; Alu+; Kali-c.
- Menses, during: *Pul.*
- One, other painful: Sil.
- Sitting cross legged, on: Alu.
- Standing long agg: Pul.
- Walking, while: *Kali-n*; Rhus-t; Sep.

One
- Motion constant, of: Bry.
- Shorter than other, as if, while walking: Cinb.

Oozing from, oedematous: *Grap*; LYC; Tarn-c.

Padded, as if: Arg-n.

Paralyzed, as if: Cup-ar.
- Dinner agg+: Tub.

Petechiae: Ap; Led; Solid.

Presses foot to floor: Ign; Med; Zin-io.

Pressure amel: Ars; Mag-p.

Red hot wire: See Hot wind or wire.

Restless: Agar; *Ars*; Carb-v; Kali-c; Med; Nit-ac; *Rhus-t*; Sul; *Tarn*; Tub; ZIN.
- Menses, during: Lac-c.
- Night, at: Ars; Caus; Med; Tarn.

Rotation agg: Bry; Cocl; Colo; Kali-c.

Separated, as if, on standing: Pho.

Severed, belonging to someone else: Op.

Shock, electric: Caus.

Shooting up: Guai; Nux-v.

LEGS

Shortened, as if: Amb; Colo; Mez; Old; Pho; Sep.
- Numb, and: Merc.

Stiff, as if: Nux-v.

Stocking, elastic, covered with, as if: Pic-ac.

Stool agg: Ap; Sec; Ver-a.

Stretch, inclination to, or must: Cina; Sul-ac.

Stretching amel: Med.

Swaying to and fro, while standing: Cyc.

Sweat: Euphr; Mang; Petr; Pod.
- Cold: Pul; Terb.

Tension, alternating with anus: Kali-m.

Tied together, as if: Syph.

Tingling: Grap; Kali-c; Lyc; Petr.

Trembling: Arg-n; Cimi; Lach; Nit-ac; Nux-v; Op; Plant.
- Coition, after: Nat-p.
- Walk, can scarcely: Cimi.

Twitching: Anac; Merc; Pho; Phys; Tarn.
- Lying agg: Meny.

Ulcers: Flu-ac; *Lach*; Sul-io.
- Climaxis, at: Polyg.
- Gangrenous: Rhus-t.

Uncovering agg: Hep; Rhus-t; Sil; Thu.

Varices: *Carb-v*; Caus; *Ham*; Lyc; *Pul*; *Zin*.
- Inflammation, after: Calc-ar.

Vexation, felt in: Nux-v.

Weak: Ars; *Cocl*; *Con*; GEL; Mang; Nat-m; Nat-s; *Nux-m*; *Nux-v*; Onos; Pho-ac; Plb; *Rhus-t*; Sep; Sul; Tarn; Zin.

LEGS, weak, descending
- Back, sprain, from: Rut.
- Descending agg: Arg-m; Sil.
- ascending, and agg: Rut.
- Hips, spot between, from: Phys.
- One, epilepsy, after: Cadm; Pho.
- Paralytic: *Cocl*; Rut+; Thu.
- pregnancy during: Agar; Plb.
- Parturition, after: Caus; Rhus-t.
- Rising from chair: Rut.
- Sciatica pain, from: Grat.
- Sitting down, when: Stan.
- Smoking, from: Clem.
- Uncertain: Mang.
- Walking agg: *Nux-m*.

Weather changes agg: Phyt.

Wind, cool, blowing on, as if: Lil-t.

Wooden sensation: Arg-n; Ars; Rhus-t.
- Walking while: *Kali-n*; *Thu*.

LENS: Euphr; *Pul*; Sil; *Sul*.

Cataract: *Calc*; Calc-f; Calc-p; CAUS; Euphr; Kali-m+; Mag-c; Naph; Pho; Sec; SIL; SUL.
- Capsular: Am-m.
- Incipient and progressive+: Chim.
- Injuries, from: Con.
- Lachrymation, with: Euphr.
- Menses absent, with: Lyc.
- Ocular lesions, from: Tell.
- Operations, after: Seneg.
- Senile: Carb-an; Sec.
- Women, in: Sec+; Sep.

LEPROSY: Ars; Crot-h; Hydroc; Sec; Sep; Sil; Sul.

LETHARGY: See INACTIVE.

LEUCOCYTHEMIA: See LEUKEMIA.

LEUCODERMA: Alu; Ars; Ars-s-fl; Calc-f; Merc; Nat-c; Nat-m; Sele; Sep; *Sil*; *Sul*.

LEUCORRHOEA: *Alu*; Ars; Calc-s; Carb-an; Caus; *Grap*; Hyds; Iod; Kali-c; *Kre*; Med; MERC; *Nat-m*; Nit-ac; Plat; *Pul*; SEP; Sil; Stan; Sul.

AGG: Chin; Kalm; Kre; Merc; Nat-m; Plat; Psor; Sep.

AMEL: Carb-v; Murx; Phyt.

Acrid, corroding: Agar+; *Alu*; Am-c+; Ars; Bor; Caul; Con; Fer; Flu-ac; Grap; Kali-bi; Kali-io; *Kre*; Lil-t; Lyc; Merc; Nit-ac; *Pho*; Pru-sp; *Pul*; Rut; Sabi; Sang; *Sec*; Sep; Sil; *Syph*.
- Albuminous: Bor; Mez.
- Children in+: Cub.
- Thighs and linen: Iod.

Blackish: Bur-p; *Chin*; Kre.

Blistering: Am-c; Kre; Med; Pho.

Bloody: Calc-s; Chin; Cocl; Murx; Nit-ac; Sep.
- Menses
  - after: Chin; Zin.
  - instead of: Chin.
- Stools, during: Murx.
- Water: Calc; Kre; Mang; Nit-ac.

Bluish: Amb.

Briny: Sanic.

Brown: Iod; *Lil-t*; *Nit-ac*; Sec; Ust.
- Stains: Lil-t; *Nit-ac*.

Burns, hot: *Bor*; Calc; Calc-s; Hep; *Kre*; Lept; Lil-t; Pul; Sep; Sul.

LEUCORRHOEA, burns
- Abdominal pain, after: Calc-p.
- Watery: Hyds.

Climaxis, at: Psor; Sang.

Coition
- After: Nat-c; *Sep*.
- Amel: Merc.

Colic, after: Am-m; Calc-p; Con; Lyc; Mag-c; Mag-m; Sil; *Sul*.

Constant: Am-m; Sec.

Copious: Am-c+; Ars; Asaf+; Calc; Caul; Flu-ac; Grap; Hyds; Merc-i-r; Sep; Sil; Stan; Sul-io; Thu+.
- Menses, like: Alu; Caus; Kre.
- Serum like discharge from anus and vagina: *Lob*.

Day only: Lac-c; Plat.

Day time agg+: Alu.

Dirty: Sec.

Exhausting: Cocl; Frax; Senec; Visc.

Flatus passing agg: Ars.

Flowing down, thighs: Alu; Lept; Lyc; Lyss; Onos; *Senec*; Syph; Tub.
- Imperceptibly: Agn.
- Warm water: Bor+; Lept.

Girls, little: Calc; Caul; Mang; *Merc*; Senec; Sep.
- Acrid: Cub.
- Infants: Cann.
- Yellow: Merc-i-f.

Glairy: Pall.

Gonorrhoeal: Nit-ac; Pul; Sabi; *Sep*.

Greenish: Asaf+; Carb-v; Merc; Merc-i-r; Nat-m; Nat-s; Nit-ac; Sep.

LEUCORRHOEA

LEUCORRHOEA, greenish
- Acrid: Merc-i-r.
- Stains: Bov; Lach; Thu.
- Water: Sep.

Gushing: Calc; Grap; Kre; Lyc; Mag-m; Psor+; Sil; Stan.
- Cramp, with: Mag-m.
- Squatting, when: Cocl.

Headache, with: Plat.
Honey coloured+: Nat-p.
Hot: See Burns.
- Water like+: Bor; Hep; Lept.

Itching, causing: Carb-ac; Helo; Hyds; Kre; Stap; Syph.
Labour like pains, with: Dros; Kali-c+.
Long lasting+: Myr.
Lumpy, curdy: Bor; Helo; Hep; Kali-c+; Psor+; Radm; Sep; Sil.
- Clear: Tarn.

Lying, while: *Pul.*
Mammae sore, with: Dul.
Masturbation, from: Canth; Plat; *Pul.*
Meat water, like: Kali-io.
Membranous: Hep.

Menses
- Before: Bov; Calc; *Grap*; Kre; *Sep*; Sul-io.
- And after: Grap; Pall; Sul-io.
- During+: Iod.
- After: Bov; Calc; Calc-p; *Grap*; *Kre*; Mag-c; Tab.
- Between: Bor; Calc; Sep.
- Instead of: Ars; Cocl; Grap; Nat-m; Nux-m; Pho; Sep; Xanth.
- Scanty, with: Calc-p: *Caus.*
- Week one, after: Kalm.

LEUCORRHOEA

Milky: Calc; Fer; Lyc+; *Pul*; Sep.
Night agg: Caus.
Offensive: Arg-m; Ars-io+; Asaf+; *Carb-ac*; Hep; *Kali-p*; Kre; Nit-ac; Nux-v; *Psor*; Sabi; Sec; Sep; Ust.
- Forceps delivery, after: Calend.
- Purulent+: Buf.

Periodical: Lyc.
Piles, suppression, from: Am-m.
Pregnancy, during: Cocl; Kali-c; Kre; Sabi+; Sep.
Puberty, at: Fer.
Purulent: Hep; Kali-p; Pru-sp; Sep.
Rising from seat agg: Plat.
Serous, fluid: Tab.

Sexual excitement
- From: Canth; Hyds; Pul; Senec.
- With: Ign.

Sitting, while: Ant-t.
Smell
- Cheese old, like+: Hep.
- Fishy+: Med.
- Green corn, like: Kre.
- Menses, like: Caus.
- Sour: Hep; *Nat-p.*
- Sweetish: Calc-p; Merc-c.

Squatting agg: Cocl.
Stains, indelibly: *Bur-p*; Mag-c; Med; *Pulex*; Sil; Vib.
Standing agg: Lac-c.
Starch boiled, like: Bor; Fer-io; Nat-m; Sabi.
Sticky, stringy: Alet+; Hyds; Kali-bi; Nit-ac; Sabi; Tarn.
Stiffens, linen: Lach.

LEUCORRHOEA
Stool
- During: Fer-io; Sanic.
- After: Mag-m; Vib; Zin.

Stooping agg: Cocl.
Stubborn: Mez.
Thick: Ars; Calc; Calc-s; Carb-ac; Hyds; Kali-bi; *Merc*; Murx; *Senec*.
- Acrid: Bov; Hyds.
- Creamy: Calc-p; Nat-p; Pul; Sec.
- Profuse, as menses: Mag-s.

Thin, watery: Fer; Grap; Lept; Lil-t; Nit-ac; Pru-sp; Pul.
Transparent, imperceptible+: Agn.
Urinary symptoms, with: Berb; Erig.
Urinating agg: Am-m; Calc; Kre; Merc; Plat; Sep; Sil.
Urinous: Ol-an.
Vagina, pressure in, with: Cinb.
Walking agg: Aur; Bov; Lac-c; Mag-m.
Washing amel: Kali-c.
White: Alet+; Bor; Calc-p; Grap; Merc; Nat-m; Sep.
- Stains linen yellow: Chel.
- Turns green: Nat-m.

Yellow: Ars; Calc; Cham; Gel; Hyds; Kre; Merc-i-f; *Murx*; Sabi+; Senec; Sep; Sul; Ust.
- Stains: Agn+; Carb-an; Chel; *Kre*; Nit-ac; Pru-sp.
  - green: Bov.

LEUKEMIA: Ars; Ars-io; Bar-io; Bar-m; Benz; Nat-m; *Nat-ar*; *Nat-s*; Pho; Pic-ac; Thu.

LEUKEMIA
Splenic: *Cean*; *Nat-s*.

LEVITATION: See FLOATING, as if.

LEWD: See LECHEROUS and LASCIVIOUS.

LICE (lousiness): Lyc; *Merc*; *Old*; Psor; Saba; *Sul*.
- Itching of: Led.

LICHEN: See ERUPTIONS, lichen.

LICKING LIPS
Agg: Val.
Tongue, with amel: Mang.

LIE DOWN
Inclination, to: See INACTIVE.
- But, thereby agg: Alu; Murx.

Must: Ap.
Will not, sits up in bed: Kali-br.

LIENTERIA: See DIARRHOEA after eating, drinking.

LIFE
Burden, is+: Alo.
Satiety, of: See SUICIDAL, disposition.
Unfit, for: Sep.
Unworthy: *Nat-s*; Plat.

LIFELESS BODY, restless mind+: Bap.

LIFTED UP sensation: Hypr; Pho; Strop.
Sleep, during: Strop.

LIFTING
Agg (See SPRAINS): ARN; BRY; *Calc*; Calc-p+; Carb-an; Caus; Con; Grap; Led; Nat-c; Onos; Pru-sp+; Psor; *Pul*; Rhus-t; Sep; *Sil*; Stro; *Sul*; Val.

LIFTING
AMEL: Spig.
Over AGG: Amb; Agn; Carb-v; Form; Grap; Lyc; Sep.

LIGAMENTS: See FIBROID TISSUE.

LIGHT as if: See FLOATING.
Body, feels: Mez.
- Onanism from or hysterical: Gel.

LIGHT
AGG: Aco+; Aesc; Ap; Arg-n; *Ars*; Bar-c; BELL; CALC; Chin; *Con*; Dros; EUPHR; *Glo*; *Grap*; Hep; Hyo; Lac-d; *Lyc*; Mag-p; *Merc*; *Merc-c*; Nat-m; *Nat-s*; *Nux-v*; Op; *Pho*; Pho-ac; Pul; *Rhus-t*; Sang; SEP; *Sil*; *Stram*; *Sul*.
- But cannot bear covering: Ap.
- Little even: Lac-d.

AMEL, darkness AGG: Am-m; BELL; Calc; Cann; Carb-an; Carb-v; *Gel*; Lyc; Plat; STRAM; *Stro*; Val.

Artificial fire, light AGG: Bell; Calc; Caus; Con; Dros; *Euphr*; Glo; Lyc; MERC; Nat-m; Pho; Rut; Sep; Stram.
- Read, cannot, in: Nat-m.

Blue AGG: Tab.
Bright, bright objects AGG: *Bell*; Buf; Canth; Stram; Thu.
Gas AGG: Caus; Glo; *Merc*; Nat-c; Nat-p.
Moon: See under MOON.
Reflected AGG: Sep.
Snow, from AGG: Ant-c; ARS; Cic; *Glo*.

LIGHT
Stained glass from AGG: Ant-c; Nat-s.
Subdued AGG: Nat-s.
Sun
- AGG: *Ant-c*; Bell; Chin; Euphr; *Glo*; Grap; Kali-bi; Lith; *Nat-c*; Sele; Sul.
- AMEL: Anac; Con; Crot-h; Iod; Kali-m; *Plat*; Rhod; *Stro*; Thu.
- Blinds: Lith.

LIGHTNING: See PAIN, shooting.
Agg+: Crot-h.

LIMBS
Upper: See ARMS.
Lower: See LEGS.
Alternating between upper and lower: See ARMS.
Bandaged: Chin; *Plat*.
Belong to her, did not: Agar, Ign; Op.
Brittle: Radm.
Clammy: Cam; Carb-v; Pic-ac.
Cold: Calc-p.
- Digestion, affection of with: Calc-p.
- Moist: Stic.
- Water, as if in: Led.

Constriction: Chin; Lyc.
Cramp: Amb; Cimi; Ran-b; Vip.
Crawling: Calc-p.
Crossing agg: See CROSSING LIMBS.
Dead, as if: Lyc.
Diarrhoea, with: *Cup*; Jat; Set.
Deep breathing agg: Cann.

LIMBS

- **Detached** (See DISLOCATED sprain, as if): Hypr.
- **Double, as if:** Petr.
- **Drawing up agg and amel:** See under DRAWING.
- **Drawn up like hedge-hog:** Colo.
- **Eating**
  - Agg: Clem; Ind.
  - Amel: Nat-c.
- **Elevating amel:** See ELEVATING LIMBS.
- **Emaciated, with plump body:** Plb.
- **Eyes alternating, with:** Kre.
- **Formication:** Lyc; Pho-ac; Rhus-t; Sec; Stro; Tarn.
  - Menses during: Grap.
- **Hanging down agg:** See HANGING down limbs agg.
- **Hard:** Radm.
- **Heated, being agg:** Zin.
- **Heavy+:** Ap.
- **Herpes, on:** Manc.
- **Immovable+:** Ap.
- **Jerks:** Phys.
  - Cough, with: Stram.
  - One, sleep in: Ant-t; Sul.
  - Spasms, during: Sil.
- **Lying agg:** Kali-c.
- **Numb:** Aco+; Ap+; Calc-p; Echi.
  - Left: Pul.
  - One more, than other: Crot-h.
- **Paralyzed, as if:** Thu.
- **Restless:** Tarx.
- **Shattered, as if:** Mez.
- **Short, as if:** Mez; Mos.
- **Tosses, from side to side:** Cina.
- **Touch agg:** *Chel*; Chin.
- **Trembling:** Merc.
- **Weak, after eating:** Clem.

LINEA NASALIS: See FACE, pale.

LINEAR PAINS: See under PAIN.

LIPS: Ars; Aru-t; *Bell*; Bry; Nat-m; *Rhus-t*; Sep; Sil; *Sul*.

Upper: Bar-c; Carb-v; Kali-c; Sul; Zin.
- Cracked: Kali-c; Nat-m.
- Hair (in women): Ol-j.
- Heavy: Caus.
- Numb, as if: Cyc.
- Red: Ars-io; Calc; Nat-m.
- Retracted: Ant-t; Cam.
- Stiff: Euphr.
- Sweat, on: Kali-bi; Med; Rhe.
- Swelled: Bar-c; *Calc*; Hep; Nat-m; Nit-ac; Psor; Sul.
  - turned up: Merc-c.
- Twitching, trembling: *Carb-v*.
- Weak: Card-m.

Lower: Bry; Ign; Pul; Sep.
- Biting of, while eating: Benz-ac.
- Cracked: Sep.
- Centre: Pul.
- Crawling, bug, as if: Bor.
- Heavy, as if: Grap; Mur-ac.
- Numb: Glo.
- Red: Sep; *Sul*.
- Swelled: Asaf; Lach; *Merc*; Sep; *Sul*.
  - as if: Glo.

LIPS, lower
- Tremble, while eating: Arn.

Abscess: Anthx.

Black: Aco+; ARS; *Chin*; Merc; Pho-ac; Ver-a.
- Blisters: Tub.

Bleeding: *Aru-t*; Bap+; Lach.

Bloated: Mur-ac.

Blue: Acet-ac; Ant-t; Arg-n; *Cam*; CUP; DIG; Hyd-ac; Lach; *Lyc*; Mos; *Nux-v*; Spo; Ver-a.
- Chill, during: Nat-m.
- Convulsions, during: Nux-v.
- Menses, during: Arg-n; Cedr.

Brown: Rhus-t.

Burning: Am-m+; Mur-ac; Saba; Thyr.
- Fire like+: Am-m.
- Smokers in: Bry.
- Touched, when: Merc.

Cancer: Ars-io+; Cic; Cist; Clem; Con; Cund; Hyds+; Sil+.

Changing colour: Sul.

Cold sores: See Herpes.

Corners
- Cold: Aeth.
- Cracked: *Aru-t*; *Cund*; GRAP; Mag-p; Merc-c; Mez; *Nit-ac*; Psor; Sil.
  - right: Merc.
- Crusty scaly: Grap; Merc; Nit-ac; Thu.
- Droop: Agar.
- Indented: Sil.
- Inflamed: Sil.
- Raw: Ant-c; Aru-t; Grap.

Cracked: Ail+; Alo+; Am-m+; ARS; *Aru-t*; Bap+; BRY; Calc;

LIPS, cracked ..
Calc-p; Carb-v; Chin; *Grap*; Ign; Lach; Meny; Merc; Mur-ac; NAT-M; Pul; Rhus-t; Sep; Sul.
- Middle: Calc; *Cham*; Hep; *Nat-m*; Pho; *Pul*; Sep.

Cramps: Ran-b.

Crawling, as of bugs: Bor.

Crusty, scaly: *Ars*; Mur-ac; Nat-m; Pho+; Pho-ac; *Rhus-t*; Sep; *Sil*; Stap.

Drawn up, retracted: Ant-t; *Cam*; Nux-v; Phyt; Tab.

Droop: Bar-c; Merc; Nux-v.

Dry: Alo+; Am-m+; Ant-c; Bry; Caus; Hyo; *Nux-m*; Pho+; *Pul*; *Rhus-t*; Sul; Thyr; Ver-v.

Egg albumin on: Ol-an; Pho-ac.

Epithelioma: Cic+; Sep.

Everted (See drawn up): *Ap*; Rhyt.
- Swollen: *Merc-c*.

Formication: Bor.
- Menses, during: Grap.

Glued, together: Cann; Stram.

Hang down: Ver-a.

Heavy: Mur-ac.

Herpes, vesicles on: *Ars*; Dul; Manc; NAT-M; Pho; *Rhus-t*; Sep; Sul-io.
- Black: Tub.
- Hard small: Calc-f.
- Inner side: Med.
- Menses, during: Sars.

Itching: Ap; Nit-ac.

Jerking, twitching: *Carb-v*; Cham; Ol-an; Senec; Tell; Thu; Vip.
- Cold air, in: Dul.

LIPS, jerking
- Convulsions, during: Sil.
- Speaking, while: Arg-n.
- Up: Tell.

Licking AGG: Val.

Licks: Agar; Alo; Ars; Kre; Lyc; Nat-m; Phys; *Pul*; Stram.
- Thirst, without+: Kre.

Move, as if speaking: Hell.

Neuralgia: Ap.

Numb: Aco; Crot-h; Nat-m; Old.

Oedema: Ap.

Pale: Ars; Fer; Hyd-ac; Kali-ar; Med.

Peeling: Aru-t; Cham; Con; Kali-c; *Lac-c*; Nat-c; *Nat-m*; Nit-ac; Nux-v; Pul; Thyr.

Picking, at: Ars; *Aru-t*; *Bry*; Hell; Kali-br; Nit-ac; Nux-v; Tarn.

Pouting, thick: Bar-c; Calc; Grap; Merc; Nat-m; Psor; Syph.
- Belly big, with: Syph.

Red: Alo; *Ars*; Bell; Merc-c; *Sul*; Thyr; Tub.

Retracted: See Drawn up.

Salty: Merc; Nat-m; Sul.

Scabby: See Crusty.

Scarlet: Strop.

Shrivelled: Am-m+; Ant-t.

Slimy: Kali-io, Stram; Zin.

Smacking, of: Amy-n.

Sordes, on: *Ars*; Colch; Hyo; Pho; *Stram*.

Sore: Lyc; Mur-ac.

Sticky: Merc-i-r; Nux-m; Zin.

Stiff: Ap; Euphr; Kalm; Lach.

LIPS

Swelled: Ail+; Ap; ARS; Aru-t; *Bell*; Bry; *Lach*; *Merc-c*; Nat-m; Nit-ac; Op; Sep.

Thickened: Med.

Tingling: Nat-m; Pic-ac.

Touch, least agg: Cadm.

Tremble
- Eating, while: Arn.
- Speaking, while: Arg-n.

Twitch, spasm: See Jerking.

Ulcerated: Bor; Stram.

Veins, distended: Dig.

Vesicles: See Herpes.

LITHEMIA: See URIC ACID diathesis.

LIVELY: See CHEERFUL.

LIVER (including right hypochondria): *Aesc*; Alo; Am-c; Am-m; Ars; AUR; Bar-c; BELL; *Berb*; *Bry*; Card-m; CHEL; CHIN; Cocl; Colch; Dios; Gel; Hyds; Iris; KALI-C; LACH; Lept; LYC; *Mag-m*; Merc; *Nat-s*; Nit-ac; Nux-m; NUX-V; PHO; *Pod*; Rhe; Sang; *Sep*; Sul; Ust+.

Abscess: Bell; Bry; *Hep*; Lach; Merc-c; Nux-v; Pul; Rut; Sep; *Sil*; Ther.
- Forming, as if: Laur.

Anger agg: Cocl.

Arm right, and: Bry; Iris.

Athophy: Aur; Calc; Hyds; Laur+; Pho.
- Acute yellow: Pho.
- Nutmeg: Laur; Lyc.

Back, of: Arn; Bor; Calc; Echi; Kali-bi; Lept; Rhus-t; Thu.

LIVER

Backward, extending to scapula: Berb; *Chel*; Dul; Lept; Merc; Myr; Sep.
- Right, to: Aco; Aesc; Aral+; Bor; *Calc*; CHEL; Dios; Grap; *Hyds*; Kali-bi; *Lyc*; Mag-m; *Nat-m*.
- cutting+: Hyds.
- Left, to: Dios; Dul; *Lept*; Myr.

Ball, lump, in: Aesc; Bar-c.
- Below: Arn; Bor; Echi; Gel; Lach; *Nat-s*; Thu; Ver-a; Zin.
- Hard, in: Nux-m.

Breathing deep
- Agg: *Bell*; Hep; Nat-s; Ptel; Sele; Ther.
- Amel: Ox-ac.

Burning, heat: Alo; Aur; *Lach*; *Lept*; Merc; Myr; Stan; Ther.
- Stool, after: Stan.

Bursting: Bry; Lept; Nat-s.

Cancer: Chel; Choles; Hyds; Myr; Ther.
- Early: Senec.
- Jaundice, with: Myr.

Cirrhosis: Card-m; Cup; Hep; Hyds; Mur-ac; Pho; Sul.
- Boils, with: Nat-p.
- Hypertrophic: Merc-d.

Coughing agg: Bry; Chin-s; Dros; Eup-p; Hep; Kali-c; Nat-s.

Cramp: Canc-fl; Mag-m; Phys.
- Menses, during: Buf.

Cutting: Berb; Dios; Hyds; Lach; Thyr.

Deep, in: Lach.

Downward: Chel.

LIVER

Enlarged, swelled: Alo; *Chin*; Chio+; Lach; *Lyc*; Mag-m; *Merc*; *Nat-s*; Nux-v; Pod; Sele; Sep; Tarx+; Vip; Zin+.
- Cardiac affections with: Mag-m.
- Children, in: Calc-ar; *Nux-m*.
- Chronic+: Mang.
- Hard and sore+: Zin.
- Pain, after anger: Cocl.
- Spleen, with+: Iod.

Epigastrium, to: Lach; Mag-m.

Eye symptoms, with: Con.

Griping: See Cramp.

Hard, small, as if: Ab-c.

Heart symptoms, with (See HEART, liver symptoms with): Myr.

Heavy: Bry; Mag-m; Nat-s; Pho-ac; Ptel.
- Aching: Phyt.

Hips, to: Vip.

Indurated, hard: Ars; Chin; Dig; *Grap*; Iod; Laur+; Mag-m; Pho; Rat; Tarx.

Inflammation: Aco; Ars; Bell; Chel; Lyc; *Mag-m*; Nat-s; Nux-v.

Jarring agg: Lach; Nat-s.

Laughing agg: Psor.

Leucorrhoea amel: Phyt.

Lung symptoms, with: Card-m; Chel; Hyds.

Lying on
- Back amel: Hyds; Mag-m; Nat-s.
- Right side agg: Chel; Dios; Hyds; Kali-c; *Mag-m*; *Merc*.

LIVER, lying on
- Left side agg: Arn; *Bry*; Card-m; Mag-m; Nat-s; *Ptel*; Sep.
- Painful side amel: Bry; Ptel; Sep.

Menses agg: Pho-ac.

Navel, to: Berb; Dul; Lept; Myr; Sep.

Nipple, to (R): Dios.

Occiput, to: Kali-c, Nux-v; Sep.

Pressure
- Agg: Bell; Bry; Carb-v; Card-m; Chin; Hep; Lach; Lyc; *Merc*; Pho; Sele.
- Amel: See Lying on painful side.

Rash, over: Sele.

Rubbing and shaking amel: *Pod.*

Shoulder, to: Kali-c; Nux-v; Sep; Vip.
- Right: Kali-bi; Med.
- Top of, and: Crot-h.

Sneezing agg: Psor.

Sore, tender: Aur-m; BELL; *Bry*; Carb-v; Chio+; Dig; Iod; Iris; *Kali-io*; *Lach*; Lept; *Lyc*; *Mag-m*; *Merc*; Mur-ac; NAT-S; *Nux-v*; *Pod.*
- Menses, with: Pho-ac.
- Vomiting, during agg+: Pod.

Spine, to: Lept; Mag-m; Sil.

Spots: See CHLOASMAE.

Sticking: Berb; Calc; Chel; Con; Lept; Mag-m; Merc; *Nux-v*; Ran-b; Sele; Sep.

Tension: Chel.

Throbbing: Crot-h; Lapp.

LIVER

Urticaria, with: Canc-fl; Myr.

Uterine symptoms, with: Mag-m.

Walking agg: Hep.

LIVES in own world +: Bell.

LIVID: See BLUE.

LOAD: See HEAVINESS and WEIGHT.

LOAFS+: Sul.

LOATHING: See AVERSION.

Herself: Lac-c.

LOCATION LOST: See BEWILDERED.

LOCHIA

Acrid: Kre.

Afterpains, with+: Xanth.

Bloody, when child nurses: Sil.

Dark: Kre, Sec.

Green: Lac-c; Sec.

Offensive, foul: Echi; Kali-chl; Kali-p; *Kre*; *Sec.*

Protracted: Carb-ac; Caul; Chin; Nat-m; Sec; Senec; Tril.
- Limbs, numb, with: Carb-an.

Scanty+: Nux-v; Radm.

Suppressed: BRY; Hep; Hyo; Mill; *Pul*; Pyro; *Sul.*
- Cold, from: Cimi; Pyro.
- Emotions, from: Cimi.
- Fright, from+: Op.

LOCK-JAW: See JAWS, locked.

LOCOMOTOR ATAXIA: *Alu*; Nux-m; Onos; Pho; Plb; Sec; Sil; Sul; Thal.

Eating amel: Nat-c.

LOINS: Canth; Plb; Rhe; Thu; Zin.
  Burning: Bar-c.
  Hollow: Pall.
  Sticking: Berb; Plb.
LONELY: See FORSAKEN.
LONGING: See CRAVING.
LOOKED AT AGG: ANT-C; Ant-t; *Ars*; Cham; *Cina*; *Nat-m*; Pul.
LOOKING
  All sides, on: Kali-br.
  Around AGG: Calc; *Cic*; CON; Ip.
  Bed, about, to find something: Ign.
  Bright, shining objects, at AGG: *Bell*; Canth; Hyo; *Lyss*; Mur-ac; Stram.
  Constantly in one direction: Bro; Hyo.
  Distant objects, at
    • AGG: Dig; Euphr; Rut.
    • AMEL: Bell.
  Down
    • AGG: Arg-n; Bor; Calc; Kali-c; Kalm; Old; *Pho*; *Spig*; *Sul*.
    • AMEL: Saba.
  Eclipse, at AGG: Hep.
  Either way, right or left AGG: *Con*; Spig.
  Everybody at her: Meli.
  Flowing water, at AGG: See Moving things.
  Intently
    • AGG (See READING agg): Cina; Mur-ac; Old.
    • AMEL: Agn; Petr.
  Knife, at: See KNIFE.
  Long, at anything
    • AGG: Aco; Aur; Nat-m; Rut; Sep; Spig.

LOOKING, long at anything
    • AMEL: Dig; *Nat-c*; Saba.
  Mirror, in AGG: Kali-c.
  Moving things, flowing water etc. AGG: Agar; BELL; Bro; Canth; *Con*; *Fer*; Hyo; Jab; Lyss; Stram; Sul.
  Others, in distress AGG: Tarn.
  Over a large surface AGG (See agarophobia): *Sep*.
  Point, at one AMEL: Agn.
  Red objects, at AGG: Lyc.
  Revolving objects, at AGG: Lyc.
  Shining objects, at: See Bright objects.
  Sideways
    • AGG: *Bell*; Merc-c; Old.
    • AMEL: Chin-s; Old; Sul.
    • On all: Kali-br.
  Sky at, without reason: Bov.
  Snow, at AGG: Ap.
  Staring agg (See EYES, staring): Cina.
  Straight forward
    • AGG: Old.
    • AMEL: *Bell*; Old.
  Through sharp spectacles, as if: Croc.
  Upwards
    • AGG: Ars; CALC; Chel; Cup; *Pho*; *Pul*; Saba; Sang; Sele; Sil; Thu.
    • High buildings at AGG: Arg-n.
    • Walking in open air AGG: Arg-n; Sep.
  White objects, at AGG: Ap; Ars; Cham; Lyc; Nat-m; Tab.
    • Yellow spots: Am-c.

LOOKING

Window, out of AGG: Cam; Carb-v; NAT-M; Ox-ac.
- For hours: Mez.

LOOSE, as if: Am-c; Bar-c; Bov; Carb-an; Caus; Chin; Croc; Hyo; *Kali-c*; Kali-m; Laur; Med; Nat-s; NUX-M; Nux-v; Psor; RHUS-T; Sec; Sul-ac; Thu.

Open, and: Sec.

LOOSE, lax: See RELAXATION.

LOQUACITY: Agar; Aur; Cann+; Cimi; Cocl; Cup; *Hyo*; *Lach*; Meph; Op; Par; Pod; Pyro; Sele; *Stram*; Ver-a; Ver-v.

Business of: *Bry*; Hyo.

Changing quickly from one subject to another: Amb; Cimi; *Lach*; Stram; Val.

Chill, during: Pod; Zin.

Cough, after: Dros.

Excited, when: Mar-v+; Sele.

Fever, during: Lach; *Mar-v*; Pod; Tub; Zin.

Hilarity, with: Ther.

Incoherent, rambling: Amb; Arg-n; Bry; Cimi; Hyo; *Lach*; Mar-v; Onos; Pho; Pod; Rhus-t; Sele; Stram; Tub.
- Headache, during: Bar-c; Lach; Stram.

Menses, during: Stram.

Precocious (child): Strop.

Rapid questioning: Aur.

Sweat, with: Calad; Cup; Sele.

LOSS OF VITAL FLUIDS agg: See DISCHARGES agg.

LOUSINESS: See LICE.

LOVE

Disappointment, unhappy, pangs: Ant-c; Aur; Cact; Calc-p; Cimi; Cof; Hell; *Hyo*; *Ign*; Iod; Lach; *Nat-m*; *Pho-ac*; Tarn; Ver-a.

Exalted: Ant-c.

Sick: Til.

LOWER LIMBS: See LEGS.

LUMBAGO: See LUMBAR BACK, pain.

LUMBAR BACK (See BACK): Aesc; Alu; ANT-T; Arg-m; *Ars*; Bar-c; *Berb*; Bry; CALC; Canth; *Caus*; Chin; *Cimi*; Dul; Eup-p; Grap; *Kali-c*; Led; Nux-m; NUX-V; Pho; Pul; RHUS-T; Sanic; SEP; Solid; *Sul*; *Vario*; Zin-ar.

Affected by everything: Kali-c; Sep.

Blowing nose agg: Calc-p; Dig.

Breaking, broken: Aese; *Bell*; Eup-p; Kali-io; *Lyc*; Nat-m; Pho; Rut; Senec.

Burning: Aeth; Pod; Terb.
- Spot: Pho.

Chest, to: Berb; Sul.

Chill, starts, in: Gel; Hyo; Lach; *Nat-m*; Stro; Sul.

Coition agg: Kob.

Coldness: Bry; Canth; Dul; *Eup-p*; Gel; *Lach*; Merc-c; Rhus-t; Sanic; Sul.
- Coughing agg: Carb-an.

Compression: Aeth; Caus; Thu.
- Tight band, as from a: *Pul.*

Coughing agg: Aco; Kali-bi; Nit-ac.

LUMBAR BACK

Craking: Sec; Sul.
- Walking, while: *Zin*.

Cramps: Ant-c; *Caus*; *Chin*.
- Buttock, and: Caus.

Crushed, as though: Berb; Chin.

Damp cloth, around as if: Lathy.

Dislocative pain: Eup-p; Lach.

Down legs: Kali-c.

Emaciation: Plb; Sele.

Exertion agg: Agar; Calc-p; Zin-ar.

Flatus passing amel: *Lyc*; Pic-ac; Rut.

Forward, in: *Berb*; Cham; *Kali-c*; Kre; SABI.
- Around pelvis: Sabi; Sep; Vib.

Groins, to: Pho; Sabi; Vib.

Heavy: Cimi; Pic-ac; Rhus-t.
- Hips, down thighs: Cimi.

Hot, iron, as if: Act-sp; Alu; Cann; Grap.
- Clothes, as if, on fire: Ars-io.

Iliac crest, to thighs+: Berb.

Injury, after: Kali-c.

Jarring agg: Thu; Zin-ar.

Lame (See Weakness): Berb; Gel; Kali-io; *Lach*; Ox-ac; *Pho*; *Rhus-t*; Sul.

Leucorrhoea gushing amel: Kre.

Lifting agg: Ant-t; Med.

Numb: Aco; Ap; *Berb*; Grap; Lapp; PLAT; Sil.

Operations after: Berb.

LUMBAR BACK

Pain (lumbago): *Aesc*; Ant-t; Bell; Berb; Bry; Caus; *Dul*; *Grap*; Kali-bi; *Led*; Mur-ac; NUX-V; Ox-ac; RHUS-T; Sec; Sele; *Sep*; Sul.
- Amel, rising on in A.M.: Fer.
- Coughing agg: Carb-an.
- Diarrhoea with: Bar-c; Kali-io.
- Efforts, repeated at rising: Aesc.
- Exertion amel: Radm.
- Headache, alternating with: Alo.
- Leucorrhoea, with: Gel.
- Menses, during: Am-c; Cimi; Lach; Nux-m; Pul; Sul.
- Motion, least agg: Buf; Chin+; Lyc.
- Night, only: Fer.
- Sick feeling, all over with: Solid.
- Urination frequent, with: Sep.
- Vertebra broken, as if: Grap.
- Vertex and occiput, with: Radm.

Paralytic: Cocl; Kali-c; Sep.
- Labour, difficult, after: Nux-v.

Pressure amel: Dul; Kali-c; Nat-m; Rhus-t; Rut; Sep.

Pubes, to: Pho; Sabi; Vib.

Pulled down, from, as if: Visc.

Radiating, from: Bap; Berb; Laur; Sep.

Raises, with the help of arms: Buf: Hyds.

Raw, as if: Nat-c.

Renal diseases, in: Calc-ar; Senec; Solid; Visc.

LUMBAR BACK

Restlessness: Bar-c; Calc-f.
- Flatus passing amel: Bar-c.

Short, tense: Am-m; Berb.

Sitting
- Agg: Agar; Arg-m; Berb; Kob; Rhus-t; Val; Zin-ar.
- Bent
  - agg+: Kali-io.
  - amel: Ran-b.
- Down, when agg: Zin.

Sleep agg: Am-m.

Sneezing agg: Con; Sul.

Standing agg: Con; Psor; *Val*; Zin; Zin-ar.

Stiff: Bar-c; Caus; Lach; *Rhus-t*.
- Thighs cannot raise: Aur.

Stitches: Agar; Berb; *Bry*; Colo; Kali-c; Lyc; Pul; Sul.
- Coughing agg: Nit-ac.

Stomach, to: Sul.

Stools agg: Bar-c; Caps.

Stooping, prolonged agg: Dul.

Straighten, cannot: Kob.

Sweat: Naj; Sil.
- Menses, before: Nit-ac.

Thighs, raising agg: Aur.

Throbbing: Bar-c; Lac-c; Sep; Sil.

Tough agg: Cimi; Lil-t.

Trembling: Benz-ac.

Upwards, from: Radm.

Urination amel: Nat-s.

Uterus, to: Nat-m.

Vertebrae, of: Kre; Stan; Zin.
- Dislocated, or, as if: Sanic.
- Gliding over each other, as if: Sanic.

LUMBAR BACK

Walking
- Agg: Aese, Murx; Psor; Sep.
- Amel: *Arg-m*; Kob; Radm; *Sep*.
- Impulse, to, with: Murx.
- With cane pressed across the back amel: Vib.

Weakness: Ars; Calc; Calc-s; Cocl; Nat-m; Pic-ac; Pul; Rhus-t; Sele; Sep; Sul; Zin.

Wind, as of a: Sul; Sumb.

LUMP: See BALL.

LUMPS, lumpy effects: Aeth; Alo; Alum; Ant-c; Calc-s; *Cham*; *Chin*; Coc-c; *Grap*; KALI-BI; Kre; LYC; *Merc*; *Merc-i-f*; PLAT; Rhus-t; Sep; Sil; Stan.
- Painful: Kali-io.

LUNGS: See under CHEST.

LUPUS: See CANCER.

LYING

AGG: Adon; *Amb*; Ant-t; Ap; Arn; ARS; AUR; Bell; *Caps*; *Cham*; Con; Dros, Dul; Euphor; *Fer*; *Hyo*; Kali-c; *Lyc*; Lycps; *Meny*; Merc; Nat-s; Pho; *Plat*; PUL; RHUS-T; Rum; *Rut*; *Samb*; Sang; Sep; Sil; Stro; Tarx; Verb.

AMEL: Am-m; Asar; Bell; BRY; *Calc*; Cham; Colo; Fer; Form; Ign; Mang; *Nat-m*; Nit-ac; NUX-V; Pic-ac; Pul; Rhus-t; Sep; *Scil*; Sil; Stan.

Abdomen, on AMEL: Acet-ac; BELL; Calc-p; Chel; Chio; Cina; COLO; Elap; Eup-p; Lach; Lept; MED; Nit-ac; Par;

LYING, abdomen on, amel ..
  Pho; Phyt; *Pod*; *Psor*; Sep; Stan; Thyr.
All troubles AMEL: Mang.
Back, on
- **AGG:** *Aco*; Am-m; Arg-m; *Ars*; Cact; *Caus*; *Cham*; Colch, Colo; *Cup*; IGN; *Iod*; *Kali-n*; Merc-i-f; Nat-s; NUX-V; *Op*; PHO; Pul; *Rhus-t*; *Sep*; *Sil*; Spig; *Sul*; Zin-chr.
- **AMEL:** Am-m; BRY; CALC; Colch; Dig; Merc-c; *Pul*; *Rhus-t*; Rut; Sang.
- Flat amel: Dig.
- Head elevated, with: See Reclining.
- Jerks the head backward, while: Hypr.
- Knees
  - drawn up and spread apart with: Plat.
  - thighs and, flexed on abdomen: Stram.

Bed in agg and amel: See BED lying in agg and amel.
Bent amel: See BENDING forwards amel.
Board, on, as if: Bap; Sanic.
Curled up on one side: Bap.
Face, on amel: Hypr.
Hands and knees on AMEL: Con; Eup-p; Euphor; *Lach*; Med; Par-b; Sep; Tarn.
Hard surface on AMEL: Kali-c; *Nat-m*; Rhus-t; Sanic; *Sep*; Stan.
Head high, with AMEL: Ant-t; Ap; Aral; *Arg-m*; ARS; Bell;

LYING, with head high amel ..
  Cact; Caps; Chin; *Con*; Gel; Glo; *Hep*; Kali-c; KALI-N; Lach; *Pul*; Samb; Sang; Spig; Spo.
Horizontal position AMEL: *Ap*; *Arn*; Bell; Con; Laur; Psor; Spo; Tab; Ther; *Ver-v*.
Ice on, as if: Lyc.
Knees on, body bent backward, with: Nux-v.
Legs
- Crossed with, cannot uncross: Bell; Ther.
- Spread aprt: Hell.

On one side one person, other side other person, as if: Pyro.
Painful side, or affected part, on agg: See PRESSURE agg.
Painless side, on AGG: BRY; *Cham*; Chin; *Colo*; Flu-ac; Ign; Nat-s; PUL; Rhus-t; Sec; *Sep*.
Quietly amel: Bry; Psor.
Reclining, on back amel: Gel; Kalm; Led; Sang; Thyr.
Side, on
- **AGG:** ACO; ANAC; Arg-n; Bar-c; BRY; Calad; CALC; CARB-AN; Cina; Con; Fer; Ign; Ip; KALI-C; Kre; *Lyc*; Merc; Merc-c; Nat-s; Par; PHO; Pho-ac; PUL; *Rhus-t*; Seneg; SIL; STAN; Sul; Thu.
- **AMEL:** Anac; *Cocl*; Lept; NUX-V; Pho; Sep.
- Right
  - AGG: Alu; Am-c; Am-m; *Arg-n*; Benz-ac; Bor; Caus; Iris; Hyds; Kali-c;

LYING, side, right agg ..
  Kalm; Lycps; *Mag-m*; Mag-p; MERC; *Nux-v*; *Pho*; Rum; Spo; Stan; Sul-io.
  - AMEL: Am-c; Ant-t; Naj; Nat-m; Pho; Sep; Sul; Tab.
  - contents of body were dragged to that side: Cinb.
  - head high with, AMEL: Ars; Cact; Spig; Spo.
  • Left
    - AGG: Aco; Am-c; Ap; *Arg-n*; *Bar-c*; *Bry*; Cact; *Carb-an*; Colch; Dig; Ip; Kali-c; Lil-t; Lyc; Naj; *Nat-c*; Nat-m; Nat-s; *Par*; Petr; PHO; Ptel; PUL; *Sep*; Sil; *Sul*; *Thu*; Tub; Vib; Zin-io.
    - AMEL: Ign; Lil-t; Mur-ac; Nat-m; Phyt; Sang; Stan.
Strange position in amel: See ATTITUDE BIZARRE.
Uncomfortably, as if: Lept; Psor; Pul; Rhus-t; Sil; Sul.
  • Aching of body, from: Lapp.
Wet surface, floor, on or sitting on moist ground AGG: Ars; Calc; Caus; Dul; *Nux-v*; Rhod; Rhus-t; Sil.
LYMPHANGITIS (See SKIN, red streaks): Ap; Bell; Buf; Lach; Merc; Pyro; Rhus-t.
LYMPHOID TISSUE: *Radm*.
LYPOTHEMIA: See MENTAL exhaustion, grief from.
MADDENING: See BESIDES HIMSELF, and HEAD, pain, maddening.

MADNESS: See INSANITY.
MAGNETISED, desires to be: *Calc*; Lach; *Pho*; *Sil*.
MAGNETISM AMEL: Calc; *Cup*; Lach; *Pho*; Sil.
MALAR BONES: *Ars-io*; *Aur*; Colo; Glo; *Kali-bi*; Kali-io; Mag-c; Mez; Ol-an; Old; Sep; Stan; Stap; Stro; Thu; Tub; Verb.
  Aching, sore: Ars-io; Aur; Glo; Merc-i-r; Phyt; Tub; Verb.
  Boring: Thu.
  Exostoses: Aur.
  Neuralgia: Stan.
    • Night amel: Cimi.
    • Running about amel: Bism.
  Numb: Plat; Sep.
  Pulled up: Ol-an.
  Stitches: Par.
  Tension, across: Ver-v.
  Tumours: Mag-c.
MALARIA: See FEVER, intermittent.
MALE (genital) organs
  In general: Agn; Arg-n; *Aur*; Cann; Canth; Cinb; CLEM; Con; *Grap*; *Lyc*; MERC; NIT-AC; *Nux-v*; Plat; PUL; *Rhod*; *Rhus-t*; Spo; Stap; *Sul*; *Thu*.
  Aching, cannot sit still: Syph.
  Briny odour, after coition: Sanic.
  Burning: *Calc*; *Canth*; Sul-ac.
    • Coition during: Kre.
  Cold: *Agn*; Caus; Gel; *Lyc*; Sabal; Sul.
  Dropsical: Grap.

MALE organs

Erection, of: See ERECTION.
Eruptions: Crot-t; Grap; Petr; Rhus-t.
Flaccid: *Agn*; Calad; *Dios*; Gel.
- Coition, during: Nux-v; Pho-ac; Sul.
- Suddenly: Grap; Lyc; Nux-v.

Formication: *Plat*; *Sec*; Tarn.
Grasping, fumbling: Aco; Bell; Buf; Canth; HYO; Merc; Stram; Zin.
Heavy: Nat-c; Psor.
Hot: Spo.
Itching: Calc; Caus; Plat; Rhus-t.
Numb: Grap.
Odour, stinking: Nat-m; Sars; Sul.
Painful: Arg-n; Arn.
- Coition, during: Arg-n.

Shrivelled: Ign; Lyc.
Spots, yellow, brown, on: Kob.
Sweat: Aur; Flu-ac; Sele; Sep; Thu.
- Offensive: Sul.
- Oily, pungent: Flu-ac.

Swelled: Arn; Rhus-t.
- Dropsical: Grap.

Tingling: Alu.
Uneasy feeling: Kali-c.

MALICE, hatred: ANAC; *Cham*; Cup; Led; Lyc; Nat-m; Nit-ac; NUX-V; Stram; Tarn.

Persons
- Who do not agree with him: Calc-s.
- Who had offended him: Aur; Nat-m.

MALIGNANCY: Ail; Am-c; Ars; Crot-h; Lach; Nit-ac; Tarn-c.

MALINGERING: Arg-n; Bell; Plb; Saba; *Tarn*; Ver-a.

MAMMAE: Bell, Bry; Carb-an; Cham; *Con*; Hyds; Iod; Lac-c; Merc; Oci-c; Phel; *Pho*; *Phyt*; Sabal; Sil; Urt.

Right: Ign; Kali-bi; *Phel*; SIL.
- Below: Carb-an; Caus; Chel; CIMI; *Grap*; Laur; Lil-t; Merc-i-r; *Pho*; *Sul*; Ust.
- Jumping alive, as if+: Croc.
- Scapula, to: Merc.

Left: Bor; Bov; *Lil-t*; *Lyc*; *Phel*.
- Arms to fingers: Ast-r.
- Below: Ap; Bry; Bur-p; Cimi; Pho; Sul; Ust.
- Pain
  - cough, with: Mos.
  - drawn back, as if+: Croc.
  - dysmenorrhoea, with: Caus.
  - head, to: Glo.
  - jumping: Croc.
  - meals, after: Rum; Stro.
  - menses
    at: Grap.
    between: Ust.
- Scapula to: Como.
- Swollen, hard: Cist.

Alternating sides: Pul.

Abdomen
- Hot water, running, from: Sang.
- To: Phel; Sang.

Abscess: Hep; Merc; Pho; Phyt; Sil; Sul.
- Threatening in old cicatrices: Acet-ac+; *Grap*; Phyt.

MAMMAE

Aching: See Sore.
- Nursing amel: Phel.

Alternating, teeth with: Kali-c.

Arms, to: Lith.

Axilla, to: Bro.

Backward: CROT-T; Laur; Lil-t; Til.
- Left: Form.
- Drawn: Croc.

Ball, below: Hura.

Bares: Cam.

Burning: Cimi; Laur; Sul.
- Below
  - right: Aeth; Pho.
  - left: Laur; Mur-ac; Rum.
- Motion amel: Ars.

Caking, milk of: Nux-v.

Cancer: Ast-r+; Aur-m+; Bad+; Bro+; Buf; Con; Cund; Grap; Hyds+; Merc; Pho; Sil.
- Itching, with: Sil.
- Stitches in shoulders and uterus, with: Clem.
- Swelling of axillary glands, with+: Goss.

Chilliness, in: Cocl; Guai.

Cicatrices, old: Carb-an; *Grap*; Phyt.
- Suppurating: Sil.

Cold: Cocl; Med.
- Agg: Sabal.
- Left: Nat-c.
  - coughing, while: Nat-c.

Congested: Aco; Ap; Fer; Pho.
- Milk with, in insanity: Bell; Stram.

Coughing agg: Con.

Cramp: Plat.

MAMMAE

Crawling (left): Ant-t.
- Cold: Guai.

Dwindled, emaciated: Ars-io; Bar-c+; Cham; Chim; *Cof*; CON; Fer; IOD; *Kali-io*; Nat-m; Nit-ac; *Nux-m*; Sabal; Sec; Sil.
- Lump hard, small, painful with: Kre.
- Ovaries, with: Bar-c.

Emptiness, after child nurses: Bor.

Enlarged, as if: Calc-p; Cyc; Sep.

Eruption: Caus; Psor.
- Herpes, in nursing women: Dul.

Erysipelas: Ap.

Everything, affects: Phyt.

Fingers, to: Ast-r; Lith.

Fistula: Pho; Sil.

Flaccid: Con; Iod.

Hard, indurated: Ast-r+; Bry; *Carb-an*; Cham; Con; Grap; Phyt; Plb; *Sil.*
- Menses absent, with: Dul.
- Nodes+: Ast-r; Nit-ac.
- Small and, during colic: Plb.

Head, to: Lac-ac.

Heavy: Bry; Chin; Iod; Lac-c; Phyt.

Hypertrophy: *Calc*; Chim; *Con*; Phyt.
- Climaxis, at: Sang.

Inflamed (mastitis): Bell; Bry; Hep; Phyt; Sil; Sul.

Inner side, arms to fingers: Ast-r.

Itching: Alu; Caus; Con.
- Warm getting, on+: Aeth.

MAMMAE

Jerks: Croc.
Large+: Chim.
Menses
- Before agg: Bry; Calc; *Con*; KALI-M; LAC-C; Lyc; Ol-an; *Phyt*; Pul.
- During agg: Con; Helo; Lac-c; Merc; Murx; Phel; Pho; Phyt; Zin.

Milk present
- Boys, in: Merc.
- Flowing in, as if: Dict; Kre; Nux-v; Pul.
- Increased+: Aco.
- Insanity, during+: Bell; Stram.
- Menses
  - absent with: Bell; Bry; Calc; Lyc; Pho; Pul; Rhus-t; Sabi; Stram.
  - during: Calc; Merc; Pall; Pul; Tub.
  - instead of: Merc.
- Virgins, non-pregnant women in: Asaf; Bur-p; Cyc; Lyc; *Merc*; PUL; Tub; Urt.

Neuralgia, left: Sumb.
Night agg: Buf.
Nodes, in: Bels; Calc-f; *Carb-an*; *Con*; Crot-t; Lyc; *Phyt*; SIL; Tub.
- Black points on skin, with: Iod.
- Girls puberty, before: Pul.
- Hard, burning+: Lyc.
- Knots in axilla, with: Merc-i-f.
- Milk, secretion of, with+: Chim.
- Movable, tender, moving arms agg: Calc-io.
- Old: Chim.

MAMMAE, nodes in
- Painful, old fat men, in: Bar-c.
- Skin, on: Iod.
- Soft, tender: Kali-m; Pul.
- Touch agg: Ars-io.
- Walnut like, in males: Bar-c; Calc-p.

Numb: Grap.
Nursing agg: Phel.
Outward, dartings: Arg-m; Clem; Ol-an.
- Menses, during: Grat.

Presses hard, with hand: Cimi; Con.
Radiating, from: Phyt.
Rivet or bullet feeling of, in region: Lil-t.
Shivering over: Cocl; Guai.
Shooting: Polyg.
Shoulder, to
- Between: Phel.
- Left: Sang.

Shuddering in, with goose flesh+: Guai.
Small, undeveloped: Iod; Lyc; Nux-m; Onos; Sabal; Sul.
- One, than other: Sabal.

Sore, painful: Arn; Bell; Bry; Calc; Cham; *Con*; Helo; Kali-m; LAC-C; Lyc; Med; Merc; Onos; Phyt; Pul; Sabal; Sil; Syph.
- Axillary glands enlargement, with: Lac-ac.
- Bath cold agg: Sabal.
- Climaxis, at: Sang.
- Dysmenorrhoea, with: Canth; Sars.
- Infants: Cham.

MAMMAE, sore
- Menses
  - absent, with: Dul; Zin.
  - at the beginning of: Tub.
  - during or other time: Grat+; Med; Murx; Syph.
- Pregnancy, during: Calc-p.
- Rubbing, hard amel: Radm.
- Sneezing agg: Hyds.
- Urination agg: Clem.
- Yawning agg: Mag-c.

Stitches: Ap; Carb-an; *Con*; Nit-ac; Sil.
- Dysmenorrhoea, with: Caus.
- Nursing, when: Calc.

Stooping, when+: Grat.

Suckling, while
- Agg: Ant-t; Bor; Bry; Crot-t; Lac-c; Lil-t; Phel; Phyt; *Pul*; Sil.
- Amel: Phel.
- Cramps: Cham.
- Pain in opposite: Bor.

Swelled: *Bell*; BRY; Con; Helo; Hep; *Pho*; PHYT; PUL; *Sil*; Sul; Urt.
- As if: Calc-p.
- Bath cold agg: Sabal.
- Climaxis, at: Sang.
- Inguinal glands, with: Oci-c.
- Lancinating pain+: Aeth.
- Leucorrhoea, with: Dul.
- Menses
  - after, secretion of milk, with: Cyc.
  - instead of: Dul; Rat.
- Milk, secretion of, with: Asaf; Cyc; Tub.
- Weaning, after: All-s; Pul.

MAMMAE
Throbbing: Bor.
Tingling: Sabi.
Tumours: See Cancer and Nodes.
Ulceration: Hep; Phyt; Sil.
Urination agg: Clem.
Uterus, with: Sil.
Warts: Cast-eq.

MANIA: See INSANITY.
Mono: Ign; Sil.
Klepto: See Steals.

MARASMUS (See EMACIATION): Abro; Bor; Iod; Mag-c; Nat-m; Nux-m; Sanic; Syph.
Feeding and medicines, in spite of: Mag-c.
Glands, enlarged with: Ther.
Infants, bottle fed: Nat-p.

MARRIAGE
Dissolve, must: Flu-ac.
Idea of, seemed unendurable: *Lach*; Nux-v; Pic-ac; Pul.
Prepartion, of: Hyo.
That he is married: Ign.
Thought of amel: Orig.

MASSETERS: Hyd-ac; Ign.
Contracted: Meny; Merc+.
Cramp: Cocl; Cup; Hyd-ac; Stram; Stry.
Stiff, hard: Ign.

MASTITIS: See MAMMAE, inflammation.

MASTODYNIA: See MAMMAE, sore.

MASTOID
Caries: *Aur*; Caps; Flu-ac; *Nit-ac*; Sil.

MASTOID
Inflammation: Aur; Calc-p; Canth; *Caps*; Fer-p; Hep; Lach; *Pho*; Sil.

Neck, to: Lith; Mur-ac.

Operations, after: Caps.

MASTURBATION
Disposion to (males): Anac; Buf; Con; Lach; Orig; Plat; Sep; Stap; Ust.

Females (See males): *Orig*; *Tub*.
- Children due to pruritus vulvae: *Calad, Orig*; Zin.
- Menses, during: Zin.

Ill effects, of AGG: Arg-m+; Arg-n+; CALC; Carb-v; CHIN; Cocl; *Con*; Dios+; Gel; Lach; Lyc; Merc; *Nat-m*; Nat-p; Nux-v; Orig; Pho; PHO-AC; Pic-ac; Plat; Pul; Sele; *Sep*; STAP; SUL; Ust.

Involuntary: Cam.

Puberty, before: Plat.

MAXILLARY JOINTS: Bell; Ign; Merc; *Rhus-t*; Thu.

Cracking, chewing when: Nit-ac; Rhus-t.

Cramp: Bell; Spo.

Dislocation, easy: Ign; Petr; *Rhus-t*; Stap.
- Laughing agg: Tab.

Tight, on chewing or opening mouth: Alu.

MEAN (See AVARICIOUS): Sul.

MEASLES: ACO; Ars; *Bry*; Cam; Cof; Dros; Euphr; Fer-p; *Kali-bi*; Kali-m; Pho; PUL; Stic.

MEASLES
Complications or sequelae of: Ant-c; *Ant-t*; *Ars*; *Bry*; Cam; Carb-v; Cup-ac; Dros; *Kali-c*; *Pul*; *Sul*; Zin.

Haemorrhagic: *Crot-h*; Fer-p.

Receding: *Bry*; Pho; Pul; Rhus-t.

Undeveloped: Bry.

MEAT WATER like: See DISCHARGES, meat water.

MEATUS
Agglutination, of: Cam; Cann; Cup; Med; Nat-m; Petros; Thu.
- Morning: Pho; *Sep*; Thu.

Burning: Berb; Sul.
- Clothes rubbing agg: Chin.

Cracks: Nat-c; Nit-ac.

Cutting: Zin.

Drop
- Clear, morning: Pho.
- Green: Merc.
- Urinating, before: Berb.
- Yellow: Flu-ac.

Eruptions, about: Caps.

Everted: Caps.

Hard: Cann.

Inflamed: Cann; Sul.

Itching: Amb; *Caus*; *Coc-c*; Petros.

Painful: Canth.
- Women: Lac-c; Sars.

Pouting: Cann; Sul; Thu.

Red: Merc; *Sul*.

Stitching: Nit-ac.

Ulcers: Merc-c; Nit-ac.

MEDICINE
Abuse of: See DURGS, abuse of.

MEDICINE

Overacts without curing: Cup; Mar-v; Pho-ac.

Refuses, to take: Calad; Cimi; Hyo.

Sensitive, to: Cup; Nux-v; Pul.
- High potency: Nit-ac.

Thinking of it agg: Asaf.

Want of susceptibility to: Carb-v; Laur; Mos; Op.

MEDULLA: Aco; Agar; Cup; Naj; Ver-v.

MELANCHOLY (See SADNESS): Ant-t+; Ars; Calc; Castr+; Cup; Grap; Helo; Hypr+; Lach; Nux-v+; Plb; Pul; Sul; Ver-a.

Brooding: Aur.

Death, fear of, with: Cup.

Eyes closed, with: Arg-n.

Financial: Mez; Psor.

Internal grief, from+: Am-m.

Parturition, after: Anac.

Puberty, during: Hell.

Religious: Kali-p+; Mez; Meli+; Psor.

MEMBRANE: See MUCOUS MEMBRANE and SEROUS MEMBRANE.

MEMORIES disagreeable recur: Amb; Am-c; Benz-ac; Calc; Cham; Hep; Hyo; Lyc; Nat-m; Nit-ac; Pho; Psor; Sep; Sul; Thu.

Old grievances, of: Glo.

MEMORY (affected in general): ANAC; Arn; Aur; Bar-c; Bell; Calc; Cann; Con; Hell; HYO; Lach; LYC; Merc; NAT-M; NUX-M; Op; Pho-ac; Rhod; Stap; Sul; Syph.

MEMORY

Active: BELL; Cof; Hyo; Lach; Op.

Bad, weak: Aco; Amb; Agn; ANAC; Arg-m; Arg-n; Ars; Art-v; Bar-c; BELL; Buf; CALC; Caus; Cocl; Colch; Con; Crot-h; Glo; Guai; Ham+; Hell; Hep; Hyo; Kali-br; Kali-p; Lach; Laur; Lyc; Med; Merc; Nit-ac; Nux-m; Onos; Petr; Pho; Pho-ac; Plat; Plb; Sep; Stap; Stro+; Syph; VER-A; Zin.
- Faces, events, names, for: Syph.
  - remembers past events: Syph.
- Naming objects, for: Chin-s.
- Vexation agg: Am-c.
- What he is doing or done: Cic; Nat-m; Nux-m.
- Suddenly from pain, fright, etc: Am-c; Anac; Arg-n; Bell; Hep; Laur; Nux-m; Pall; Pru-sp; Pul.

Lost: BELL; Cic; HYO; VER-A.
- Objects, naming for: Chin-s.
- Past life: Nux-m.

MENIERE'S DISEASE: Arn; Benz-ac; Caus+; Cheno; Chin-s; Eucal; Kali-m; Nat-sal; Radm; Sal-ac; Sil; Tab; Thyr.

Sea sick, as if: Tab.

MENINGITIS: See CEREBRO-SPINAL axis.

MENOPAUSE: See CLIMAXIS.

MENSES

Before
- AGG: Bov; Calc; Calc-p; Cimi; Cocl; Cup; KALI-C;

MENSES

MENSES, before, agg..
LACH; *Lyc*; Nat-m; PUL; *Sep*; Spo; *Sul*; *Ver-a*; Vib; *Zin*.
- AMEL: Murx.
- Queer feeling: Bro.

At start of AGG: Aco; Calc-p; *Hyo*; Jab; Kali-c; Lac-c; Lach.

Before and after agg: Bor; Calc; Fer; *Grap*; Kali-m; *Kre*; *Lac-c*; *Lach*; Lil-t; Mag-c; *Nat-m*; Pall; Thu.

During
- AGG: Aco; AM-C; *Arg-n*; Bov; Castr; Caus; *Cham*; Cimi; Cocl; GRAP; HYO; Ign; Kali-c; Lac-c; *Mag-c*; MAG-M; Nux-m; Nux-v; PUL; Sec; *Sep*; Stap; *Sul*; Thu; *Zin*.
- AMEL: Cyc; Kali-c; *Lach*; Mos; Murx; Senec; *Zin*.

After
- AGG: Bor; Carb-an; Grap; Kre; Lac-c; Lach; Lith; Lyc; *Nux-v*; Sep; Tarn.
- Old symptoms of AGG: Nux-v.

Distubrances, of (in general): Aco; BELL; *Calc*; *Cham*; Cocl; Fer; *Grap*; Ip; *Kali-c*; Kre; Lach; Mag-c; Nat-m; NUX-M; Nux-v; Pho; Plat; PUL; *Sabi*; Sec; Sep; *Sul*.

Abdomen, pressure on amel: Mag-c.

Absent, amenorrhoea, suppressed: Aur; Bell; Cimi; *Con*; Cup; Cyc; *Dul*; *Grap*; Hell; Helo; *Kali-c*; Lac-d; Lach; *Lyc*; Nat-s; Pho; PUL; *Senec*; Sep; Sil; *Sul*; Tub; Xanth+.

MENSES, absent
- Abdomen, bloated, with: Apoc.
- Asthma, with: Spo.
- Bath, from: Nux-m.
- Careworn, tired women, in: Ars.
- Cause without: Ust.
- Chagrin, from: Colo.
- Cold, from: Hell; Senec.
- Concomitants, with: Senec; Ust.
- Dancing, excessive, from: Cyc.
- Deafness, with: Nat-c.
- Diabetes, in: Uran-n.
- Dropsy, with: Ap; Apoc; Kali-c; Senec.
- Emigrants, in: Bry; *Plat*.
- Emotions, from: Cimi.
- Foot sweat, suppressed, from: Cup.
- Fright, from: Op.
- Functional: Senec.
- Girls, young+: Senec.
- Grief, from: *Ign*.
- Hands putting in cold water from: Lac-d.
- Indignation, from+: Stap.
- Jaundice, with: Chio.
- Liver, affections, with: Lept.
- Love, disappointed, from: Hell.
- Mammae, scirrhus of, with: Bro.
- Milk in breast, with: Pho; Rhus-t.
- Months, for: Lyc; Sil.
- Neuralgic pain in body, with: Kalm.

MENSES, absent
- Ophthalmia, with+: Euphr.
- Puberty of+: Ap; Sep.
- Rheumatism with: Bry; Cimi; Lach; Rhus-t.
- Suddenly: Aco.
- Tuberculosis, in: Solid; Ust.
- Weaning, after: Sep.
- Wet, getting feet, from: Pul; Rhus-t.

Acrid: Kali-c; Lach; Nit-ac; Sil; Stram.

Ammoniacal: Lac-c.

Awkward, during: Alu.

Bathing amel: Kali-c.

Between, periods: Amb; Bov; Calc; Cham; Ham; Helo; Hyds; Ip; Lyc; Mang+; Pho; Rhus-t; Sabi; Sil.
- Day time, only: Ham.
- Sexual excitement, with: Amb; Sabi.

Black: Chin; Croc; Cyc; Ham; Helo; Kali-m; Kali-n; Lach; Mag-p; Plat; Pul; Ust; Xanth.
- A.M. only: Carb-an.
- Sticky: Coc-c.

Bladder symptoms, with: Canth; Erig; Sabal.

Breathing, difficulty with: Flu-ac.

Brown: Bap; *Bry*; Carb-v; Iod; Thu.

Burning, hot: Arn; *Bell*; Kali-c; Kre; Sabi; Sil; Sul.
- Like fire: Lac-c.
- Lying, cease when: Scil; Sil.

Childbirth, after: Tub.

Choleric symptoms, with: Am-c; Sil.

MENSES

Clotted (See DISCHARGES lumpy): Am-c; Apoc; Bell; Calc; Calc-p; Chin; Coc-c; Cyc; Ip; Kali-m; Kre; Lach; Mag-m; Med; Murx, Pul; Sabi; Zin.
- Dark: Am-c; Bell; Cham; Coc-c; Croc; Med; Sabi; Vip.
- Fluid, blood, with: Apoc; Bell; Sabi; Sec; Ust; Vip.
- Gelatinous, bright blood with: Laur.
- Serum, and: Lyc; Ust.
- Urinating, while: Coc-c.

Coition agg: See FEMALES, coition after.

Cold bath agg: Ant-t.

Collapse, at: Merc.

Copious, profuse, excessive: Apoc; *Ars*; *Bell*; Bov; *Calc*; Calc-p; Cham; *Chin*; Cocl; *Croc*; Cyc; Erig; *Fer*; Ham; Helo; Ip; Kali-n; Kre; Mag-m; Med; *Mill*; Murx; *Nat-m*; *Nux-m*; NUX-V; PHO; *Plat*; Rat; SABI; *Sec*; Senec; *Stram*; Tril; Ust; Vinc; Zin.
- Abortion, after: Ust.
- Bathing amel: Kali-c.
- Climaxis, during: Apoc; Aur-m+; Calc; Lach; Sep; Sul; Tril; Vinc.
  - long, after: Vinc.
- Clots, large with: Apoc; Coc-c; Murx; Zin.
- Dancing, after: Croc; Cyc.
- Erotic, spasms with: Tarn.
- Faintness, with: *Ip*; Tril.
- Forceps delivery, after: Calend.

MENSES, copious
- Icy coldness of body, with: Sil.
- Labour, hasty, after: Caul.
- Labour like pains with+: Alet.
- Mania, with: Sep.
- Moon, new and full agg: Croc.
- Nausea, with: Apoc; Caps; *Ip*.
- Night agg+: Bad.
- Obstinate, continuous: Nux-m; Vinc.
- Old Maids+: Mag-m.
- Short duration: Lach; Plat; Sil; Thu.
- Tenesmus of bladder and rectum, with: Erig.
- Urination, hot, with: Fer.
- Vomiting, with+: Ver-a.
- Widows, young+: Arg-n.
- Women young, in: Kali-br.
  - sedentary habits, of: Colo.

Curetting agg: Bur-p; Nit-ac.

Day only: *Caus*; Cof; Cyc; Ham; PUL.

Delayed, in girls at puberty: Ap; Caus; Grap; *Kali-c*; Lac-d; *Lyc*; Mang; Nat-m; *Pul*; SENEC; Sep; Sul+.
- Feels distrubed, if slightly: Flu-ac.
- Mammae undeveloped, with: Lyc.
- Milk, drinking much, from: Lac-d.

Diarrhoea agg: Am-m; Bov; Castr; Kre; Mag-c.

Early: *Amb*; Ars; BELL; Bor; *Bov*; CALC; Calc-p; Carb-an; *Carb-v*; Caul; CHAM; *Cocl*; Cyc; *Fer*; Fer-p; *Ip*; Kali-c; Lac-c; Mag-m; Mag-p; *Mang*;

MENSES, early ..
Nat-m; Nux-m; NUX-V; *Pho*; PLAT; Rat; *Rhus-t*; *Sabi*.
- Black clots, preceded by blindness+: Dict.
- Profuse, and: Alet+; Kali-c; Sep; Stan; Ver-a+; Xanth+.
- Scanty, and: Alu; Lept; Nat-m.

Evening only: Coc-c; Cof; Phel.

Exertion agg: *Amb*; Bov; *Calc*; *Erig*; Kre; Nit-ac; Tril.

Exhaustion+: Alu.

Faints at: *Ip*; Lach; Nux-v; Sep.

Fearsome: Nat-m.

Feel like coming: Carb-an; Lil-t; Mos; Onos; Pho; Pul; Senec; Vip; Zin-chr.
- Diarrhoea with: Kali-io.
- Frequently: Plat.
- Uterine spasms, with: Kali-c.

Fever, septic agg: Pyro.

Foul: Bell; Bry; Carb-v; Croc; Helo; Kali-p; Kre; Sabi; Syph.
- Putrid meat, like: Alu-sil; Cham; Lachn; Med; Psor; Syph.

Green: Grap; *Lac-c*; Med; Pul; *Sep*; Tub.

Grief, brings on: Ign.

Gushing (See HAEMORRHAGE gushing): Ip; Lac-c; Pho; Sabi.
- Tip toe standing on: Cocl.
- Wakes her from sleep+: Coca.

Heart symptoms, with: Cact.

Hot: See Burning.

Indelible: Bur-p; Culex: Mag-c; Mag-p; Med; Pulex.

Inky: Kali-n.

MENSES

Intermittent, reappearing: Amb; Arg-n; Bov; Coc-c; Fer; Ham; *Kre*; *Lach*; Mang; Nux-v; Pho; Pul; Saba; Sabi; Sil; Ust.
- Abortion, after: Plat.
- Blood, black: Elap.
- Daytime, only: Ham.
- Girls young, in: Polyg.
- Interval of one day: Ap.
- Old Maids, in: Mag-m.
- Parturition, after: Acet-ac.
- Sexual excitement, with: Amb; Sabi.
- Sometimes stronger, sometimes weaker: Saba.
- Women, childless or young widows, in: Arg-n.

Irregular: Cimi; Cocl; Con; Ign; Iod; Kali-p; *Nux-m*; *Sec*; Senec.
- In time and amount: Cimi; Coc-c; Ign; Nux-m; Plat.
- Palpitation, with+: Phys.

Itching, causing: Petr; Sul; Tarn.

Joints, pain, with: Sabi.

Jolting, from: Ham.

Lactation, during: Calc; Calc-p; Pall; Sil.

Late: Caul; *Caus*; Con; Cup; *Dul*; *Grap*; *Kali-c*; LACH; *Lyc*; *Mag-c*; *Nat-m*; Nux-m; PUL; Saba; *Sep*; *Sil*; SUL; Vib.
- First menses: See Delayed.
- Scanty, and: Kali-c; Sep; Vib.

Leucorrhoea, with: Kre; Sep.

Lifting agg: Kre.

Lumbar pain with: See LUMBAR BACK, pain.

MENSES

Lying
- Back, on agg: Cham.
- Ceases, on: Cact; Caus; Lil-t; Sabi.
- More, on: Kre; Mag-c; Pul.

Mammae agg (See MAMMAE): Bry; Calc; Lac-c.

Membranous: Bor; Cham; Cyc; Lac-c; Mag-p; Phyt; Vib.
- Puberty, at: Cham.

Mental excitement agg: CALC; Tub.

Molasses like: Mag-c.

Month, alternate: Bur-p; Syph.

Moon full or new agg: Croc.

Morning
- More: Bor; Bov; Carb-an; Sep.
- Rising, on: Mag-c.

Motion
- Agg: Croc; *Erig*; Helo; *Ip*; Sabi; Sec.
- Amel: Bov; Cyc; Kre; Mag-c; *Sabi*.
- Only, during: Cact; Caus; *Lil-t*; Manc; Nat-s; Sec.

Night only: Am-c; Am-m; Bov; Coc-c; Mag-c; Mag-p; Nat-m.

Nursing agg: Pall; Pho; Sil; Vip.

Offensive: See Foul.

Painful, dysmenorrhoea: Bell; Cact; *Calc*; Calc-p; Caul; CHAM; *Cimi*; Cocl; Con; Cup; Dios; *Grap*; Kali-c; Lyc; Med; Nux-m; Plat; PUL; Psor; Sep; SUL; Tub; Ver-a; VIB; *Xanth*; Zin-val.
- Abortion, after: Senec.
- Barren women, in: Phyt.

MENSES, painful
- Bending
  - back amel: Lac-c.
  - double must: Op.
- Blood
  - black, with: Elap.
  - gray, serum like+: Berb.
- Blotches, all over, body with: Dul.
- Climaxis, at: Psor.
- Colic, after: *Kali-c.*
- Convulsions, with: Caul; Nat-m.
- Emotions, from: Cham.
- Eructations, with: Vib.
- Fainting, with: Kali-s; *Lap-a*; Lyc; Nux-m.
- Feet, pressing against support, amel: Med.
- Few drops of blood, with: Castr.
- First day: Gnap; Lach.
- Flatulence, with: Vib.
- Flow
  - amel: Mag-p.
  - scanty, with: Caul; Gnap; Grap.
- Frightful: Tub.
- Gnawing: Thyr.
- Jerks, with: Plat.
- Lying
  - back on with legs stretched amel: Sabi.
  - hard pillow, over amel: Mag-m.
- Mental excitement agg: Calc.
- More flow, more pain: Cann; *Cimi*; Pho; Tarn; Tub.
- More pain less flow: Lach.

MENSES, painful
- No relief, in any position: Xanth.
- Over whole body: Nux-v; Xanth.
- Prolapsus, with: Ver-a.
- Retracted nipples, with+: Sars.
- Sexual desire, with: Cham.
- Shrieks, with: Plat.
- Strangury, with: Ver-v.
- Sweat, cold, after: Castr.
- Thighs, down: Cham; Chel; Cimi; Kali-c; Rhus-t; Sep; Zin-val.
- Urination frequent, with: Med.
- Washing amel: Kali-c.

Pale: *Fer*; *Grap*; *Nat-m.*

Pregnancy, during: Asar; Cham; Cocl; Croc; Ip; Kali-c; Lyc; *Nux-m*; Pho; Rhus-t; Sabi; Sec.

Pressure on
- Abdomen amel: Mag-c.
- Back while sitting amel: Kali-c; Mag-m.

Protracted, too long: *Calc*; Carb-an; Carb-v; *Cup*; Fer; Kali-c; *Lyc*; *Mill*; *Nat-m*; NUX-V; Pho; *Plat*; Psor; Pul; Radm; Rat; Rhus-t; Sabi; *Sec*; Senec; Sil; Vinc; Vip.
- Labour, hasty after: Caul.
- Replaced by smarting leucorrhoea: Pho.
- Scarcely recovers form one, when another begins: Bur-p.
- Sexual desire, with: Kali-br.

Puberty, before: Calc; Cina; Sabi; Sil.

MENSES

Putrid, meat like: Lachn; Syph.
Rectum symptoms, with: Erig.
Return in old women: Calc; Plat.
Scanty: *Am-c*; Calc-p; *Con*; Cyc; *Dul*; *Grap*; *Kali-c*; *Lach*; Mag-c; Mang; Nat-m; Pho; PUL; Seneg; Sep; SUL.
- Dyspnoea, with: Arg-n.

Semen, odour like, strong: Stram.
Serum, like, gray: Berb.
Short: Am-c; Lach; PUL; *Sul*.
- Few hours: Vib.
- Leucorrhoea, bloody, followed by: Radm.
- One day only: Alu; Ap; Arg-n; Euphr; Radm; *Sep*.
  - or appear at the interval of one day: Ap.
- One hour: Euphr; Psor.

Shreddy: Phyt.
Sitting
- Agg: Mag-m.
- Amel: Kre.

Skin symptoms, with: Bor; Carb-v; *Dul*; *Grap*; Kali-c; Mag-m; *Nat-m*; Sang; Sars; Sep; Stram; Ver-a.
Stain indelibly: See Indelible.
Standing
- Agg: Am-c; Cocl; Mag-c; Psor.
- Tiptoe on agg: Cocl.

Stools
- During, after agg: Hep; Iod; Lyc; Murx.
- Hard, from: Amb; Lyc.

Stooping amel: Mag-c.

MENSES

Suppressed: See Absent.
- Agg: Aco; Bry; Caul; Cimi; Cup; Glo; Hell; Lyc; Mill; Mos; Pho; Pul; Senec; Sil; Sul.

Tarry: Kali-m; Mag-c; Mag-m; Mag-p.
Throat agg: Bar-c; Calc; Gel; Lac-c; Mag-c; Sul.
Urinary symptoms, with: Berb.
Vicarious (See DISCHARGES, vicarious): Bry; Fer; Grap; LACH; Pho; *Pul*; Sec; Senec; Sul; Ust; Zin.
Watery, thin: Aeth; Alum; Dul; Fer; Goss; Nat-m; Pul; Ust.
Weeks
- Every two: Bov; Bro; Calc-p; Cean; Lyc; Mag-c; Pho; Tril.
- Every three: Fer-p.

MENTAGRA: See under ERUPTIONS.

MENTAL

Alternations: See ALTERNATIONS.
Depression: See SADNESS.
Exertion AGG: Agar; Anac; Arg-m; *Arg-n*; Aur; CALC; Calc-p; *Ign*; Kali-p; *Lach*; Lyc; Nat-c; *Nat-m*; NUX-V; Pho; Pho-ac; *Pic-ac*; Pul; Rhus-t; Sele; *Sep*; *Sil*; Stap; *Sul*.
Exaustion, prostration (See BRAIN FAG): *Agar*; *Anac*; Arg-m; Aur; *Bar-c*; Con; Cup; Kali-p; Lach; *Lyc*; Nat-c; Nat-p; Nit-ac; NUX-V; *Pho*; PHO-AC; PIC-AC; *Plb*; Pul; Sep; Sil; *Stap*; Sul; Tab.

MENTAL, exhaustion
- Grief, from: Ign; Nux-m.
- Menses, after: Alu.

MERCURY, ill effects of: See under DRUGS, Abuse of.

MESENTERY: Bar-c; Calc; Iod; Sul-io; Tub.

METALLIC TUBE, breathes through as if: Merc-c.

METASTASIS (See ALTERNATING STATES): Abro; Carb-v; Cup; Pul.

Milk suppression, from: Agar.

MICTURITION: See URINATION.

MIGRAINE (See HEAD, one sided): Chio; Gel; Ip; Kali-bi; Lac-d; Nat-m; Nat-s; Onos; Psor; Rob; *Sang*; Spig; Sil; Ther.

Cerebral Origin+: Stan.

Face, pale with: Amy-n; Ars.

Nausea, vomiting, with+: Ip.

Prolonged: Cyc; Lac-d.

Polyuria with+: Ol-an.

Sleepy, before: Sul.

Sunset amel: Lac-d.

Vomiting amel+: Stan.

MILDNESS: See PLACID.

MILIARY: See ERUPTIONS, miliary.

MILK: See under LACTATION.

Agg and amel: See under FOOD.

Crusts: See HEAD EXTERNAL.

Leg: See PHLEGMASIA ALBA DOLENS.

MILKY: See DISCHARGES, milky.

MIND

Affections in general: *Aco*; *Ars*; Aur; BELL; Bry; *Calc*; Cham; Chin; HYO; *Ign*; LACH; Lil-t; *Lyc*; Nat-c; *Nat-m*; NUX-V; Op; *Pho*; Pho-ac; Plat; PUL; Sep; STRAM; *Sul*; Val; *Ver-a*.

Acute: *Cof*; *Op*.
- Weakness, physical, with: Sil.

Admonition agg: Bell; Pall; Plat.

Anger, suppression of agg: Ign; Lyc; *Stap*.

Anticipations agg: See ANTICIPATIONS.

Blank: Cor-r; Hell; Stan.

Childish, body grows: Buf.

Diarrhoea amel: Cimi.

Digestive affections, with: Arg-n.

Eating, little amel: Bell; Tarn.

Evening amel: Tarn.

Exertion physical
- Agg: Plb.
- Amel: Calc; Iod; Tarn.

Eyes, closing
- Agg: Carb-an; Mag-m.
- Amel: Kali-c; Zin.

Fickle+: Bism.

Filthy: Merc.

Heart, alternating with: Lil-t.

Laughing agg: Ther.

Leucorrhoea, appearing amel: Murx.

Menses
- Before
  - agg: Stan.
  - amel: Cimi.
- During agg: Nat-m; Stan; Stram.

MIND, menses

- Suppressed agg: Plat.

Narrating her symptoms agg: Calc; Pul.

Nose blowing amel: Kali-chl.

Pain agg: Cham; Sars; Ver-a.

Rheumatism agg: Cimi.

Shaving agg: Calad.

Soles, rubbing amel: Chel.

Stools amel: Bov; Cimi; Nat-s.

Syphilis agg: Asaf; *Aur*; Hep; Lach; Merc; Nit-ac; Phyt.

Tension+: Mos.

Tranquil, haemorrhage with+: Ham.

Uterus, alternating with: Arn; Lil-t.

Vacant+: Am-c.

Waking on agg: Calc; LACH; *Lyc*; STRAM; Zin.

Walking in open air agg: Glo; Nux-m; Petr.

Washing
- Face amel: Ars; Pho.
- Feet agg: Nat-c.

Weak, spasms after: Sec.

Yawning amel: Bry.

MINER'S DISEASE: Carb-s; Card-m; Nat-ar.

Coal: Sul.

MISCARRIAGE: See ABORTION.

MISCHIEVOUS: Anac; Calc; Cann; Nux-v.

MISDEEDS of others AGG: Colch; *Stap*.

MISERABLE: Flu-ac; Grap; Iod; Kre; Saba; Sep; Stan; Tab; Zin.

MISERABLE

Makes himself, by brooding over imaginary wrongs and misfortunes: Naj.

MISERLY : See AVARICIOUS.

MISFORTUNE: See FEAR, future.

Consolation, refuses for his own: Nit-ac.

Others of agg: Colo.

MISTAKES IN

Calculating+: Am-c.

Reading+: Sep.

Speech etc: Alu; *Calc*; *Chin*; Grap; Hep; Kali-br; Lac-c; LYC; Nat-c; *Nat-m*; Nux-v; Sep; Thu.

Writing: Am-c+; Hypr+; Lach; Lyc; Sep+; Thu.

- Omits words+: Benz-ac.

MOANING, groaning: Aco; Bell; *Bry*; Cann; Cham; *Cic*; Grap; Kali-c; Mang; Merc; *Mur-ac*; Zin.

Anxiously: Calad.

Breath, every, with: Bell.

Children: Lach; Mill.

Continuous+: Kre; Mang.

Fever, in: Arn; *Pul*.

Head, holds and vomiting when: Cimi.

Impulse, to: Grap.

Involuntarily: Alu; Cham.

Loudly, persistent: Mur-ac.
- Sleep, in: Calad.

Menses
- During: Ars.
- After: Stram.

Pain, with: Eup-p; Sil.

Sleep, in: Aur; Carb-an; Lach; Pod; Stan.

MOBILITY: Cam; Croc; Stram.

MOCKERY: *Lach*; Nux-m; Tarn.

MOISTNESS increased: See DISCHARGES, increased.

MOLASSES like: See DISCHARGES, molasses like.

MOLLITIS OSSIUM: See Bone, curvature.

MONOMANIA: Ign; Sil.

MONS VENERIS: Nat-m; Rhus-t; Sil.
  Eruptions: Sil.
  Itching: Eup-p.

MONTH: See DAY, every 28th.

MOODS CHANGING: See CHANGING MOODS.

MOON LIGHT
  AGG: Ant-t; Sep; *Sul*; Thu.
  AMEL: *Aur*.
  Blindness: Bell.

MOON PHASES, full moon etc.
  AGG: ALU; Bry; *Calc*; *Cina*; Cup; *Lyc*; Nux-v; *Pho*; Saba; SIL; Sul.
  AGG and AMEL: Clem; Phel; Tarn.
  Every alternate, full agg: Syph.
  New AGG: Caus; Cup; Kali-br; Nux-v; Rhus-t; Saba; Sep; Sil.
  First quarter agg: Ars; Bry; Nat-m.
  Full AGG: Bov; Calc; Cina; Grap; Nat-m; *Pho*; Psor; Saba; Sep; Sil; Sul.
  Increasing agg: Thu.
  Last quarter agg: Lyc; Sep.
  Waning agg: Daph.

MORAL PERVERSIONS: *Anac*; BELL; Buf; HYO; Nux-v; Op; Pho-ac; *Plat*; STRAM; Tarn; VER-A.
  Sense blunted+: Cocain.

MORBID: Stap.

MORBUS COXARIUS: See HIP JOINT, tuberculosis.

MORNING AGG: See under TIME.
  One day, evening other day: Eup-p; Lac-c.

MOROSE AND SULLEN: Anac; Ant-c+; Aur; Bry; Lyc+; NUX-V; Pul; *Sang*; Sil; Sul-ac; Tab+; Tub.

MORPHINISM: Avena; Nat-p; Passif.

MORTIFICATION, chagrin, vexation and agg from: *Aco*; Alu; Am-m; Anac; Aur-m+; Bell; *Bry*; Caus; Cham; *Colo*; Gel; *Ign*; Lyc; Merc; NAT-M; *Nux-v*; Op; Pall; *Petr*; Pho-ac; Plat; Stop; Ver-a; Zin.

MOTION: See GAIT.
  Absent: *Bry*; Cocl; Gel; Hell; Rhus-t.
  Agile: See Active.
  Angular+: Agar.
  Automatic: See AUTOMATIC ACTS.
  Averse, to: Aco; Ars; Bell; BRY; *Calad*; Calc; Calc-s; Caps; Chel; *Guai*; *Lach*; Nat-m; NUX-V; Rut; Sil; Sul.
    • Seated, after being: Kali-p.
  Difficult: Bell; *Bry*; Caus; Lyc; Petr; Rhus-t; *Sep*.

MOTION

Disorderly: Stram.
- **Paralytic parts, of:** Merc.

Erratic: Tarn; Ver-v.
Exaggerated: Agar; Ign.
Graceful: Pho; Stram.
Incessant, but walking agg: Tarn.
Irregular: Agar.
Oscillatory: Agar; Elap; Stram.
Rhythmic: Elap; Stram.
Side, one, only: Stro.
Tumultuous: Aco; Glo; Tab.
Uncertain+: Agar.

MOTION, WALKING etc. (See also WALKING)

AGG: Aesc, *Arn*; BELL; Bism; BRY; Calad; *Calc*; Calc-s; Caus; Chel; Chin; *Cocl*; COLCH; Colo; Con; Guai; *Kali-c*; Kalm; Led; Merc; *Nat-m*; Nit-ac; NUX-V; Pho; Phyt; Pic-ac; Pod; Pyro; Radm; Ran-b; Rhus-t; Sabi; Sep; SIL; SPIG; Stan; *Sul*; Sumb; Tab; Tarn; Tril; Tub; Vib; Zin-chr; Zin-val.

AMEL (rest AGG): Ant-t; *Arg-n*; *Ars*; *Aur*; CAPS; *Con*; Cyc; DUL; EUPHOR; *Fer*; *Flu-ac*; Gel; Helo; Iod; Kali-c; *Kali-io*; Kali-s; Kre; Lil-t; *Lyc*; Mag-c; Mag-m; Merc-c; PUL; Pyro; *Rhod*; RHUS-T; *Saba*; *Samb*; *Sep*; *Sul*; Tarn; *Tarx*; *Val*; Zin.

After AGG: *Agar*; ARS; *Cann*; *Pul*; RHUS-T; SEP; Spo; *Stan*; Sul-ac; *Val*.

Air open
- **AGG:** Ars; Caus; Cocl; Mag-p; Nux-v; Sele; Spig; *Sul*.

MOTION
- **AMEL:** *Alu*; *Arg-n*; Dios; *Flu-ac*; Iod; *Kali-io*; Kali-s; Lil-t; Lyc; Mag-c; Mag-m; *Pul*; *Rhus-t*.

Arms, of AGG: See ARMS, motion agg.

Beginning AGG, continued AMEL: *Amb*; Anac; *Calc-f*; Caps; Con; Euphor; Fer; Ign; Kalm; Kob; Lyc; Pho; *Pul*; Radm; RHUS-T; Sep; Syph.

Distant parts of agg: Ap; *Bry*; Cocl.

Feet of AMEL: Ars; Rhus-t; *Zin*.

Gliding AMEL: Nit-ac.

Rapid, violent etc.
- **AGG:** *Ars*; *Bry*; Sil; Sul; Symp.
- **AMEL (running dancing etc):** Am-m; *Ars*; Aur-m; Bro; Bur-p; Flu-ac; Grap; Ign; Nit-ac; Scop; *Sep*; Stan; Sul-ac; Tarn; *Tub*.

Slightest AGG: *Bry*; Buf; Cadm; Latro; Lob; Ther.

Slow, gentle AMEL: Agar; Alu; Amb; *Aur*; Caus; Colo; FER; Glo; *Kali-p*; Mag-m; PUL; Sumb; Syph; Tarn.

Sudden
- **AGG:** Cocl; Fer; Kali-c.
- **AMEL:** Rhod; Saba.

Wrong
- **AGG:** Bry; Lyc.
- **AMEL:** Am-m.

MOTTLED, patchy: AIL; Ars; Bap; Bell; *Carb-v*; Con; CROT-H; Glo; Kali-bi; Kali-m;

MOTTLED
LACH; Led; Lil-t; Manc; *Nat-m*; *Nux-v*; Ox-ac; Pho; Rhus-t; Sars; Syph; *Thu*; Ver-v.

MOULDY: See MUSTY.

Forming body over, as if: Sil.

MOUNTAIN climbing AGG:
Arn; Ars; Coca.

MOUTH
Affections in General: See THROAT.

Agg and amel: See THROAT.

About: Ars; Bry; Cina; Kali-n; *Kre*; Nat-m; Rhus-t; Sep; Stap; *Sul*.
- Bluish: *Cina*; Cup; Ver-a.
- Cobweb: Rat.
- Eruptions: Kali-m.
  - coryza during: Mez.
  - pimples: Ant-c; Ast-r.
- Muscles seem contracted: Gel.
- Pale: Aru-t; Bell; Cic; Cina; Merc-c; Stram.
- Sweat: Rhe.
- Trembling, twitching: Ign; *Op*; Senec; Thu.
- Yellow: Nux-v.

Angles
- Droop: Agar.
- Jerks, with pain: Tell.

Aphthae (See ulcers): Ant-c; *Ars*; *Bap*; *Bor*; Caps; Carb-v; Kali-bi; Kali-chl; Kali-m; Lach; Med; MERC; Merc-c; Mur-ac; Nux-v; Plb; Rhus-t; Sanic; *Sul*; *Sul-ac*; THU.
- Chewing gum, from: Merc.
- Children: Bor; Merc, Sul-ac.
- Diarrhoea, lienteric, with: Hell.

MOUTH, aphthae
- Eye affections, with: Bro.
- Mother's, nursing: Bap; Hyds.
- Pregnancy, during: Kre.
- Small and sore: Med.
- Sour and salty food, after: Bor.
- Suckling, of+: Bap.

Bitter: Menis; Zin.

Bleeding: Chin; Crot-h; Hep; Pho.

Brown-red: Lyc.

Burning, heat, raw, smarting: ARS; *Aru-t*; *Bell*; *Bor*; Cham; Iris; Manc; Med; Mez; Sang; Sul; Sul-io.
- Cold, not amel by: Merc.
- Sneezing, with: Ver-v.
- Thirst, with: Hypr.

Burnt, scalded, as if: Iris; Mag-m; Pul; Sep.

Clammy: Bell; Dios; Lach; Onos.

Close, cannot, at night: Chim.
- Desire to keep: Kob.

Cold: Ars; Cam; Carb-v; Kali-n; Tell; Ver-a.
- Corners: Aeth.

Covers it: Am-c; Arg-n; Cor-r; Cup; Ip; Kali-bi; *Lach*; Rum; Thu.

Cracked: Cocl; Pho; Pho-ac.
- Corners+: Cund; Mez.

Crawling: Zin.

Crusts: Myr.

Distorted: Con; Dul+.

Drawn to
- One side+: Dul.
  - left: Pho; Ver-v.

MOUTH

Dry: *Aco*; *Ars*; BELL; Berb; Bry; Chin; Lach; Lyc; *Merc*; Mur-ac; Nat-m; Nux-m; *Nux-v*; *Pho*; *Pho-ac*; Rhus-t; *Sep*; Stram; Stro; *Sul*; Sul-io; Tub; Ver-a; Ver-v.
- Anterior: Ars; Bry; Nux-v.
- But no thirst: Ap; Bry; Calad; Cocl; Kali-c; Lach; Lyc; NUX-M; *Nux-v*; *Pul*; Spig.
- Chewing, food, on: Thu.
- Chill, during: Petr.
- Cough, with, as if: Phyt.
- Food seems too, while eating: Calad; Chin; Fer; Ign; Kali-io; Ox-ac; Raph.
- Posterior: Mez; Thu.
- Rinse, must: Cinb.
- Saliva increased, with: Alu; Aral; Colch; Kali-c; Lyc; Mag-m; *Merc*; Nat-m; Plb.
- Scraping: Seneg.
- Sleep, in: Nux-m.
- Wakes from sleep: Cinb.
- Water, no amel+: Chio.

Eating amel: Benz-ac.

Fingers in, children put: Calc; Cham; *Ip*.

Foam, froth: Bell; Cham; Cic; Cup; *Hyo*; Ign; Laur; Sec; Stram; Ver-v.
- Chill, shaking during: Ther.
- Constant chewing, from: Asaf.
- Milky: Aeth.
- Reddish, bloody: Crot-c; Ign; Lach; Sec; Stram.
- Talking, while: Lac-d.
- White, rises from throat continuously: Mag-m.
- Yellow green: Sec.

Food escapes from, during chewing: Arg-n.

Furred, as if: Ther.

Gangrenous: Lach.
- Children, in: Ars.

Grasps, at: Sil.

Greasy: Iris; Ol-an.
- Rancid: Euphor.

Hairy sensation, in: Ther.

Herpes in, after sea-bathing: Zin.

Hot, as if: Hypr.

Induration inside cheek: Caus.

Inflammation: Kali-chl; Merc; Nit-ac; Petr.

Itching: Merc; Phyt; Rhus-t.

Loose skin, in: Phys.

Milk covered with, as if: Kali-io.

Motion of
- Sucking, as of: Bell.
- Talking: See TALKS himself to.

Mucous
- Adhesive: Myr.
- Foul: Myr; Rhe.
- Sleep after: Rhe.

Numb: Bap; Bar-c; Bell; Bov; Kali-br; Mag-m; Stro; Ther.
- Prickling, with: Nat-p.

Odour from, bad breath: See BREATH, Offensive.

Open, hangs, jaws drop: *Ail*; Ars; Bap; Bar-c; Carb-v; Colch; Gel; Hell; Hyo; *Lach*; LYC; Merc-c; Mur-ac; Naj; Nat-c; Op; Rhus-t; *Sul*; Zin.
- Cannot, or difficult: Caus; *Lach*; Merc-c; Nux-m; Pho.

MOUTH, open
- Convulsions or epilepsy
  - before: Buf.
  - during: Cup.
- Involuntarily: Ther.
- Night, at: Chim.
- Rapid succession, in: Myg.
- Remains
  - cannot close: Ther.
  - sleep, during: Nat-c.
  - yawning after: Ant-t.

Opening
- AGG: Aru-t; Bry; Caus; Cocl; *Lach*; *Merc*; Merc-c; Nux-v; Pho; Saba; Spig.
- AMEL: Mez.

Peppery: Coca.
Pins, needles, full of, as if: Spig.
Plate of teeth agg: Alum; Bor.
Raw: See Burning.
Rinsing agg: Coc-c.
Salt water, in: Carb-an; Verb.
Scalded, as if+: Ver-v.
Sleep, after: Rhe.
Sticky (See Clammy): *Aesc*; Berb; *Caps*; Chel; KALI-BI; Kali-c; Lach; Merc; Myr; Pul; Rhus-t; Tub.
Swelled: Kali-chl; Merc; Nit-ac.
Tongue, protruding agg: Cist.
Tumours: Calc; *Lyc*; *Nit-ac*.
- Painless: Calc; *Nit-ac*.

Twists, face, with: Lyc.
- One side to, when speaking: Cub.

Twitches: Op.
Ulcers (See Aphthae): *Ars*; Iod; Kali-io; Lach; Mur-ac; *Nit-ac*; Phyt.

MOUTH, ulcers
- Extending from mouth, to intestines: Terb.

Varicose veins: Thu.
Vesicles: Ars.
- Burning: Ars.

Warm, biting in, sneezing on: Ver-v.
- Unusually: Cimi; Croc.

Wipe, must: Kali-bi; Sec.
Yellow: Plb.
- Red: Lyc.

MOVEMENTS: See MOTION.
MUCOUS COLITIS: See STOOLS, mucus and COLITIS MUCOUS.
MUCOUS MEMBRANES: Aco; Ant-t; Ap; *Arg-n*; *Ars*; *Bell*; Bor; Bry; Caps; Cep; *Cham*; *Dul*; Eucal; Euphor; Hep; Hyds; Ip; Kali-bi; Kali-c; *Merc*; *Nux-v*; Pho; *Pul*; Rum; Saba; Sang; Scil; Senec; Seneg; *Stan*; *Sul*; Syph; Terb; Thu.

Dark: Aesc; Bap; Carb-v; Ham; Lach; Merc-i-r; Mez; Pho.
Dry: Alu; *Bell*; Bry; Caus; Kali-c; Nux-m; Sang; Stic.
Pale: Ars; Chin; Fer; Kali-c; Mang; Pho.
Patches: Arg-n; Lach; Merc-i-f; Nit-ac; Phyt; Pul.
Raw: Aru-t; Nux-v.
Red bright: Aco; Bell; Canth.
Secretion, altered: See DISCHARGES, mucous, altered.
Shrivelled: Bor.
Spongy: Caps; Phyt.
Ulcerated: Arg-n; Ars; Hyds; Kali-io; Kre; Merc-c; Nit-ac;

MUCOUS MEMBRANE,
  ulcerated: Phyt; Sil; Sul-ac.
  Vesicles: Ap; Bor; Canth; Carb-v.
  Wrinkled: Ars; Elap; Merc.
MUDDLED: See CONFUSION.
MUMPS (See PAROTIDS): Bell; Cham; Con; Jab; Lach; Merc; *Phyt*; *Rhus-t*; Sil.
  Fever, without: Kali-m.
  Limits, duration of+: Jab.
  Measles, after: Dul.
  Metastasis to
   • Mammae: *Pul.*
   • Testes: Ars; Carb-v; *Pul*; Rhus-t; Stap.
  Right, side+: Kali-bi.
  Septic: Anthx; Lach; Syph.
  Typhoid fever, in: Mang.
MUSCAE VOLITANTES: See under VISION.
MUSCLES: Agar; Anac; Arn; Ars; BELL; BRY; *Calc*; CAUS; Cimi; Cocl; Con; *Eup-p*; Gel; Hell; Hyo; Kali-c; *Mur-ac*; Nux-v; RHUS-T; Sec; Til; Val; *Ver-a*; Zin.
  Aching+: Bap.
  Atrophy: Ars; Calc; Caus; Plb; Thal; Thu.
   • Progressive: Crot-h; Kali-p; Mang; Pho+; Phys; Plb; Ver-v+.
  Belly, of: Cimi; Thu.
  Control, uncertain+: Caus.
  Cramps: Anac; Bell; *Calc*; Cina; Con; CUP; *Lyc*; Merc; *Nux-v*; Plat; Sep; Tab.
  Heavy+: Bap.

MUSCLES
  Increased ability to exercise, without fatigue+: Flu-ac.
  Indurated: Calc-f; Sil.
   • Neuralgia, after: Bry.
  Jumping: Colch; Dios; Hyds; Pul.
  Knots: Cup; Phyt; Senec; Syph.
  Lax, flabby: *Aeth*; Ant-t; Calc; Caps; Carb-ac; *Chin*; Cocl; Colch+; *Gel*; *Lyc*; Mur-ac; Pho+; Pho-ac; Stram; Sul.
  Obey feebly: Anac; Ast-r; Gel; Hell; Phys; Tarn.
  Rigidity+: Phys.
  Short: See CONTRACTIONS.
  Sore, from dancing etc: Cimi.
  Stiff: Terb.
  Stitches, burning, in: *Ap*; Asaf; Cocl; Glo; Mez; Nux-v; Rhus-t; Stap; Sul-ac; Thu.
   • Pressive, in: Sars.
  Tense: Aco; Lach; Nit-ac; *Nux-v*; Pho; Sep.
  Undeveloped: Nat-m.
  Undulating: Asaf.
  Weak (See WEAKNESS): Calc; Cimi; Cocl; Gel; Kali-c; Phys; Radm; Sil; Sul-ac; Ver-v.
MUSIC
  AGG: Aco; Amb; Buf; *Calc*; *Cham*; Croc; Dig; Grap; Kre; Lyc; Med; *Nat-c*; Nat-m; NUX-V; *Pho*; *Pho-ac*; Sabi; SEP; Sumb; Tarn; Tub; Vio-o.
  AMEL: Aur; Tarn.
  Menses during agg: Nat-c.
  Sad amel: Mang.

MUSTY, MOULDY: Bor; Crot-h; Mar-v; Rhus-t; Sanic; Stan; Stap; Thu; Thyr.

MUTINISM of childhood: Agrap; Lyc.

MUTTERING: See DELIRIUM, muttering.

  Himself, to: Tarx.

MYOPIA: See VISION, near sight.

MYXOEDEMA: Ars; *Thyr*.

NAEVI: See BIRTH MARK.

NAGGING: Lyc; Nux-v; Plat.

NAIL: See PLUG.

NAILS: Ant-c; Grap; Merc; *Sil*; *Sul*; Thu; Ust.

  Around: Psor.

  Base: Calc-p; Caps.

  Bites: Aco; Ars; Aru-t; Cina; Lyc; Med; Senec; Stram.

  Bood, oozing from: Crot-h.

  Blue: Aur; Chin; Dig; Nit-ac; *Nux-v*; Ox-ac; Sil; *Ver-a*.

  Brittle, crumbling: Alu; Clem; Flu-ac; Grap; Lept; Merc; *Psor*; Scil+; Senec; Sil; Sul; Thu.

  Burning: Sars.

  Corner, of: Lach.

  Crippled+: Sep.

  Curved: Nit-ac.

  • **Consumption, in:** Med; Tub.

  Cutting: Petr; Sars.

  Deformed, thickened etc: Alu; Ant-c; Calc-f; Flu-ac; *Grap*; Saba; Sep; *Sil*; Sul; Syph; Thu.

  Depressed: Med.

  Discoloured: Grap; Nit-ac; Thu.

  Edge of: Calc-p; Radm.

NAILS

  Falling: Grap; Hell; Scil; Sil; *Ust*.

  Fly, off: Pyro.

  Fold, remains attached to the growing: Osm.

  Gnawing: Alu; Berb; Lach; Lapp.

  Grey: Merc-c.

  Grow, quickly: Flu-ac.

  • **Do not:** Ant-c; Radm.

  • **Interrupted:** Kali-s.

  Hang nails: Calc; *Nat-m*; Nat-s; Rhus-t; *Sul*.

  Hypertrophy: Calc-f; Laur.

  Ingrown: Flu-ac; *Grap*; Hep; *Mag-p-aus*; *Mar-v*; Nit-ac; *Sil*; Sul-io.

  • **Pain, motion amel:** Mar-v.

  Knotty+: Laur.

  Loose, as if: Ap; Pyro; Ust.

  Painful: Caus; Grap; Merc; Nit-ac; Sil; Sul.

  Pricking, under: Elap.

  Ribbed: Flu-ac; Thu.

  • **Transversely:** Ars.

  Run around: See FINGERS, felon.

  Scaling: Alu.

  Soft: Lept; Plb; Thu.

  Splitting: *Ant-c*; Flu-ac; Lept; Rut; Scil+; *Sil*; Thu.

  Spotted: Nit-ac; Sil.

  • **White:** Alu; Nit-ac; Sil.

  Thick: See Dformed.

  Thin: Lept.

  Tingling, in: Colch.

  • **Under:** Sil.

  Ulcer: Sil.

NAILS
Under: Alu; Berb; Bism; Sars; Sep.
- Growth: Ant-c.
- Irritable feeling: Am-br.
- Splinter: Calc-p; Coc-c; Flu-ac.

Yellow: Con; Nit-ac; Sep; Sil.

NAKED, wants to be: Bell; *Hyo*; Pho; Sec; Tarn.

NAPE: See Under NECK.

NAPS amel: See SLEEP, short amel.

NARCOTICS agg: See Under DRUGS, abuse of.

NARRATING her symptoms agg: Calc; Cic; Mar-v; Pul.

NARROW: See FORCED through narrow opening.

NASO-PHARYNX (posterior nares): Cinb; Elap; Hyds; *Lyc*; *Merc*; *Merc-c*; Merc-i-r; *Nat-c*; *Nat-m*; Pho; Rum; Sep; *Spig*; *Stap*; Sul; Ther; Thu; Zin-io.

Bleeding: Cor-r; Spig.

Discharges, from: Arn; Coc-c; Cor-r; Mag-c; Nat-c; Phyt; Syph; Ther.
- Bloody: *Hep*; Saba; Tell.
- Drips: Cep; Hyds; Merc-c; Spig.
- Lumpy: Calc; Cimi; Mar-v; Merc-i-f; Sep; Syph.
- Sticky: Caps; Kali-bi.

Dry: Rum.

Expansion, sensation of: Flu-ac.

Food, sensation of: Nit-ac; Sil.

Hot, dry: *Aco*; Aesc; Lyc; Sep; Zin-io.

Itching: Ail; Kali-p; Nux-v; Ran-b.

NASO-PHARYNX
Lump, as of, a: Aesc; Cist; Hyds; Kali-bi; *Lach*; Mar-v; Nat-m; Pho; Sep; Spig; Stic; Sul; Zin.

Mucus drops into: Cinb; Cor-r; Lith; Med.

Raw, sore: Aco; CARB-V; Kali-n; Sep.

Stuffed, up: Elap.

NATES: See BUTTOCKS.

NAUSEA:
AETH; ANT-C; ANT-T; Arg-n; ARS; Bell; BRY; *Carb-v*; *Cham*; Chin; COCL; *Colch*; *Cup*; *Dig*; Dul; Hell; *Hep*; *Ign*; *Ip*; Kali-c; Lac-d; Lob; *Lyc*; Nat-m; *Nit-ac*; *Nux-v*; Petr; *Pho*; *Pul*; *Rhus-t*; Sang; *Sep*; Sil; *Sul*; Sul-ac; Tab; Val; VER-A; Zin.

Abdomen, felt in: Cimi; Polyg.

Alcoholism, from: Cimi.

Amorous caresses, from: Ant-c; Sabal.

Anus, burning in, with: Kali-bi.

Anxiety, with deathly: Ant-c; Ant-t; Cocl; *Crot-h*; *Ip*; LOB; Pul; *Tab*.

Ascending rapidly, on: Glo.

Chest, felt, in: Ant-t; Calend.

Chill, with: Cocl; Echi; Eup-p; Kali-m; Sul-ac.

Coffee
- Agg: Caps.
- Amel: Alet.

Coition
- During: Saba; Sil.
- After: Kali-c; Mos.
- Thought of: Sep.

Cold, when: Cadm; *Cocl*; Hep.

NAUSEA

Concomitant, as a: Nat-s.
Continuous: IP; Iris; *Nux-v*; Sil; Vib.
- Eating amel+: Vip.

Convulsions, before: Hyd-ac.
Cough, during: Ip; Kali-p; Pul.
Crowd, in: Sabi.
Deathly: See Anxiety, with.
Descending agg: Nat-s.
Diarrhoea, with: Cist.
Dinner amel: Alet.
Dream, in: Arg-m.
Drinking
- After: Calc; Cocl; Pul.
- Amel: *Bry*; Lob; Pho.
- Ice water amel: Calc.

Drowsiness, with: Apoc.
Ear, felt in: Dios.
Eating
- Amel: Arg-n; Fago; Lac-ac; Mez; Phyt; Radm; Sang; Sep; Vib.
- While: Ver-a.

Erection, with: Kali-bi.
Eructation
- During: Cimi; Kali-c; Nit-ac.
- Amel: Caus; Kali-p; Lac-c; Rum.

Excessive, vanishing of sight; with+: Crot-t.
Excitement, after: Kali-c.
Eyes
- Closing
  - agg: Lach; Ther.
  - amel: Con.
- Using agg: Jab; Pul; Sars; Sep; Ther.

NAUSEA

Faint like: Cocl; Lach; Nux-v.
Fasting, while: Calc; *Lyc*.
Fatty food agg: Dros.
Fever, during: Nat-m.
Fish, after: Nat-m.
Flatus passing
- Agg: Ant-t.
- Amel: Bell.

Food: See Odour.
- Thought of agg: Cocl; Colch; Mos.
  - eaten, of: Sars.

Fruits agg: Ant-t; Ip.
Hawking agg: Stan.
Headache during: Ant-c; Caus; Cocl; Con; Ip; Iris; Sang; Stro.
- Trembling of body, with: Bor.

Head, felt in: Colch.
Heat of body, with: Kali-bi.
Hiccough, with: Lach.
Hot
- Drinks amel: See Warm drinks.
- Stove, near agg: Laur.

Hunger agg: Ign; Petr; Val; Ver-a.
Ice
- Creams, from: Rhus-t.
- Drinks, from: Laur.

Indigestible things, amel+: Ign.
Itching with, before urticaria: Sang.
Lips, touching on: Cadm; Nux-m.
Looking at
- Moving objects: Asar; Cocl; Ip; Jab.

NAUSEA, looking at
- One object steadily: Ther.

Lying on
- Side amel: Ant-t; Nat-m.
- Right side agg: Bry; *Cann*; Crot-h; Iris; Sang; Sul-ac.

Menses
- Agg: Bor; Cocl; Grap; *Nux-v*; Symphor.
- After: Crot-h.
- Profuse, with: Caps.

Midnight
- After: Ran-sc.
- At: Fer.

Milk amel: Chel.

Morning: Calc; Carb-v; Cimi; Grap; Lac-ac; Med; *Nux-v*; PUL; *Sep*.
- Early: Lob.
  - continues whole day: Cact.

Motion, least agg: Tab; Ther.

Night agg: Carb-an; Lob.

Noise, from: Ther.

Nose, blowing agg: See Sneezing.

Odour
- Any, from: Vario.
- Food, of, cooking etc. agg: Ars; Cocl; COLCH; Dig; Ip; Merc-i-f; Sep; Stan; Vario.
- Of his own body: Sul.

Operation on abdomen, after: BISM; Stap.

Pain
- During: Cadm; Chel; Ip; Kalm; Sep; Spig.
- Abdomen in, from: Colo; Nux-v.

NAUSEA
Palpitation, with: Arg-n; Bro; Myg; Sil.

Pessary in uterus, from: Nux-m.

Pregnancy, during: Asar; Cimi; Kre; Lac-ac; Mag-m; Nux-v; Sep; Stap; Tab.

Pressure
- Abdomen, on: Tub.
- Downward in intestine with: Agn.
- Forehead, in+: Alet.
- Neck, on: Cimi.
- Painful spot, on: Nat-m.
- Spine, on: Cimi.
- Throat, on: Lach.

Prickling, all over, with: Lob.

Putting hands in warm water: PHO.

Quiet amel: Cadm.

Rectum, felt in: Rut.

Renal origin, from: Senec.

Respiratory symptoms, with: Lob.

Rinsing mouth, on: Bry; *Sep*; Sul-ac.

Room, closed, in: Lyc; Nat-c; Tab.

Saliva, swallowing on: Colch.

Salt, thinking of: Nat-m.

Sewing, while: Lac-d; Sep.

Shivering, with: Kali-m; Sul-ac.

Singing, while: Ptel.

Sleep, before going to: Lach.

Smoking
- Agg: Carb-an; Clem.
- Amel: Sanic.

NAUSEA

Sneezing, while: Hell; Lach; Sang; Sul.
Sour things amel: Arg-n.
Speaking agg: Ther.
Spitting agg: Led.
Standing amel: Tarx.
Stomach, felt in: Cocl; *Ver-a.*
Stool, loose
- After: Aco.
- Amel: Terb.
- Urging, with: Dul.

Stooping amel: Petr.
Stove near: Laur.
Sudden, when eating: Rut.
Sun, heat of, agg: Carb-v.
Swallowing
- Empty, on: Colch.
- Preventing: Arn.

Sweets agg: Arg-n; Cyc; *Grap;* Ip; Merc.
Thinking
- Food he has eaten, about: Sars.
- Hard, when: Bor.

Throat
- Dryness, with: Cocl.
- Felt, in: Aral; Cyc; Mez; Pho-ac; Stan; Val.

Trembling, with: Ars; Bor; Plat.
Uncomfortable: Ars-io.
Uncovering amel+: Tab.
Urination
- Agg: Dig.
- Amel: Nat-p.

Urticaria, then: Sang.
Vision dim, with: Myg.

NAUSEA

Vomiting
- Amel: Phyt; Pyro.
- Does not amel: Dig; Ip; Sang.
- Purging, and, with+: Ver-v.

Warm drinks amel: Pyro; Ther.
Washing, while: Bry; Ther; Zin.
Water
- From: Apoc; Ars; Calc; Ver-a.
- Iced
  - agg: Lach.
  - amel: Calc.

Waves, in: Ant-t.
Worm, rising in throat, as if with: Spig.
Yawning, while: Arn; Nat-m.

NAVEL AND REGION:
Bry; *Colo;* Dios; *Dul;* Ip; Kre; Lept; Nux-v; *Pho-ac; Rhus-t;* Spig; *Ver-a;* Verb.

Aching, headache, with: Lept.
Back, to: Plat.
Bladder, alternating with: Terb.
Bleeding from, in new born: Abro; *Calc-p.*
Bloated: See Inflated.
Breast, to: Pall.
Bubbling: Aeth; Hypr.
Burning: ACO; Bov; Kali-io; *Lach;* Lyc; Phyt; Plb; Sep.
- Oesophagus, to: Hyd-ac.

Cramp, colic: Clio; *Colo;* Dios; Ip; Nat-s; Rhod; Senec; Stro.
- Directions, to all, stool amel: Senec.

Creeping: Rum.
Cutting: Colch; *Colo;* Dul; Ip; *Nux-v;* Ver-v.

NAVEL, cutting
- Breathing deep agg: Mang.
- Leucorrhoea, with: Am-m; Sil.
- Stools amel: Benz-ac.

Drawn, in: Chel.
Empty: Flu-ac; Kob.
Eruptions, about: Dul.
- Eczema: Sul.

Festers: Abro; Calc-p; Nux-m.
Flatus amel: Mag-c.
Groins, to+: Ver-v.
Hard: Pul.
Hernia: See under HERNIA.
Hunger, felt in: Val.
Inflated: Calc; Phys.
Lump at, as if: Kre; Nux-v; Rhus-t; *Sep*; Spig; Verb; Zin.
- Behing: Ran-sc.
- Falling to back, from: Laur.
- Hard, below: Bism.

Moisture, at: Calc-p.
Motion, as of, expiration, on: Card-m.
Painful, children with worms+: Spig.
Pelvis, to: Pall; Rum; Sep.
Pouting: Dul.
Proud flesh: *Calc*; Kali-c; Nat-m.
Radiating, from: Benz-ac; Senec.
Rectum
- From: Colo; Lach.
- To: Alo; Ars; Crot-t; Dios; Fer-io; Lyc.

Red: Phys.
- Streak, curved above: Par.

Retracted: Calc-p; *Plb*; Pod; Pul; Stan; Tab; Ver-a; Zin.
- Colic, with: Nat-c.

NAVEL
Rumbling: Tarx.
- Pinching, and+: Strop.

Sickening pain, after stools: Pho-ac.
Sitting agg: Symp.
Sore: Nux-m; Phys; Thu+.
Stools
- Agg: Lept.
- Amel: Senec.

Suppurating: Pho.
Swelling, painful: Caus.
Throbbing: Kali-c.
Turns and twists+: Plat.
Twisting, at: Cina; Verb.
Ulceration
- Above: Ars.
- Infants: Petr.
- New born: Ap.

Urine oozing, from: Hyo.
Uterus, to (See Pelvis to): Ip.
Yellow discharge, from suppressed gonorrhoea: Nat-m.

NEAR SIGHT: See VISION, near.

NECK AND NAPE: Aco; Bar-c; *Calc*; Cimi; Gel; *Nux-v*; Phyt; Pul; Rhus-t; Sanic; Sep; Sil; Stap; Tub.

Abscess: Sul-ac.
Aching: *Bry*; Chin; *Cimi*; *Gel*; Guai; Hyds; Kali-p; Kalm; Lach; Lachn; Lil-t; Lyc; Lyss; Onos; Par; *Phyt*; Sil; Ver-v.
- Nape: Cocl; Gel; Pho-ac; Pic-ac; Stro.

Alternating sides: Calc-p; *Pul*.
Arms, to: *Kalm*; *Lach*; Nat-m; Nux-v.

NECK

Ascending from nape: Meny; Sul.
Bending head, forward AGG: Cimi; Lyss; Radm.
Blow, as of: Naj.
Blowing nose agg: Kali-bi.
Bluish nape: Lach; Rhus-t.
Boils: Kali-io; Sil; Sul; Sul-io.
• Nape: Pic-ac; Sul.
Breathing deeply agg: Chel.
Brown: Sanic.
Bubbling+: Lyc.
Burning, heat: Lach; Merc; Pho-ac.
• Swallowing, when: Petr.
Carbuncle: Lach; Sil.
Chewing agg: Form.
Chloasmae: Caul; Sanic.
• Greasy: Lyc; Petr.
Clothes agg (See CLOTHES, pressure about neck agg): Caus.
Cold: Con; *Sil*; Spo.
• Icy, Nape: Chel.
Constriction
• As of a band: Bell; Glo; *Lach*; Nux-m; Sep; Spo.
• Cord, as from: Chel; Spo.
Contracted, rigidly: Ran-b.
• Speaks by moving shoulders up and down: Ran-b.
Cracking: Chel; Cocl; Nat-c; Petr; Sul.
Cramp: Calc-p; *Cic*; Cimi; Naj; Phyt; Plat; Spo; Ver-v.
• Nape: Hyd-ac; Nux-v.
Curvature: Calc; Syph.
Cutting: Kali-bi.

NECK

Cysts, both sides, on: Bro.
Draft, air on agg: *Calc-p*; Hep; Lach; Merc; Psor; Sanic; *Sil*; Stro.
Drawing: Chel; Cimi; Thu.
Emaciated: Calc; Lyc; Mag-c; NAT-M; Sanic; *Sars*.
Eruption: Arn; Sil; Sul-io.
Exertion
• Agg: Arg-n; *Calc*; Lil-t; *Sep*.
• Mental agg: Par; Zin.
Face, to: Kalm.
Fingers, to: Par.
Formication: Nux-v; Sec.
Full: Glo.
Gargling agg: Form.
Gnawing: Nat-s; Thu.
Hand
• Motion of agg: Cimi.
• Seized by, as if: Grat.
Hawking agg: Form.
Head could not support, as if: Fago.
Heavy: Par; Rhus-t.
• Nape: Meny; *Nux-v*; Par; *Rhus-t*.
Injury, concussion: Mez.
Itching: Alu; Nat-m; Sul.
Jerking, muscles, in: Aeth; Colo; Sep.
• Convulsions, before: Buf.
Lame nape (See Weak): Zin.
Large, too, as if: Kali-c.
Left head or shoulder, to: Spig.
Lifting agg: Calc.
Looking up agg: Grap.
Neuralgia: Hyds.

NECK

Numb: Chel; Plat.
Pressing: Bell; Par; Pho.
Prickling: Carb-an.
Pulsation: See Throbbing.
Red: Bell; Crot-h; *Grap*; Pho; Rhus-t; Ver-a.
Short: Alu; Bell; Cic; Cimi; Syph.
- Nape: Ign; Nat-m; Tub.
Shooting: *Nat-m*; Sul-ac.
Shoulder, and: Crot-t; Guai; Lachn; Stic; Sul; Ver-v.
- Right: Nux-v; Zin.
Sitting erect, amel: Radm.
Sneezing
- Agg: Am-m; Arn.
- Amel: Calc.
Sore: Nat-s; Pho-ac; Sil; Stic.
Spondylitis: Pho-ac.
Standing amel: Radm.
Stiff: Agar; Anac; Arg-m; Bar-c; *Bell*; Bry; Calc; Chel; *Caus*; Cimi; Glo; Ign; *Kali-c*; Lachn; Lachn; Lyc; Mag-c; *Merc*; Merc-i-r; *Nit-ac*; Nux-v; Pho; Phyt; Rhus-t; Sep; Sil; Spig; Stic; Sul; Tub.
- Back, down: Anac.
- Bending head forwards agg: Kali-bi.
- Cracks, moving when: Petr.
- Headache, with: Sil.
- One side: Colo; Guai; Stic.
- Right: Agar; Caus; Nat-m.
  - temples, to: Chel; Spig.
- Left: Bell; Carb-an; Chel; Colo; Glo; Guai; Kre; Lyc.
  - spine, with: Adon.
  - temples, to: Spig.

NECK, stiff, left
- yawning, on: Nat-m.
Stools amel: Asaf.
String around (See constriction+): Chel.
Swallowing
- Agg: Calc-p; Colch; Zin.
- Amel: Spo.
Sweat: *Calc*; Chin; Lach; Mang; *Pho-ac*; Sanic; STAN; Sul.
- Cold, nape: Con.
Swelling
- Fatty: Am-m.
- Nape: Bar-c.
Temple
- Right, to+: Chel.
- Left, to+: Spig.
Tense: Con; Sep; Sul; Tub.
- Numbnes, with: Plat.
Thick growing: Con; *Iod*; Pho.
- Talking, while: Iod.
Throbbing, pulsation: Ap; *Bell*; Op; Pyro; Spig; Ver-v.
- Menses
  - before: Nit-ac.
  - during: Nit-ac; Ver-v.
Touch agg: Lach.
Tumours
- Cystic; Bro.
- Fatty: Bar-c; Thu.
- Malignant: Calc-p.
Turning agg: *Bell*; Bry.
Uncovering amel: Sars.
Uneasy, nape: Aeth.
Veins, swollen: Op.
Vertebrae
- Crack: Chel; Ol-an.
- Sore: Ham.

NECK

Vertex, to: Kalm.

Weak, tired: Abro; *Aeth*; Ant-t; Bap+; Calc-p; Caul; *Cocl*; Nat-m; Par; PLAT; Sanic; Sep; Sul; *Ver-a*; Ver-v.
- Headache, with: Fago.
- Head falls, forwards: Nux-m.
- Then, stupor: Hyo; Zin.

Wrinkled, skin: Sars.

Writing agg: Carb-an; Lyc; ZIN.

Wry, torticollis: *Bell*; Cimi; Dul; Glo; Hyo; Lachn; Lyc; Nux-v; *Pho*; *Rhus-t*.
- Right: Cup; Lyc.
- Left: *Bell*; *Lyc*; Nux-v; *Pho*.
- Chronic: Bar-c.
- Shock, from: Nux-v.
- Throat, sore, with: Lachn.

Yawning agg: Cocl; Nat-s.

NECROSIS (See BONES): Calc-io; Radm.

NEEDLES: See PAIN, stitching.

Cold: *Agar*; Ars.

Hot (See HOT, iron): Ars; Lith; Ol-an; Vesp.

NEGLECTED

Appearance, his own: Coca.

He is: *Arg-n*; PALL.

His duty, he has: AUR; Ign; *Lyc*.

NERVOUS patients, nerves etc:
Aco; Arg-n; Asaf; Aur; *Bell*; Bor; Castr; Caul; *Caus*; Cham; *Chin*; Cimi; *Cocl*; *Cof*; *Con*; Cup; *Hyo*; IGN; Iod; Jab; Kali-p; LACH; *Lil-t*; Mag-c; Mag-m; Mag-p; Merc; *Mos*; Nat-m; *Nit-ac*; Nux-m; NUX-V; *Pho*; Pic-ac; Pru-sp; PUL; Sabal;

NERVOUS ..
Senec; Sep; SIL; Stap; Stic; *Stram*; *Sul*; *Tarn*; Ther; Thyr; Vib; Visc; Zin; Zin-val.

Activity: Vio-o.

Coughing, when: Cimi.

Disorders, from suppressed eruptions: Asaf.

Paralysis: Pru-sp.

Prostration, neurasthenia: Agar; Ars; *Calc*; Gel; Ign; Kali-p; *Lach*; Lecith; Lyc; Nat-m; Nux-v; Ol-an; Onos; Pic-ac; Pho; Plat; SEP; SUL; Vio-o.
- Grief, from: Phys.
- Prostatic: Thu.
- Sexual: Calad; Onos; Sabal; Stap.
- Unmarried perons, of: Agn.
- Urinating, when: Cimi.

NETTED: See BIRTH-MARK.

NETTLE RASH: Dul; Urt.

NEURALGIA: See PAIN.

Brachial: Kalm; Terb; Ver-a.
- Cervico: Chel; Nux-v.

Caries, from: Stap.

Ciliary+: Mez; Pru-sp; Rhod.

Coffee, abuse of+: Grat.

Coition after (male): Ced.

Coldness, along nerve, with: Terb.

Crural: Stap.

Diaphragmatic: Stan.

Injury, from: Hypr.

Intercostal: See PLEURODYNIA.

Lumbo-abdominal: Aran.

Menses during: Amy-n; Aran.
- Suppressed from: Kalm.

NEURALGIA

- **Operation, surgical, after:** Cup.
- **Orbital:** See ORBITS.
- **Palpitation, with:** Lach.
- **Paralytic weakness and trembling with:** Kalm.
- **Periodical:** Cact.
- **Peripheral:** Arg-n.
- **Phrenic:** Bell.
- **Prodrome, as a:** Nux-v.
- **Sepsis, from:** Crot-h.
- **Shingles, after:** Caus; Dol+; Kali-chl; Kalm; Mez; Plant; Pru-sp; Ran-b; Vario; Zin.
  - Touch
    - agg: Petr.
    - amel: Zin.
- **Stump, of:** Am-m; Arn; Asaf; Cep; Hypr; Pho-ac; Stap; Symp.
  - Breathing, deep Amel: Pho-ac.
- **Subscapularis:** Terb.
- **Suppressed agg:** Stan.
- **Veins, pressure from distended:** Sec.

NEURASTHENIA: See NERVOUS prostration.

NEURITIS

- **Injury, after:** Cep; Hypr; Stram.
- **Multiple:** Ars; Bov; Con; Morph; Stro; Thal; Vip.
- **Numbness, and tingling with:** Bov.
- **Optic:** Plb.
- **Retrobulbar:** Chin-s; Iodf.
- **Touch amel:** Sang.

NEUROMA+: Cep.

NEVER WELL since: Carb-v.
- **Abortion:** Sec.

NEVER WELL since
- **Burns;** Caus.
- **Chest affections:** Sul.
- **Climaxis:** Lach.
- **Diphtheria:** Lac-c; Phyt; Pyro.
- **Infectious diseases:** Psor.
- **Influnza:** Gel.
- **Pneumonia:** Kali-c.
- **Puberty+:** Pul.
- **Septic fever:** Pyro.
- **Typhoid:** Carb-v; Mang; Psor; Pyro.

NEVUS: See BIRTH MARK

NEW
- **All objects seem:** Hell; Stram.
- **Cannot do anything:** Agar.
- **Growth:** See Growth, New.

NEWS
- **Bad:** See BAD NEWS.
- **Glad:** See Joy.

NIBBLING: See APPETITE, nibbling.

NICTALOPIA: See NIGHT blindness.

NIGHT: See under TIME.
- **Blindness:** Bell; *Chin*; Hell; *Lyc*; Nux-v; Phys; Stram.
- **Mare, terrors:** See AWAKES, fright.
- **Sees, better, at:** Fer.
- **Sweats, phthisis, of:** Ars; Bry; Calc; Carb-v; Chin; Fer; Pho; Pho-ac; Samb; Sep; Sil; Stan; Sul.
  - All night: Pho.
  - Amel: Kali-io.
  - Awaking on: Samb.

NIGHT, sweat
- First sleep
  - after: Lach.
  - in: *Ars*.

Watching agg (See SLEEP amel, loss of agg): Caus; *Cocl*; Cup; *Nit-ac*; Sele; Zin.

NIPPING: See Pain, twinging.

NIPPLES: *Arn*; Cham; Grap; Lyc; Pul; Rat; *Sul*.

Left: Nat-s; Pyro; Rum.
- Under: Ascl; Rum.
  - palpitation, with: Ascl.

Abscess: Merc; Sil.

Air, from: Cyc.

Backward, from: Crot-t; Phel.
- Left: Sul.
- Nursing, when: Crot-t.

Bleeding: Buf; Ham; Lyc; Merc; *Sep*; Sil; Sul.

Bloody water, from: Lyc; Phyt.

Burning: Agar; Grap; Lyc; Sil; *Sul*.
- Left: Senec.
- Look angry, during pregnancy+: Alu.
- Sore, and: Pho.

Cold: Med.

Cracked: Aesc; Carb-an; Cast-eq; *Caus*; GRAP; PETR; *Phyt*; *Rat*; SARS; Sep; Sul.
- Herpes, around with: Caus.
- Nursing women+: Hyds.

Crawling: Sabi.

Cutting, scapula, to (male): Tell.

Deformed: Merc.

Dryness: Cast-eq.

Erect: Lach.

NIPPLES

Excoriated: Arn; *Caus*; *Flu-ac*; *Phyt*; Sul.

Glandular swelling, about: Merc-c.

Hanging: Cast-eq.

Hot: Pho.

Indurated, hard: Bry; Calc; Carb-an; Merc.

Inflammation: Cadm; Cham; Pho; Sil.

Inverted: See Retracted.

Itching: Grap; Onos; Petr; Sep; Sul.
- Menses, during: Hep.
- Pimples, around: Psor.
- Voluptuous: Sabi.

Mealy, covering, on: Petr.

Milky water, from (right): Bur-p.

Neuralgia: Plant.

Numb: Sars.

Oozing: Med.

Outward going pains: Berb; *Bry*; Gel; Kali-bi; Lapp; Lyc; Mez; *Ol-an*; Spig; Stan.

Red: Psor.

Retracted, inverted: Con; Grap; Hyds; Lach; *Nat-s*; Phyt; *Sars*; Sil; *Thu*; Tub+.
- Dysmenorrhea, with: Sars.

Scapula, to: Crot-t.

Sore, tender: Arn; Bap; Caus; Crot-t; Flu-ac; Ham; Helo; Lach; Lyc+; Med; Pho; Pyro; Sil.
- Constantly: Lac-c.
- Menses, during: Helo.
- Touch of clothing agg: *Cast-eq*; Con; *Crot-t*; Helo; Oci-c.

NIPPLES, sore
- Under: Sang.

Stitches: Con; Nat-m.
- Breath deep agg: Con; Ign.
- Walking agg: Con.

Swelling: Merc-c.
- Glandular, about: Merc-c.
- Right: Flu-ac.

Ulceration: Cast-eq.

White spot in centre: Nux-v.

NIPS: See PAIN, twinging.

NODES: *Ant-c*; CALC; Carb-an; Caul; Caus; Cinb; Dul; *Grap*; Guai; Iod; Kali-s; Lach; Lyc; Mag-c; Mez; *Pul*; Rhod; Rhus-t; Rut; Sars; Sil; Stap; *Sul*; Ther.

Gouty, sore+: *Sars.*

Hard: Mag-c.
- Burning: Hep.
- Joints, around: Form.
- Painful: Phyt.
- Red, sore: Petr.

Red: Med.

Shin, bones, on: Cinb.

Site of an old boil: Lyc.

NOISE

AGG (sensitive to): Aco; Asar; BELL; Bor; CHIN; Chin-ar; *Cof*; Con; Kali-c; *Mag-c*; Mag-m; *Nit-ac*; NUX-V; Op; *Sep*; *Sil*; Tarn; *Ther*; Tub; Zin.

AMEL: Grap.

Bell, of AGG: Ant-c.

Labour pains, during: Cimi.

Menses, during: Kali-p.

Penetrating AGG: *Asar*; Bar-c; Chin; Cocl; Con; Fer; Iod; Lept; Lil-t; Lyc; Manc; Mur-ac; Sabi; *Ther.*

NOISE

Rattling, shrill agg: Calc; Nit-ac.

Slightest AGG: Asar; Buf; Calad+; Cof; Fer+; Nux-v; Op; Sil; Ther.
- But not loud: Bor.
- Greatly accentuated: Bad.

Strikes, painful part: Ther.

Sudden agg: Bor; Calad; Cocl; Nat-c; Nat-m.

Talking of several persons AGG: Petr.

Water, splashing of AGG: Bro; LYSS; NIT-AC; Stram.

NOISY: Aco; Bell; Cham; Cic.

NOMA: See CANCER, cancrum oris.

NOSE: Aco; Aesc; Alu; *Ars*; *Aur*; Calc; Grap; Hep; Hyds; Ign; Iod; KALI-BI; *Kali-io*; *Lyc*; *Merc*; Merc-i-f; *Nat-m*; Nit-ac; Nux-v; Pho; PUL; Saba; *Sep*; SIL; Spig; *Sul*; Zin-chr.

One side: Am-m; Hep; Ign; Nux-v; Pho; Phyt; *Saba*; Sinap; Sil.
- Right: Con; Mar-v; Spig.
  - hot swollen, coryza in: Merc-i-r.
- Left: Carb-v; Nat-m; Rhod; Sep.
- Alternating between: Kali-io; Lac-c; Lach; Mez; Nux-v; *Pho*; Phyt; Rhod; *Sinap*; Sul.

Aching, in: Dul.

Acne: Ars.

Air, open amel: Aco; *Cep*; Hyds; Iod; Nux-v; *Pul*; Tell.
- Feels cold, in: Hyds.

NOSE, air
- Inspired
  - agg: See AIR, inspiring agg.
  - feels cold: Lith.

Alae: See NOSTRILS.
Behind: Merc-c.
Bleeding (See EPISTAXIS): *Pho*; Vip.
Blowing
- Agg: See BLOWING NOSE.
- Lumps, of: Merc-d.
- Painful, on: Mang.
- Tendency for: Am-m; Bor; Hyds; Kali-bi; Lyc; Mang; *Mar-v*; *Stic*.
  - but no relief: *Kali-bi*; Lach; *Mar-v*; Psor; *Stic*.

Boils, small, painful inside: Ap; Tub.
Bones: Aur; Kali-bi; *Merc*; Pho; Rhus-t.
- Caries: Aur; Nit-ac.
- Painful: Aur; Hep; Kali-bi; Rhus-t; Sil.
- Two loose bones rubbing together as if+: Kali-bi.

Boring into, with fingers picking at, itching: Anac; *Aru-t*; Aur; Carb-v; Caus; CINA; Hep; Lyc; Mar-v; Merc; *Nat-m*; Nat-p; Pho; *Pho-ac*; Saba; *Sil*; Spig; Stro+; Sul; Thu; Zin.
- Brain symptoms, in: Cina; Sul.

Bridge: Pho-ac; *Sep*; Thu.
- Bones: Kali-bi; Rhus-t.
- Painful: Cinb; Thu.
- Squeezing: Chio; Lachn.

Brown, across: *Carb-an*; *Lyc*; Op; Sanic; SEP; Sul; *Syph*.
Bubbling sensation: Sars; Sul.

NOSE
Burning, sore: Led.
- Inspiring, cool air, on: Aesc.
- Throbbing: Kali-io.

Cancer, flat: Euphr.
Catches, of passing strangers: Merc.
Cold: Ap; Arn; *Cam*; *Caps*; *Carb-v*; *Lac-c*; Meny; Murx; VER-A.
- Agg: Sul.
- Inspiration, during: Cor-r.
- Knees, hot with: Ign.
- Sores: Ars.

Congestion, from high blood pressure: Iod.
Cracked: Aru-t; Carb-an.
Crawling, formication: Mar-v; Merc; Nat-m; Ran-b.
- Blows and hawks, to relieve: Ran-b.
  - until tears flow: Cham.

Crusts, scales from: Alu; Aur; Bov; GRAP; *Kali-bi*; Kali-c; Merc; Nit-ac; SEP; *Stic*; Sul; *Thu*; Tub; Zin-chr; Zin-io.
- Bloody: Stro+; Thu.

Cutting: Kali-bi; Nit-ac.
Desquamation: Carb-an.
Dirty: Med; Merc.
Discharges
- Acrid: *Ars*; *Ars-io*; Aru-t; Hyds; Merc; Merc-c; Nit-ac.
- Bluish: Am-m; *Kali-bi*.
- Burning, hot: Aco; Ars-io; Cep; Iod; Nat-m; Pul.
- Changing: Stap.
- Cold: Ambro; Ichthy; Kali-io; Lach.

NOSE, discharges
- Coryza, without: Agar; Terb.
- Cough agg: Agar; Lach; Nat-m; Nit-ac; *Scil*; Sul; Thu.
- Crusts: See Crusts.
- Dark: Cinb; Merc-d.
- Dinner after: Tromb.
- Dripping: Am-c; *Ars*; Ars-io; Aru-t; Calc; *Cep*; Eup-p; Euphr; Grap; Kali-io; Nit-ac; Nux-v; Pho; Rhus-t; Saba; Scil; Sul; Tab.
  - diphtheria, in: Nit-ac.
- Eating on: Carb-an; Clem; Nux-v; Plb; Sanic; Sul; *Tromb*.
- Expectoration, with: Sabal.
- Fish-brine: Elaps; Thu.
- Frothy: Merc; Sil.
- Glutinous: Hep; *Kali-bi*; Merc-c.
- Grey: Amb; Lyc.
- Green: Ars-io; Kali-bi; Kali-io; Lac-c; Merc; Nit-ac; PUL; Sep.
  - blood streaked: Pho.
  - stains pillow, in sleep: Lac-c.
- Gummy: Sumb.
- Gushing fluids: Agar; Dul; Euphr; Flu-ac; Hyds; Kali-bi; Lach; *Nat-c*; NAT-M; Pho; Scil; Sele; *Thu*.
  - morning: Scil.
- Lips, upper, reddening: Ars-io.
- Lumpy: Alu; Cinb; KALI-BI; Mar-v; Merc-d; Pho; Sele; Sep; Sil; Solid; Zin-io.
- Musty: Nat-c.
- Night: Lac-c; Nat-s.
- Offensive: See OZOENA.

NOSE, discharges
- Orange coloured: Pul.
- Purulent: Aur; *Calc*; Con; Hep; LACH; *Merc*; *Pul*; Zin-chr.
- Reading aloud, when: Verb.
- Salty: Aral; Cimi; Nat-m.
- Singing, when: Cep.
- Stool, during: Thu.
- Talking, while: Kali-bi; Nat-c.
- Urinous odour: Pul.
- Watery, without coryza: Agar; Terb.
- Yellow-green: Kali-bi; Kali-c; Merc; Ther.
  - stains, pillow at night: Lac-c.
  - watery, suddenly: Plant.

Dry: Ars; Ars-io; Bar-c; *Bell*; Bry; Calc; Carb-v; GRAP; *Kali-bi*; Lyc; *Nat-m*; *Nux-m*; Pho; Saba; Samb; *Sep*; SIL; Sinap; Spo; *Stic*; *Sul*; Thu; Thyr; Zin-io.
- As if: Petr; Sil.
- Breathe through mouth, must: Meli.
- Indoors: Nux-v; Thyr.
- Painful: Grap.
- Sensation, on blowing nose: Bar-c.

Dyspnoea in (See Obstructed): *Ars*; Kre; Lach; Merc; Pho; Pul; Saba; Sul.

Ears, to: Elap.
- Swallowing agg: Elap.

Eczema: Cist.

Eruption, on (lower): Caus.

Excoriated: ARS; Ars-io; Aru-t; Caus; *Cep*; Gel; Grap; Iod; Kali-io; Kre; *Merc*; Merc-c; Nat-m; Nit-ac; Nux-v; Pho; Sinap.

NOSE

External: *Aur*; Carb-v; Caus; Kali-c; *Merc*; Nat-c; Pho-ac; Pul; *Rhus-t*; Sep; Spig; Sul.
- Heat, burning: Agar; Saba.
- Itching: Carb-an; Caus; Cina; Saba; Sul.
- Pimples: Carb-an.

Face ache, with: Spig.

Flows
- Coryza without: Agar; Terb.
- Obstruction, with: Ars; Aru-t; Bry; Calc; Kali-bi; *Lach*; Merc; Nux-v; Onos; Pul; Sil.

Foreign body, plug, as if in: Psor; Rut; Sep.
- Upper part, in: Am-m.

Foetor, foul: See OZOENA.

Fullness: Bap; Kali-io.

Hard: Carb-an; Kali-c.

Heat, burning: Ars; Carb-an; Chin; Kali-io; Merc; Sang; Sil.
- Fever, in: Arn.
- Sneezing, when: Como.

Heavy: Kali-bi; Merc; Phyt.
- Stooping, on: Am-m; Sil.
- Weight, as if, hanging: Kali-bi.

Hot: Saba.
- Water flowing from, as if: Aco; Gel.

Itching: See Boring into.
- Child starts out of sleep, and rubs: Lyc.
- Eating, when: Jat; Lach.
- Menses, after: Sul.
- Pharynx, to: Rum.
- Rubs constantly: Cina.
- Violent, rubs+: Arg-n.

Liquids, food return through, when swallowing: Aru-t; Cocl; Gel; Kali-per; Lac-c; Lach; *Lyc*; Merc; *Pho*; Sul-ac.

Lying agg: Pul.

Numb: Aco; Bell; Vio-o.
- Epistaxis, with: Aco; Bell; Med.
- One side: Nat-m.

Obstructed: Ars; Ars-io; ARU-T; Aur; *Calc*; Caps; Carb-v; Caus; Con; *Grap*; Hep; *Kali-bi*; Kali-c; *Lyc*; Mang; *Mar-v*; Med; *Nat-c*; Nat-m; NIT-AC; NUX-V; Pho; Pul; *Samb*; Sil.
- Air open amel: Kali-c; Pho; Pul; Sul.
- Alternately: Lac-c; Pho; Phyt; Rhod; Sul.
  - lachrymation, with: Bor.
- Blood pressure, high from: Iod.
- Blow, desires to+: Am-m.
- Breathes through mouth: Am-c; Kali-c; Lyc; Mag-c; Mag-m; Nux-v; Samb.
  - adenoids, removal after: Kali-s.
- Children in (snuffles): Amb; Am-c; Apoc; Aur; Kali-bi; *Lyc*; Med; *Nux-v*; Osm; Pho; Saba; *Samb*; *Syph*.
  - new-born+: Nux-v.
- Chronic: *Calc*; Con; Sars; Sele; Sil; Sul.
  - obstinate: Sars.
  - years, for: Sars.
- Diphtheria, in: Kali-m; Lyc; Merc-cy.

NOSE, obstructed
- Fluent discharge, with: Aru-t.
- Foetid discharge, with: Aru-t.
- Fresh air, in: Dul.
- High, in: Nat-m.
- Hot wet application amel: Dul.
- Lachrymation with: Bor.
- Lying agg: Bov; Caus; *Nux-m.*
- Menses, before: Mag-c.
- Night, at: Amb; Am-c; Lyc; Nux-v; Zin-io.
- Pus, with: Calc; Lyc; *Sil.*
- Room, in amel: Dul.
- Speaking, reading aloud while: Kali-bi; Mar-v; Sil; Verb.
- Stooping, on: Agar.

Odours, in: Calc; Pul; Zin-chr.
- Eggs, rotten: Meny.
- Fishy: Thu.
- Remains for a long time: Dios.
- Sweetish: Nit-ac.

Oily: Hyds; *Iris.*

Operations, after: Fer-p.

Pain, in: Aur; Grap; Hep; Kali-bi; Kali-io; Merc; Pul; Sil.
- Saddle: Cinb; Thu.

Parchment sensation, as if: *Kali-bi*; Sul.

Peeling: Nat-c; Nat-m; Nit-ac; Pho.

Pinched: Cam; Kali-bi; Lyc; Spo.
- As if: *Kali-bi*; Spo.
- Blue, and+: Ver-v.

Plug: See Foreign body.

Pointed: Ars+; Cam; Nux-v; *Ver-a.*
- Point, cracked+: Alu.

NOSE

Polypus: Cadm; CALC; Kali-bi; *Mar-v*; Merc-i-r; Pho; Sang; Thu; Zin-chr.

Pressure of glasses AGG: Arg-n; Chin; Cinb; Con; Cup-ar; Flu-ac; Kali-bi; *Merc*; Pho.

Prickling, tears, with: Nat-p.

Pulled, as if: Nat-c.

Pulls, strangers, of: Merc.

Pulsation: Ars; Kali-io.

Raw (See excorated): Aral; Aru-t; Caus; Nat-m.

Red: Agar; ALU; Ap; *Aur*; Bell; *Calc*; Cann; *Caps*; Carb-an; Chel; Iod; Kali-io; *Lith*; Merc; Nit-ac; Pho; Rhus-t; SUL.
- Across: Lapp.
- Anger, from: Vinc.
- Knobby: Aur.
- Pimples, on: Kali-c; Lach; Psor.
  - white: Nat-c.
- Swollen: Lith; Mag-m.
  - across: Poth.
- Young women: Bor.

Root and above: Aco; Ars; Calc; Chio; Cimi; Cup; Gel; *Hep*; *Hyo*; Ign; Iod; Kali-bi; Kali-io; Merc; Par; Pho; *Pul*; Sang; Sars; Sil; Stic; Ver-v; Zin.
- Abscess: Pul.
- Cramp: Mang; Plat.
- Fullness, stuffy: Stic.
- Heaviness+: Bism.
- Jerks, suddenly: Hyo.
- Painful: Hep; Kali-bi; Ther.
  - vomiting, after: Dig.

NOSE, root
- Pressure: Cinb; Sep; Stic; Zin.
  - epistaxis with: Rut.
- Pulsation: Kali-bi.
- Sore: Ant-t; Nit-ac.
  - operation, after: Fer-p.
- Swelling: Sars.
- Tension: Ant-t; Cep; Kali-bi; Kali-io.
- Twitching: Hyo; Mez.

Rosaceae: Carb-an; Kali-io; Rhus-t; Sars.

Rum blossom: Agar; Lach; Led.

Sensitive to inspired air: Aco; Aur; Bro; Cam; Cimi; Cist; Cor-r; *Ign*; Med; Nux-v.

Septum
- Boil: Anthx.
- Crusts: Thu.
- Deviated: See Obstructed.
- Perforated: Kali-bi; Kali-io; Merc; Merc-c; Sil; Syph.
- Sore: Kali-bi.
- Ulcers: Aur; Kali-bi; Sil.

Shiny: Pho.

Sinuses: Cinb; Hyds; Kali-bi; Kali-io; Lach; Merc; Pho; Syph.
- Burning, throbbing: Kali-io.

Smoke, as if, in: Bar-c.

Snuffles: See Obstructed, in Children.

Sunken: Aur; Psor.

Sweat
- About: Rhe.
- On: Rut; Tub.
  - cold: Chin.

NOSE

Swelled, thick: Ap; Arn; Aur; *Bar-c*; Bell; *Calc*; Caus; Hep; Iod; *Kali-c*; Kali-io; Lyc; *Merc*; Merc-c; Nat-c; *Pho*; Pho-ac; Pul; Rhus-t; Sars; *Sep*; *Sul*; Zin.
- Knobby: *Ars*; *Aur*.
- Shiny: Bor.

Syphilitic: Aur.

Tension: Aco; Ham; Kali-io; Petr; Senec; Thu.
- Skin, in: Petr; Pho.

Tingling, in: Arn; Saba.
- Cobweb, as from: Bro.
- Spreading to whole body: Saba.

Tip: Carb-an; Carb-v; Caus; *Sep*.
- Abscess, boil: Aco; Am-c.
- Cold: Alo+; Ap; Calc-p; Med.
- Cracked: *Alu*.
- Drips, water: Rhus-t.
- Eruptions: Aeth.
  - pimples: Caus.
- Hot: Caps.
- Itching: Med; Petr; Sil.
- Knobby: Aur.
- Numb: Gel; Vio-o.
- Painful: Cist.
- Red: Nit-ac; Rhus-t.
  - drunkards, in: Agar; Lach; Led.
- Scurfy: Nit-ac.
- Sensitive: Rhus-t.
- Shiny: Bell; Pho; Sul.
- Sore: Bor; Cist; Lith.
- Swelling: Bry+; Caus; Chel.
- Tremulous, twitching: *Bry*; Chel.
- Tumour: Carb-an; Sul.

NOSE

Twitching: *Amb*; Am-c; Aur; *Calc*; *Chel*; *Con*; *Hyo*; *Kali-bi*; Nat-m; Phys; *Plat*.
Ulcer: Ars; Merc; Nat-m; Pul.
• Menses, instead of: Euphr.
Uneasy feeling around: Ail.
Warts on: Caus.
Weather changes agg: Ars.
Winter agg: Am-c; Ars; Sul.
Wrinkled, skin: Cham.
Yellow, across: Sep.

NOSTALGIA: See HOMESICK.

NOSTRILS

Alae (wings): Lyc; Thu.
Agglutinated: AUR; Lyc.
Cracks: Ant-c+; Merc; Thu.
Crusty: Ant-c+; Bor.
Dark, sooty: Ant-t; Colch; Crot-h; Hell; Hyo.
Dilated: Ant-t; Ars; Cup; Hell; Iod; Lyc; Spo.
• As if: Iod.
Dirty: Merc.
Drawn, in: Aeth; Cina.
Eczema+: Ant-c.
Gummy: Bor.
Hair, in: Kali-bi.
Itching: Syph.
Motions, flapping: *Ant-t*; Ars; Bap; Bell; Bro; *Chel*; Cup; Diph; LYC; PHO; Pyro; Rhus-t; Spo; Sul-ac; Zin.
• Palpitation, with: Lyc.
• Snoring, with: Diph.
Sore: Ant-c+; Nux-v.
Water, hot, flowing as if: Gel.
White: Stram.

NOSTRILS

Wide apart, as if+: Iod.

NOTHING

Ails him, says: Ap+; Arn; Iod; Op.
Seems right: Phys.

NUMBNESS insensibility: ACO; *Anac*; Ap; *Aran*; Ars; Berb; Cadm; Carb-v; Caus; Cham; COCL; *Con*; Crot-h; Diph; Gel; Glo; GRAP; Hyo; *Kali-c*; *Kalm*; Lapp; LYC; Mag-c; Med; Nat-m; Nux-m; Nux-v; *Old*; *Op*; *Pho*; *Pho-ac*; Pic-ac; *Plat*; *Plb*; PUL; Radm; RHUS-T; *Sec*; *Stram*; Sul-io; Tarn; Tell; Thu; Xanth; Zin.

Affected part, of: *Cham*; Cocl; *Con*; *Kali-n*; Led; Lyc; Old; PLAT; Plb; Pul.
Bad news, after: Calc-p.
Brain affections, in: Flu-ac.
Coldness, with: Plat; Sumb.
Diagonal: Thyr.
Epilepsy, before: Buf.
Extreme heat or cold, to: Berb.
General, whole body: Acet-ac+; Ascl; Bar-m; Cedr; Chel; *Kali-br*; Ox-ac.
• Headache, during: Cedr.
• Lying, on: Zin.
• Morning: Amb.
Grasping objects agg: Cocl.
Internal: *Gel*; Op; *Plat*.
Lower half: Spo.
Lying down agg: Zin.
One sided: Ars; Caus; Chel; Nat-m; Pho; *Pul*.
• Right: Caus; Elap; Naj.

NUMBNESS, one sided
- Left: Ars; Sumb; Xanth.

Pain, from: Asaf; Cham; *Colo*; Gnap; Hypr; Kalm; Mez; Nat-m; Plat; Pul; Rhus-t.

Part
- lain, on (See DIRECTIONS, side lain on): Am-c; Arn; Calc; *Carb-v*; Chin; Mag-c; Nat-m; *Pul*; *Rhus-t*; Sil.
- Not lain, on: Flu-ac.

Partial, single parts: Aran; Bar-c; Cadm; Carb-an; Cocl; Croc; Grap; Kali-c; Kali-n; Lyc; Merc; Plat; Pul; Rhus-t; Sil.

Places, changing: Raph.

Prick, pain, heat, etc: Kre; *Plb*; Thu.

Prickling, with: Tarn.

Radical nerve, along: Pho-ac.

Spinal affections, in: Flu-ac.

Spots, in: Amb; Buf; Lyc; Plat; Sul-io.

Stretching part agg: Old; Radm.

Ulnar nerve, along: *Aran*.

Upper half: Bar-c.

Waking, on: Aran; Cham.

Wooden feeling: Kali-n; Petr; Thu.

NUTRITION affected: Abro; BAR-C; *Bor*; CALC; *Calc-hyp*; CALC-P; *Grap*; *Lac-c*; LYC+; NAT-M; Sanic; SIL.

NYMPHOMANIA: See FEMALE, sexual desire, violent.

OBESITY: Am-m; *Ant-c*; Bell; Buf; CALC; CAPS; *Fer*; *Grap*; Kali-bi; Lac-d; Lith; Phyt; Pul; Rum; Seneg; Sul; Thyr.

OBESITY
Atrophy, limbs of, with: Plb.
Body fat, legs thin: Am-m.
Old people: Bar-c; Kali-c.

OBSCENE: See LECHEROUS.

OBSTINATE: See STUBBORN.

Says, there is nothing the matter with him: Ap; ARN.

OCCIPUT: Bell; *Bry*; Calc; *Carb-v*; Chin; CIMI; Cocl; GEL; Ign; Nat-s; *Nux-v*; Onos; *Petr*; *Phyt*; Sep; SIL; Sul; Vario; Ver-v; Zin; Zin-ar.

Right: Bell; Chel; Sang.

Left: Kali-bi; Lyc; Nat-m; Nux-v; *Onos*; Sep; Spig; Sul.

Alternating sides: Sep.

Aching, waves in, from spine: Crot-h.

Air cold, as agg: Sanic.

Ascending through: Arg-n; *Bell*; *Calc*; Carb-v; *Cimi*; GEL; *Glo*; *Kali-bi*; Lac-c; Lach; Lil-t; Onos; *Par*; Petr; Pho; Saba; SANG; Sep; SIL; *Spig*; Sul; Ver-v.
- Warm water, as if: Glo.

Band, constriction: Arg-n; Grap.
- Sensation, of: Grap.

Bathing, cold amel: Calc-p.

Bending backwards amel: Cocl; Murx.

Blow on, as if: Ap; Bap; Bell; Cimi; Crot-h+; Kali-m; Lach; *Naj*; Tab; Tarn; Zin.

Bone sinks, marasmus in: Mag-c.

OCCIPUT

Burning, heat: Aur; Med+; Pho; Zin.
Bursting: Gel; Lach.
Cold: Calc-p; Chel; Dul; Pho+.
Confusion, in: Amb.
Coughing agg: Fer; Pul.
Cutting: Sul.
  • Night: Syph.
Depression, at: Calc-p.
Downward: Calc-p; Pho; Pic-ac+; Val; Zin.
Drawing: Arn; Bry.
Empty: Stap; Sul.
Enlarged, swelled, as if: Bry; Cocl; Dul; Med.
Eruption: Caus; Sil; Sul.
Exertion agg: Onos.
External: Carb-an; *Carb-v*; *Petr*; *Sil*.
Eyes, to: Med; Sars.
Eye strain agg+: Onos.
Finger pressing, as if: Meph.
Formication: Sep.
Forward, from: Sang; Sil.
  • Right, to: Bell; Gel; Sang; Sil.
  • Left, to: Arg-n; Cimi; Lach; Lil-t; *Spig*; Thu.
Hand, putting on amel: Murx.
Heat: See Burning.
Heavy: BELL; Calc; *Carb-v*; CHEL; Kali-m; Merc-i-r; Mur-ac; NAT-M; *Petr*; *Pic-ac*.
  • Looking intently agg: Mur-ac.
  • Sitting bent, while: Con.
  • Waking, on: Lach.
Legs, weak with: Zin.
Lying on agg: Bry; Cact; Carb-v;

OCCIPUT, lying on, agg .. COCL; Kali-p; Nux-v; PETR; Pho; *Sep*; Spig.
Nose, root of, to: Sars.
Numb: Flu-ac; Kali-br; Stap.
  • Prickling: Ox-ac.
  • Spine, down: Phys.
Opens and shuts: Cocl.
Pillow on, agg: Buf; Glo.
Pressure, outward: Aesc; Calc; Gel; Sul.
Pupils dilated, with: Ver-v.
Screwed, as if: Onos.
Shocks: Pho.
Shoulder, to: Kali-bi; Onos; Stic.
Sinciput, to: Senec.
Sore, bruised: Cimi; Eup-p; Gel; Nux-v; Pru-sp; Stap.
Sprained, as if: Amb.
Stools amel: Asaf.
Sweat, on: Sanic.
Swollen: Bar-c.
Tension: Lyc.
Throbbing, pulsating: Bell; Bry; Cann; Lyc; *Pho*; *Sep*.
  • Hot if, agg: Lyc.
  • Night agg: Lyc.
  • Standing amel: Cam.
  • Stools, during: Ign.
Twitching: Mag-m; Spig.
Ulcer: Sil.
Uneasy: Aeth.
Up and down, from: *Onos*; Sep.
Vision dim, with: Ver-v.
Vomiting agg: Ip.

OCCUPATION AMEL (See ACTIVE amel and BUSY when amel): Cup; Hell; Ign; Kali-br;

OCCUPATION amel..
  Merc-i-r; Nat-c; Nux-v; Pip-m; *Sep*.
OCCUPATIONAL DISEASES: Arn; Caus; Gel; Mag-p; Nux-v; Pic-ac; Sil; Zin.
ODOURS, smells (See also SENSITIVE, NAUSEA) **AGG:** Ars; Aur; Bell; Cof; COLCH; Eup-p; Grap; Ign; Lyc; *Merc-i-f*; Nux-v; Op; Pho; Saba; Sang; SEP; Stan; Sul; Ther; Vario.
Camphor AGG: Kali-n.
Dirty clothes AGG: Carb-an.
Eggs on AGG: Colch.
Fish, of AGG: Colch.
  • Smells, foul: Par.
Flowers AGG: Cep; Grap; Lac-c; Nux-v; Pho; Saba; Sang.
Food, of cooking etc: See under FOOD.
Foul AGG: Anthx; Kre; Pyro.
  • Bread: Par.
  • Milk: Par.
  • Remains for a long time: Dios.
  • Sensitive, to: Par.
Imaginations of: See under Smell, Illusory.
Mice, of AGG: Saba.
Musk, of AMEL: Mos.
Peach, skin of AGG: Cep.
Sour AGG: Alu; Dros.
Stools of AGG: Dios; *Sul*.
Strong AGG: Anac; Cof; Sele.
Sweet, agreeable AGG: Arg-n; Aur; Nit-ac; Sil.
Takes away, her breath: Pho-ac.

ODOURS
Tobacco agg: Bell.
  • Addicted, though+: Lob.
Wood agg: Grap.
OEDEMA: See DROPSY.
Affected part, around: Crot-h.
Angio-neurotic: Agar; *Ap*; Ars; Hell; Hep; *Rhus-t*; Urt.
Injury, after: Bels.
Joints of, fractures, after: Bov.
Neonatorum: Ap; Carb-v; Dig; Lach; Sec.
Red: Ap; Como.
Saccular: Ap; Ars; Kali-c.
Sprain, after: Bov.
Sudden: Kali-n.
OESOPHAGUS
Bubbling, in: Chel.
Burning: Canth; *Merc-c*; Pho; *Sang*; Ver-v.
  • Eating agg: Pho.
  • Pregnancy, during: Hell.
  • Typhoid, in: Ars; Bell; Bry; Nux-v; Pho; Rhus-t; Sul.
Choking: Cact; Ign; Kali-c; Merc-c.
Clucking, in: Cina.
Cold: Meny.
  • Hot and/or ascending: All-s.
Cramp, eructation, on: Colo.
  • Palpitation, with: Colo.
  • Swallowing, on: Op.
Cutting: Vinc.
Distended, as if: Hypr; Op; Ver-a.
Drinking water, runs out side, as if+: Ver-a.
Drinks, roll audibly+: *Laur*.

OESOPHAGUS

Dry: Cocl; Lach; Mez; Naj; Sep; Sul.

Food
- Feels, going through: Alu.
- Lodged in, as if: Ars; Bar-c; Calc; Caus; Chin; Gel; Kali-c; Pul.
- Whole length: Alu.

Foreign body in, as if: Gel; Lyc.

Gurgling in, drinking while: Ars; Hyd-ac.

Hot risings, after fright: Hypr.

Inflamed: Ars; Rhus-t; Ver-v.
- Corrosive things, swallowing, from: Rhus-t.

Injury, fish bone etc. agg: Cic.

Lump, in: Chel; Pod.
- Hard: Lyc.

Paralysis: Con; Elap; Hyd-ac.

Rough: Nat-c.

Spasm, constriction: Asaf; *Bap*; Bar-c; *Bell*; *Ign*; Lach; Laur; Merc-c; *Naj*; Nux-v; Ran-b; Ver-v.
- Can swallow liquids only: *Bap*; Bar-c; Plb.
- Food, suddenly arrested, then falls heavily in stomach: Elap.

Split, as if, on eructation: Coca.

Spongy: Elap.

Stricture: Am-m; Ars; Bap; *Bar-c*; Cic; Cund; Kali-c; Nat-m; Pho; Stro; Zin.
- Old: Pho; Zin.

OFFENDED

Easily: Anac+; Ars; Calc; Caps; Cocl; Ign; Lyc; *Nux-v*; Pall; Plat;

OFFENDED, easily.. *Pul*; Sars+; Sep+; *Stap*.

At everything+: Colo.

OFFENSIVENESS, foetor: Ail; Arn; *Ars*; Asaf; *Bap*; Bry; Carb-ac; Carb-an; *Carb-v*; Con; Crot-h; Grap; Hep; Kali-chl; Kali-p; Kre; LACH; Med; *Merc*; Mur-ac; Nit-ac; Osm; Pho; Pod; PSOR; Pyro; Rhus-t; Sabi; Sec; Sep; *Sil*; Sul; Sul-ac; Tell; Thu; Tril; Ust.

Body, of: Bap; Guai; Hep; Kali-io; Kali-p; Med; Nit-ac; *Psor*; *Pyro*; Sep; Sil; Stan; *Sul*; Syph; Thu.
- Can not wash it off: Lac-c; Med; Psor+.
- Cheese, old, like: Sanic.
- Menses, during: Psor; Stan.
- Unclean: Guai.
- Urinous: Ust.

OIL application of amel: Euphor.

OILY: See Greasy.

OLD AGE, senility: Amb; Ant-c; Arn; Ars; AUR; BAR-C; Caps; Carb-an; Carb-v; Chin; *Con*; Flu-ac; Hyds; *Kali-c*; LACH; LYC; Nit-ac; OP; Pho; Sanic; Sars; Scil; *Sec*; Sele; Seneg; Sil; Sul-ac; Sumb; Syph; Tub; Ver-a.

Athletes: Coca.

Early, premature: Amb; Arg-n+; Bar-c; Berb; Con; Flu-ac+; Kali-c; *Lyc*; *Sele*; Sumb.

Look: See FACE.

Maids: Bov; Cocl; Con; Lil-t; Mag-m; Plat.

Men: Sabal.

ONANISM: See MASTURBATION.

ONIONS, smell like: Bov; Kali-io; Kali-p; Lyc; Petr; Tell.

ONYCHIA: See FINGERS, felon.

OPENING AND SHUTTING, as if: *Cact*; Calc; CANN; *Cimi*; COCL; Cup; Glo; Lil-t; *Lyc*; Sep; Spo; Tarn.

OPERATIONS, surgical
  After AGG (See INJURIES): Arn; Bels; Calend; Cep; Echi; Ham; Hypr; Pho-ac; Rhus-t; Stap; Stro; Sul-ac; Zin.
  Abdominal+: Bism.
  Adhesions, after: Calc-f; Sil.
  Fistula, after: Calc-p.
  Orifices, on: Colo.
  Skin is drawn tight over the wound: Kali-p.
  Stones, for: Mill.

OPISTHOTONOS (See TETANUS): Abs+; Ign; Stram+; Ver-v.
  Diarrhoea, after: Med; Ver-v.

ORBITS: *Ap*; Asaf; Aur; Bar-c; Cinb; Kali-bi; Merc; Merc-i-f; Mez; Rhus-t; Spig; Syph; Val; Zin-s.
  Cellulitis: Phyt; Rhus-t.
  Herpes, around: Hep.
  Neuralgia, of: Ars; Ced; Chin-s; Kali-bi; Kalm; Nat-m; Spig; Stan.
   • Coition agg: Ced.
   • Screaming and unconsciousness, with: Kali-cy.
   • Testes, of, with: Lycps.

ORDEALS: See under FEAR.

ORGASMS: See WAVES.
  Sexual, easy: Stan.

ORIFICES
  Affections of: *Aesc*; Alo; *Bell*; *Caus*; Grap; Ign; Kali-c; Lach; Lyc; *Merc*; Mur-ac; Nat-m; NIT-AC; NUX-V; Pho; Pod; Rat; *Sep*; *Sil*; SUL.
  Cracked: Nit-ac.
  Red: Alo; Nit-ac; Pyro; Sul.
  Swelled: Nit-ac.

OSCILLATIONS: See EYES, and MOTION.

OSTEOMALACIA (See BONES softening): *Iod*; Merc-c; Pho-ac.

OSTEOMYELITIS: Arn; Calc; Pho.

OVARIES: AP; *Bell*; Canth; *Colo*; Guai; LACH; Lil-t; Lyc; Mag-p; Pod; Pul; Sabal; Stap; THU; Ust; Zin-val.
  Right: Bell; Lyc; Pall+; Pod.
   • Lying on side amel: Ap.
  Left: Arg-m; Lach; Thu; Ust; Zin.
   • Heart, to+: Naj.
   • Lying on side amel: Kali-p; Pall.
  Alternating between (See GENITALS, alternating): Cimi; Colo; Lac-c; Lil-t; Onos; Ust.
  Atrophy: Bar-m; Con; *Iod*.
  Back, to, right: Rum.
  Ball, like a heavy, right: Carb-an.
  Bed
   • Turning, in agg: Lyc.
   • Warmth of agg: Ap; Merc.
  Bending back amel: Lac-c.
  Breast
   • To: Lil-t; Murx; Senec.
   • With: Sabal.

OVARIES

Burning (R): Ust.
Coition after agg: Ap; Plat; Stap; Syph.
Congested: Ap.
Continence agg: *Ap*; Kali-br.
Cutting: Con.
- Coition, during: Syph.

Cystic: Ap; Apoc; Arg-m+; Aur; Bov+; Form; Kali-br; Iod; Lyc.
Drawing: Med.
Feet, moving amel: Ars.
Head, with: Sabal.
Heavy: *Ap*; Plat; Sep.
Hydatid, of: Buf.
Indurated, hard: Ap; Bro; *Con*; *Grap*; Lach.
Inflamed: Ap; Bell; Lyc; Merc; Pho; Pod; Sabi.
Insufficiency, of: Lecith.
Left, heart, to: Bro; Cimi; Lac-c; Lach; Lil-t; *Naj*; Sul; Vib.
Limbs, to: Lil-t.
Menses
- Before agg: Thu.
- Checked, suddenly+: Aco.
- During and after AGG: Zin-val.

Numb: Ap.
Painful: Naj.
- Love sick girls, in: Ant-c.

Parturition, after: Lach.
Pinching: Plat.
Pressure
- Agg: Stap.
- Amel: Med.

Pulsations: Bell; Cact; Lach; Onos.

OVARIES

Raising
- Arms agg: Ap.
- Legs agg: Lyc.

Sexual desire during, agg: Kali-br.
Shoulder, to: Pod.
Sitting bent agg: Ars.
Sore: Ap; *Lil-t*; Sep.
- Rectum, with: Onos.
- Uterus, with: Ust.

Stooping agg: Ap.
Stretching legs
- Agg: Pod.
- Amel: Plb.

Swelled, enlarged: Ap; Bell; Con; Lach; Lil-t; Lyc.
Tearing: Plat; Thu.
Thighs, to: Colo; Grap; Lil-t+; Pod; *Stap*; Ust; Xanth; Zin-val.
Tumours: Ap; Lach; Lyc; Pod.
Uterus, to+: Iod.

OVEREXERTION+: Bov.

OVERLIFTING: See under LIFTING agg.

OVERPOWERED, as if (under superhuman power): Anac; Lach; Naj; Op; Plat; Thu.

OVERSTRAIN mental, physical+: Cocl; Con.

OVERSTUDY+: Nat-c; Sele.

OVERUSE+: *Arn*; Con.

OXALURIA: See under URINE, oxalic acid.

OZOENA: Asaf; AUR; CALC; Grap; *Hep*; *Kali-bi*; Kali-io; *Merc*; Nat-c; Nit-ac; Nux-v; Psor; PUL; Sep; Sil; *Sul*; Syph+; Ther.

OZOENA
Acrid: Lyc; Mag-m.
Crusty: Mag-m.
Menses, during: Grap.
Syphilitic: Aur; Hep; Nit-ac; Sil.

PAIN
In general, nueralgia: ACO; ARS; BELL; *Bry*; *Caus*; *Cham*; Chin; Cimi; Cof; COLO; Dios; Gel; Hypr; IGN; *Iris*; *Kali-bi*; Lach; *Lyc*; *Mag-c*; *Mag-p*; Merc; Nat-m; *Nux-v*; Pho; *Psor*; Pul; Ran-b; *Rhus-t*; Rum; *Sang*; *Spig*; Stan; *Sul*; Sul-ac; Thu; *Ver-a*; Verb.

Absence, of (in affections which are usually painful): Am-c; Ant-t; *Hell*; OP; STRAM.

Aching: Agar; Arn; *Bap*; Bels; Bry; Carb-v; *Chin*; Cimi; Dul; Echi; Erig; *Eup-p*; *Gel*; Hyo; Ign; Kalm; Lach; Lapp; Lept; Merc-i-f; Nux-v; *Onos*; *Phyt*; Pyro; Radm; Rhus-t; Rut; Terb; Vario; Ver-v.
- Heavy: Carb-v.

Associated: See SYNALGIAS.
Bearing down: See Pressing.
Begins
- On one side, goes to other and there agg: Arg-n; Fer; Iris; Lac-c; LYC; Mang; Nat-m; Tub.
- Sleep, in: Nit-ac.
  - disppears on waking: Sul-ac.

Biting, raw, smarting: ARG-M; Aru-t; Berb; Calc; *Canth*; Carb-v; CAUS; Cist; Euphr; Flu-ac; *Grap*; *Hep*; Hyds; *Ign*; Iod; Kre; *Lach*; Led; *Lyc*; Meli;

PAIN, biting ..
Merc; NUX-V; Nit-ac; Ol-an; Petros; *Pho*; Polyg; *Pul*; Ran-sc; Sang; Sep; Stap; Stan; *Sul*; *Sul-ac*; Zin.
- Burning: See under BURNING.
- Internal: Bro; Carb-v; Nux-m; *Nux-v*; Pho; Sang.

Boring, grinding: ARG-N; Asaf; *Aur*; *Bell*; Bism; *Colo*; Dios; Hep; Lach; Mag-p; Med; *Merc*; *Mez*; Plat; Plb; *Pul*; *Ran-sc*; *Spig*; Xanth; *Zin*; Zin-chr.

Breaking, broken: *Arn*; BELL; Calc; Calc-p; Chel; *Cocl*; EUP-P; Grap; Guai; *Lyc*; Merc; Nat-m; Nux-v; Pho; Ran-b; Rhus-t; *Rut*; Sil; Sul; *Thu*; Val.

Bruised, soreness: *Ap*; ARN; Aur; *Bap*; *Bell*; Bels; BRY; Canth; *Carb-v*; *Caus*; *Chin*; Chio; Cimi; *Con*; EUP-P; Gel; Ham; Hep; Hypr; Kalm; *Lach*; Lapp; *Lith*; *Mill*; *Nit-ac*; NUX-V; Ol-an; Onos; Plant; Pho; Phyt; *Pul*; *Pyro*; Ran-b; RHUS-T; RUT; SIL; *Sul*; Terb; Til.
- Body all over+: Gamb.
  - when touched+: Mang.
- Coition, after: Sil.
- Deep: Mang.
- Excessive exertion, as if, from: Chel; Clem.
- Internally: Bels; Cann; Pul.
- Menses, during: Nat-c.
  - scanty, with: Carb-v.
- Pains, after: Aco; *Arn*; Chin; Cimi; Gel; Glo; Grap; Mez; Onos; *Plat*; Sele; Tell.

PAIN, bruised
- Parts
  - bleeding: Arn; Fer.
  - lain, on: Arn; Nux-m; Pyro; Rut.
- Spots: *Arn*; Glo; *Kali-bi*; Lith; Merc; Pho; Ran-b; *Saba*; Sul.
  - blows, fall, as from: Lith.
  - trifles, every from: Terb.
- Waist, about: Visc.

Burning: See BURNING.
- Hot irons: See HOT IRONS.
- Stinging: See BURNING, stinging.

Bursting, splitting: Act-sp; BELL; BRY; Calc; Caps; Carb-ac; *Chin*; Eup-p; *Glo*; Ham; *Ign*; Kali-m; Lac-c; Lept; Lil-t; Lyc; *Merc*; NAT-M; *Nux-v*; Ran-b; Rat; Senec; Sep; *Sil*; Spig; Stan; Sul; Thyr; *Vip*.

Cannot stand: See SENSITIVE, and BESIDES HIMSELF.

Come and go: See Fleeting.

Cold: Arn; Med; Syph.

Colicky: See Cramp.

Constricting: See CONSTRICTION.

Cramps, griping, colic: Agar; *Bell*; Cact; CALC; Caus; *Cham*; Cocl; COLO; CUP; *Dios*; Dul; *Grap*; Hyo; *Ign*; Lach; *Lyc*; Mag-m; Mag-p; *Nit-ac*; NUX-V; *Plat*; Plb; Rhe; Scop; Sec; Sil; Stan; Stap; SUL; Ver-a; Ver-v+; Vib.
- Coition agg: Colo; Cup; Grap.
- Every where: Hyd-ac; Old.
- Exertion prolonged, on: Mag-p.

PAIN, cramps
- Menses, after: Chin; Cup; Pul.
  - with: Mag-m.
- Nursing agg: Cham.
- Pains, after: Sec.
- Paralysis, then: Tab.
- Radiating over whole body: Dios; Lyc; Nux-v.
- Stiffness
  - then: Sec; Sele.
  - with: Ver-a.
- Transfixion: Cup.

Cutting: Aco; BELL; Bry; *Calc*; Calc-p; Calc-s; *Canth*; COLO; *Con*; Dios; Hyo; KALI-C; Kali-m; Lyc; Merc; *Nat-m*; Nit-ac; *Nux-v*; Petr; Plant; Polyg; Pul; Rat; Sabal; Sil; *Sul*; Tell; Ver-a; Zin.
- Smarting: Canth.
- Squeezing: Thu.

Darting: See Shooting.

Drawing: Arn; *Bry*; Carb-v; *Caus*; Cham; *Chel*; Chin; Cimi; Colo; Grap; Kali-bi; Kali-c; Lach; Lil-t; Lyc; Merc; Nit-ac; Nux-v; Pul; Rhod; RHUS-T; Sep; Sil; Sul; *Val*.

Extend from original site: Ther.

Fine: See Stitching, needle like.

Fits and starts, in: Bar-m; Cup; Mez.

Fleeting, come and go: Nit-ac; Nux-m; Pall; Phyt; Poth; Sabal; Stro; Tell; Val.
- Attacks repeated in: Bell.

Flesh, torn from body as if+: Nit-ac.

Fluid, forcing its way, as if, with: Coc-c.

PAIN

Gnawing, eating, festering: Agn; Am-m; Berb; Bry; Cham; Colo; Grap; Guai; Ign; Kali-s; Kre; *Lach*; Lyc; Mag-m; Nat-s; Nit-ac; Old; Ox-ac; *Pho*; *Plat*; PUL; *Ran-sc*; Rhus-t; Rut; Sec; Sep; SIL; Spo; Stap; Sul; Sul-ac; Thu; Ver-a; Zin-chr.
- Burning: Rut.
- Grinding: Zin-chr.

Goes to
- Parts, recenlty lain, on: Pul.
- Side
  - lain, on: Ars; *Bry*; Calc; *Kali-c*; Merc; *Nux-v*; *Pho-ac*; PUL; Sep; Sil.
  - not lain, on: Bry; Cup; Flu-ac; Grap; *Ign*; Kali-bi; Pul; Rhus-t.

Girdle: Lach; Sul.

Gradually increase, decrease etc: See DIRECTIONS, symptoms.

Grinding: See Boring.

Growing: See GROWING PAINS.

Hacking like hatchet: Am-c; Ars; Aur; Clem; Kali-n; Lyc; Pho-ac; Rut; Stap; Thu.

Heat agg: Tab.

Insensitive, to+: Bap.

Itching, alternating, with: Stro.

Jerking: Asaf; Bell; Calc; Caus; CHIN; *Ign*; Kali-c; Meny; Nat-m; Nit-ac; NUX-V; PUL; *Rhus-t*; Sil; Sul; *Tarx*; Thu; Val.
- Part affected: Merc.
- Shock, sudden from: Pod.

Labour: See Under LABOUR.

Lightning: See Shooting.

PAIN

Linear: Bell; Buf; Caps; Caus; Cep; Fago; Ox-ac; Pyro; Syph; Tell.

Maddening: See BESIDES, HIMSELF.

Many: Med; Mez; Naj; Rum.

Nail, Clavus: See PLUG.

Needle like: See Stitching.

Nerves, along: Terb.

Nips: See Twinging.

Operations, after: Hypr.

Paralytic: See PARALYSIS.

Paralyzed parts, in: Agar; Ars; Cact; Caus; Cocl; Kali-n; Latro; Plb.

Pecking: Chin; Rut.

Persistent: Syph.

Piercing: Ap; Mill; Nat-s.

Pinching: See Squeezing.
- suddenly, as if: Arg-n.

Pressing, bearing down: *Agar*; *Ap*; *Bell*; CANTH; *Castr*; *Cimi*; *Con*; LIL-T; MERC-C; *Nat-m*; NUX-V; Pall; Pho; *Plat*; *Pul*; Rhus-t; Rut; SEP; Sil; Stan; SUL; Thyr.
- Blunt instrument, as from: Lith.
- Coldness, with: Sec.
- Inward: Anac; Plat; Stan.
  - deep, with instrument as if: *Bov*; Ign; Ver-a.
- Outward: Asaf; Bry; Cimi; Pul; Sul.
- Together: Asar.

Prickling: Aco; Ap; Bry; Ham; Kali-p; Lob; Lyc; Nat-m; Nat-p; *Plat*; Ran-sc; Rhus-t; Sul; Symp; Tarn; Urt; *Ver-v*; Xanth.

PAIN, prickling
- All over: Lob.
- Numbness, with: Tarn.

Pulling: See Drawing.

Quick: See Shooting.

Radiating: See under DIRECTIONS.

Raging: Led.

Rawness: See Biting.

Rheumatic: See RHEUMATISM and JOINTS.

Shifting: See Wandering.

Shingles, before: Stap.

Shocks in: Cina; Zin-chr.

Shooting, darting, quick, lightning: Aco; *Agar*; Alu; Arg-n; Ars; BELL; *Berb*; *Cimi*; *Colo*; Cup; Dios; Fer; Hyd-ac; Hyo; Hypr; Kali-bi; Kali-c; Kali-m; Kalm; Mag-c; Mag-m; *Mag-p*; Mez; Nit-ac; Nux-v; Ox-ac; Paeon; Plb; Pru-sp; Radm; Ran-b; Rhus-t; Rum+; Sabi; Sep; Spig; SUL; Tell; Xanth; Zin.
- Burning: Sul-ac.
- Laming: Colch; Iris.

Sleep
- Felt in: Nit-ac.
- Waking amel: Sul-ac.

Smarting: See Biting.

Sore: See Bruised.

Splinter: See Stitching, needle like.

Spots, in: See Bruised, spots.

Squeezing, pinching, compression: Alu; Anac; *Ant-t*; Asar; Bels; Berb; Bry; *Cact*; Calc; Carb-v; Cimi; *Cocl*; COLO;

PAIN, squeezing
Grap; Ign; Kali-io; Kalm; Meny; *Merc*; *Nat-m*; Nat-s; Nit-ac; Old; PLAT; Rut; Stap; Thu; Val; Verb; Zin.

Sticking: See Stitching, needle like.
- Point, one to: Merc.
- Smarting: Stap.

Stinging: Aco; AP; *Ars*; Berb; Bry; Kali-c; Lyc; Merc; Nit-ac; *Pho*; Pul; Sabal; *Sep*; SIL; *Sul*; Ther; Zin.
- Burning: See BURNING, stinging.

Stitching: Aco; Ars; Asaf; Bell; Berb; Bor; BRY; Caus; Colch; KALI-C; Kali-m; Kali-s; Led; Merc; *Nit-ac*; Pul; Ran-b; *Rhus-t*; Sep; *Sil*; Spig; Strop; SUL; Symp; Zin-chr.
- Crawling: Arn.
- Jerky: Cina; Nux-v.
- Motion, impeding: Zin-chr.
- Needle like, fine splinter: Agar; Alu; Ap; ARG-N; *Ars*; Bry; Caps+; Cep; HEP; Kali-bi; *Kali-c*; Nat-m; NIT-AC; Paeon; Rhus-t; Saba; SIL; Sul; Syph; Tarn; Val; Ver-a.
- Tensive: Spig.
- Wounds, healed, in: Symp.

Strangling: Caps; Sul; Val.

Stumps, in (after operation): Am-m; Arn; Asaf+; Cep; Hypr; Pho-ac; Symp.

Sympathetic (See SYNALGIA): Tarn.

Takes the breath away: See RESPIRATION, pain agg.

PAIN

Tearing, very severe, violent: Aco; Anac; *Arn*; Ars; Bell; Bry; *Calc*; Caps; *Carb-v*; *Caus*; Cham; Chin; Colch; Con; Kali-c; *Lyc*; Merc; Nat-c; *Nit-ac*; *Nux-v*; *Plat*; Pul; *Rhod*; RHUS-T; Sep; Sil; Stap; Stro; Sul; Vip; Xanth; Zin.
- Paralytic: Carb-v; Chin; *Kali-c*; *Stap*.
- Pressive: Carb-v; Stan.
- Stitching, prickling: Anac; Calc; Colch; Guai; Led; Mang; Merc; Pul; Stap; Thu; *Zin*.
- Twitching, jerking: Chin; *Pul*.

Throbbing, pulsating: See PULSATION.

Trembling and paralytic weakness, with: Kalm.

Tugging, pulling: See Drawing.

Twinging, nips: Am-m; Laur; Mos; Plb.

Twisting: Ars; Bell; Calc; Cina; Colo; DIOS; Ign; *Nux-v*; Pul; Rhus-t; *Sil*; VER-A.

Ulcerative: See Gnawing.

Undulating: Anac; Asaf; Colo; Zin-io.

Violent: See Tearing.

Voluptous: Lach.

Wakened, by: Aco; Ars; Chin; Kali-c; Lach; Nux-v; Sil; Sul.

Wandering, shifting: Arn; Berb; *Caul*; Cimi; Colch; Cup; Fer; KALI-BI; Kali-n; Kali-s; Kalm; Lac-c; *Led*; Mag-p; Merc-i-r; Nux-m; Plant; Pru-sp; PUL; Rhod; Rhus-t; Rum; Sil; Thu; Zin-chr.

PAIN, wandering
- Rheumatic: Merc-i-r.
- Suddenly: Amb; Arn; Colch; Radm; Rhod.
- Zigzag: Rhod.

PAIN during AGG: Ars; Cham; Cimi; Colo; Ign; Lyc; Nat-c; Onos; Rhus-t; Sars; Sep; Thu; Ver-a.

PAINLESSNESS: See NUMBNESS and PAIN, absence of.

PALATE

PALATE: *Aur*; Bell; Crot-h; *Merc*; *Nux-v*; Pho.

Hard: Bell; *Nit-ac*; Nux-v; *Pho*.
- Cancer: Hyds.

Soft: Merc.
- Rim: Merc-i-f.
- Ulcer, eating, uvula: Hep.

Abscess: Pho.

Aphthae: Agar; Bor; *Kali-bi*; Sars.

Bleeding: Crot-h; Lach; Pho.

Bluish, red: Aco; Ap; Cham.

Burning: Cam; Mez; Polyg.

Chewing agg: Bor.

Crawling: Ars; Carb-v; Pho; Polyg; Ran-b; Sil.

Dry: Nux-m; Pho; Pho-ac; Sul; Ver-a.

Excoriated: Caus.

Greasy: Asaf; Card-m; Kali-p; Ol-an.

Hair, on: Kali-bi.

Heat: See Burning.

Indurated: Mez; Phyt.

Itching: Aru-t; Kali-p; Mar-v; Merc; Nux-v; Pho; Polyg; Saba; Stry.
- Ear, with: Mar-v.

PALATE
Node: Asaf; Mang.
Numb: Bap; Ver-a.
Oedema: Ap; Kali-io.
Pressing: Carb-v.
Raw, sore: Aru-t; Bell; Caus; Iris; Lach; Merc; NIT-AC; Nux-v; *Pho*; Phyt.
Scalded, as if: Sang; Sanic.
Shrivelled: Bor; Cyc.
Skin, loose, on: Phys.
Stiff: Crot-h; Grat; Nat-m.
Swelled: Arg-m; *Lach*; Sul.
Vesicles: Mag-c; Nat-s.
White: Fer; Merc; *Nat-p*.
Wrinkled: *Bor*; Pho.
Yellow, creamy: *Nat-p*.
PALMS: Anac; Grap; Petr; Ran-b; Sele; Spig.
Abscess: Ars; Cup; Flu-ac; Sul; Tarn-c.
Contractions, in: Caus; Grap; Guai; Nat-m; Ver-a.
Cracks: Calc-f; Kre; Merc-c; Merc-i-r; Ran-b; Rhus-t; Sul.
- Moist: Merc-i-r.

Cramps: Naj; Sabi.
Desquamation: Elap; Grap; Rhus-t; Sep; Sul.
- Tender, and, as if: Merc-c.

Dry: Ars; *Bism*; Cham; Diph; Lyc; *Nux-m*; Rhus-t; Sul.
- Crusts: Sele.

Eczema: Sul; Vario.
Gnawing (L): Ran-sc.
Hot, burn: *Ap*; Crot-h; Diph; Ip; Lach; Med; Ol-j; Pho; Rhus-t; Sang; Stan; *Sul*.

PALMS, hot
- Climaxis, at: Sang.
- Flushed, in: Phys.
- Soles, and: Bism; Lil-t; Lyc; Petr; *Pho*; Sang; Stan; Sul.
- Washing agg: Rhus-t.

Itching: *Anac*; Fago; Kre; Ran-b; *Sul*; Tub.
- Janudice, in: Ran-b.
- Night, at: Anac.

Moist, sweaty: Cratae; Dul; Ign; Naj; Nux-v; Sep; Sil; Sul; Vio-o.
- Clammy: Anac.
- Cold: Con.
- Cough, with: Naj.
- Putting them together, when: Rhe; Sanic.
- Warm: Ign.

Nodes: Caus; Rut.
Peeling of skin: See DESQUAMATION.
Pricking, grasping, when: Rhus-t.
Psoriasis: Petr; Pho; Sele.
Red: Flu-ac.
Sore: Rhus-t.
Stiff, writing, while: Kali-m.
Vesicles: Anthx; Buf; Kali-c; Kre; Merc.
Warts, on: Anac; Dul; Nat-m+; Rut; Sul.
Washing agg: Rhus-t.
Withered: Diph; Sang.
Yellow: Chel; Sep.
- Ascites, with: Chel.

PALPITATION: See under HEART.
PANARIS: See FINGERS, felon.

PANCREAS: Chio; Con; Iod; *Iris*; Merc; *Pho*; *Spo*.
  Cancer: Calc-ar.
  Induration: Bar-m; Carb-an.
PANNUS: Arg-n; Aur-m; Hep.
PAN OPHTHALMITIS: Hep; Rhus-t.
PARADOXICAL: *Ign.*
PARALYSIS (paralytic pain): Ant-t; Arn; *Ars*; Bell; Carb-v; CAUS; Chin; *Cocl*; Colch; Con; Dul; *Gel*; Hell; Helod; Hyo; Kali-p; *Lach*; Lyc; Mang; NUX-V; *Op*; Phys; PLB; RHUS-T; Sang; Sec; Sil; Stap; Sul; Verb; Zin-p.
  Agitans: *Agar*; Ant-t; *Arg-n*; Bar-c; Buf; Con; *Gel*; Hyo; Kali-br; *Lil-t*; Lol-t+; Mag-p+; Mang; MERC; Nux-v; Phys; Plb; Rhus-t; Stram; Zin.
  Apoplexy, after: *Arn*; *Bell*; Cocl; Lach+; Nux-v; Pho; Stan; Zin.
  Ascending: Ars; Con; Mang; Ox-ac; Pho; Pic-ac; Vip.
  Cold bathing amel: Caus; Con.
  Coldness, of parts, with: Caus; Cocl; Dul.
    • Icy; Ars; Dul; Grap; Nux-v; *Rhus-t.*
    - body of, with: Bar-m.
  Contraction of limbs, with: Ars; Cheno; Old; Sec; Val.
  Convulsions, then: Tarn-c.
  Cramps, after: Tab.
  Descending: *Bar-c*; Merc; Zin.
  Diphtheritic: Ap+; Arg-n; Caus; *Cocl*; Diph; Gel; Lac-c; *Lach*; *Rhus-t.*

PARALYSIS
  Emaciation of part rapid, with: Sec.
  Emotions, from: Gel; Ign; Lach; Nat-m; Stan; Stram.
  Epilepsy, after: Cur; *Hyo.*
  Extensor muscles, of: Alu; Ars; Cocl; Crot-h; Cur; *Plb.*
  Flaccid: Plb.
  Flexor muscles, of: Caus; Mez; Nat-m.
  Formication, with: Cadm; Pho; Sec.
  General, of insane: Cann; Crot-h; Pho; Phys; Stram.
  Gradual: Caus; Syph.
  Haemorrhage, with: Plb.
  Heat in paralyzed part, with: Alu; Pho.
  Hyperaesthesia of well side: Plb.
  Hysterical: Arg-n; Asaf; Cham; Cocl; *Ign*; Nux-m; Pho; Plb; *Tarn*; Val.
  Infantile: Bung; Calc; Caus; Gel; Kali-p; Lathy; Plb; Vip.
    • Dentition, during: Kali-p.
    • Paresis, after: Old.
  Infectious diseases, after: Caus.
  Internal, sense of: Lyc; Nat-m; Pho.
  Limbs, of: Agar; Alu; Buf; CAUS; COCL; Nux-v; Plb; Rhus-t; Rut; Sec; *Sil*; Sul.
    • One arm or one leg only: Both.
    • Sensation, of: Grap.
    - walking, while: Rhus-t.

PARALYSIS

Localized, single parts, organs: Ant-t; Bar-c; Bell; CAUS; Dul; Gel; Hyo; Nux-v; Op; Pho; Pul; Sec; Sil; Sul.
Moistness, with: Stan.
Motion disorderly, with: Merc.
Muscles, isolated, of: Cup.
Numbness, with: Sec.
One side: See HEMIPLEGIA.
Pain
- From: Nat-m.
- With: Cadm.

Painless: Cann; Cocl; Con; Gel; Hyo; Lyc; Old; Plb; RHUS-T.
Paraplegia: Agar; Arg-n; Ars; Bap; Mang; Nat-m; NUX-V; Plb; Rhus-t; Rut; Sec; Sul; Thal; Vip.
- Atrophy, with: Ars.
- Diphtheria, after: Ars.
- Exertion, after: Nux-v; Rhus-t.
- Fever, after: Rhus-t.
- Hunger, with: Cina.
- Hysterical: Cocl; Ign; Tarn.
- Parturition, after: Caul; Caus; Plb; *Rhus-t.*
- Progressive: Mang.
- Rigidity of muscles, with: Chel.
- Sensation, of: Aesc; Aur.
- Sexual excess, after: Rhus-t.
- Spastic: Gel; Hypr; *Lathy*; Nux-v; Sec.
- Vaccination, after: Ars.

Pseudo-hypertrophic: Cur; *Pho*; Thyr; Ver-v.
Rheumatism, after: Bar-c; Chin; *Fer*; *Rut.*

PARALYSIS

Runs forward, when attempting to walk: Mang.
Sexual excess, from: Nat-m; Rhus-t.
Spasms
- After: Cocl; Cup; Cur; Elap; Hyo; *Sec*; Stan; Vib.
- Then: Tarn.
- With: Nux-m.

Sphincters, of: Gel.
Spine, diseased, from: Med.
Supressions
- After: *Caus*; Hep; Lach; Sul.
- Foot sweat, after: Colch.

Tingling of affected part, with: Cann.
Touch, sensitive to: Plb.
Tremors, after: Plb.
Twitching: Stram.
Typists: Stan.
Typhoid, in: Agar; Lach; Rhus-t.
Unilateral: See HEMIPLEGIA.

PARAPLEGIA: See under PARALYSIS.

PARCHMENT LIKE: Anac; *Ars*; BAR-C; Calc-f; Lyc; Petr; Sil; Sul.

PAROTIDS (See MUMPS): Calc-f; Cham; Iod; Merc; Phyt; Pul.

Enlarged, ear affections, in: Ail+; Sil.
Fistula+: Calc.
Hard, but warm: Bro.
Hypertrophy, after mumps: Sul-io.
Swollen+: Carb-an.

PAROXYSMS, repeated (See also CONVULSIONS and RELAPSES): *Agar*; *Ars*; *Bell*; Calc; *Caus*; CHAM; *Chin*; COCL; COLO; Cup; *Dios*; Gel; Ign; Lach; MAG-P; NUX-V; Plat; Plb; Pul; SEP; Stan; Sul; Tab.

PASTY: See DISCHARGES, Sticky.

PATCHY: See MOTTLED.

PATELLAE: Bell; Con.

Bursa, enlarged, over: Sil.

Dislocated, as if: Gel.
- Upstairs, going, on: Cann.

Gurgling: Asar.

Hygroma: Arn.

Pain, impeding walking: Nit-ac.

Plug under: Cham.

Pulsation: Spig.

PECKING, hacking: See under PAIN.

PEDICULOSIS: See LICE.

PEDUNCULATED: See FUNGUS GROWTH.

PEELING of skin: See DESQUAMATION.

PEEVISH, petulent: Aco; Am-c+; *Ant-c*; Ant-t+; Aur+; *Calc*; Calc-p+; Caps+; *Cham*; CINA; Clem+; Cocl; Cop+; Kali-c; Lyc; Old+; Rat+; Stap; Sul; Syph+; Zin+.

Childish, old person: Sul.

PELLAGRA: Ars; Bov; Gel; Hep; Sec.

PELVIS

Around: Sabi; Sep; Vib.

Bones
- Loose, as if: Murx.
- Painful, sitting on: Carb-an.

PELVIS

Cellulitis: Pyro.

Disorders: Med.

Heavy: Alo; Gnap; Helo; Lil-t; Pall; Tarn; Vib.
- Dragging, dysuria, with: Lil-t.
- Standing agg+: Pall.

Menses, amel: Vib.

Organs, upside down+: Vib.

Peritonitis: Pall.

Sore
- Above: Ver-v.
- Spot, something pressing on, as if: Murx.

Thighs, to: Thyr; Vib.

Throbbing: Jab.

PEMPHIGUS: See under ERUPTIONS.

PENIS: Arn; *Cann*; Canth; Clem; Dul; *Merc*; Thu.

Absent, as if: Coca.

Atrophy: Ant-c; Arg-n; Berb; *Ign*; *Lyc*; Stap.

Bubbling: Grap; Kali-c.
- Erection, during: Kali-c.

Burning: Mez; Spo.
- Coition, during: Clem; Kre.

Cold: Agn; Lyc; Onos; Sul.
- Small, and: Agn; Lyc.

Condylomata, head of+: Sep.

Constriction: Kali-bi.
- By string, as if: Plb.

Contracted, small: Ign.

Drawing: Iod.

Eczema, back of: Alum; Radm.

Erections: See Erections.

Flaccid: Agn; Lyc.

Formication: Sec.

PENIS
Gangrene: Canth; Lach.
Induration, old men, in: Berb.
Injury: Mill.
Itching: Caus; Plat.
Jerking, sleep in: Cinb.
Long, as if: Calad.
Needles at: Asaf.
Neuralgia: Tab.
Numb: Merc.
Oedema: Rhus-t.
Pulsation: Cop; Ign.
Red, spots on: Caus.
Retracted: See Contracted.
Rigid, tenesmus, with: Thu.
Sensitive: Tab.
Stiff, emission, after: Grat.
Swelling: Arn.
- Hard, dorsum: Sabi.
- Lymphatic vessels, along: Merc.
- Painless: Mez.

Twitching: Thu.
Upwards, bends+: Berb.
Vesicles: Crot-t; Nit-ac.
Warts: Ant-t; Med; Thu.

PERCEPTION CHANGED (mental or visual):
Aco; Arg-n; *Ars*; Bar-c; BELL; Calc; *Cann*; HYO; Kali-br; Lac-c; *Lach*; Merc; Nux-m; Op; Pho; Pho-ac; Plat; Pyro; STRAM; Sul; Ver-a.

PERFORATION:
Kali-bi; Merc; Merc-c; Sil; Tub.

PERICARDIUM
Effusion+: Ascl.
Hydro+: Colch.
Inflammation+: Colch.

PERINEUM:
Agn; Alu; Carb-an; Carb-v; Chim; Cyc; Ol-an; Paeon; Sanic; Sul.
Abscess: Crot-h; Hep; Merc; Sil.
- Anus in and around, as if: Cyc.

Ball, lump: Cann; CHIM; Kali-m; *Ther.*
- Sitting on, as if: Chim.

Burning: Rhod.
- Coition, after: Sil.

Bursting: Sanic.
- Stools, after: Sanic.

Drawing: Cyc; Kali-bi.
Erection, during: Alu.
Eruptions: Petr; Sul.
- Herpes: *Petr.*

Excoriated: Lyc.
Fistula: Thu.
Fullness: Chin.
Genitals, to: Bov.
Heavy, weight: *Con*; Med; Ther.
Injury, penetrating: Symp.
Itching: Petr; Sul.
- Stools, after: Tell.

Lacerated: Stap.
Moist: Carb-an; Carb-v; Paeon; Thu.
Pain: Caus.
- Coition, after: Alu.
- Erection, during+: Alu.

Penis, to: Phyt.
Pinching: Pul.
Pressing: Berb; Cyc; Ol-an.
Pulsation: Caus.
Rectum, to: Bov.
Sitting agg: Cyc.
Stitching, and extending to penis: Calc-p.

PERINIUM
Stools agg: Sanic.
Swelling, suture of: Thu.
Tubercle: Thu.
Walking agg: Cyc.
Wriggling: Chel.

PERIODICITY, periodically
In general AGG: Alu; Aran; Arg-m; ARS; Cact; *Cedr*; CHIN; Chin-ar; *Chin-s*; *Eup-p*; *Gel*; Hep; *Ip*; Kali-c; Lach; Lyc; NAT-M; Nit-ac; *Nux-v*; Pul; Rhus-t; Sep; Sil; Spig; Sul; Tarn.

At the same hour AGG: Ant-c; Aran; Ars; Bov; *Cedr*; *Chin-s*; Cina; Ign; Lyc; Nat-m; *Saba*; Verb; Tarn.
- Neuralgia, every day: *Kali-bi.*

Exact: Aran; Ars; Cedr; Chin-s; Nat-m; Tarn.

Yearly AGG: Am-c; *Ars*; Crot-h; Echi; Elap; Lach; Lyc; Naj; Psor; Rhus-t; Tarn; Urt; Vip.
- Half: Lach; Sep.

PERIOSTEUM: See under BONES.

PERISTALSIS, reversed: Asaf; Elap; Nux-v; Rhus-t; Ver-a.

PERITONITIS: See ABDOMEN, inflammation.

PERSECUTION, ideas of: Anac; Chin; Con; Cyc; *Dros*; Hyo; Lach; Thyr.

PERSEVERE cannot: Alu; Asaf; Bism+; Grat; Lac-c; Lach; Nux-m+; Nux-v; *Sil*; Sul.

PERSPIRATION: See SWEAT.

PERVERSITY with tears (children)+: Bell.

PETECHIAE: See ECCHYMOSIS.

PETIT MAL: See EPILEPSY, minor.

PETULENT+: See PEEVISH.

PHAGEDENA, slough: ARS; Carb-v; Caus; Chel; Crot-h; Hep; *Lyc*; *Merc*; Merc-c; Merc-cy; Mez; NIT-AC; *Petr*; SIL; *Sul.*

PHANTASY: See IMAGINATIONS.

PHARYNX
Burning: Bell; Carb-v.
- Menses, during: Nat-s.

Chronic conditions: Aesc; Cinb; Rum; Sep.
Dry: Bell; Nux-m.
Fissured: Elap; Kali-bi.
Glistening: Ap.
Inflamed: Bell; Merc.
Scraping: Mez; Sang.
Tickling: Stic.
Tightness of, to stomach+: Alu.

PHILOSOPHER: Sul.

PHIMOSIS, para phimosis: Ap; Canth; Colo; Guai; *Merc*; Merc-c; *Nit-ac*; Rhus-t; Thu.
Friction, from: Arn.

PHLEBITIS: See BLOOD VESSELS, inflammation.

PHLEGMASIA ALBA DOLENS (white milk leg): Ap; Ars; Bell; *Bry*; CALC; Ham; *Lach*; Lyc; Merc; *Pul;* *Rhus-t*; Sul; Vip.

Forceps delivery, after: Cep.
Touch agg: Crot-h.

PHLYCTENAE: See CONJUNCTIVA.

PHOTOMANIA: See LIGHT, amel.

Delirium, with: Calc.

PHOTOPHOBIA: See LIGHT, agg.

Chronic: Aeth.

Inflammation, without: *Con*; Hell.

Masturbation, after: Cina.

Operations, after: Stro.

Spring season, in: Kob.

Warm room agg: *Arg-n*.

PHTHISIS: See CONSUMPTION.

PHYSICAL EXERTIION agg: See EXERTION, Physical agg.

PHYSOMETRA: See VAGINA, flatus from.

PIANO PLAYING agg (See FINGERS, working with agg): Nat-c; Sep.

  Body, heaviness of, after: Anac.

PICKING: See CARPHOLOGY.

PIECES, IN: See DUALITY.

PIERCING: See Under PAIN.

PILES, haemorrhoids: AESC; ALO; Ars; Carb-an; Carb-v; *Caus*; *Coll*; *Grap*; *Ham*; *Kali-c*; *Lach*; Lyc; Merc-i-r; MUR-AC; NIT-AC; NUX-V; Paeon; Pho; Pul; Sep; SUL.

  Alternating, with: Abro; Coll; Sabi.

  Bathing cool
- Amel: Alo; Bro; Kali-c; Nux-v; Rat.
- Warm, or agg: Bro.

PILES

Bleeding: Am-c; Bar-c; Caps; Coll; *Fer*; Hypr; Kali-c; Nat-m; *Pho*; Pho-ac; Psor; *Pul*; Sabi; Sep; Sul.
- Amel: Aesc.
- Easy+: Nit-ac.
- Flatus passing, while: Pho.
- Menses, during: Am-c; Am-m.
- Removal, after: Nit-ac.
- Slight, exhausts: Hyds.
- Stools
  - during: Am-c; Ham; Nat-m; Pho.
  - after: Am-c.
- Walking, while: Sep.

Blind: Aesc; Nux-v.
- Smarting+: Led.

Bluish: Aesc; *Carb-v*; *Lach*; Mur-ac.

Bunch of cherries, like: Alo; Calc; Dios; Mur-ac.

Burning+: Caps.

Bursting: Ham.

Chronic: Aesc; Coll; Merc-i-r; Nux-v; Sul.

Climaxis, during agg+: Aesc.

Cough agg: Caus; Ign; *Kali-c*; Lach.

During agg: Coll.

Dysmenorrhoea, after: Cocl.

Foul, offensive: Carb-v; Med; Pod.

Hot application, heat amel: *Ars*; Lyc; Mur-ac; Petr; Pho; Zin.

Large, impeding stools: Caus; Paeon+; Sul-ac.
- Ulcerated+: Paeon.

PILES

Leucorrhoea, suppressed agg: Am-m.
Lifting agg: Rhus-t.
Lying agg: Pul.
Menses agg: Am-c; Lach.
Milk agg: Sep.
Moisture, oozing, from: Calc-p; Sul-ac.
Operations, after agg: Coll; Croc.
Painful: Mur-ac; Nit-ac; Paeon; Stap.
- Stand, cannot: Plant.

Parturition, after: Kali-c; Lil-t.
Pendulous: Nit-ac.
Pregnancy during: Mur-ac; Sep.
Protruding: Abro; Alo; Am-c+; Calc; Kali-c; Mur-ac; Sep; Sul; Zin.
- Bleeding, with: Lach; Lept.
- Flatus passing, while: Bar-c; *Mur-ac*; Pho.
- Lying, when: Pul.
- Menses, during: Pul.
- Stool
  - during: Calc-p; Rat; Sil.
  - after+: Am-c.
  - preventing: Caus+; Sul-ac; Verb.
- Urination, during: *Bar-c*; Kali-c; Mur-ac.
- Walking agg: Am-c+; Sep.

Reflex, from: Coll.
Riding amel: Kali-c.
Sitting
- Agg: Caus; Grap; Thu.
- Amel: Calc; Ign.

PILES

Sneezing agg: See Cough agg.
Standing agg: Caus.
Stepping, wide agg: Grap.
Sticking: Sep.
- Cough, during: Ign; *Kali-c*; Lach; Nit-ac.

Stricture, from: Bap.
Suppressed agg: Coll; Lycps; Mill; Nux-v; Sul.
Thinking of it agg: Caus.
Touch agg: Bell; Caus; Mur-ac; Rat; Sul; Thu.
Ulcerate: Carb-v; Sil; Zin.
Urinating agg: Kali-c.
Walking
- Agg: Aesc; Bro; Carb-an; Caus; Mur-ac; Sep; Sul; Zin.
- Amel: *Ign*.

White: Carb-v.

PIMPLES: See ERUPTIONS.

PINCHING: See PAIN, Squeezing.
Amel: Ap; Ars.

PINING: *Aur*; *Lyc*; Nat-m; Pho-ac; *Tub*.

PINK EYE: Euphr.

PINWORMS: See under WORMS.

PITCHY: See DISCHARGES, tarry.

PLACENTA

Adherent, retained: Canth; Hyds; Ign; *Pul*; Sabi; Sec; Sep.
- Habitual: Hyds.

Previa: Erig; Ip.
Septic: Sec.

PLACID, tranquil: Ap; Arn; Chin; *Hell*; *Op*; *Pho*; PHO-AC; SEP; Stap; Sul.
  Anger, after: Ip.
PLAGUE: Ars; Crot-h; Ign; Lach; Pho; Pyro; Tarn-c.
PLAINTIVE: Crot-h.
PLETHORIA, full blooded: *Aco*; Aur; BELL; Bry; Calc; *Fer*; Hyo; Kali-bi; Lyc; Nat-m; *Nux-v*; PHO; *Pul*; Sep; Sil; *Sul*.
PLEURISY: See under CHEST.
PLEURODYNIA: Aco; Arn; Ascl; Bor; Bry; Chin; Cimi; Fer; Fer-p; Lach; Nux-v; Pul; Ran-b; Saba; Sul.
PLICA POLONICA: Grap; Vinc; Vio-o.
PLUG, nail, wedge, clavus: Agar; *Anac*; Arn; Asaf; *Cof*; Hep; *Ign*; Lith; Mos; *Plat*; *Ran-sc*; Rat; *Rut*; Spo; Sul; *Sul-ac*; THU; Val.
  Blunt: Rut; Sul-ac.
  Rough: Rut.
PNEUMONIA: See under CHEST.
POISON, fears: See under FEAR.
POISONED, feeling: Lac-c; Lach; Naj; Vip.
POLLUTIOINS: See SEMINAL EMISSIONS.
POLYPI (See FUNGUS GROWTH): Calc; Calc-p; Coc-c; Con; Form; Mar-v; Pho; Sang; Stap.
POLYURIA: See URINE, profuse.
POMPOUS, important: Bell; Calc; Cup; *Lyc*; Pho; PLAT; *Ver-a*.

POPLITAE: Bell; Con; Mez; Nat-c; Nat-m; Onos; Pho.
  Aching: Mez.
  Bending knee agg: Calc-p; Chin; Rhus-t.
  Bubbling, heels, to: Rhe.
  Contraction: Caus; Guai; Nat-m; Tell.
  Excoriation: Amb; *Sep*.
  Extending leg agg: Carb-an; *Rhus-t*.
  Fibroids, recurrent: Calc-f.
  Heel, to: Alu.
  Itching: Lyc; Mez; Sep; Zin+.
  Motion agg: Nat-c; Plb.
  Numb: Onos.
  Painful: Caus; Lyc; Nat-c; Phys; Radm.
  Sitting agg: Berb.
  Standing agg: Grap; Par; Rum.
  Stiff: Caus.
   • **Stooping, on:** Sul.
  Sweat, on: Bry; *Carb-an*; Con; Dros; Sep.
  Swelling: Mag-c.
  Weakness: Val.
POSITION
  Awkward, strange: See ATTITUDE BIZARRE.
  Change of amel: See CHANGE OF POSITION agg and amel.
  Odd amel: Rhe.
  Rest, cannot, in any: Lyc; Pip-m; Ran-b; Rhus-t; Sanic; Sul; Syph; Xanth.
   • **Sleep, during:** Caus.
  Wrong, in agg: Ars; Bry; Lyc; Tarx.

POWER

Higher, under, as if: Anac; Lach; Naj; Thu.
- Therefore powerless: Anac.

Lack, of: See Control.
- Will: Op.

PRAISE AMEL: Pall.

PRAYING: Ars; *Aur*; Bell; *Pul*; Stram; *Ver-a*.

PRAYS, curses, shrieks, in turns+: Ver-a.

PRECOCIOUS: Lyc; Merc.

Loquacious (children): Strop.

PREGNANCY, child-bed affections of or since AGG: *Aco*; Alet; Arn; Bell; *Bry*; Calc; Caul; Cham; Cimi; Cocl; Con; *Gel*; Helo; Ign; Ip; *Kali-c*; *Kre*; Mag-c+; Nux-m; NUX-V; Plat; PUL; Pyro; *Rhus-t*; Sabi; Sec; SEP; Stram; Sul; Tab; Ver-a; Vib.

Abdomen, lying on amel: Pod.

Bilious complaints, during: Chel.

False: *Caul*; Croc; Nux-v; *Thu*.

Feverish restlessness, during last month: Colch.

Itching: Sabi; Tab.

Late: Bell.

Looks, as if+: Vario.

Strange, notions, desires: Lyss.

Toxaemia, of: Kali-chl.

Troubles, many, during+: Pod.

Walk about, must at night: Rat.

PREMOTION: See FEAR, future.

PREPUCE: Ap; Calad; Merc; Rhus-t.

PREPUCE

Burning: Nit-ac.

Cold: Berb.

Cracked: Hep; Merc; Sep; Sul; Sul-io.

Eruptions: Nit-ac.

Excoriation: Merc.
- Coition after: Calend.
- Easy: Nat-c.

Gangrene+: Kre.

Haemorrhage+: Kre.

Hard, like leather: Sul.

Herpes, on: Pho-ac; Sars.

Inflammation: Cinb; Merc.

Itching: Caus; Cinb; Con; Ign; Nit-ac; Petr; Rhus-t.

Numb: Berb.

Oedema: See Swelling.

Phimosis: See PHIMOSIS.

Red, scurfy, spots on: Nit-ac.

Retracted: Calad; *Nat-m*.

Rubbing, slight agg: Cyc.

Scurf, inside: Caus.

Slough: Thu.

Swelling: Calad; Cinb; Merc; Nit-ac; Rhus-t; Thu; Vesp.
- Itching, with: Vio-t.

Thickened: Lach.

Ulcers: Aur-m; Merc; Merc-c.

Varices: Ham; Lach.

Warts: Cinb; Sep; *Thu*.

PRESBYOPIA: See VISION, far sight.

PRESENTIMENTS: See FEAR, future.

PRESSING: See PAIN, pressing.

PRESSURE

AGG: (lying on painful side or affected side agg): Aco; *Agar*; Ap; Arg-n; Ars; *Bar-c*; Bell; Bry; Calad; Calc; Carb-v; *Cina*; Dros; *Hep*; IOD; Kali-c; Kali-io; LACH; Laur; Lil-t; *Lyc*; Mag-c; Mag-m; Merc-c; Nat-s; Nux-m; *Nux-v*; Pho; Pho-ac; Psor; Rut; Saba; SIL; Spo; Tarn; Tell; Ther; Thu; Vib; Zin-chr.

AMEL (lying on painful or affected side amel): Am-c; Arg-n; BRY; Calc; Caps; Castr; Cham; Chel; *Chin*; COLO; Con; Cup-ar; Dios; *Dros*; IGN; Lil-t; *Mag-m*; *Mag-p*; Meny; Nat-c; *Plb*; *Pul*; Pyro; *Rhus-t*; Sep; Sil; STAN; Vib.

Boots, shoes, of AGG: Bor; Paeon.

Clothes of agg: See CLOTHES, pressure agg.

Hard over edge
- AGG: Rut.
- AMEL: Bell; *Chin*; COLO; Con; Ign; *Lach*; Mag-m; Meny; Nux-v; Psor; Samb; Sang; Stan; Zin.

Hat, cap, of AGG: Carb-v; Nit-ac; Sil; Val.

Opposite side on AGG: Vio-t.

Painless side on agg: See LYING, on painless side agg.

Sharp: Ign.

Simple, sense of: Bell; Bry; Lach; Lyc; *Nat-m*; Nit-ac; *Nux-v*; *Pul*; *Sep*; Sil; Stan; SUL.

Spine, on AGG: Agar; Arn; Bell; *Chin*; Kali-c; *Phys*; Sep; SIL; Ther.

Steady AMEL: Nit-ac; Spig.

Support, and AMEL: Murx.

PRIAPISM: See ERECTIONS, painful.

PRICKINGS: Crot-h; *Nit-ac*.

PRICKLING: See under PAIN.

PRICKLY HEAT: Ant-c; Urt.

PRIDE, arrogance: Lil-t; Lyc; PLAT; Sul; *Ver-a*.

Over weening: Grat.

Wounded+: Nux-v; Pall; Plat; Ver-a.

PRIM: Plat.

PRODROME: Chel; Chin; Corn; Eup-p.

PROFANITY: ANAC; Lil-t; Lyc; Nit-ac; Stram; Tarn; Ver-a.

PROLAPSE, falling: Alo; Arg-m; Arg-n; Aur; *Bell*; Bor; *Calc*; Gel; Helo; *Ign*; Kali-cy; Lach; Lil-t; *Merc*; *Mur-ac*; Nat-m; Nux-v; Pall; Pho; Plat; Pod; *Pul*; *Rhus-t*; Sep; Stan; *Sul*.

PROPHYACTICS

Catheter fever: Cam-ac.

Cholera: Ars; Cup-ar; Ver-a.

Diphtheria: Ap; Diph; Merc-cy.

Erysipelas: Grap.

Hay fever: Ars; Kali-p; Psor.

Hydrophobia: *Bell*; Canth; Hyo; Lyss; Stram.

Influenza+: Eucal.

Intermittent fever: Ars; Chin-s.

Labour, pains, false: Caul.

PROPHYLACTICS
Measles: *Aco*; Ars; Pul.
Mumps: Trif.
Plague+: Ign.
Pus infection: Arn.
Quinsy: Bar-c.
Scarlet fever: Bell; Eucal.
Tetanus: Hypr; Phys.
Variola (small-pox): Maland; Vacci; Vario.
Whooping cough: Dros; Vacci.
Yellow fever: Ars.

PROPORTION sense of, disturbed: Agar; Calc; Cann; Onos; Plat; Stram.

PROSOPALGIA: See FACE, pain.

PROSTATE GLAND: Ap; Bar-c; Chim; CON; Crot-h; Dig; Lyc; Med; Par-b; Pho; Polyg; PUL; *Sabal*; *Sele*; Sep; Solid; *Stap*; Sul; THU.
Abscess: Sil.
Ball, sensation on sitting: Chim; Sep.
Burning: Caps.
Cancer: Crot-h.
Coition AGG: Alu; Cep; Psor.
Emission of prostatic fluid (prostatorrhea): Con; Lyc; Pho-ac; SELE; *Sep*; Stap.
- Cause, without: Zin.
- Easily discharged, with even passing flatus: Mag-c.
- Emotions, from: Con.
- Fondling women: Agn; CON.
- Lascivious thoughts, with: Con; Nit-ac.
- Sitting, while: Sele.

PROSTATE GLAND, emission
- Sleep, in Sele.
- Stools
  - with: Con; Hep; Nat-c; Nux-v; Pho-ac; Sele; Sep.
  - difficult, with: Nit-ac; Pho-ac; Sil; Sul.
- Talking to a young lady, while: Nat-m; Pho.
- Tobacco agg: Daph.
- Urination, After: Hep; Nat-c; Sul.
- Walking, while: Sele.

Enlarged: Apoc; *Bar-c*; *Calc*; Cann; Chim; *Con*; *Dig*; Med; Ol-an; Par-b; Pic-ac+; *Pul*; Sabal; Senec; Sil; Ther.
- As if: Ther.
- Piles, with: Stap.
- Pressure in perineum, with: Berb.
- Senile: Bar-c; Dig; Fer-pic; Sabal; Sele.

Hard, indurated: Con; Iod; Senec; Sil; *Thu*.
- As if: Senec.

Heavy: Med.

Inflamed: Ap; Aur; Chim; Fer-pic; Pul; *Sabal*; Solid; *Thu*.
- Suppresed gonorrhoea, from: Merc-d; Nit-ac; Thu.

Masturbation, complaints after: Tarn.

Pulsation, painful: Polyg.

Rectal troubles, with: Pod.

Sore: Chim.

Stitches
- Urging to stool, or urination, with: Cyc.
- Walking, when: Kali-bi.

PROSTATE GLAND
Swelled: Chim.
- As if: Senec.

Urethra, extending, to: Stap.
Urination agg: Lyc; Polyg; *Pul.*
Walking agg: Cyc; Kali-bi.

PROSTATORRHOEA: See PROSTATE GLAND, emissions of.

PROSTRATION: See WEAKNESS and NERVOUS.

PROTRUSION, also sense of internal parts as eyes, hernia etc: *Aco*; Aur; *Bell*; *Cocl*; Fer; *Glo*; Hyo; Iod; LACH; *Lyc*; Lycps; NUX-V; Op; Spig; Stram; Sul-ac.

PROUD: See PRIDE.

PROUD FLESH (See FUNGUS GROWTH): Alu.

PRURIGO: See ITCHING.

PRURITIS senilis: See ITCHING, old people in.

PRYING: Sul.

PSORA: Ars; Bar-c; *Calc*; Grap; Hep; Iod; Merc; Pho; *Psor*; Sil; *Sul*; Tub.

PSORIASIS: See under ERUPTIONS.

PTERYGIUM: Cann; Rat; Sul; Tell; Zin; Zin-s.
Cornea, over: Nux-m.
Pink: Arg-n.

PTOMAINE POISONING: ARS; Carb-v; Crot-h; *Cup-ar*; Kre; Lach; Pul; Pyro+; *Ver-a.*

PTOSIS: See PROLAPSE, and EYELIDS, heavy.

PUBERTY and affections of youth: *Ant-c*; Bell; *Calc-p*; Caus; Cimi; Croc; Fer; *Fer-p*; Guai; Hell; Kali-br; *Kali-c*; Kali-p; *Lach*; Nat-m; PHO; Pho-ac; PUL; Senec; Vio-o.
Dried and wrinkled girls+: Alu.
Slow in girls: Calc-p.

PUBES
Aching over, during menses: Radm.
Backward to lumbar region, from: Calc; Pho; Sabi.
Gurging: Scil.
Plug, wedge, weight between coccyx and: Alo; Cact; Sep.
Pulsation, constant, behind: Aesc.

PUDENDUM
Itching: Amb+.
- Menses
  - before: Grap.
  - during: Hep.

Pulsation: Pru-sp.
Urine burns: Caus; Scop.

PUERPERAL SEPSIS (See BLOOD SEPSIS): Arn; Ars; Echi; Lach; *Lyc*; *Op*; Pho; *Pul*; *Pyro*; RHUS-T; Sec; SUL.
Lochia, suppressed, from: Lyc; Sul.

PUFFINESS (See also SWELLING): Ap; ARS; Bov; CALC; Caps; *Fer*; *Flu-ac*; *Kali-c*; Kre; Led; Lith; Med; Nat-c; Nux-m; Op; Pho; Phyt; RHUS-T; Rum; Rut; Ust.

PULLED UP: Ol-an.

PULSATION, throbbing: Aco; Ast-r; BELL; *Bels*; Bry; *Calc*; Chin; Coc-c; Fer; GLO; Jab; Kali-c; Kre; Lach; Lil-t; Meli; Nat-m; *Pho*; Polyg; PUL; *Sep*; Sil; Strop; Sul.

Arteries, in: Bell; Chin; Glo.
- Carotid+: Pru-sp.
- Large, in: Iod.

Fever, in: Urt.
- Sudden: Pyro.

General, all over body: Aco; Alu; Amb; *Ant-t*; *Bell*; Calc; Calc-hyp; *Carb-v*; Fer; GLO; *Grap*; *Kali-c*; *Kre*; Lach; Lil-t; Lyc; Nat-m; PHO; PUL; Sang; Sele; *Sep*; *Sil*; Sul; Ver-v; Zin.
- Breath holding agg: Cact.
- Eating agg: Sele.
- Sleep, preventing: Sele.
- Sweat, with: Jab.

Hard: Asaf.

Localised+: Am-m.

Lying agg: *Glo*; Sele.

Motion agg: Sil.

Numbness, with: Glo.

Odd places, in: Cact.

Painful: Aco; Am-m; *Bell*; *Fer*; *Ign*; Polyg; Sep.
- Wandering: Polyg.

Single parts in: Kali-c; Mur-ac.

Sitting agg: Sil.

Veins, in: Glo.

Violent: Sabi.

PULSE

Changeable, variable: Cina; Dig; Laur; Naj.

Dicrotic: Gel; Kali-c.

Fast: See Rapid.

PULSE

Flowing: Fer-p; Gel; Syph; Ver-v.

Pluttering: Nux-v.

Full: Aco; *Ant-t*; Bell; Berb; *Bry*; Calc; Canth; Chel; Colo; Dig; Fer; FER-P; *Gel*; *Glo*; Grap; Hep; *Hyo*; Kali-n; Merc; Mez; *Nux-v*; *Op*; Pho; *Ran-sc*; Spo; *Stram*; *Sul*; VER-V.
- Right: Kali-chl.
- Strong, and: Aco; Bell; *Bry*.
- Weak, and: *Fer-p*; Gel; Ver-a.

Hard: Aco; Am-c; *Bell*; Berb; *Bry*; Canth; Chel; Chin; Colch; Colo; Fer; Grap; Hep; *Hyo*; Ign; Iod; Mez; *Nit-ac*; *Nux-v*; Pho; *Plb*; Sil; *Stram*; Sul.
- Cord like: Tab.
- Single beats: Aur; Cact; Lach; Lil-t; Zin.

Imperceptible: Aco; Carb-v; Colch; Cup; Sil; Tab+; Ver-a.
- Almost: Aco; Cam; Gel.

Intermittent: Adon; Ars; Carb-v; Chin; *Dig*; Kali-c; Lycps; Merc; Mur-ac; *Nat-m*; Pho-ac; Sec; Sep; Spig; Tab; Terb+; Ver-a.
- Every
  - third beat: Mur-ac; Nat-m; Nit-ac.
  - third or fourth beat: Cimi.
  - third to seventh beat: Dig; Mur-ac.
  - fourth beat: Calc-ar; Nit-ac.
- Long interval, exciting fear of death: Nux-m.

Irregular: Aco; Adon+; Ant-c; Ars; CACT; Cann; *Chin*; DIG; Fer; Glo; *Kali-c*; Lach; Myr;

PULSE, irregular ..
NAT-M; *Op*; Pho-ac; Sec; SPIG; Stram; Strop; VER-V.
- Forceps delivery, after: Cact.

Large: Aco; *Fer-p*; Lycps; Manc; Pho; Syph; *Ver-v*.

Rapid, quick, fast: ACO; Adon+; ANT-T; Ap; Arn; ARS; Aur; BELL; Bry; Coll; Con; Crot-c; Cup; Dig; Fer-p; Gel; *Glo*; Iod; LACH; Merc; Nat-m; NUX-V; Op; PHO; Pho-ac; Pyro; *Rhus-t*; Sil; Spig; *Spo*; Stan; Stram; SUL; Thyr; VER-V; Zin.
- Eating agg: Lyc.
- Evening agg: Lyc.
- Morning, in: Ars; Grap; Sul.
- Out of all proportion to temperature: Lil-t; *Pyro*; Thyr.
- Tumultuously: Aco; Amy-n; Lycps.
  - sweat, with: Coca.

Sharp: Rhus-t.

Slow: Berb; Cann; Cic; Cup; DIG; Gel; *Kalm*; *Myr*; Naj; Ol-an; Op; Scil; Sep; Stram; *Ver-v*.
- Day, during: Grap.
- Hard: Scil.
- Heartbeat violent, with: Ver-v.
- Neuralgia, with: Kalm.
- Puberty, at: Dig.
- Rapid
  - alternately: Chin; Dig; *Gel*; Iod; Strop.
  - than heart beat: Dig; Kali-n; Spig.
- Sinks to 40 beats: Cann; Naj; Plb.
- Vertigo, with: Ther.

PULSE
Small: *Aco*; *Ars*; Cam; Carb-v; *Cup*; Dig; Guai; Hell; *Rhus-t*; Scil; Sec; Sil; Stram; Strop; *Ver-v*.
- Left: Kali-chl.

Soft: Ant-t; Carb-v; Cup; Dig; *Fer-p*; *Gel*; Lach; Mur-ac; Op; Stram; Syph; Terb; *Ver-v*.

Synchronise, does not, with heart: Lycps.

Temperature, discordant: Pyro.

Thready: Ars; *Calc*+; Colch+; Tab; Terb+; Ver-a.

Tremulous: Ant-t; Calc; Cimi+; Kalm+; Naj+; *Spig*.

Unequal: Agar; Hyd-ac; Ign; Kali-chl; Op.

Venous: Glo.

Weak: Aco; *Ant-t*; *Ars*; Aur; Berb; Cam; *Carb-v*; Cimi+; Colch; Crot-h; Gel; Kali-c; Kalm+; Lach; Laur; Merc; *Mur-ac*; Naj; *Pho-ac*; *Rhus-t*; Ver-a.

PUNCTURED wounds (See INJURIES): Led; Plant.

PUPILS
Adherent: Nit-ac.

Contracted: Aco; *Chel*; Cocl; Jab+; *Op*; Sep; Sil; Sul; Thu; *Ver-a*.

Dilated: Agn+; Ail+; Arg-n; BELL; Bro+; Buf+; CALC; Chin; Cina; Gel; *Hyo*; Mang; Op; Sec; Spig; Stram; Ver-v+.
- Contracted and alternately: Bar-c; Hell; Lach; Phys; Strop.

PUPILS, dilated
- Convulsions, before: *Arg-n*; Buf.
- One: Nat-p.
- Reading agg: Pho-ac.

Insensible to light, fixed: Arn; *Bell*; Carb-v+; *Cup*; Hyo; OP.

Irregular: Aur+; Dig+; Merc; Sul.

Mobile: See Dilated, contracted, alternately.

Unequal (one smaller than other): Colch; Hyo; Tarn.

PURGATIVES agg: See under DRUG, abuse, of.

PURGING
AMEL: Abro; Nat-s; Zin.
With vomiting: See VOMITING with purging.

PURPLE: See BLUISH.

PURPURA: See ECCHYMOSIS.

PURSUED, as if: Anac; Hyo; Kali-br; Lach; Rhus-t; Stram.
Animals, by: Nux-v.

PUS (See DISCHARGES)
Acrid: Ail; *Ars*; *Bels*; Bro; Echi; Euphr; Gel; *Kali-io*; *Nit-ac*; Ran-b; Saba; Sanic; Sars; *Sul*.
Air bubbles, in: Sul.
Bloody: Calc-s; Merc; Nit-ac; Pho; Rhus-t.
Burrowing (See FISTULAE): Arn; Asaf+.
Foul, offensive: *Ars*; Asaf; Bap; Calc-f; *Carb-v*; Hep; *Lach*; Led; Mag-m; Nit-ac; Pho; *Psor*; *Pyro*; Sep; Sil; *Sul*; Syph.
- Asafoetida like: Carb-v.

Green: Sec; Syph; Tub.

PUS
Hair, destroying: Bels; Lyc; Merc; Rhus-t.
Plugs, of: Kali-bi; Nit-ac.
Profuse: Ars; Asaf; *Calc*; Dul; Hep; Kali-io; *Merc*; Nat-m; Nux-v; Pul; Sep; *Sul*.
Salty: Iod; Kali-io.
Scanty: Aco; *Bry*; *Hep*; Lach; Sil.
Slimy: Merc.
Sour: Sul.
Suppressed: *Bry*; Dul; *Lach*; Pul; Sil; Stram; *Sul*.
Tenacious: Bor; Coc-c; Con; Hyds; Kali-bi.
Thick: Arg-n; *Calc-s*; Euphr; *Hep*; *Kali-bi*; *Pul*; Sanic.
Thin: Ars; *Asaf*; Caus; *Flu-ac*; Mag-m; Merc; Nit-ac; Pho; *Sil*; *Sul*.
Unhealthy: Asaf; Hep; Merc; Pho; *Sil*.
Yellow: Calc-s; Euphr; Mag-m; Mez; Pul; Sanic.
- Bloody: Arg-n; Hep.
- Green: Ars-io; Kali-bi; *Kali-s*; Merc; Pul.

Watery: Asaf; *Merc*; Sil.

PUSHED
Down: Lyc; Psor.
Forward: Fer-p.

PUSTULES: See ERUPTIONS, pustulating.

PYEMIA (See BLOOD SEPSIS): Ars-io; Chin; Lach; Pho; Pyro.

PYELITIS: Berb; Calc-s; Kali-s; Merc-c; Hep; Rhus-t; Sul-io; Terb.
Coma, with: Bap.

PYLORUS
Cancer: Acet-ac; Grap.
Constriction: Chin; Nux-v; Pho.
Relaxation: Fer-p; Pho.
Wall, indurated: Sil.

PYORRHOEA: See GUMS, suppuration.

PYREXIA: See FEVER.

PYROSIS: See WATERBRASH.

PYURIA: See URINE, purulent.

QUALMISHNESS: Ars; Caus; Nat-s; Sul.

QUARRELSOME: See ABUSIVE.

QUESTIONS, speaks in, continuously: Aur.

QUICK
Pains: See Pains, shooting.
To act: Cof; Ign; Lach.

QUIET AMEL: *Bry*; Cadm; Colch; Nux-v.

QUININE, ill effects: See under DRUG Abuse.

QUINSY: See TONSILS, suppuration.

QUIVERING: Agar; *Asaf*; *Bell*; *Con*; Hyo; Kali-c; Mez; Nat-c; Stram; *Sul*; Tarn; Thyr+; Tub; Zin.
All over: Lyss.
• Vetigo, followed by: Calc.
Lying, while: Clem.

RADIATING: See DIRECTIONS.

RADIUS broken: Gymn.

RAGE: See DELIRIUM, maniacal.

RAGS
Are silk of beautiful, thinks: Sul.
Body torn into, as if: Phyt.

RAINS, when agg: Aran; Plat.

RAINY SEASON
Agg: See DAMPNESS agg.
Amel: See AIR, dry clear agg.

RAISING
Arms agg: See under ARMS.
Up
• AGG: *Aco*; Bell; *Bry*; Cadm; Cham; Cocl; Fer; Ign; *Merc-i-f*; Nat-m; Nux-v; Op; Pho; *Phyt*; Pul; Rhus-t; Sil; Sul; Ver-v; Vib.
• AMEL: Am-c; Ant-t; Aral; ARS; *Calc*; Dig; Glo; Kali-c; *Samb*; *Sep*.

RANCID, taste, odour etc: Alu; Carb-v; *Pul*; Tell; Thu; Val.

RANULA: Amb; Calc; Flu-ac; Merc; Mez; Nit-ac; *Thu*.
Chewing, talking agg: Mez.

RASHNESS: See RECKLESS.

RATS sees (See also VISION, illusions, of): Aeth; Ars.

RATTLING: Am-m; ANT-T; Cact; Calc-s; *Chin*; *Cup*; HEP; IP; Kali-s; Lob; *Lyc*; Op; Scil; Sil; Sul; Ver-a.

RAW: See PAIN, biting.
Scratches, himself: Aru-t; Psor.

RAWNESS, feeling+: Meli; Nux-v.

RAYNAUD'S DISEASE: Ail; Ars; Cact; Fer-p; Sec.

REABSORBENT: See ABSORBENT, action.

REACHING high AGG: Sul.

REACTION, lack of, poor: Aeth; Amb; Am-c; Ant-t; *Calc*; *Caps*; *Carb-v*; Castr+; Con; CUP; Dig;

REACTION, lack of ..
Fer; Gel; Hell; Hyd-ac; Kali-bi+; *Laur*; *Med*; Mos; Old; OP; Pho-ac; PSOR; SUL; SYPH; Tarn; Ther; Tub; Val; ZIN.

Genito-urinaty, sphere, in: Senec.

Violent: Bell; *Cup*; *Nux-v*; Zin.

READING, eye strain, AGG: Arg-n; *Calc*; Cina; Con; Croc; Kali-c; Lil-t; *Lyc*; Mang; Naj; NAT-M; Onos; Pho; Pho-ac; Phys; Radm; Rhod; Rhus-t; RUT; *Seneg*; Sep; Sil; Sul.

All symptoms of, AGG: Carb-ac.

Aloud
- AGG: Amb; *Carb-v*; Pho; Sele; Verb.
- AMEL: Nat-c.

Difficult, artificial light in: Nat-m.

Fine print
- Difficult: Cadm; Mang; Meph; Nat-c.
- more distinctly+; Cof.

Someone, after her: Mag-m.

RECKLESS, rashness (See boldness): Aur; Cic; Tub.

RECLINING AMEL: See under LYING.

RECOGNIZE, does not
Her own children: Acet-ac.
His relatives: Bell; Hyo.

RECOVERY, despair of: See DESPAIR.

RECTUM: Aesc; Alo; Calc; *Ign*; Lyc; Mag-m; *Merc-c*; Nat-m; *Nux-v*; Pho; *Pod*; Rat; Sep; *Sul*.

RECTUM

Abscess (peri-rectal): Calc-s; Rhus-t; Sil.

Aching: *Aesc*; Coll; Grap; Lyc; *Rat*.

Ankles, to: Alu.

Ball
- Big, as if in+: Sul-ac.
- Sitting on, as if : Cann.

Bladder (urinary) with: Amb; *Canth*; Caps; Erig; *Merc-c*; Lil-t; Pyro; Sabi.

Bleeding (See PILES): Bism; Rat.
- Clots, large: Alu; Alum.
- Constant in drops, no blood with stool: Kob; Pul.
- Flatus, passing on: Pho.
- Menses, during: *Am-m*; Grap; *Lach*.
- Piles, removal after: Nit-ac.
- Standing agg: Crot-h.
- Stools
  - after: Echi.
  - hard, from: Flu-ac; Kali-c; *Nat-m*; Tub.
  - soft, with: Hep.
- Walking, while: Alu; Crot-h; Sep.
- Women, old: Psor.

Boring: Bry.

Burning: *Ars*; Caps; Carb-v; Cep; Iris; Kali-c; Lyc; Merc; Stro; Sul.
- Cold application, amel: Alo; Kali-c; Terb.
- Continuous: Kali-c; Lyc.
- Pregnancy, during: Caps.
- Pressure amel: Kali-c.
- Standing agg: Crot-h; Lach.

RECTUM, burning
- Stools
  - after amel: Ver-v.
  - during and after+: Am-m.
- Urination, after: Nit-ac; Rhus-t.

Cancer: Alum; Laur; Phyt; Rut; Sang.

Chilliness, before stool: Lyc.

Coition agg: Caus; Merc-c; Sil.

Cold, passing flatus or stool during: Con.

Constriction, spasm: Caus; IGN; LACH; Lyc; *Merc-c*; NIT-AC; *Nux-v*; Op; Plb; Rat; Sep; Sil.
- Itching, alternating, with: Chel.
- Lying amel: Mang.
- Standing agg: Arn; Ign.
- Stools
  - during: Nat-m; Nit-ac; Plb; Rat; Sil.
  - after: Colch; Ign; Lach; Nit-ac.
  - hard, from: Fer.
  - preventing: Lyc.
- Urination, during: Caus.
- Uterine cancer, from: Kre.
- Walking, preventing: Caus.

Coughing agg: Ign; *Lach*; Nit-ac; Tub.

Crawling (See ANUS): Sul.

Cutting: Alu; Nux-v; Sil.
- Diarrhoea, during: *Ars*.
- Flatus or passing stools, amel: Canth.
- Standing agg: Lach.

Dragging, heavy: Aesc; Alo.

Dry: Hypr; Nat-m.

RECTUM

Electric shock, stool, before: Ap.

Enema, water of, escapes: Syph.

Faeces, remained in, as if: Grap; Lyc; *Nat-m*; Nit-ac; *Sep*; Ver-a.

Fistula (See ANUS): Calc-p; *Sil*; Sul.
- Pulsating: Caus.
- Vagina, and: Thu.

Fluid, dark, from: Med; Merc-i-f.

Fullness: Aesc; Alo; Ham; NIT-AC; *Sul*.
- Urination, frequent, with: Fer-pic.

Genitals, to: Chin; Lil-t; Rhod; Sil; Zin.

Heat, glowing: Cep.

Heavy: See Dragging.

Hot applications amel: Rat.

Itching: See Anus.

Laughing agg: Lach.

Narrow: Nat-m.

Neuralgia: Plb.

Numb+: Caus.

Orange coloured fluid from: Kali-p.

Pain
- Continuous: Kali-chl; Nit-ac; Phyt.
- Diarrhoea, in: Kali-chl.
- Long, after stool: Aesc; Agar; Alo; Alum; Am-c; Am-m; Calc; *Colch*; *Grap*; *Ign*; Mur-ac; Nit-ac; *Paeon*; Rat; Sil; Stro; Sul.
  - must walk about: Paeon.

RECTUM

Painful, knife sawing up and down+: Aesc.
Paresis, piles removal, after: Kali-p.
Parturition, after: Gel; Pod; Rut.
Passing out, something, as if: Lept.
Plug, lump: Anac; Cann; Crot-t; Kali-bi; *Lach*; Lil-t; Nat-m; *Plat*; SEP; Sul-ac.
- Menses, during: Sil.
- Stool
  - before: Lach.
  - not amel, by: Sep.
- Urination, urging, with: Lil-t.

Pockets: Polyg.
Polypus: Kali-br.
Pressed, asunder, as if: Op.
Pressing down, on: Crot-t; Pod; *Sul*.
Pressure on navel
- Agg: *Crot-t.*
- Amel: Kali-c.

Prolapsed: *Alo*; Ap; Calc; Coll; Gel; *Ign*; Lyc; Merc; *Mur-ac*; Nux-v; Pho; *Pod*; Radm; Rut; Sep.
- Acute: Ars; Bell.
- Bleeding, from: Ars.
- Contracted: Mez.
- Coughing, on: Caus.
- Diarrhoea agg: Dul; Merc; Nux-v; Pod.
- Easy, without straining: Grap; Kali-c; Rut.
- Flatus, passing: *Mur-ac*; Val.
- Mental excitement from: Pod.

RECTUM, prolapsed

- Paralysis, with: Plb.
- Parturition, after: Gel; Pod.
- Pregnancy, during: Pod.
- Replacing, difficult: Mez.
- Sitting agg: Ther.
- Smoking on: Sep.
- Sneezing, on: Pod.
- Stool
  - before: Pod; Rut.
  - during: Ign; Lyc; Pod; Sep.
  - after: Merc; Pod.
  - urging, with: Rut.
- Straining without, easy: Grap; Kali-c; Rut.
- Urinating, while: Mur-ac.
- Vomiting, while: Mur-ac; Pod.
- Walking, after: Arn.
- Washing body, amel: Arn.

Shooting: Ign.
Sneezing agg: Lach.
Sore, sensitive, smarting: Bell; Carb-v; Grap; *Mur-ac*; Nit-ac; Onos; Pul; Radm; Sul.
- Ovaries, with: Onos.

Standing erect agg: *Petr.*
Sticks, burr, splinter: AESC; Caus; Grap; Hell; Iris; Nit-ac; Nux-v; *Rat*; Sanic; Sul.
- Flatus passing amel: Colo; *Mag-c.*
- Menses, during: Ars.
- Vomiting, on: Agar.

Stooping
- Agg: Caus; Rut.
- Amel: Chel.

Stricture: Rut; Syph.
- Piles, from: Bap.

Tearing: Tub.

RECTUM

Tenesmus (See CONSTIPATION): Erig; *Merc-c.*
- Dysentery, after: Calc.
- Stools, during and after Amel: Ver-v.

Tension: Sil.
Testes, to: Sil.
Thighs, to: Alum.
Throbbing, pulsation: Lach.
Tingling: Carb-v; Colch.
Ulcers: Cham; Sil.
Upward, in: Grap; *Ign*; Lach; Pho; *Sep*; Sul.
Urging constant, not for stool: Lach.
Urinating agg: *Mur-ac*; Val.
Vomiting agg: Mur-ac; Pod.
Wrists, alternating with: Sul.
RECURRING: See RELAPSES.
RED, redness (skin, discharges etc.): ACO; *Ap*; *Arg-n*; Ars; BELL; *Bry*; *Cham*; Chin; Fer; Jab; Lach; Meli; *Merc*; *Nux-v*; Op; Pho; *Rhus-t*; Sabi; *Sang*; Sep; SUL.

Bluish, dark: Bap; Phyt; Rhus-t.
Body, whole: Op.
Fiery: Bell; Cinb; Med; Stram; Sul.
Orifices: See ORIFICES.
Parts become pale+: Fer.
Rosy: Ap; Pyro; Sil.
Spots: Merc; Pic-ac; Rhus-t; Stic; Sul.
- Blood: Cor-r; Pho.
- Elevated: Mang.
- Fiery: Med.

RED, spots
- Pink: Colch.
- Small, all over body: Scil.
- Wine: Cocl; *Sep.*

Streaks: Bell; Bry; Buf; Myg; Pyro.
Turn, white: Bor; Hell; Merc; Val.
- Yellow or green: Con.

REELING, tottering, staggering, feeling (See GAIT): Ars; Bell; Bry; Caus; Gel; Ign; *Lach*; Nux-v; Op; Rhus-t; Stram; Sul; Ver-a; Ver-v.

Coition, after: Bov.

REGURGITATION

Aeth; Ant-c; Ant-t; Arn; Asaf; *Bry*; Carb-v; Chin; Fer; Fer-p; Lach; Merc; NUX-V; PHO; Pho-ac; *Pul*; Sars; *Sul*; Sul-ac; Vario.

Astringent: Merc-c.
Bitter: Lyc; Nat-c.
- Food: Lyc; Nat-s.

Coughing after: Raph.
Eating
- Immediately, after: Mag-p.
- Hour, after: Aeth.

Fluids, of: Asaf; Kali-bi; Pul; Sul-ac.
- Painless, diphtheria in: Carb-ac.

Ingesta, of: Bry; *Pho*; Pul.
Milky: Sep.
Mouthful, by: Fer; *Pho.*
Mucous, of: Hyds.
- Frothy: Sep.

Salty: Kali-c.
Sour: Mag-c.
Stooping, while: Pho.

REGURGITATION

Vexation, after: Fer-p.

Walking, while: Mag-m.

Wants, to: Vario.

Watery: Ap.

RELAPSES, recurrences, recurrent attacks (See also PAROXYSMS repeated):
Aco; Ars; Bar-c; Bar-m; Bell; Chin; Colo; Cup; Dios; Hep; Kali-io; Lyc; Mag-p; Mez; Nat-m; Pho; *Psor*; Sul; Tub; Val; Verb.

Easy: Asaf; Cup.

RELAPSING FEVER: See under FEVER.

RELAXATION, flabby feeling (See INACTIVE):
Aeth; Alet+; Alo; Ant-t; Ars; Bov; *Calc*; Caps; CAUS; Chin; Cocl; *Colch*; GEL; Grap; Hell; *Hyo*; Lob; LYC; *Mag-c*; Merc-cy; MUR-AC; Nat-c; Nat-m; Op; PHO-AC; Seneg; Sep; *Spo*; Ver-a.

AMEL: Tarn.

Internal: Calc; Kre; SEP.

RELIGIOUS ideas, minded:
Ars; *Aur*; Hyo; *Lach*; Lil-t; *Lyc*; Pul; *Stram*; *Sul*; VER-A; Zin.

Children, in: Ars; Calc; Lach; Sul.

Sexual excitement, alternating with: Lil-t; *Plat*.

Want, of, feeling: See IRRELIGIOUS.

REMITTENCY: Gel.

REMITTENT FEVER: See under FEVER.

REMORSE: See GUILT, sense of.

Complaints, from: Arn.

Trifles, about: Sil.

RENDING: See PAIN, shooting.

REPEATED: Lach; Lyc; Stan; Zin.

Same action: Cheno.

REPENTENCE, ill effects of+: Arn.

REPRIMANDS AGG: Colo; *Ign*; Op; Stap.

Laughs, at: Grap.

REPROACHES

Himself: Aur; Cyc; Kali-br; Stram.

Others: *Aco*; *Ars*; Chin; Mez; *Nux-v*.

REPUGNANCE to everything: Ant-c; Merc; Pul.

REPUTATION, loss of AGG: Kali-br.

RESERVED: Lyc; Nat-m.

Anger+: Stap.

Displeasure: Aur; Ign; Ip; Nat-m; *Stap*.

RESPIRATION

Affections in general: Aco; Ant-t; *Ap*; ARS; *Bell*; Bry; Carb-v; Cup; Dig; Dros; Grind; Hep; IP; *Kali-c*; LACH; Lob; *Lyc*; Nat-s; OP; PHO; PUL; Ran-b; *Samb*; SPO; Stan; SUL; Tarn; Vib.

Abdominal: *Ant-t*.

Air, open
- Agg: Psor.
- Amel: Ant-t; Ap; Nat-m; Pul; Sul.

RESPIRATION

Anxious: ACO; Ars; Bar-m; Chel; *Ip*; Nat-m; *Pho*; Pru-sp; *Pul*; Ran-b; *Scil*; Sec; Spo; Stan.

Arms
- Apart amel: Lach; Laur; Nux-v; Psor; Spig; Tarn.
- Exertion, amel: Nat-m.
- Motion of raising agg: Am-m; Berb; Lach; Spig; Tarn.

Arrested: See Difficult.
- Children, on being lifted: Bor; Calc-p.
- Coughing or drinking, on: Anac.

Ascending
- Amel, walking on level ground agg: Ran-b.
- Stairs agg: Iod; Merc.

Asthmatic: See ASTHMA.

Back touching agg: Adon.

Bending
- Backwards agg: Cup; Psor.
- Head, backwards amel: Hep; Lach; *Spo*; Ver-a.

Breathe, again cannot: See BREATHE AGAIN, cannot.

Cardiac (See Difficult): Cratae; Strop.

Cheyne-stokes: Bell; Carb-v; Coca; Grind; Op; Sul; Sul-ac.

Choking: See Difficult.

Clothing agg: Ars; Chel; Lach.

Coition, emission agg: *Amb*; Cedr; Dig; Pho; Stap.
- Desire for, with: Nat-c.

Colic agg (See Pains during agg): Arg-n; Berb.

RESPIRATION

Consumption, in: Carb-v; Ip; Pho.

Cough agg: Am-m; Ant-t; Ars; Cup; *Dros*; Ip; Just; Merc-cy; Naj; Nux-v; Op; *Pho*; Stan; Tarn; Tub.
- Alternating, with: Ant-t.
- Before: Ant-t; Caus.

Covering nose or mouth agg: Arg-n; Cup; Lach.

Deep: Arg-n; Aur; *Bry*; Calc; *Caps*; Carb-v; Coca; Hep; IGN; *Ip*; *Lach*; Lil-t; Nat-s; *Op*; Pho; Plat; *Sele*; *Sil*; Sul.
- Breath
  - agg: Thu.
  - amel: Caps; Sul.
  - enough, cannot get: Aur; Crot-t; Lach; Pru-sp; Radm.
  - excites, cough: Arg-n; Bro; Bry.
  - inability to take: Stry.
  - wants: Arg-n; Aur; Bro; Bry; Cact; Calc; Caps; Cup; Dig; Hyd-ac; *Ign*; *Lach*; Lil-t; Mos; Nat-s; Op; Sele; Sul; Xanth+.
- Yawns to force it down: Pru-sp.

Difficult, suffocating choking: Aco; Anac; *Ant-t*; Ap; ARS; *Bro*; *Bry*; Cact; Carb-v; Caus; Chel; Chin; *Chlor*; Cina; Crot-t; *Cup*; Cup-ar; Fer; *Hep*; Ign; *Iod*; IP; Kali-ar; *Kali-c*; *Kali-io*; Kali-m; LACH; Laur; Lob; Lyc; Meph; Merc-c; *Naj*; Nat-m; *Nat-s*; Nux-m; *Op*; *Pho*; PUL;

RESPIRATION, difficult ..
Rum; *Samb*; Scil; Sele; SPO; *Stan*; SUL; *Sumb*; *Tarn*; *Ver-a*; Ver-v; Vib.
- Anger from
  - adults: Ran-b.
  - children: Arn.
- Ankles, swelling around with: Hep.
- Athletes, aged, in: Coca.
- Coryza, with: Ars; Ars-io; Calc; Ip; Nit-ac; Pho; Sul.
- Crowd, in: Arg-n.
- Crowded room, in+: Lil-t.
- Diseased condition of distant parts not involved in respiration: Berb; Pul.
- Dropsy, in: Eup-pur.
- Epilepsy, before: Am-br.
- Exhalation (See EXHALATION agg): *Chlor*; Kali-io; Med; Meph; *Samb*.
- Eyes, closing on+: Carb-an.
- Falling down, on: Petr.
- Flatulence, from: Arg-n; Zin.
- Formication, preceded by: Cist.
- Fright, from: Samb.
- Gastric pain, with+: Arg-n.
- Haemoptysis, with: Arn.
- Hiccough, with: Aeth.
- Inhalation: Bro; Caus; Samb.
- Itching, with: Saba.
- Knocked down, when: Petr.
- Labour pain, each, with: *Lob*.
- Lips, redness of, with: Spig.
- Menses
  - during: Colo.
  - after: Am-c.

RESPIRATION, difficult
- Metrorrhagia, with: Flu-ac.
- Motion, rapid amel: Lob.
- Nausea with: Ip; Kali-n.
- Nervous: *Arg-n*; Ars; Carb-an; Lob; Mos.
- Nose
  - felt, in: See NOSE, dyspnoea, in.
  - itching, after: Saba.
- Pregnancy, during: Vio-o.
- Pricking, with: Lob.
- Sitting up, agg+: *Laur*.
- Sleep
  - falling to, on: Bap; Dig; Grap; *Grind*; *Lach*; *Op*.
  - after: Sep.
- Sneezing
  - with: Ars-io; Pho.
  - agg: Naj; Pho.
- Standing amel+: Sep.
- Sweat, with: Bap.
- Ulcer, with: Kali-n.
- Uremia, with: Solid.
- Uterine displacement, from: Nit-ac.
- Vertigo, with: Kali-c.
- Wakes him+: Am-c.
- Yawning agg: Bro.

Drawing shoulders back amel: Calc; Calc-ac.
Dust agg: Ars-io; Bro; Dul; Nat-ar; *Poth*; *Sil*.
Eating
- Agg: Kali-p; Lach; Nat-s; *Pho*; Pul; Zin-val.
- Amel: Amb; *Grap*; Iod; Med; *Spo*.

Emphysema agg: Am-c; Sars.

RESPIRATION

Epigastrium, or stomach, from: *Ars*; Chin; Cocl; Guai; Lach; Nat-m; *Pho*; Rhus-t; Sul.

Eructations amel: Amb; Ant-t; Aur; *Carb-v*; Mos; *Nux-v*.

Exertion
- Agg: Ars; Calc; Coca; Ip; Lach; Lob; Lyc; Lycps; Nat-m; Spo.
- Least agg: Calc; Con; Kali-c; Nat-s.

Expectoration amel: *Ant-t*; Aral; Grind; Hypr; Ip; Lach; Sep; Zin.

Eyes, closing agg: Carb-an; *Carb-v*.

Fanned, wants to be: Carb-v; Med; Naj.

Gasping: Ap; Carb-v; Cor-r; Hyd-ac; Kali-n; Latro; Laur; Lob; Lyc; Meph.
- Chorea, with: Laur.
- Haemorrhage, with: Ip.
- Spasms, before, during, after: Caus; Laur.

Hands, using on: Bov.

Hang down legs amel: Sul-ac.

Heart symptoms or pain with: Cact; Carb-v; *Kalm*; Spig; Spo; Strop; Sumb; Tarn.
- And overian troubles with: *Tarn*.
- And urinary troubles with: *Laur*; Lycps.

Heat, with or overheated agg: Ap; Kali-c.

Heavy: Glo; Ver-v.

Hissing: See Whistling.

Holding to something amel: Grap.

Hot: See BREATH, hot.

Humid air agg: Aur; Bar-c; Nat-s.

Hysterical (See NERVOUS): *Arg-n*; Ars; Nux-m; Val.

Injury, from: Petr.

Inspiration double: Led.

Intermittent: See Unequal.

Irregular: Ail; BELL; *Cup*; Dig; Hyd-ac; Op; Sul.

Itching, with: Saba.

Jerky: Bell; *Ign*; Laur; Ox-ac; Tab.

Kneeling amel: Caus.

Kyphosis, in: Aco; Ant-c; Asaf; Aur; Bar-c; Bell; Bry; Calc; Cam; Cic; Clem; Colo; Dul; Hep; Ip; Rhus-t; Rut; Sabi; Sep; Sil; Stap; Sul; Thu.

Last breath, cease as if: See BREATHE AGAIN cannot.

Laughing agg: Aur; Cup.

Light: See Shallow.

Lips red, with: Spig.

Long: Lil-t.

Loud, noisy: Calc; CHAM; *Chin*; Kali-bi; Lach; Pho; *Samb*; SPO; Sul; Ver-a.

Lying
- Agg: Ap; Ars; Carb-v; Grap; Kali-c; Lob; Tub.
- Amel: Calc-p; Chel; Dig; Hell; Kali-bi; Laur; Nux-v; *Psor*; Terb.
- Back on
  - agg: Lyc.
  - amel: *Cact*; Kalm.

RESPIRATION, lying
- Head low with, agg: Ap; Cact; Chin; Kali-c.
- Side on
  - agg: Ars; Pul.
  - amel: Alu.
  - right
    amel: Naj; Spig.
    with head high amel: Cact; Spig; Spo.
  - left
    agg: Merc.
    amel: Castr.

Motion
- Agg: Ars; Bry; Calc; Chin; Kali-c; Spig; Spo; Stan.
- Amel: Arg-n; Aur; Bro; *Fer*; Lob; Pho; Pul; Samb.
- Quick agg: Merc.

Night
- Agg: Ars; Kali-ar; Lach; Naj; Ox-ac; Pho; Samb; Sul; Vib.
- Mid-night agg: Ars; Fer; Grap; Samb.

Odours agg: Ars; Pho-ac; Sang.

Oppressed: ACO; Am-c; Ap; Apoc; ARS; Ars-io; *Bell*; *Bry*; Cact; CARB-V; Chin-s; Colch; *Cup*; Fer; *Ign*; IP; Kali-c; Kali-m; Nat-s; Nux-m; *Nux-v*; Op; PHO; PUL; Sele; Seneg; *Sep*; SUL; Tub; *Ver-a*.
- Epilepsy, before: Am-br.
- Fever, during: Bov; Kali-c.
- Room, crowded, in: Lil-t.
- Spasms, alternating with: Ign.
- Talking agg: Caus.
- Walking rapidly agg: Meli.

RESPIRATION

Pain
- During agg: *Ars*; Bry; Carb-v; Cocl; Kalm; Nat-m; Pru-sp; *Pul*; Ran-sc; Sep; Sil; Sul.
- Gastric agg: Arg-m; Arg-n; Berb.

Painful: Bry; *Ran-b*.

Palpitation, with: Aur; Kalm; Mer-i-f; Pul; Spig; Ver-a.

Panting: Bry; Calad; *Ip*; Nit-ac; Pho; Stram; Ver-v.
- Reading, when: Nit-ac.
- Running rapidly, as from: Hyo.
- Stooping on: Nit-ac.

Puffing, stertorous: Am-c; Cheno; Naj; Op

Quick: ACO; Ant-t; Ars; *Bell*; Bry; *Carb-v*; Chel; *Cup*; Gel; *Ip*; *Lyc*; *Pho*; *Sep*; SUL.

Rattling: Am-c; ANT-T; Apoc; Ars; Cact; *Carb-v*; Caus; Chin; *Cup*; Dul; HEP; IP; Kali-s; Lob; *Lyc*; Pho; Pul; *Scil*; *Seneg*; Sil; Stan.
- But no expectoration+: *Ip*; Lob.
- Cold drinks agg: Pho.

Reading agg: Nit-ac.

Running amel, slow motion agg: Sep.

Shallow: *Bell*; Chin; *Laur*; Nux-m; *Pho*.

Shrill: Bell; Gel; Ign; Mos.

Short: See Difficult.

Sighing: Bry; Calad; Calc-p; Carb-v; Dig; IGN; Ip; *Lach*; Op; Sec; Sele; *Sil*; Stram.

RESPIRATION, sighing
- Cough, after: Led.
- Leucorrhea, with: Phys.
- Sleep, in: *Aur*; Calc.
- Unconsciousness, with: Glo.

Singing, when agg: Arg-m.

Sitting
- Erect amel: Aco; *Kali-c*; Lach; Laur; Lyc; Nat-c; Seneg; Terb.
- Head bent forward on knee, with amel: Kali-c.

Sleep falling to, on agg (See also Difficult): Am-c; *Ars*; Cadm; Carb-v; Gel; *Grind*; Kali-c; *Lach*; Pho; Spo; Sul; Tab.

Slow: Bell; Hyd-ac; *Op*; Ver-v.

Smoke, vapour, fumes, as of: Ars; Bar-c; Bro; Chin; *Ign*; Lach; Lyc; Pul.

Sneezing
- Agg: Naj; Pho.
- Amel: Naj.
- With: Ambro; Ars-io; Pho.

Snoring: Hyo; Merc-c; Nat-m; Op.
- Adenoids, removal after: Kali-s.
- Children, in: Mez.

Sobbing: See Sighing.

Spine, pressing on agg: Chin-s.

Standing amel: Bap; Cann; Sil; Spig.

Stomach, from: See Epigastrium.

Stool amel: Poth.

Stooping agg: Calc; Nit-ac; Sil.

Summer agg: Arg-n; Syph.

RESPIRATION

Swallowing agg: Bell; *Bro*; Calc; Cup.

Sweat, with: Samb.

Talking
- Agg: Lach; Spo; Sul; Thu.
- Amel: Fer.
- Fast agg: Caus.

Tongue, red, with: Mos.

Unequal, intermittent: Ant-t; Nit-ac; Op.

Urinating agg: Chel; Dul.

Water, standing in agg: Nux-m.

Wet weather agg: Aran; Nat-s.

Whistling, hissing, wheezing: Ars; Aur; Caus; Chin; Hep; *Ip*; Kali-c; Kali-io; *Samb*; Seneg; Spo; Stram.

Yawning amel: Croc.

RESPONSIBILITY

Inabillity to realize: Flu-ac.

Unusual agg: Aur.

REST

Agg: See MOTION, amel.

Cannot, in any position: *Lyc*; Pip-m; Ran-b; Rhus-t; Sanic; Sul; Syph; Xanth.
- Sleep, during: Caus.
- When things are not in proper place: Anac; *Ars*.

RESTLESSNESS, anxious: ARS; Calc; Cimi; Iod; Kali-ar; Kali-c; Merc; Nat-c; Pho; *Tarn*.
- Lying down amel: Mang.

General, physical: ACO; Anac; Ap; Arg-n; ARS; Bap; *Bell*; Calc; Calc-p; Cam; *Cham*; Cimi; Cina; Cof; Colo; Cup; Fer; HYO; Lyc; Mag-p; Mar-v;

RESTLESSNESS, physical ..
MERC; *Pho*; Plb; Pul; RHUS-T; Sec; SEP; Sil; Stap; Stram; *Sul*; TARN; Val; Vib; *Zin*.

Afternoon agg: Bor.

Alone, when+: Pho.

Compelling, rapid walking: Arg-n; *Ars*; *Tarn*.

Constant walking+: Pru-sp.

Convulsions
- Before: *Arg-n*; Buf.
- After: Oenan.

Exertion, least, agg: *Merc*.

Eyes, closing on, at night: *Mag-m*; Sep.

Hands, clutching, tightly amel: Med.

Internal: Ars; Rhus-t; Sil.

Menses, before: Kre; Sul.

Sitting, while: Lyc.

Sleep, loss of, from: Lac-d.

Sunlight agg: Cadm.

Thunderstorm, before: Psor.

Tossing about, in: Aco; Ars; Bell; Cham; *Cof*; Cup; Fer; Rhus-t; Tarn.

Walking in air open amel: Lyc; Pul.

Weeping, with+: Rhod.

Working, while: *Grap*.

RETCHING AND GAGGING:
Bell; Bry; Cham; Colch; Dros; Eup-p; *Ip*; *Nux-v*; Phyt; *Pod*; Pul; Rhus-t; Sul; Tab; Ver-a.

AGG from: Asar.

Constant: Pod.

Coughing, when: Cina; Hep; Nit-ac; Stan.

RETCHING

Dyspnoea from: Am-c.

Eating
- When: Ver-a.
- Amel: Ign; Nat-c.

Emotions, from: Op.

Empty: Asar; Sec.

Epilepsy, before: Cup.

Expectorating, when: Carb-v; Sil; Tarn.

Food, thought of: Merc-cy.

Happy surprise, from: Kali-c.

Hawking agg: Arg-n; Nux-v.

Menses, during: Pul.

Stool, diarrhoea, during: *Arg-n*; Cup; Pod.

Swallowing empty, on: Grap.

Violent: Phyt.

Vomiting, after: Colch.

Warm drinks amel: Ther.

Yawns, then: Tell.

RETENTION sense, of: Tell.

RETICENT: See TACITURN.

RETINA

Anaemia: Lith.

Anaesthesia, looking at eclipse, from: Hep.

Detachment, of: *Aur-m*; Dig; *Gel*; Naph; Pho.

Embolism, central artery of: Op.

Exudation: Kali-m.

Haemorrhage: Arn; Both; Crot-h; Ham; *Lach*; Led; Pho.

Hyperaesthesia+: Ox-ac.

Images, retained, too long: Gel; *Jab*; *Lac-c*; Nat-m; TAB; Tub.

RETINA

Inflammation: Aur; Merc; Merc-c; Plb; Sul.
- Albuminuric: Gel; Merc-c; Pho+.
  - pregnancy, during: Kalm.
- Diabetic: Sec.
- Eyes, overuse from: Sul.
- Haemorrhagic: Merc-c.
- Pigmentary (retinitis pigmentosa): Nux-v; Pho.

Injuries: See Haemorrhage.

Oedema: Ap; Kali-io.

Thrombosis, degeneration: Ham; Pho.

RETINITIS: See RETINA, inflammation.

RETRACTION, drawn back:
Ast-r; Cic; Clem; Crot-t; *Cup*; Hyds; Lach; *Merc*; Nat-m; Nux-v; Op; Par; *Phyt*; PLB; Sars; Sil; Thu; *Zin*.

REVENGEFUL, spiteful:
Calc; Lach; Nat-m; Nit-ac; *Nux-v*.

REVERBERATIONS: See HEAD, noises in, and HEARING, illusory sounds.

REVERY: See DREAMINESS.

RHEUMATISM (See JOINTS):
Aco; Arn; Ars; *Bell*; Benz-ac; BRY; *Caus*; Cham; Chel; *Colch*; Fer-p; Form; Kali-io; Kalm; Led; *Lyc*; *Merc*; Med; *Phyt*; PUL; Rhod; RHUS-T; Sang; Sars; Stic; *Sul*; Thu.

Acute articular+: Tub.

Alternating
- With: Kali-bi; Lapp; Urt.
- Mental symptoms, with: Cimi.

RHEUMATISM, alternating
- Urinary affections, with: Benz-ac.

Asthma, with: Benz-ac.

Chronic
- Ankylosis, with: Kali-io.
- Rigidity, with: Ol-j.

Cold amel: Am-c; Guai; *Led*; *Pul*; *Sec*.

Diarrhoea
- With: Stro.
- After: Abro; Cimi; Dul; Kali-bi.

Dyspepsia, with: Nat-c.

Eruptions, with: Dul.

Gonorrhoea, checked, from: Thu.

Hives, with: Urt.

Hot weather, heat agg: COLCH; Kali-bi; Kali-s; Rhod.

Inability to move limbs: Abro.

Kidney affections, with: Radm; Terb.

Paralytic: Colch.

Recurrent: Nat-s; Senec.

Tonsilitis, after: Echi; Guai; Lach; Phyt.

RHUS POISON: Rhus-t.

RHYTHMIC: Agar; Lyc; Stram.

RIBS

Along: Ap.

Ball, round moving to and from, as if: Cup.

Below: Ap; Chin; Sul; Terb.
- Balls, round: Cup.

Dislocated, broken, as if: Agar; Caps; Kali-bi; Naj; Petr; Psor; Stram.

Exostosis: Merc-c.

RIBS

Fifth and sternum
- Right: Mag-c; Thu.
- Left: Ox-ac.

Floating: Benz-ac.
- Right: Berb.
  - undulating pain, along: Zin-io.
- Left: Ther.
  - aching, backward, along: Amy-n; Arg-n.

Last, left: Arg-n.
- Boil, near: Arg-m.

Lung, sticking to, as if: Kali-c.

Neuralgia, lower left: Arg-m.

Plug between: Anac; Aur; Caus; Cocl; *Lyc*; *Ran-sc*; *Ver-a*.

Sore: Carb-v.

Stepping agg: Rat.

Upwards, from: Ap.

RICKETS: *Calc*; *Calc-p*; Kali-io; Pho; Sil; Sul.

RIDICULED, is being+: Bar-c.

RIDING on horse back (See JARRING)

AGG: Ars; Bell; Bor; Bry; Grap; Lil-t; Mag-m; *Nat-m;* Rut; SEP; Sil; Spig; *Sul-ac*; Tab; Val.

AMEL: Bro; Calc; Lyc; Tarn.

Car, in agg and amel: See CAR SICKNESS.

RIGIDITY: See STIFFNESS.

RINGING NOISES: See HEARING, illusory sounds.

RINGWORM: See ERUPTIONS.

RISING

Arms, uses for: Hyds.

Efforts at: Aesc; Agar; Petr; Rut; Sul.

Sitting, seat from
- AGG: Aesc; Agar; Ant-t; Berb; BRY; Calc; *Caps*; *Caus*; *Con*; Kali-bi; Led; *Lyc*; *Nat-s*; Petr; PHO; *Pul*; *Rhus-t*; Rut; Sep; *Spig*; Stap; SUL.
- AMEL: Kob; Rut.
- Bed from amel: See BED.
- Body feels heavy, sore: Spig.

Stooping, from AGG: Lyc; *Pho*; Pul.

Then falling: See Directions, up and down.

Turns, to right, when: Kali-c.

RIVET FEELING: Lil-t; Sul.

ROAMING, roving: Lyss; Nux-v.

Aimless: Ver-a.

ROARING: See HEAD, noises in, and HEARING, illusory sounds.

ROBUST habit: Aco; Asaf; Bell; Caps.

Emaciating, suddenly: Samb.

ROCKING

AGG: *Bor*; Carb-v; Cocl; Thu.

AMEL: Carb-an; Cham; Cina; Kali-c; *Merc-c*; Pul; Pyro; Rhus-t; Sec.
- To and Fro: Bell; Hyo.

ROLLING, rools on the floor: Calc; Cic; *Op*; Paeon; Tarn.

Or turning over, as if: Am-c; Ars; BELL; Cact; Crot-h; Cup; Gel; *Grap*; Kali-c; LACH; Lyc; Pho; Pul; Rhus-t; Saba; SEP; Tarn.

Filth, in his own: Cam.

Side to side: Am-c; Ars; Lach; Tarn.

ROMANTIC: Cocl.
  Sensitive girls+: Cocl.
ROOM IN
  AGG: See AIR, open amel.
  AMEL: Chin; Cocl; Tarn.
  Close AGG: Amy-n; Just; Lil-t; Med; *Tub*; Vib.
  Full of people AGG: Arg-n; Lil-t; Lyc; Pho; Plb; Sep.
  Lights many with, AGG: Nux-v.
  Shut AGG: Arg-n; Lac-d.
  Too many things in AGG: Phys.
ROSEOLA: See under ERUPTIONS.
ROTATION AGG: Bry; Cocl; Colo; Kali-c.
ROUGH, scratchy, as of a rough body: Aesc; *Alu*; Amb; Am-m; Arg-n; *Berb*; Calc-f; Carb-v; Grap; Kali-bi; Mang; Naj; Nat-m; *Nux-v*; Par; Pho; *Phyt*; Rut; *Sul*.
RUBBING, stroking
  AGG: *Anac*; *Con*; *Old*; *Pul*; *Sep*; *Stro*; Sul.
  AMEL: *Calc*; *Canth*; Cina; *Cup*; Dros; Mag-p; Merc; Mos; NAT-C; Ol-an; Pall; PHO; PLB; Pod; Rhus-t; Rut; Sep; Sil; Tarn; Thu; Val; Zin; Zin-val.
  Abdomen amel: Nat-s; Pall; Pod.
  Clothes, of agg: Old.
  Gently
    • **AGG:** Mar-v.
      • **AMEL:** Crot-t; Form; Dios; Lil-t; Lyss; Med.
  Hand warm, with AMEL: Lil-t.

RUBBING
  Hard AMEL: Med; Radm.
  Soles AMEL: Chel.
  Together, as if: Cocl; Kali-bi; Sul.
RUBELLA: See under ERUPTIONS.
RUDE: See INSOLENT.
RUMBING: See ABDOMEN, and HEARING, illusory sounds, roaring.
RUNNING: See CREEPING, and MOTION, rapid.
  Backward: Bry.
  Better, than walking: Tarn.
  Forwards, when trying to walk: Mang.
  Impulse, for: Iod; Orig; Ver-a.
    • **Menses, before:** Lach.
  Recklessly, in room: Saba.
RUNS about (See ESCAPE): Hyo; Stram; Ver-a.
  Menses, before: Lach.
RUN ROUND: See FINGERS, felon.
RUPIA: See under ERUPTIONS.
RUSTY: See BROWNISH.
SACRUM and region: Aesc; Agar; Gel; Grap; Hep; Hypr; Mur-ac; Pul; Rhus-t; Sep.
  Breathing agg: Merc.
  Bruised: Aesc; Rut.
  Burning: Kre; Pho; Pod; Terb.
  Cold, icy, near: Arg-m; Benz-ac; Dul.
  Coughing agg: Bry; Chel; Tell.
  Crawling: Grap.
  Damp cloth, on: Sanic.

SACRUM

Dragging: Helo.
- Buttocks, to: Helo.

Exostoses: Rhus-t.
Feet, to: Kali-m; Kob.
Forceps delivery, after: Hypr.
Heavy, weight: Arg-n; Chin.
- Genitals, in, with: Lob.
- Sitting, while: Rhus-t.

Laughing agg: Tell.
Leucorrhoea
- Agg: Aesc; Psor.
- Amel: Murx.

Lying
- Agg: Berb.
- Amel: Agar.

Menses
- Before agg: Nux-m+; Sabi+; Spo.
- At start of agg: Asar.
- Instead, of: Spo.

Numb: Calc-p; Grap.
- Legs and: Calc-p; Grap.

Paralysed, as if: Pho.
Parturition, after: Hypr; Nux-v; Pho.
Piles, due to, pain in+: Abro.
Prickling: Mez.
Pulsating: Nat-m.
Riding in car agg: Nux-m.
Sensitive to touch of clothes: Lob.
Sitting
- Agg+: Rhod.
- Erect agg: Lyc.

Solid, as if: Sep.
Sprained, as if: Ol-an.
Standing, erect agg: Petr.

SACRUM

Stools pressing at, agg: Tell.
Stooping agg: Kali-bi.
Sweat, cold, on: Plant.
Thigh into
- Right: Colch; Tell.
- Left: Kali-c.

Touch, slight agg: Lob.
Urinating agg: Grap; Sul.
Uterine, disease from+: Sep.
Weak: Pho; Sep; Sil.
Wood, stretched across, as if: Nux-m.

SADNESS, low spirits, mental depression: Abro+; Aco; *Ars*; AUR; Calc; CARB-AN; Caus; Cham; *Chin*; *Cimi*; Colch; Gel; GRAP; Helo; IGN; Lod; Kali-br; Kali-io; *Kali-p*; Lac-c; Lac-d; *Lach*; Lept; Lil-t; *Lyc*; *Med*; Merc; Mill+; Murx; *Mur-ac*; NAT-C; NAT-M; *Nat-s*; NIT-AC; Plat; PSOR; PUL; *Rhus-t*; Sele; Sep; STAN; Sul; Syph; Tarx; Thu; Ver-a; Zin; Zin-p.

Causeless: Nat-m; Pho; Sars+; Stap; Tarn.
Children, in: Ars; Calc; Lach.
Climaxis, at: Manc.
Coition agg: Nat-m; Sep; Sul.
Company, society
- Agg: Euphr.
- Amel: Bov.

Continence agg: *Con.*
Domestic affairs, over: Sep.
Eating
- Agg: Grap; Nux-v.
- Amel: Tarn.

SADNESS

- **Elation, alternating with:** Cof; Senec.
- **Emission, from:** *Nux-v*; Pul.
- **Enjoys:** Ign; Nat-m.
- **Everything viewed, in sad light+:** Alu.
- **Fear, from:** Sec.
- **Flatulence, with+:** Scop.
- **Flowers, smell of, from:** Hyo.
- **Girls, before puberty:** Ars; Hell; Lach.
- **Grief, from+:** Nux-m.
- **Happy, on seeing others:** Cic; Helo.
- **Health, over one's:** Sep.
- **Horrid:** Syph.
- **Indifference, alternating with:** Sep.
- **Joy, alternating, with:** See Elation, alternating.
- **Light, subdued agg:** Nat-s.
- **Love, unhappy, from:** Dig.
- **Masturbation agg:** Con; Nat-m; *Pho-ac*; Plat.
- **Menses**
  - Before: Nat-m; Pul; Stan.
  - Suppressed: Con.
- **Music**
  - Agg: *Aco*; Dig; Nat-p; Nat-s; Sabi.
  - Distant agg: Lyc.
  - Sad amel: Mang.
- **Pain, from:** Sars.
- **Parturition, after:** Thu.
- **Perspiration, during:** Con.
- **Pregnancy, in:** Lach; Nat-m.

SADNESS

- **Puberty**
  - At: Ant-c; *Hell*; Manc; Nat-m.
  - Girls, before: Ars; Hell; Lach.
- **Sad stories, from:** *Cic*.
- **Sexual**
  - Erethism, with: Manc.
  - Loss of power, from: Spo.
- **Society:** See Company.
- **Sterility, from:** Aur.
- **Sunshine agg:** Stram.
- **Sympathy agg:** Con.
- **Thunderstorm amel:** Sep.
- **Trifles, about:** Dig; Grap.
- **Waking, on:** Alu; Coc-c; Lach.
- **Walking, only while:** Pho-ac.
- **Weep cannot:** Am-m; Gel; *Nat-m*.
- **Weeping amel:** Dig; Med; Pho.

SALIVA: Merc; Sul.

- **Acrid:** Aru-t; Kre; Merc; Merc-c; Merc-i-f; *Nit-ac*.
- **Bitter:** Ars; *Chel*.
- **Bloody:** Buf; Crot-c; Mag-c; Merc; NIT-AC; *Pho*; Rhus-t.
  - Menses, before: Nat-m.
  - Sleep, during: Rhus-t.
  - Taste
    - disgusting, with: Kali-io.
    - sweetish, with: Kali-io.
- **Blue:** Plb.
- **Cold:** Asar; Bor-ac; Cist.
- **Convulsions, with:** Bar-m; Kali-bi; *Oenan*.
- **Cottony:** See Frothy.
- **Dark:** Merc-d.
- **Diminised, scanty:** *Bell*; Kali-bi; Merc-c; Nux-v; Nux-v; Pho; Stram; Sul; *Ver-a*.

SALIVA

Dries on palate and lips, becomes tough: Lyc.
Egg, white of, like: Calad; Jab+.
Foul foetid: Iod; Lach; Manc; MERC; Merc-d; *Nit-ac*; Petr.
- Hot: Daph; Saba.

Frothy, cottony, foamy: Ap; Bell; *Berb*; Caul; Dul; *Ign*; Iod; Kali-m; Lach; *Nux-m*; Ol-an; Pho; Pho-ac; Pic-ac; *Pul*; Sabi; Spig.
Green: Grap; Sec.
Gushes, of: Carb-v; Ign; Nat-m.
- Suddenly: Ign; Nat-m.
- Colic, with: Led.

Increased (salivation): Am-c; Aru-t; Bar-c; Bor; *Dig*; *Dul*; Flu-ac; Ip; *Iris*; Kali-c; Lyss; *Manc*; MERC; Merc-c; Merc-i-r; Nat-m; *Nit-ac*; *Nux-v*; Pho; *Pul*; Ran-b; RHUS-T; Stram; VER-A.
- Accompaniment, as a: Lob.
- Colic, with: Led.
- Coryza, with: Kali-io.
- Cough, with: Am-m; Lach; Thu; Ver-a.
- Dark, putrid+: Merc-d.
- Dentition, during: Helo.
- Diarrhoea, with: Rhe.
- Diphtheria, during: Lac-c.
- Dryness, with: Calad; Lyc; *Merc*; Nat-m.
- Dyspnoea, with: Lob.
- Headache, with: Epiph; *Merc* Nat-s.
- Heat, all over, with: *Cic*.
- Hiccough, with: Lob.
- Hunger, wth: Lob.

SALIVA, increased

- Larynx, pressure on, as if, with: Tarx.
- Menses
  - before: Pul.
  - during: Merc; Nux-m; Phyt; Pul; Pulex+.
  - after: Cedr.
- Nausea, with: Lob.
- Nauseous, taste, with: Sul.
- Night, sweetish taste+: Cham.
- Pain, colic, etc. agg: Cocl; Epiph; Gran; Helo; Led; Mang; Merc; Pho; Plant; Rhe.
- Paralysis, in: Mang.
- Pregnancy, in: Ant-t; Cof; Helo; Kre; Lob; Zin-s.
- Retching, with: Lob.
- Sleep, during: *Bar-c*; Cup; Ign; Ip; Lac-c; Lach; MERC; Nit-ac; *Pho*; *Rhus-t*; Syph.
- Sneezing, with: Flu-ac.
- Spit, desire to+: Cocl.

Oily: Aesc; Cub.
Onion, odour of: Kali-io.
Pasty: Lach.
Ropy: Coc-c; *Iris*; Saba; Sul.
Salty: Ant-c; Cyc; Sanic; Ver-a.
- Water: Verb.

Soapy (See Frothy): Bry.
Sour: Con; *Ign*.
Sticky: Bell; *Kali-bi*; *Lach*; Plb.
Stooping, when: *Grap*.
Swallow, must: Ip; Merc.
Sweet: Canth; *Cham*; Iris; Pho; Plb; PUL.
- Disgustingly: Canth.

SALIVA, sweet
- Meals, after: All-s.

Talking, while: Iris; Lach; Mang.

Viscid, thick: Chel; *Cimi*; Dul; Glo; *Kali-bi*; *Lach*; Lyc; Lyss; Merc; Merc-c; Nux-m; Phys.
- A.M. in: Glo.
- Dribbles: Stram.

Watery: Cyc; Sul-ac.

Yellow: Gel; Manc; Merc; Merc-c; Phyt.
- Blood, as from: Gel.

SALIVARY GLANDS: Calc-f; Cham; Iod; Merc; Nit-ac+; Phyt; Pul.

SALIVATIOIN: See SALIVA, increased.

SALPINGITIS: See FALLOPIAN TUBES.

Serum or pus, escapes from uterus: Sil.

SALT AGG: See under FOOD.

SALTY, saltiness: *Ars*; Calc; Carb-v; Flu-ac; Grap; Iod; Kali-io; *Lyc*; MERC; Merc-c; Nat-c; Nat-m; *Pho*; *Pul*; Sanic; *Sele*; SEP; Tell.

SALVATION: See RELIGIOUS Ideas.

SAND as if: Ap; Ars; Berb; Bov; Cist; Coll; Thu.

SARCASM, satire: Ars; *Lach*.

SARCOCELE: *Aur*; Calc; Iod; Merc-i-r; Pul; Rhod; Spo.

Indolent: Tarn.

SARCOMA: See under CANCER, and FUNGUS GROWTH.

Cutis: Calc-p; Sil.

SATYRIASIS: See SEXUAL desire (males) increased.

SAWING, as if: Aesc; Bro; Hypr; Pho; Spig; Spo; Sul; Syph; Tarn.

SCABIES: See ERUPTIONS, itch like.

SCABS: See CRUSTS.

SCALDED: See BURNT, as if and BURNS.

SCALES: See DESQUAMATION.

SCALP: See under HEAD EXTERNAL.

SCAPULAE (and region): Chel; Chin; Dul; Kali-c; Kre; Merc; Rhus-t; *Sep*; Tell.

Right: Bry; *Chel*; Ol-an; Pod; Rum.

Left: Cimi; Zin-chr.

Between: Am-m; Ars; Calc; Calc-p; Caps; Helo; Nit-ac; Pho; Rhus-t; Sep.
- Aching: Carb-ac; Helo; Rhus-t; *Sep*; Sul.
  - breathing, impeding: Calc.
- Air, blowing, on: Caus; Hep.
- Broken, as if: Crot-c; Lil-t; *Mag-c*; Nat-m; Plat; Ver-a.
- Burning: *Ars*; *Lyc*; Med; *Pho*; Rob; Sul.
- Coldness: Ars; *Caps*; Caus; Nat-c; Pyro; *Sep*.
  - icy: Am-m; Lachn.
- Colic, with: Am-c.
- Cramps: Grat; Pho; Ver-a.
  - motion, during: Ip.
- Cutting: Canth; Nat-s; Zin.
- Epigastrium, to: Bry.
- Eructation amel: Zin.

SCAPULAE, between
- Fluttering: Cup.
- Heart, to: Bry; Sul.
- Heaviness: Calc; Chin; Gran; Lach; *Nux-v*; Rhus-t.
- Lump: Chin; Lyc; Mag-c; Nux-v; Rhus-t.
- Numb: Bry.
- Soreness: *Chin*; Cimi; Ham; Hypr; *Pho*; Sep.
  - spot, in (R): Berb; Chel.
- Sprain: Am-m.
- Stitches: Lac-c; Nit-ac; Petr.
- Swallowing agg: Kali-c; Rhus-t.
- Throbbing: Plant; Sul.
- Weakness: Agar; Alu; *Ap*; Bur-p; *Cocl*; Kali-io; *Nat-m*; Radm; Raph; Sars; Sul-ac.

Aching (R): Ol-an.
Adherent: Ran-b.
Boring, left: *Aur*; Dig; Hypr; Meny; Mez; Nat-c; *Pho-ac*; Rut; Spig.
Breathing agg: Am-m.
Bruised, right: Calend; Kali-c; Kre.
Bubbling, at: Lyc.
- Beneath+: Scil.

Burning: Bar-c; Echi; Med; Merc.
- Right: Lycps.
- Left: Med.

Crawling
- Right: Hep.
- Left: Med.

Cutting: Lac-c; Med; Spig.
- Edge, of: Ran-b.

Fingers, using agg: Ran-b.

SCAPULAE
Forward, from: Bar-c; Pho; Sul.
- Right: Merc.
- Left: Mez; Pho; Ran-b.
  - heart, to: Bry.

Itching, left: Caus.
Lump, left: Pru-sp.
Pressure amel: Ol-an.
Sore: Ham.
- Inner edge (L): Ran-b.

Throbbing, left: Mag-m.
Underneath: Calc; *Gel*; Merc; Myr.
- Right: Chel; Colo; Pod; Rum+.
  - hot, ache: Lycps.
- Left: Cratae; Gel.
  - burning: Echi.
  - buzzing: Kali-m.
- Bubbling: Scil.
- Chilly, cold: Cam.

SCARLATINA: See under ERUPTIONS.
SCARLET: Am-c; Bell; Croc; Merc.
SCARS: See CICATRICES.
Remaining after eruptions+: Kali-br.
Unsightly+: Carb-an.

SCIATICA: Ars; Bry; Buf; COLO; Dios; Grap; Ign; Iris; Kali-bi; Kali-io; Mag-p; *Nux-v*; RHUS-T; Rut; Sele; Sep; Sul; *Tell*; Zin.

Ascending: *Led*; Nux-v; Rut.
Atrophy, of parts, with: *Calc*; Caus; Ol-j; Plb.
Bed, turning in agg: Nat-s.
Blowing nose agg: Grap.
Boring: Lach.

SCIATICA

Brown, spots, wih: Sep.
Coughing
- Agg: *Caps*; Caus; Sep; *Tell.*
- Alternating, with: Stap.

Chronic: Ran-b.
Day, during amel: Rut.
Deep, pain: Kali-bi; Rut.
Descending: Am-m; Rut.
Feet, tender, with: Mag-p.
Flexing leg
- Amel: Ars; Gnap; Kali-bi; Kali-io; Val.
- Abdomen, on amel: Colo; Glo; Gnap.

Formication, with: Gnap.
Hang down, leg
- Agg: Val.
- Over sides of bed agg: Ver-a.

Heat
- Agg: Fer; Guai; *Led*; Merc; Visc.
- Amel: ARS; Lyc; *Mag-p*; Rhus-t.

Heels, localized, in: Sep.
Injury, after: Arn; Hypr.
Jarring agg: *Bell*; Nux-m; Tell.
Knees, to: Ind.
Laughing agg: Tell.
Limb, gives way with pain: Grat.
Lying
- Agg: Gnap; Kali-io; Nat-m; Rut; Tell.
- Amel: *Am-m*; Bry; Dios.
- Back of amel: Pho.
- Painful side on agg: See Pressure agg.
- Right side on amel: Pho.

Mental exertion agg: Mag-p.
Motion least agg, must lie still: Colo; Lach.
Move, must: Bry; Caus; Lyc; Mag-c; *Rhus-t*; Val; Zin-val.
Muscles, jerking with: Kali-c.
Numbness, with: Aco; Caus; Cham; Colo; Grap; Phyt; Rhus-t.
- Burning, with: Dios.

Otorrhoea, with: Visc.
Pain, all over the body, with: Petr.
Pregnancy amel: Sep.
Pressure agg: Kali-bi; Kali-c; *Kali-io*; *Lyc*; *Rhus-t.*
Shooting pain: Aco; *Colo*; Iris; Mag-c.
Sitting
- Agg: *Am-m*; Bell; Hypr; Ind; Lept; Lyc; Val.
- Chair, in amel: Gnap.
- Prolonged agg: Hypr.
- Rising, from agg: Nat-s.

Sneezing agg: Fer; Sep; Tell.
Spine, painful with: Petr.
Sprained agg: Tell.
Standing amel: Bell; Mag-p; Stap; Tell.
Stepping, agg: Gnap.
Stools, agg: Rhus-t.
Stooping agg: Tell.
Stretchng limbs, standing while agg: Val.
Sudden, soreness with: Sele.
Summer
- Agg: Xanth.
- Amel: Ign.

SCIATICA

Touch agg: CHIN; *Chin-s*; Cof; *Lach*; Plb; Visc.
Uncovering agg: *Mag-p*; SIL.
Urination amel: Tell.
Uterine: Bels; Fer; Gnap; Merc; *Pul*; Sep; Sul.
Vertebral origin: Nat-m; Sil.
Walk
- Amel: Val.
- Must: Ars; Sep; Sul.

Wetting, after: Dul; *Rhus-t.*
Winter agg: Ign.
Yawning agg: Zin.

SCIRRHUS: See under CANCER.
SCLERODERMA: Radm; Thyr.
SCLEROSIS: Aur; Aur-m; Bar-m; Plb.
Coronary: Aur.
Disseminated: Acet-ac; Arg-n; Ars; *Hyo-hydr.*
Multiple: Arg-n; Bar-m; Crot-h; Lathy; Plb; Tarn.

SCLEROTITIS: Ars; Merc-c; Spig; *Thu.*

SCOLDING: See ABUSIVE.
AGG: Agar; Stap; Tarn.
Angry, without being: Dul.
Herself: Merc.

SCOOPED OUT (cupped): Thu; Vario.

SCORBUTIC symptoms: Am-c; Carb-v; Kali-m; *Merc*; Mur-ac; *Nux-v*; Stap; Sul.

SCORCHED: See BURNT, as if.
SCORN: See CONTEMPTUOUS.
SCORPIONS sees: Op.

SCRAPED, as if: Bro; Dros; Nux-v; Pul; Sul; Ver-a.
SCRATCH, desire to: Arn.
SCRATCHES
Hands, with: Stram; Tarn.
Himself, raw: Aru-t; Psor.
Lime of the walls: Arn; Canth.

SCRATCHING
AGG: *Anac*; *Ars*; Asar; Caps; Grap; Kali-c; Lach; Old; PUL; RHUS-T; SUL.
AMEL: *Asaf*; *Calc*; *Cyc*; *Mur-ac*; *Nat-c*; *Pho*; Rut; *Sul.*

SCRAWNY: Calc-p; Nux-m; Rat; Sec.
SCREAMS: See CRIES
SCREWED together: Aeth; *Colo*; Elap; Naj; Onos; Ox-ac; Sars; Stro; Zin.

SCROFULA (psora of childhood): Bar-c; *Calc*; Calc-p; Cist; Hep; Iod; Lyc; *Merc*; *Sil*; Sul.
Erethistic: Calc-p; Psor; Tub.
Torpid: Calc; Sul.

SCROTUM: Arn; Crot-t; *Petr*; Rhus-t; Sul.
Blue: Ars; Mur-ac; Pul.
Bubbling: Stap.
Cold: Berb; Caps; Merc.
- Shrivelled, and+: Caps.

Elephantiasis: Sil.
Eruptions, on: Grap; Hep; Petr.
- Eczema: Alum; Crot-t; Pho-ac.

Excoriated: Ars; Hep; Polyg; Sil; Sul.
- Between, and thighs: Lyc; Merc; Nat-c; Petr.

Fistula: Spo.

SCROTUM
Heat, burning: Calc; Chel; Spo.
Indurated: *Rhus-t*; *Sul.*
Itching: Rhod.
- Perineum, and +: Sars.
- Spots: Sil.
- Voluptuous: Anac; Stap.

Moisture: Cinb; Petr; Rhod; Sul.
- Between, and thighs: Hep.
- Spots, on: Sil.

Nodules, hard, brown, on: Nit-ac; Syph.
Numb, knees, up to: Bar-c.
Oedema: Ap; Ars; Colch+; Flu-ac; Grap; Rhus-t.
Scaly: Calc.
Sensitive: Stap.
Shiny: Grap; Merc.
Spots: Sil.
Sweat+: Ign.
- Cold: Plant.
- Strong smelling+: Dios.
- Warm, profuse+: Gel.

Swelling: Rhus-t.
- Painless: Mez.

Thin: Pyro.
Wrinkled: Rhod.

SCURFS: See SKIN, scaly.
SCURVY: See SCORBUTIC symptoms.

SEA
AGG: *Ars*; Bro; Mag-m; Nat-m; Nat-s; *Rhus-t*; *Sep*; Syph.
Air AMEL: Bro; Med.
Bathing AMEL: Med.
SEARCHING on the floor: Ign; Plb; Stram.

SEASICKNESS: See CAR SICKNESS.
Feeling, of: Tab.
Nausea, without: Kali-p.

SEASONS
Autumn, summer etc: See different headings.
Change of: See CHANGE, Temperature.

SECRETIONS: See DISCHARGES.
SECRETIVE: Dig; *Ign*; Lyc; Nat-m.

SEDENTARY living
AGG: Alo; Asar; NUX-V; *Sul.*
Burning spots, from: Ran-b.

SEEING: See LOOKING.
Alive things: Cocl.
Faces: Amb; *Bell*; Calc; *Op*; Tarn.
- Mirror, in, except his own: Anac.

Imaginary objects: Med.
Others in misery AGG: Tarn.
Same person, in front and behind: Euphor.
Thinks, someone else is, for him: Alu.

SELF
Accusation: Hell; Op; Stram.
Angry, with: Ign.
Antagonism: See ANTAGONISM.
Centered: Senec.
Contempt: Agn; Aur.
Criticism: Aur.
Confidence, want of: *Anac*; Arg-n; Ars; *Lyc*; Old; Pic-ac; *Sil*; Ther.
Knows not, what to do, with her: Stan.

SELF

Loathing: Lac-c.
Odd, at: Anac; Bar-c; Cann.
Over estimation of: Cic.
Pity: Agar; Nit-ac.
Reproaches: See REPROACHES.
Torture: *Aco*; *Ars*; Bell; *Lil-t*; Plb; Tarn; Tub.
SELFISH: Agar; Ars; Pul; Senec; Sul; Tarn.

SEMEN

Bloody: Canth; Caus; Flu-ac; Merc; Led; Lyc; Petr; Pul; Sars.
Cold, coition during: Nat-m.
Dribbling: Calad; Pic-ac; Sele.
Hot: Agar; Calc; Tarn.
Odourless: Sele+; Sul.
Offensive: Thu.
- Pungent: Lach.
- Urine, stale like: Nat-p.

Thick: Sabal.
Watery: Led; Nat-p; Sele; Sul.

SEMINAL DISCHARGE

Difficult: Lach; Zin.
Failing, during coition: Calad; *Grap*; Lyc; Lyss; Psor.
Painful: Cann; Canth; Sabal; *Sul*.
- Cutting: Con.

Premature, too quick: Agar+; Agn; Calc; Carb-an; Chin; *Grap*; *Lyc*; Pho; Sele; ZIN.
- During coition, followed by roaring in head+: Carb-v.

SEMINAL EMISSION (nightly): Bar-c; Bor; Calc; *Chin*; *Con*; Dig; Dios; *Fer*; *Gel*; Kali-p; Lyc; Nat-c; Nat-m; Nat-p;

SEMINAL EMISSIONS .. Nux-v; PHO; PHO-AC; Plb; *Sele*; Sep; Stan; Stap; Sul.

Agg (See COITION agg and MASTURBATION agg): Kob.
AMEL: Calc-p; Lach; Zin.
Afternoon, sleep: Alo; Ther.
Atonic+: Dig.
Aware, wihout being: See Involuntary.
Caressing or frolicking with women, while: Arn; CON; Gel; *Pho*; Sars; Sele; Sul.
Coition, after: Am-c; *Nat-m*; Pho-ac.
Diarrhoea, during: Ars.
Dreams
- Lascivious+: Pho-ac.
- Urination of, after: Merc-i-f.
- Vivid, with: Vio-t.
- Without: Anac+; Arg-n; Dios; Guai+; Pic-ac.

Erection
- Feeble, with: Sele.
- Painful, then: Grat; Kali-c.
- Without: Dios; Gel; Grap; Kob.

Erotic: Scil.
Exertion, over, from: Fer.
Frequent: Nux-v; Pho-ac; Stap.
- Old man, in: Bar-c; Caus; Nat-c.

Involuntary: Dios; Ham; Nat-p; Sele; Sep.
Leaning the back against anything, on: Ant-c.
Night, every+: Ust.
Old symptoms agg: Alu.

SEMINAL EMISSIONS
Pain or colic, during: Plb.
Painful: Kali-c; Nat-c; Sabal.
Spasms, with: Art-v; Grat; *Nat-p*.
Stools
- Difficult, with: Petr.
- During: Sele; Vio-t.
- Straining, when: Ol-an.

Urination, after: Daph; Kali-c.
Vertigo, during: Sars.
Voluptuous: Vio-t.
- Thrill long after: Sele.

Women
- caressing when: See Caressing.
- In the presence of: *Nux-v*; Salix; *Ust*.

SEMINAL VESICLES: Merc; Pul.
SENILITY: See OLD AGE.
SENSES, SPECIAL
Acute: Aco; Ars; Asar; Bell; Cimi; *Cof*; Lyss; Nux-v; Op; Pho.
Blunt, dulled: Anac; Bell; *Calc*; Caus; Gel; Hell; Hyo; Laur; Lyc; Merc; *Nat-m*; Nit-ac; Nux-m; Pho; PUL; *Sil*; *Sul*.
Perverted: Arg-n; Op.
Vanishing
- As if (See FAINTING): Alu; Calc; Cann; Carb-an; *Cup*; *Plat*; Stram.
- Pains, from: Plb.

SENSITIVE (susceptible to noise, light, pain, odour, touch, trifles etc.): *Aco*; *Amb*; Arg-n; Arn; Ars; *Asaf*; Aur; BELL; Bor; *Cham*; CHIN; Chin-s; Cic; Coc-c; *Cof*; Colch; Croc; Cup; Fer; Gel;

SENSITIVE ..
Hep; Hyo; *Ign*; LACH; Lyc; Lyss; Mag-c; Mang; *Mar-v*; Med; Nat-m; *Nit-ac*; NUX-V; Paeon; *Pho*; *Plat*; Plb; Psor; Pul; Ran-b; Sep; *Sil*; Sul; Sul-io; Tarn; Tell; Terb; *Ther*; Tub; Val; Vip; *Zin*.
Diffused, around affected part: Kali-io.
Everything, to: Sul-io.
Morbidly: *Stap*.
What, others say about her, to: Stan; Stap.

SENSORIUM depressed: Bap; *Hell*; Pho-ac; Pyro; Rhus-t.
SENTIMENTAL (See DREAMINESS): *Ant-c*; *Ign*.
Diarrhoea, during: Ant-c.
Menses, before: Ant-c.
Twilight, in: Ant-c.

SEPERATED, as if (See DUALITY): Agar; Arg-n; Calc-p; Cocl; Daph; Dul; Hypr; *Psor*; Sabi; Sep; Stram+; Tril; Ver-a.
SEPSIS: See BLOOD SEPSIS.
Adynamic: Elap; Pyro.
SEPTICEMIA (See BLOOD SEPSIS): Ars; Carb-v; Crot-h; Lach; Pyro.
SERIOUSNESS, alternating with buffonery+: Sul-ac.
SEROUS MEMBRANE: Aco; Ap; Ars; BRY; CANTH; Colch+; *Hell*; Kali-c; Lyc; Ran-b; Seneg; Scil; Sil; Sul.
SEWING
AGG: See FINGERS working with.
AMEL: Lach; *Nat-m*.

SEXUAL

Affections, disturbances in general: Agn; Bar-c; Calc; CANTH; Chin; *Con*; Grap; *Lil-t*; LYC; *Nux-v*; PHO; Pho-ac; Pic-ac; Plat; Sele; *Stap*; Stram; Sul.

Desire (males)
- Abnormal, from agg: Lyss.
- Absent, in fleshy persons+: Kali-bi.
- Decreased, weak: Agn; Bar-c; CAUS; Grap; Kali-bi; Kali-br; *Lyc*; ONOS; *Pho-ac*; Sabal; Sil; Stap; Sul.
- Increased: Calc; Calc-p; Cam; Cann; CANTH; Carb-v; Con; Flu-ac; Lyc; Lyss; Mos; *Nux-v*; Onos; PHO; PIC-AC; PLAT; *Pul*; *Sil*; Stap; Stram; *Tub*; Zin.
  - emission after: Nat-m; Pho-ac.
  - erection, without: Am-c.
  - excessive, maniacal: PHO; *Stram*; Tarn; *Zin*.
  - old men, in: Flu-ac; Lyc; Sele.
  - paralysis, with: Sil.
  - physical weakness, with: Calad; Calc; Con; Grap; *Kali-c*; *Lyc*; Nat-m; *Pho*; Sele.
  - priapism, with: Nat-m; Sil.
- Perverted: Agn; Nux-v; Plat; Stap.
- Suppressing
  - ill effects from AGG: Ap; *Cam*; *Con*; Kali-br; Lyss; Pho; *Pul*.
  - AMEL: Calad.

SEXUAL

Enjoyment absent (males): Agar; Anac; Calad; Grap; Nat-m; Sep.
- Emission, during: Psor.

Erethism (children): Alo.
- Climaxis, at: Manc.
- Puberty, at: Manc.

Excitement
- Easy: Pho; Sumb; Zin.
- AGG: *Buf*; LIL-T; Plat; Sars; Senec; Tarn.
- Uneasy feeling in body, with: Ant-c.

Exhaustion, excess, after agg (See COITION agg): Calad; Con; Grap; Lil-t; *Lyc*; Nat-p; Nux-v; Onos; Pho; Pho-ac; Sec; Stap; Sul; Symp.

Female: See FEMALE

Minded: Sep; Stap.

Neurotics: Sabal.

Restlessness: Canth; Kali-br; Raph.

Thoughts: Grap; Pho; Plat; Stap.

Tough, mere agg: Con; Grat; Nat-c; Plat.

Urge, unsatisfied, futile: Stap.

SHADE in agg and amel: See TWILIGHT agg and amel.

SHAKING agg: See JARRING agg.

SHALLOW: See RESPIRATION and ULCERS.

SHAMELESS (See AMATIVE), **exposes the person:** *Hyo*; Pho; Phyt; Sec; Tarn.

SHAMS+: Op.

SHATTERED, flying into pieces, explosions, as if: Aeth; Ars;

SHATTERED ..
  Bell; Bry; Carb-an; *Cof*; Dig; Glo; *Mur-ac*; *Nit-ac*; *Nux-v*; PUL; RHUS-T; Sil; *Stan*; Stap; Sul; Ver-a.

SHAVING
  AGG: Caps; *Carb-an*; Cic; Ox-ac; Pho; Pho-ac; Plb; PUL; Radm.
  AMEL: Bro.

SHIFTING: See WANDERING.

SHINGLES: See ERUPTIONS, Zoster.

SHINING, shiny: See GLISTENING.
  Objects agg: See GLISTENING, objects agg.

SHIVERING: See SHUDDERING and CHILLY.
  Concomitant, as a: Saba.

SHOCKS (through body): Amb; Arg-m; *Ars*; Bell; Cic; Cocl; Colch; Cup; Kre; Lyc; Nux-v; Op; Pod; Ran-b; Sil; Stro; Thu; Val; *Ver-a*; Zin; Zin-chr.
  Electric like: Arg-m; Arg-n; Ars; Buf; Cimi; Mag-m; Nat-p; Radm; Ver-a; Ver-v.
  • AGG: Pho.
  • Sleep, during: Ant-t; Arg-n; Ars; Cup; Mag-m; Nat-m; Nat-p; Nux-m; Nux-v; Radm.
  • Wide awake, when: Mag-m; Nat-p.
  Injury, from: See Nervous and Traumatic.
  Mental (See also INJURIES): Aco; Ap; *Arn*; Mag-c; Nit-ac; Nux-m; Pho-ac; Pic-ac.

SHOCKS
  Nervous: Aco; Amb; *Arn*; Cam; Carb-v; Cof; Gel; Hyo; Hypr; *Ign*; Iod; Op; Ver-a.
  Pain, from: Arg-n; Cina; Lyc; Plat; Pod; Sul-ac.
  Painful: Zin-chr.
  Sleep, on going to: Arg-n; Ars.
  Sudden: Cic; Ign.
  Surgical: Aco; Cam; Carb-v; Stro; Ver-a.
  Touching anything: Alu.
  Traumatic: (See also INJURY and CONCUSSION) Aco; ARN; Cam; *Hypr*; *Lach*; Op; Ver-a.
  Violent: Stro.
  • Pain, as from: Plat.

SHOOTING: See PAIN, shooting.

SHORT, too, as if: Alu; *Am-m*; *Caus*; *Colo*; Dig; Dios; Grap; Guai; Lach; Merc; Mez; Nat-m; Nux-v; *Rhus-t*; *Sep*; Syph.

SHOULDERS (and region): Aco; Bry; Fer; Fer-p; Kali-c; Kalm; Mag-c; Phyt; Pul; Rhus-t; Sang.
  Right: Fer; Kali-m; Kalm; Phyt; *Sang*; Stic; Stro.
  Left: *Fer*; Fer-p; Led; Mag-c; Nux-m; Rum; Sul.
  • Neck, to: Spig.
  • Night agg: Pho.
  • Right, to: Lyc.
  Abducting arm agg: Chel.
  Alternating: Lyc.
  Ankylosis: Cup.
  Arm
  • behind him agg: *Fer*; Rhus-t; Sanic.
  • Hanging, down amel: Pho.

SHOULDERS, arm

Chest, to: Fer-p.
Chill, between+: Tub.
Chilliness: Lept.
Cold: Caus; Kali-bi; Kre; Vio-o.
Constriction: Cact.
Contraction: Mag-c.
Cough agg: Dig; Fer; Lach.
- **Right:** Pyro.
- **Left:** Rum.

Cramp: Naj.
Emaciation: Plb.
Fingers, along, with: Fago; Flu-ac.
Fluttering, between: Cup.
Heaviness: Anac; Chin; Lach; Pho; Pul; *Rhus-t*; Stap; Sul.
- **Right, under:** Kali-m.

Higher, as if, left: Hell; Merc.
Joint: Calc; *Fer*; *Fer-p*; Ign; Kali-c; Nat-m; Pul; Rhus-t; *Sang*; Sep; Stap; Sul.
- **Cracking, in:** Calc; Cic; Croc; Kali-c.

Lump, between: Mag-s.
Menses agg: Mag-c.
Night agg: Flu-ac; Sang; Ust.
Numb, fingertips, to: Ox-ac.
Pulsation: Led.
Raising arm
- **Agg:** Led; Phyt; Rum; Sang; Sanic.
- **Amel:** Pho-ac.

Sensitive: Ap.
Shrugging agg: Calc.
Singing agg: Stan.
Sprained, as if: Alu; Rhus-t.

SHOULDERS

Stiff: Calc-s; Rhus-t.
Swelling: Colo.
Talking agg: Pyro.
Uneasy: Ascl.
Wind blowing on, as if: Lyc.
Wrist, to: Fer-p.

SHRIEKING: See CRIES.

Help, for: Plat.

SHUDDERING (nervous): *Aco*; Am-m; ARN; Ars; Bell; Cham; *Cimi*; Cina; Cocl; Dios; Gel; Glo; Hell; *Hypr*; *Ign*; Led; Mez; Mos; Nat-m; NUX-V; Phys; Pul; Ran-b; Rhe; Rhus-t; Sep; Sil; Spig; Thu; Zin.

Affected, part, of: Ars.
Air, cold, from: Mos.
Coition, after: Kali-c.
Contradiction, from: Elap.
Deformed persons, on seeing: Benz-ac.
Disagreeable things, thinking on: Benz-ac; Pho.
Draft agg: Phys.
Drinking, when: Caps.
Emotions agg: Asar.
Eructations, with: Dul.
Flower, smell, from: Lac-c.
Internal: Canc-fl.
Menses, before: Sep.
Pain
- **After:** Glo.
- **From:** Ars; Bar-c; Caps; Dios; Ign; Mez; Ran-b; Sep.

Part touched: Spig.
Sleep, falling to, on: Tub.
Stools, after: Canth; Rhe.

SHUDDERING
Urination
- Desire, with: Hypr.
- During: Stram.
- Urging for, when not attended: Sep.

Vomiting, with: Dul.
Yawning, when: *Cina*; Old.

SHUT PLACES AGG: See FEAR, narrow or shut places.

SHY, timid, mild (See ANTHROPOPHOBIA): Alu+; Bar-c; Bor; Calc; Calc-s; Coca; Cocl; Con; Crot-h; Gel; Grap; *Kali-c*; Kali-p; Lyc; Nat-c; Petr; Pho; Plb; PUL; Sep; Sil; Sul.

SICK
Feeling: See ILL feeling.
Says he is not: See NOTHING ails him.
Suddenly: Con.

SICKLY: See DELICATE.

SIDE: See DIRECTIONS, and PAIN, goes to side lain on.
Stitches: Abro; Aco; Bry; Pul; Ran-b; Sang; Sul.
- Right: Chel; Kali-c; Nat-s.

SIGHS, groans, takes deep breath (See also RESPIRATION wants deep; sighing): Apoc; Arg-n; Calc-p; *Cimi*; IGN.
Involuntary: Calc-p+; Hell.
Leucorrhoea, during: Phys.
Menses, before: *Ign*; Lyc.
Sweat, with: *Bry.*

SILENT: See TACITURN.
SILLY: See CHILDISH.

SINGING, sings: Cic; Cocl; Fer-p; Hyo; Mar-v; Sang; *Spo*; STRAM.
AGG: Arg-m; Aru-t; Carb-v; Dros; Fer-p; Hep; *Nux-v*; PHO; Sang; Sele; Stan; Verb.
Menses, during: Stram.
Sleep, during: Bell; Croc; Pho-ac; Sil.

SINGLE parts, effects: Agar; Alu; Bar-c; Caus; Con; Dul; Kali-c; Ol-an; Plb; Rhod; Sec; Sul-io; Val.
Turn white and insensible: Sul-io.

SINKING
Down: See PROLAPSE.
Hollow feeling: See Empty.
Sensation: Alu; *Bry*; Chin-s; Cup; Dul; *Glo*; Hell; Hyd-ac; Kali-c; *Lach*; Laur; Lyc; Nat-m; *Pho*; Rhus-t; Tab; Ver-a; Xanth.
Through floor: Benz; Hyo; Pho.
Unconscious: Glo; Hyd-ac.

SINUS
Affections, of: See NOSE, sinuses.
Painful to inhaled air+: Syph.

SIT
Aversion to: Iod; Lach.
Inclination, to: *Ars*; Caps; *Carb-v*; CHIN; *Cocl*; CON; GRAP; *Guai*; Lil-t; Merc; *Nat-m*; NUX-V; PHO; *Pul*; *Scil*; Stan.

SITS
Bed, in
- Suddenly, and lies down: *Hyo.*
- Will not lie down: Kali-br.

SITS

Bent forward, straightens with difficulty: Lathy.
Breaks, pins and sticks: Bell; Calc.
Elbows and knees, on: Lob.
Hands, supporting the body, with: Berb; Sul.
Legs crossed, cannot uncross: Bell; Ther.
Meditating: Calc-s.
- **Misfortunes, imaginary over:** Calc-s; Lil-t.

Mops, sadness with: Cimi; Psor; Pul.
Quite stiff: Cham; Hyo; Kali-m; Sep; Stram.
- **For a long time:** Nat-p.

Silently+: Flu-ac.
Speechless, in a corner+: Hep.
Still: Bro; Cocl; Flu-ac; Gel; Hell; Hep; Plat; *Pul*; Sep; Ver-a.
- **As if wrapped in deep and sad thoughts:** Cocl; Plat; *Pul*; Ver-a.
- **Ground, looking at:** Stram.
- **Moody silence, in:** Mag-p.
- **Thinks about little affairs:** Calc.

Thought, in as if+: Arn.
Weeping: Amb.
With knees drawn up, resting her head and arms on knees: ARS.

SITTING

AGG: *Agar*; Am-m; Ap; Ars; Asaf; CAPS; CON; CYC; DUL; EUPHOR; Fer; Kob; Laur; LYC; Mag-m; Mur-ac; *Nux-v*; Pho; PLAT; PUL; *Rhus-t*; *Rut*; *Sep*; *Sul*; Tarx; *Val*; VERB; Vio-t; ZIN.
AMEL: BRY; Cocl; COLCH; Cup; Hyo; *Nux-v*; Scil; Sep.

Bent
- **AGG:** Ran-b.
- **AMEL:** Lach.

Chair, low agg: Syph.
Crooked AMEL: Sul.
Down on first
- **AGG:** *Am-m*; Ant-t; *Spig*.
- **AMEL:** *Caps*; *Con*.

Elbows, knees, on AMEL: Kali-c.
Erect
- **AGG:** *Kali-c*; Nat-m; Sul.
- **AMEL:** ANT-T; Ap; Aral; Ars; Bell; Con; DIG; Gel; *Hyo*; Kali-bi; Kali-n; Nat-m; *Nat-s*; Pho; Pul.
- **Hand, folded across chest, with:** Ox-ac.

Supports weight on hands, with: Sul.
Up in bed amel: *Kali-c*; Samb.
Wet surface, moist floor etc. Agg: See LYING, wet surface.
SIZE: See PROPORTION, disturbed.

SKIN

Affections in general: Ap; Amb; ARS; Bell; Bry; Calc; Caus; Grap; Hep; *Lach*; *Lyc*; MERC; Mez+; Nit-ac; Petr; Pho; Pul; Ran-b; Ran-sc; RHUS-T; Saba; Sars; Sep; Sil; SUL; Thu; Thyr; Ust; Vio-o; Vio-t.

SKIN

Alternating, with: Ant-c; Ars; Calad; Grap; Hep; Stap; Sul.
- Digestive symptoms, with: Grap.
- Internal symptoms, with: Ars; Crot-t; Rhus-t.
- Joint pains, with: Stap.

Biting: *Euphr*; *Led*; *Pul*; Syph.
- Scratching, after: Lach; Old.

Black and blue spots: See ECCHYMOSES.

Bleeds, scratching, on: Aru-t; Lyc; Psor.

Bluish: See BLUISH
- Eruptions, after: Abro.

Branny (See DESQUAMATION): Calc-p; Sanic; Thyr.

Brownish: See BROWNISH.

Bubbling: Calc.

Burning, heat (See BURNING): ACO; Ap; ARS; BELL; Bry; Flu-ac; Kali-bi; *Lach*; Lyc; Pho; *Radm*; Rhus-t; Sil; *Sul*; *Terb*; Ust.
- Coldness, with: Ver-v.
- Fever, without: Grap; Lach.
- Mustard, plaster, like: Kali-c.
- Sparks, as from: Calc-p; *Sec*.
- Spots: Pho-ac; Sul.
- Touch, on: Canth; Fer.

Burnt, scorched, as if (See BURNT, scalded): *Ars*; *Canth*; Ran-b; Ver-a; Ver-v.

Chaffed, easily: Old; Rut.

Clammy: Aeth; Pho.

Cold (See COLDNESS): Cam; Carb-v; Kali-chl; Kali-n; Latro; Med; Mos; Sec; Tab; *Ver-a*.

SKIN, cold

- Agg: Agar; *Hep*; Lac-d; Petr; *Psor*; *Rhus-t*.
- Bathing agg: *Ant-c*; Thu.
- Dry, and: Cam; Nux-m.
- Icy: See Coldness, Icy.

Contracted: Rhus-t.

Cracks: See CRACKS.
- Deep, bloody: Nit-ac; Petr.
- Itching: Petr.
- New skin cracks and burns: Sars.
- Painful: Grap.
- Washing, after: Calc; Sep; Sul.
- Winter in: Calc; Carb-s; Petr; Sep; Sul.
- Yellow: Merc.

Dirty colour: *Ars*; Fer; Fer-pic; Merc; Petr; Pho; *Psor*; Sec; Sul.

Dry (See DRYNESS): *Ars+*; *Cam*; Diph; Flu-ac; GRAP; Iod; Kali-c; *Lyc*; Nat-c; *Nat-m*; Nit-ac; *Plb*; Rhus-t; Sang; Sec; Thyr; *Tub*; Vio-o.
- Cracking, as if: Murx.
- Hot: Ust.
- Jaundice, in: Sang.
- Sweat, gushing, alternating with: Ap.

Dusky: Ars-io; Calc-p; Merc.

Edges: Grap; Hep; Nat-p; Nit-ac; Petr; Psor; *Sul*.
- Itching: Amb; Caus; Petr.

Excoriated, denuded, raw: *Arn*; ARU-T; *Aur*; Bar-c; Calc; Calc-s; *Carb-v*; CHAM; *Chin*; GRAP; *Hep*; IGN; LYC; *Merc*; Nit-ac; *Petr*; *Psor*; PUL; Rhus-t; *Sep*; Sul.

SKIN

SKIN, excoriated
- Scratching, after: Grap; Petr.

Exhalation, foul (See SWEAT offensive): Stram.

Filthy: Psor; Sul.

Flabby: Abro; Calc; Ver-a.

Folds, flexures: Ars; Calc; Carb-v; GRAP; Hep; Lyc; Merc; *Nat-m*; Ol-an; *Petr*; PSOR; Pul; Sele; Sep; Sil; Sul.
- Cracked: Mang.
- Pimples, at: Cup.
- Rough: Mang.
- Soreness+: Caus.

Formication (See FORMICATION): Lyc; Pho-ac; Rhod; Rhus-t; Sec; Sul; Tarn.
- Between flesh, and: Cadm; Pho; Sec; Zin.
- Paralysed parts, in: Cadm; Pho.

Fragile: Petr.

Friction
- Clothes, of agg: Bad; Old.
- Constant agg: Sep.
- Slight agg: Sul; Vinc.

Frozen, as if+: Agar.

Hairy: See HAIR, body over.

Hard: *Ant-t*; Calc-f; Cist; Clem; Dul; Grap; Petr; Pho; *Rhus-t*; Sars; *Sep*; Sil.

Heal won't, vulnerable, suppurates, unhealthy (See HEALING DIFFICULT): Ant-c; *Arn*; *Ars*; Bor; Calc; Calc-s; *Cham*; Con; Grap; *Hep*; Kali-bi; *Lach*; Lyc; Merc; Mez; Petr; *Sil*; *Sul*; Thu.
- Joints, around: Mang.

Hide bound, as if: Crot-t.

SKIN

Inactive: *Anac*; CON; *Kali-c*; Kali-p; *Lyc*; *Pho-ac*.

Indented: Ap; Ars; *Bov*; Caps; Pho; Ver-a.

Inelastic: Bov; Cup; Rhus-t.

Inflamed: *Cham*; *Hep*; Merc; Petr; Pul; Rhus-t; *Sep*; *Sil*; Sul.
- Malignant, with oedema: Como.

Injury, slight agg: Alu.

Irritable: Radm.

Jumping out, as if: Thu.

Loose: Carb-an; Pho.
- Torn, bones from, as if: Ol-an.

Menses agg: Bor; Calc-p; Carb-v; *Dul*; *Grap*; Kali-c; Kali-m; Mag-m; *Nat-m*; Sang; Sars; Sep; Stram; Ver-a.
- Scanty agg: Con.

Moist: Carb-v; *Grap*; Lach; *Lyc*; *Rhus-t*.

Moon, full and new+: *Alu*.

Mottled (See MOTTLED): Ail; Lach; Pul; Sars; Sul; Syph; Thu.

Nodes, on (See NODES): Con; Iod; Pho; Sep.
- Hard: Kali-io; Nat-s; Sil.
- Under: Alu; Kali-ar; Mag-c.

Numb, insensible (See NUMBNESS): *Anac*; Arg-n; Con; Nux-v; Old; Sec.
- Scratching, after: Old.
- Spots, in: Buf.

Oily (See GREASY): Psor+; Thu.

Oozing: *Calc*; *Grap*; *Lyc*; *Merc*; *Petr*; *Sul*.

SKIN

Painful: See SENSITIVE.
- Cold, to: Agar; Aur; Plb; Rhus-t.
- Pressure amel: Ign.
- Scratching, after: Bar-c; Sil; Sul.

Parchment like: *Ars*; Calc-f; Lyc; Petr; Sil.
- Dry: Saba.

Peeling off (See DESQUAMATION): Elap; Thyr; Vip.
- As if: Agar; Bar-c; Lach; Pho; Pho-ac; Phyt; Rhus-t; *Sul*.

Pinch, remains raised: Caps.

Pressure, slight agg: Sul.

Prickling, tingling (See PAIN, prickling): Ham; Kali-c; Lob.

Prurigo: See ITCHING.

Puffed, bloated: Ant-c; *Ap*; Calc; Caps; Cup; Fer; Syph.

Quivering, twitching: Mang; Pho; Sec; Tab.

Rough, ragged: Ars; Bell; *Calc*; Calend; Flu-ac; *Grap*; Iod; Nit-ac; *Petr*; Phyt; Psor; Saba; *Sep*; *Sul*; Tub.
- Knots, small, as from: Hypr.

Scaly, scurfy (See DESQUAMATION): *Ars*; Calc; Dul; Kali-m; Kre; Lyc; Manc; Med; Nat-c; Nit-ac; Pho; Rhus-t; Sep; *Sil*; *Sul*; Thyr.

Scorched, as if: See Burnt.

Sensitive: Ars; Asaf; Bell; Calc; Carb-v; Chin; Coc-c; *Cup*; *Hep*; Kali-c; *Lach*; *Merc*; Mang; *Nit-ac*; *Nux-v*; Nat-m; Old; *Pho-ac*; Plant; Rut; Sil; *Sul*; Tub; Ver-a.
- Spots, in: Fer; Hep.

SKIN

Shiny: Ap; Bell.

Shrivelled: See Withered.

Soft, boggy: Ars; Caps; Kali-c; Lach; Sil; Thu.

Soggy: See Withered.

Sore: See Sensitive and BED sores.
- Feeling: Cimi; Eup-p; Hep; Merc; Sep; Zin.

Spots
- Blue, brown etc: See under BLUISH, BROWNISH.
- Every tint of: Crot-h.
- Itching: See Itching.
- Pigmented: Iod; Lyc; Sep.
- Pink+: Colch.
- White: See LEUCODERMA, and WHITE.

Sticky: Pho.

Stiff: Kalm; *Rhus-t*; Ver-a.

Stinging (See PAIN, stinging): Asaf; Ham; Stap; Ther; Thu; Urt.

Stripes, streaks, on: *Bell*; Buf; Carb-v; Cep; *Hep*; Merc; Myg; *Pho*; Sabi; Sil.

Strophulus (dentition during): Bor; Cham; Merc; Sul.

Swelled: Syph.

Swelling, on (See NODES): Ant-c; Arg-m; Ars; Bar-c; Grap; Thu.

Swollen, as if: Bell; Pul; Rhus-t.

Tanned: Tub.

Tense: Cact; Caus; Meny; Nit-ac; *Pho*; Stro.

Thick: Ant-c; Cast-eq; Cist; Dul; *Grap*; Hydroc; Petr; Radm;

SKIN, thick ..
   Rhus-t; *Sep*; Sil; Sul.
   • Purple: Sep.
   • Scratching, after: Rhus-t.
   Under: Aco; Aesc; Agar; Alu; Bell; *Bro*; Cic; Coca; Euphor; Lach; Pho; *Sec*; Thu; *Zin*.
   • Crawling, like a bug or worm: Calc; Cocaine; Oenan; Stram; Vario.
   • Clothes, touch agg: Oenan.
   • Heat: Terb.
   • Nodules, small: Kali-ar.
   • Thin cord, as if: Euphor.
   • Worm, moves away, when touched+: Coca.
Urinary affections, with: Vio-t.
Washing, bathing agg: Ars; *Sul.*
Wind agg (See WIND agg): Psor.
Wine coloured: Sep.
Winter agg: Alu.
Withered, shrivelled: Abro; Ars; Bor; *Calc*; *Chin*; *Cocl*; Cup; *Iod*; Lyc; Phyt+; Rum; *Sec*; Sil; *Ver-a.*
Worms: Ars; Coca; Merc; Nat-c; Nit-ac; Sele; Sil; Sul.
Wrinkled: *Calc*; Cam; Pho-ac; Sars; *Sec*; Sep; Ver-a.
Yellow (See YELLOWNESS): *Merc.*

SKULL: See under HEAD EXTERNAL.

SLEEP
   Afternoon AGG: Bry; Lach; Pul; *Stap*; Sul.
   Before AGG: *Ars*; BRY; CALC; Carb-v; *Lyc*; *Merc*; *Pho*; Pul; *Rhus-t*; Sep; Sul.

SLEEP
   During AGG: *Aco*; Arn; *Ars*; Bell; Bor; Bry; Cham; Cina; Con; Hep; Hyo; LACH; Merc; Op; *Pul*; *Sil*; *Stram*; *Sul*; Zin.
   Falling to, or first
   • AGG: Aral; Ars; Bell; *Bry*; Carb-v; Crot-h; *Grind*; Kali-c; LACH; Op; Pul; Samb; *Sep*; Sul.
   • AMEL: Merc.
   • Waking or both AGG: Stan.
   Half asleep, when
   • AGG: Cam; Nic-ac; Saba; Val.
   • AMEL: Sele.
   AMEL, loss of AGG: Ars; Calad; Carb-v; Cimi; *Cocl*; Cof; Colch; Cup; Kali-p; Lac-d; Laur; Med; Merc; Myg; Nit-ac; *Nux-v*; Pall; PHO; Pul; Sang; Sele; Sep; Zin
   After waking from agg: See AWAKENING after agg.
   Anxious: Aco; Ars.
   Broken: See Unrefreshing.
   Cannot fall to: Laur; *Pho.*
   • Unless legs are crossed+: Rhod.
   Cat naps, in: See AWAKES, frequently.
   Chattering, during: Pul.
   Comatose, deep: Aeth; *Ant-t*; Arg-n; Arn; *Bap*; Bell; Chin; Con; *Croc*; Grap; *Hell*; Kre; *Nux-m*; *Nux-v*; OP; *Pul*; VER-A.
   • Chill, violent, during: Op.
   • Menses, during: *Nux-m*; Pho.
   • Old people in: Op.
   • Snoring, with (Children): Chin.

SLEEP — SLEEPINESS

SLEEP, comatose
- Spasms, during: Op.
- Vomiting, after: Aeth.
- Yawning, with: Cimi.

Eyes
- Half-open+: Ip.
- Open, with: Cadm.

Jerks, starts, on falling to: Aco; Ars; *Bell*; Bor; Bry+; Calc; Cham; Cina; Ign; Kali-c; *Lyc*; Nit-ac; Op; *Pul*; Sep; Sil; Stram; Zin.
- Air, wanting, as if from: Calc-s.
- During: Carb-v; Dig; Hell; Hyo; Kali-c; Op; Rhe.
- Fear, with: Sabal.

Laughs and weeps+: Lyc.

Light, hears every sound: Aco; Alu; Alum+; Am-c; Ars; Cof; Ign; Lach; Merc; Op; Pho; Sele; Sul.

Little, enough: Rhe.

Pains, during: *Ars*; Aur; Bell; Carb-an; Cham; Grap; Lyc; Merc; *Nit-ac*; Nux-m; Rhus-t; Sul; Sul-ac; Til.
- Abdomen, in: Ant-t.
- After: Phyt.

Restless, tossing about: Aco; *Ars*; *Bar-c*; BELL; Carb-an+; *Chin*; Cina; Cocl; Cup; Grap; Lyc; Op; *Pul*; RHUS-T; SIL; *Sul.*
- Heat of body, from: Bar-c; Mag-m+.
- Sexual thoughts, from: Aur+; Canth; Kali-br; Raph.
- Shocks, from+: Mag-m.
- Voluptous dreams, from+: Bism.

SLEEP, restless
- Whining and Crying+: Rhe.

Roused from AGG: Spo.

Short
- AGG: Aral.
- AMEL: Calad; Flu-ac; Kali-bi; Meph; Nux-v; Pho-ac.
- Seems too long but amel: Med.

Side, not lain on, as if: Flu-ac.

Sobs, during+: Aur; Hyo; Nat-m.

Starting, up: See Jerks.

Stupid: See Sleep, Comatose.

Talks+: Carb-an.

Unrepreshing, awakes tired: Bry; Chin; Con; Hep; *Lach*; *Mag-c*; Mag-m; Nit-ac; Op; Pho; Rhus-t; Sul; Zin.
- Though sound: Pic-ac.

Walking, in: See SOMNAMBULISM.

SLEEPINESS (by day): Aeth; Am-c+; *Ant-c*; ANT-T; Ap; Ars; *Bap*; Bell; Calc; Carb-v; Caus; *Chel*; Chin; Clem; *Croc*; *Fer-p*; *Gel*; Grap; Lach; Lept; Merc-c; Mos; NUX-M; NUX-V; OP; Pho; *Pho-ac*; Pic-ac; Pod; *Pul*; *Sul*; *Terb*; Thu.

Accompanied, by: Ant-t; Nux-m; Pul.

Afternoon: Chin; Nux-v; Rhus-t; *Sul.*

Caused by other complaints: Ant-t; Nux-m; Op; Rhus-t; Ver-a.

Coition, during: Bar-c; *Lyc.*

Consciousness, losing, as if with: Phys.

SLEEPINESS

Coughing
- With: *Ant-t*; Ip; Kre.
- After: Anac; *Ign*.

Eating, on: Agar; Calc; Caps; Chin; *Kali-c*; Nux-v; Pho; Rhus-t; *Sul*.

Exertion
- Agg: Ars; Bar-c; *Nux-m*; Sele.
- Mental agg: Ars; Gel; Hyo; Kali-c; Nux-m; Pho-ac; Saba; Sele.

Evening: Amb; Am-m; Ars; *Calc*; Calc-s; *Kali-c*; NUX-V; Pul.

Fever
- During: Ant-t; Calad; Eup-p; Gel; Lach; Lyc; Mez; *Nat-m*; Pho; Pho-ac; Pod; Samb.
- Paroxysms after: Pod.
- Septic: Stram.

Forenoon: Ant-t; Saba.

Intoxicated, as if: Led; *Nux-m*.

Laughing, after: Pho.

Lying, left side, on: Thu.

Menses
- During: Kali-c; Mag-c; *Nux-m*; Pho; Sul.
- Absent, with: Senec.

Migraine, then: Sul.

Morning: Calc; Calc-p; Con; Grap; Nux-v; Sep; Sul.

Morose, and +: Cyc.

Occupation, literary amel: Croc.

Overpowering: Nux-m; Op; Phys.

Pains
- During: See under SLEEP.
- After: Phyt.

SLEEPINESS

Parturition, after: Phel.

Pneumonia, in: *Ant-t*; Chel; Op; Pho.

Pregnancy, during: Helo; Nux-m.

Reading, while: Bro; Colch.

Sewing, while: Fer.

Sitting, while: Fer; Nat-p; Nux-v.
- Sleepless, lying when: Cham.

Sleepless, at night: Fer; Mag-c; Mos; Op; Pho-ac; Pul; Rhus-t; Sul.

Standing, at work while: Phel.

Stool, after: Aeth; Nux-m; Sul.

Student, in: Fer; *Gel*; Mag-p.

Sudden: Rum.

Sweat, with: Rhus-t.

Talking, speaking while: Chel; Mag-c; Plb.

Twilight: *Am-m*.

Urine, retention, with: Terb.

Vomiting, after: Aeth; Ant-t; *Ip*; Sanic.

Writing while: Pho-ac.

SLEEPING SICKNESS: Ars; *Atoxy*; Gel; Nux-m; Op.

SLEEPLESSNESS (insomnia):
Aco; Anac; Arg-n; ARS; *Bell*; Bels; Bry; Cact; *Calc*; *Cham*; Chin; Cocl; COF; Hep; HYO; *Kali-c*; *Lach*; *Merc*; Merc-c; Mos; NUX-V; *Op*; Ox-ac; *Pho*; Plb; PUL; *Rhus-t*; Senec; *Sep*; *Sil*; Stan; Stap; SUL; Syph; Thu; Zin-val.

SLEEPLESSNESS
Aching
- Body, from: *Stap.*
- Bones, from: Daph.

Alternate, night: Anac; Lach.

Although sleepy: Ap; *Bell*; Cham; Chel; Hep; Op; Pho; Pul; Sep.

Caused by: Ars; Bry; Calc; *Cham*; Chin; Cof; Merc; Pho; Pul; Rhus-t; Sep.
- Horrible dreams+: Adon.
- Nervous excitement: Scut.
- Rambling thoughts+: Adon.

Conversation, after: *Amb.*

Drugs and liquor habitues: Sec.

Drunkards: Lach; Nux-v; Op.

Exhaustion agg: Avena; Chlo-hyd; Coca; Cocl; COF.

Eyes won't stay shut: Pho.

Grief, from: Ign; Kali-br; *Nat-m.*

Hearing, acute, from+: Op.

Heart symptoms, from: Cratae; Tab.

Homesickness, from: *Caps.*

Ideas, fixed, from: Calc; Grap; Pul.

Lasting several nights: Anac.

Lying on left side: Card-m; Thu.

Menses, during: Agar; Senec.

Midnight
- Before (Sleeps after): Amb; *Ars*; *Bry*; *Calc*; Calc-p; *Carb-v*; *Chin*; Cof; Con; *Grap*; Kali-c; Lyc; Mag-m; *Merc*; Nat-c; *Nux-v*; *Pho*; Pic-ac; PUL; *Rhus-t*; *Sep*; Sil; Sul.

SLEEPLESSNESS, midnight
- After (Sleeps before): Ars; *Caps*; *Cof*; Hep; *Kali-c*; NUX-V; Pho-ac; SIL.
  - 1 A.M.: Bels; Mag-c; Nux-v; Sep.

Nervous excitement, from: Aco; Calc; Chin; COF; Gel; Hyo; Lach; Lyc; Mar-v; Mos; *Nux-v*; *Plat*; Stic.

Neuritis, multiple, from: Con.

Nicotinism, chronic, from: Plant.

Old age: Bar-c.

Once awakening, on: Ars; Lach; *Nat-m*; *Nux-v*; Sil.

Operation, surgical, after: Stic.

Persistent+: Thu.

Prodrome, as a: Chin.

Restlessness, from: Aco; Ars; Cham; Iod.

Retiring, after, but sleepy before: *Amb.*

Rush of ideas, from: Ars; Calc; Cof; Gel; Hep; Hyo; Ign; Nux-v; Op; Pul.

Sexual: Canth; Kali-br; Raph.

Twitchings, from: *Ars*; Bell; Ign; Pul; Sul.

Uterine complaints, from: Senec.

Weaning of child, from: Bell.

Yawning, with: Cimi.

SLEEPS
Abdomen, on: Bell; Colo; Med; Stram.

Arms
- Abdomen on: Cocl; *Pul.*

SLEEPS, arms
- Apart: *Cham*; Plat; Psor.
- Head
  - over: Ars; Cimi; Lac-c; Nux-v; *Pul.*
  - under: Ars; Bell; Plat.

Back, on: *Bry*; Colch; Merc-c; *Pul*; *Rhus-t*; Stram.
- Knees drawn up, with: Bry; Hell; Lach; Merc-c; Stram+.
- and spread apart: Plat.

Curled up like a dog: Ars; Bap; Bry.

Knees, chest, on: Med.

Odd position, in: Plb.

One leg stretched out, and the other drawn up, with: Lac-c; Stan.

Side on: *Bar-c*; Colch; Pho.
- Not lain, as if: Flu-ac.

Sits up and, again: Hyo.

Strange position, in: See ATTITUDE BIZARRE.

SLIDES down in bed: See BED.

SLIGHT CAUSES AGG: Amb; Amy-n; Carb-an; Cocl; Kali-p; Mag-c; Nit-ac; Nux-m; Pho.

SLIMY: See DISCHARGES.

SLOUGH: See PHAGEDENA.

SLOVENLY: See INDOLENT, gait.

SLOW

Comprehension, thinking etc.: Amb; Anac; Ars; BAR-C; Bry; *Carb-v*; Cocl; *Con*; Echi; HELL; Kali-bi; Kali-m; Lycps; Old; Onos; Op+; Pho; *Pho-ac*; Plb; Pul; SUL.

Motion: Cocl; Pho.

SLOWED DOWN everything+: Aesc.

SLUGGISH: See Indolent.
Organs and functions+: Eup-p.
Processes: Sil.
Responses+: Hell.

SLY: *Tarn.*

SMALL as if (object, rooms etc.): Berb; Carb-v; Cyc; Merc-c; Nat-c; Plat.

SMALLER, seems
Body, limbs etc.: Agar; Cact; Calc; Carb-v; Croc; Glo; Kre; Saba; Tab; Tarn.
Cranium: Chel; Glo; Grat.

SMALL POX: Ant-t; Ars; Bap; *Merc*; *Pul*; *Rhus-t*; Sul; *Thu*; *Vario.*

SMARTING: See PAIN, biting.

SMEGMA
Foul: Sul.
Increased: Canth; Caus; Nux-v.

SMELL (See also ODOUR)

Affections in general: Aur; BELL; Calc; *Colch*; Grap; Hep; Lyc; Nat-m; NUX-V; PHO; *Pul*; *Sep*; *Sil*; SUL.

Acute: Aco; *Ars*; *Aur*; *Bell*; Carb-ac; *Chin*; *Cof*; COLCH; *Grap*; Ign; *Lyc*; NUX-V; Op; PHO; Saba; *Sep*; SUL.

Diminished, wanting, weak: Anac; *Bell*; *Calc*; Calc-s; Cyc; *Hep*; Hyo; Mar-v; Merc; *Nat-m*; Plb; Pho; PUL; Sang; *Sep*; SIL.
- Epilepsy, with: Plb.
- Taste, and: Anac; Crot-t; Just; Mag-m; *Nat-m*; *Pul*; Sil.

SMELL, diminished
 - Coryza
   with: Med.
   after: Mag-m.
Illusory: Anac; Bell; Calc; Manc; Par; Sul; Val.
- Agreeable: *Agn*; Pul.
- Burnt feathers: Bap.
- Cabbages: Benz-ac.
- Catarrh, as of: Grap; Pul; *Sul.*
- Cheese, like old +: Nux-v.
- Dung: Manc.
- Dust: Benz-ac.
- Earth, as of: Calc; Ver-a.
- Foul: *Bell*; Benz-ac; Kali-bi; Meny; *Par*; Pho; *Pul*; *Sul.*
- Gun powder: Manc.
- Onions, roasted, like: Sang.
- Sulphur, as of: Nux-v.

Preverted: Anac; Mag-m; Mag-p; Sang.

SMILE
Does not: Alu; Amb.
Foolishy: Bell.
Sleep, in: Cadm.

SMOKE
AGG: Ars; Chin; Euphr; Kali-bi; Lyc; Pho; Sep; *Spig.*
Tobacco, inhalation agg: Bro.

SMOKE
As of: See VAPOUR and RESPIRATION, smoke.
Hot, coming through all orifices, as if: Flu-ac.
SMOKING agg: See TOBACCO.
SMOOTH: Alu; Pho; Terb.
SNAKES, imagines: Lac-c; Tub.

SNAPPISH: Lil-t; *Stap.*
SNEEZING
AGG (See JARRING): Ars; Bell; Bry; Kali-c; *Lyc*; Pho; Rhus-t; SUL; Verb.
AMEL: Chlo-hyd; Lach; Mag-m; Naj; Thu.

SNEEZING (remedies in general): *Ars*; Ars-io; Bry; CARB-V; CEP; *Cina*; Coc-c; Eup-p; *Gel*; Ign; Ip; Kali-io; Kali-p; Merc; *Nat-m*; NUX-V; Pul; RHUS-T; Rum; *Saba*; Sang; Scil; Senec; Seneg; *Sil*; SUL.

Abortive: Ars; Calc-f; *Carb-v*; Nux-v; *Saba*; Sil.
- Agg sneezing: Carb-v.

Blowing, nose agg: Carb-v.
Combing or brushing the hair, from: Sil.
Coryza, without: Agar; Calc; Cic; Merc; Nit-ac; Stap.
Cough
- Before: Ip.
- Whooping, with: Cina.
- With: Agar; Bad; Bell; Just; Psor; *Scil.*

Dizzy, until: Seneg.
Ear, itching in, with: Cyc.
Eyes
- Closed, with: Gamb.
- Opening, on: Am-c; Grap.

Head thrown backwards while: Lyss.
Larynx, irritation, from: Carb-v.
Morning
- Agg: Am-c; Cam; Caus; Kali-bi; Nat-m; *Nux-v*; Sil.

SNEEZING, morning
- Waking on: Am-c; Grap+.

Mucous secretions profuse with: Solid.
Night, at: Aru-t.
Nose, burning in, with: Senec.
Odours, from: Pho.
Painful: Dros.
Persistent: Cyc; Saba; Sang.
- For hours, with weakness: Petr.

Putting hands in water, on: Pho.
Rapid and continued: Ver-v.
Salivation, with: Flu-ac.
Sleep, in: Bar-m; *Nit-ac*; Pul.
Sunshine, in: Agar; Aur; Merc; Sang.
Talking, prevented: Rhus-t.
Throat pain, with: Pho.
Two A.M.: Kali-p.
Unconvering least, on: Hep; Nux-v; Pyro; *Rhus-t*; Sil.
Unsatisfactory: Ars-io.
Violent: Agar; Cep; Kali-io+; Nat-c; Nux-v; Rum; Saba; Scil; Seneg.
- Day time only+: Gamb.

Wakes him from sleep: *Am-m*.
Wind, cold, from every: Hep.
Yawning, with: Bry; Cyc; Lob.

SNOW
Air AGG: Agar; Calc; *Con*; Form; Lyc; Mag-m; Pho; Pho-ac; Pul; Rhus-t; *Sep*; Sil; Sul; Urt; Vib.
Light AGG: Aco; Cic; Glo.

SNUFFLING (See NOSE obstructed): Kali-bi; Med; Merc; Osm; *Samb*; Vib.

SOBBING like a child+: Lob.

SOCIETY
Social functions
- AGG: Coca; Pall.
- AMEL: Bov.

Girls, modern: Amb.
Ill at ease in: Coca.
Prefers+: Lil-t.

SOLES: Cup; Pho-ac; Pul; Tarx.
Aching: Rhus-t; Sul-io; Zin-ar.
- Standing, when: Sul-io; Zin-ar.
- Tired, when: Zin-ar.
- Walking, while: Rhus-t.

Boils: Rat.
Burning: Calc; *Lach*; Lyc; Psor; Sang; Sanic; SUL; Sul-io.
- Bed, in: Cham; Sul.
- amel: Nat-c.
- Itching: Psor.
- Walking agg: Nat-c.

Callosities: *Ant-c*; Ars; *Bar-c*; Grap; Sep; SIL; Sul.
Cold, icy: Nit-ac.
- Bed, in: Sul.

Cracks: Ars; Merc-c.
Cramps: *Calc*; Carb-v; Caus; Cup; Nux-v; Sil; Stro; *Sul*; Ver-v.
Desquamation: Manc.
Dry: Bism; Manc.
Formication: Caus.
Itch: Cimi; Hydroc; Med; Tarn.
Knees, to: Lith.
Needles, at: Bry; Nat-c.
Numb: *Cocl*; Raph; Sep.
Painful (See Aching): Caus; *Kali-c*; Kali-p; Led; *Lyc*; Med; Pul; Syph; Thu.

SOLES, painful
- Contractive feeling, with: Syph.
- Feet, swollen, with: Saba.
- Pavement, walking on agg: Alo.

Pressure amel: Zin-ar.
Rubbing amel: Chel.
Soft, furry: ALU; Ars; Cann; Cocl; Helo; *Xanth*; Zin.
Sticking: Bor.
Swelled: Fer; *Lyc*; Pul.
Tender, sore: Alu; *Ant-c*; Bar-c; Calc; *Led*; MED; *Nat-c*; Sul-io; Thu; Zin.
- Balls of: Med.

Thick skin: *Ars*.
Tingling: Sil.
Vesicles: Kali-bi; Manc; Merc; Nat-c; Nat-s.
Vibrations: Old.
Withered+: Ant-c.
Wooden sensation: Ars.

SOMEONE ELSE: See DUALITY.

SOMNAMBULISM (walking in sleep):
Aco; Art-v; Bry; Dict; Kali-br; Kali-p; Nat-m; *Pho*; Op; Sil.

Children, in: Kali-br.
Emotions, suppressed, from: Zin.
Honour wounded, from: Ign.

SOOTY: See NOSTRILS.
SORE: See PAIN, Bruised.
SORROW (See GRIEF): Aco; IGN; *Nat-m*; Pho-ac; *Pul*; Stap.
SOUR, sourness, acidity: CALC; Chin; *Grap*; Hep; Iris; Kali-c; Kob; Lapp; Lith; *Lyc*; *Mag-c*; Merc; Nat-c; Nat-m; Nat-p; Nat-s; NUX-V; Ox-ac; *Pho*; Pho-ac; Pul; Rhe; Rob; Sep; Sil; SUL; Sul-ac; Tarx.

All over: Mag-c; Rhe.
Bitter: Iris; Nux-v.
Body of+: Sul-ac.
Food
- All turns: Lapp.
- Tastes, good+: Radm.

Kraut agg: See FOOD.
Smells, sensitive, to+: Dros.
SPASMS: See CONVULSIONS.
SPARKS, sensation: See ELECTRIC sparks.

SPEAKING, talking
AGG: Aco; Alu; Amb; Am-c; *Anac*; Arg-n; *Arn*; *Ars*; Aru-t; *Calc*; Cann; Chin; COCL; Dros; *Ign*; Iod; Mang; *Nat-c*; *Nat-m*; Nux-v; PHO; *Pho-ac*; *Rhus-t*; *Sele*; *Sep*; Sil; *Spo*; *Stan*; SUL.

Long agg: Nat-m.

SPEECH
Affected (See also VOICE): Arg-n; *Bell*; *Caus*; Coll; Crot-c; *Gel*; *Glo*; *Hyo*; Kali-br; Kali-io; LACH; Lyc; *Merc*; Merc-c; Nat-c; Nat-m; Nux-m; *Nux-v*; Pho; Stan; STRAM.

Babbling: Hyo; Lyc.
Chorea, in: Caus.
Development, retarded: Pho.
Difficult: Bell; Cocl; Dul; Gel; Kali-br; Lac-c; Lach; Lol-t; Nat-m; Op; Stan; Stram.
- Menses, during: Cedr.

SPEECH, difficult
- • Though, she tries: Cimi.
- **Faltering, hesitating:** *Arg-n*; Nux-m.
- **Foreign tongue, in:** Lach; Nit-ac; *Stram*.
- **Hasty:** Ars; Bell; Cocl; Hep; Hyo; Lach; Lyss; Merc.
- **Indecent+:** Cam.
- **Indistinct:** Cocl; Glo; Lyc.
  - • Excitement, from: Laur.
- **Jerky:** Agar; Caus; Myg.
- **Lisping:** Ars; Ver-a.
- **Lost, wanting:** Bar-c; Bell; Both; Caus; Cheno; Cup; Kali-cy; Laur; Lyc; Merc; Naj+; Nit-ac; Old; Onos; Plb; Stram.
  - • Amnesic: Kali-br; Plb.
  - • Fright, from: Hyo.
  - • Inteligence, intact+: Kali-cy.
  - • Stomach pain, from: Laur.
  - • Typhoid like fevers, in: Ap; Ars; Op; *Stram*.
  - • Uterine displacement, in: Nit-ac.
- **Nasal:** Bar-m; Bell; *Kali-bi*; Lac-c; Lach; Pho-ac.
  - • Tonsils, enlarged, with: Stap.
- **Plaintive:** Crot-h.
- **Rapid+:** Ars.
- **Slow:** Thu.
  - • Hunts, for words: Thu.
- **Spasmodic+:** Mag-p.
- **Strammering:** Agar; *Bell*; Bov; Buf; *Caus*; Cocl; *Hyo*; Kali-br; Merc; Nux-v; Spig; *Stram*; Ver-a.
  - • Children: Bov.
  - • Coition, after: Cedr.

SPEECH, stammering
- • Every word, loudly: Hyo.
- • Last word: Lyc.
- • Suddenly: Mag-c.
- • Talking
  - - fast, when: Lac-c.
  - - strangers to, when: Dig.
- • Typhoid, in: Arg-n; Lyc; Ver-a.
- **Stuttering+:** Cann.
- **Thick:** Agar; Bap; Caus; Dul; GEL; *Lach*; Nux-v.
  - • Blundering: Lach.
- **Tries to, but cannot:** Cimi
- **Understand, cannot, but can speak:** Elap.
- **Utters every word loudly:** Hyo.
- **Whispers+:** Ol-an.
- **Word/s**
  - • Cannot
    - - form rightly: Aesc.
    - - find right+: Dul.
  - • Convulsive motions of head and arms, with every: Cic.
  - • Roll out, tumbling over each other: Hep.
  - • Says, not intended+: Cup.
- **SPERMATIC CORD:** Berb; Ham; *Pul*; Rhod; Spo.
- **Abdomen, to:** Rhod.
- **Aching:** Clem; Sars.
- **Burning:** Berb; Pul; Spo.
- **Coition, emission agg:** Mag-m; Nat-p; Sars; Ther.
- **Heat in, with seminal discharge:** Sabal.
- **Indurated, hard:** Pho-ac; *Syph*.
- **Inflammation:** Pul; Spo.
- **Nodes:** Syph.

SPERMATIC CORD
Painful, sore: Berb; *Clem*; Ham; Kali-c; Ox-ac; *Phyt*.
Riding, carriage amel: Tarn.
Swelled: Pul; Spo.
- Inguinal glands, with: Clem.
- Sexual excitement, after: Sars.

Tension: Clem; Pul; Sul.
Thickening: *Clem*; Rhus-t; Sul.
Thighs, to: Rhod.
Tubercles: Pul; Sil; Spo.
Twitching: Mang.
Urination agg: Polyg.
SPHINCTERS: Laur; Sil; Stap.
  Relaxed+: Pod.
SPINA BIFIDA: Bry; *Calc-p*; Psor; Tub.
SPINAL CORD: Med; Ox-ac; Pic-ac; Plb; Sec.
  Calcareous deposits in: Vario.
  Spasms from: Pic-ac.
SPINE (See BACK): Par; Ther; Val; Vario.
  Aching: Agar; Lac-c; Nux-m; Syph; Tell; Zin.
  Air
  - Cannot bear a draft of: Sumb.
  - Warm streaming up, into head: Ars; Sumb.

  Along, legs down: Kob.
  Breathing deep agg: Chel; Rut.
  Burning: Alu; Ars; Cocl; Glo; Kali-bi; Lach; *Lyc*; Med; *Pho*; Pho-ac; Phys; Pic-ac; Sec; Tab; Zin.
  - Right, side+: Kali-c.

  Coition agg: Nit-ac.

SPINE
Coldness (interscapular): Agar; *Am-m*; Arg-n; Caps; Helo; Hyo; Lachn; Med; Petr; Rhus-t; Sec.
- Creeping up: Ox-ac.

Concussion: See Injuries.
Congested: Gel.
Cracking: Agar; Sec.
Curvature: Aur; *Calc*; Calc-f; Calc-s; *Lyc*; *Merc*; Merc-c; Pho-ac; PUL; Sil; SUL.
- Lies on back, with knees drawn up: Merc-c.
- Painful: Aesc; *Lyc*; *Sil*.

Cutting, up: Elap; Nat-s; Polyg.
Down: Pic-ac; Tab; Tell.
- Epileptic Aura: Lach.
- Feet, to: Kob.

Eating agg: Kali-c.
Eructation amel: Zin.
Formication: *Aco*; *Agar*; Ars; Lach; Nux-v; Pho-ac; Sal-ac.
Hot irons: *Alu*; Buf; Cam.
Injuries, concussion: Arn; Bels; Con; HYPR; *Nat-s*; Nit-ac; Sil; Zin.
- Lies on back, jerking head backwards: Hypr.
- Lifting, from: *Calc*; *Rhus-t*.
- Old: Ign.
- Spasms, from: Zin.
- Wounds: Rut; Symp.

Jarring agg: *Bell*; Grap; Sil; *Ther*; Thu.
Lower bulged backwards, as if: Aur.
Needles, icy, in: Agar; Cocl.
Numbness, creeping down: Phys.

SPINE

Pain in
- Relieves the headache: Kali-p.
- Sciatica, during: Petr.

Paralytic: AESC.

Pressure
- Agg: Bell; Lac-c; Tarn.
- Amel: Ver-a.
- Pain in remote parts, on: Sil; Tarn.

Pulsating: Arg-n; *Lach.*

Sensitive, sore: AGAR; *Bell*; *Chin*; CHIN-S; *Cimi*; Grap; *Hypr*; *Ign*; Kali-p; LACH; Lyss; Med; *Nat-m*; Nat-p; *Nux-v*; *Pho*; Phys; Rut; Sil; Stram; Tarn; Tell; *Ther*; *Zin.*
- Fever, during: Chin-s; Cocl.
- Leaning against chair agg: *Agar*; *Ther.*
- Pressure, slight agg: Stram.
- Stretching agg: Med.

Sexual excess agg: Calc; Croc; *Nux-v*; *Pho-ac*; *Sele.*

Short, as if: Agar; Sul.

Shuddering along haematuria, with: Nit-ac.

Sitting
- Agg: Pho-ac; Rut; Zin.
- Amel: Mur-ac.

Spots, in: Agar.

Standing
- Agg: Nit-ac; *Pho-ac*; Zin.
- Amel: Mur-ac.

Stooping agg: Agar.

Swallowing agg: Caus.

Tickling: Sumb.

Trembling: Lil-t.

Tumour, of: Tarn.

SPINE

Up and down: Gel; Phyt.
- Occiput, to: Petr.

Vertebra
- Absent, as if: Mag-p.
- Cracking, in: Ol-an.
- Rub against, each other as if: Ant-t.
- Single, heat, sensitive to: Agar.
- Tuberculosis of, Pott's disease (See BONES, caries of): Aur; Calc-p; Iod; Pho; Pho-ac; Stan; Syph; Tub.
  - lies on back, with knees drawn up: Merc-c.

Walking
- Agg: Grap; Mur-ac; Rut; Sul.
- Amel: Gel; Hyds; Pho-ac.

Weak: See BACK.
- Sitting agg: Calc; Sul; Zin.
- Standing, impossible: Sul-ac.
- Support body, cannot: Ox-ac.
- Typhoid fever, after: *Sele.*

SPITEFUL: See REVENGEFUL.

SPITTING, spits: Ant-t; Bar-c; Cam+; Lyss; Stram; *Tab*; Zin-chr.

Agg: Led; Nux-v.

Bile, of: Sang.

Complaints, other, with: Tab.

Constant desire+: Coc-c.

Constantly+: *Lyss.*

Food: Fer.

In face of people: *Bell*; Calc; Cup; Pho; Stram; Ver-a.

On the floor and licking it up: Merc.

Spasmodic: Lyss.

SPLASHING, swashing, as of water: Ars; *Bell*; Carb-ac; Carb-an; *Chin*; *Crot-t*; Dig; Glo; *Hep*; *Hyo*; Kali-c; Nat-m; Pho-ac; *Rhus-t*; *Spig*.

Hot: Chin; Hep; Sumb.

SPLEEN (left hypochondria): Alu; Arn; Ars; Asaf; *Carb-v*; Cean; CHIN; Con; Flu-ac; Ign; Iris; Helian; Kali-bi; Naj; *Nat-m*; *Nat-s*; Nit-ac; Ran-b; Rut; Scil; *Sul*; Ther.

Breathing, deep agg: Card-m; Kob; Sul.

Bulging: Tub.

Burning, heat: *Asaf*; Coc-c.

Chest, to: Bor.

Coughing agg: Bell; Card-m; *Chin-s*; Scil; Sul-ac; Sul.

Enlarged: Ars; Bro+; *Cean*; *Chin*; Chin-s; *Iod*; Mag-m; Nat-m; Scil; Sul-ac.

Gurgling: Verb.

Hard, indurated: Ars+; Bro+; *Chin*; Sul-ac.

Heavy: Kali-io; Sul.
- Walking, when: Mag-m.

Inflammation: Chin.

Painful: *Cean*; *Chin*; Scil.
- Chill, during: Chin-s; Pod.
- Diarrhoea, with: Cean.
- Dyspnoea, with: Cean.
- Fever, during: *Carb-v*; Nat-m; Nux-v.
- Menses
  - profuse, with: Cean.
  - suppressed, with: Cean.

Sore, tender: *Chin*; *Rhus-t*.

SPLEEN

Stitching: Agar; *Ars*; Card-m; *Cean*; Sil; Sul.
- Eating, while+: Am-m.
- Headache, with: Urt.
- Lumbar region, to+: Kali-bi.
- Running agg: Agar; Tub.
- Walking, fast agg: Rhod.

Swelling: Chin.
- Painful: Rut.

SPLINTER: See PAIN, stiching, needle like.

To promote expulsion+: Anac.

SPLITTING: See PAIN, bursting.

As if: Thyr.

SPOKEN to or addressed AGG: Cham.

SPONDYLITIS cervical: Pho-ac.

SPOONERISM (See SPEECH): Caus; Chin.

SPOTS (symptoms, sensations occur in general): Agar; *Alu*; Arg-m; Ars; *Berb*; Buf; *Calc-p*; Caus; *Cist*; Colch; *Con*; Flu-ac; Glo; Hep; Ign; KALI-BI; LAC-C; Lil-t; *Nat-m*; Nux-m; Ol-an; Ol-j; *Ox-ac*; *Pho*; Rhus-t; Sars; Sele; *Sep*; Sil; SUL; Thu; Zin.

Cold: Calc-p; Petr; Sep; Tarn; *Ver-a*.

Hectic: See FACE, hectic spots.

Moist: Petr.

Painful, sore: Arn; *Glo*; Kali-bi; Lith; Merc; Pho; *Ran-b*; *Saba*; Sul.

SPRAINS and STRAINS (See LIFTING agg): Agn; Arn; Bels; Calc; Calc-f; Carb-an; Con; Grap; Kali-m; Lach; Mill+;

SPRAINS ..
   Onos; Petr; Rut.
   Chronic: Am-m; Nat-m; Stro.
   Easy: Carb-an; Pho; Rhus-t.
   Lameness, after: Rhe; Rut.
   Parts, lain on: Mos.
SPRING (season) AGG: Amb; *Bell*; Bry; Calc; Calc-p; Carb-v; Cep; Con; Crot-h; *Gel*; Iris; Kali-bi; LACH; *Rhus-t*; Sars; Ver-a.
SQUATTING AGG: Calc; *Colo*; Grap; Syph.
SQUEEZING: See PAIN, Sqeezing.
SQUINT: See under EYES.
SQUIRMS: Val.
STAGE FRIGHT: See FEAR, appearing in public.
STAGGERING: See REELING and GAIT, staggering.
STAINS: See under DISCHARGES, MENSES, LEUCORRHOEA, URINE, and STOOL.
STAMMERING: See under SPEECH.
STANDING
   AGG: Alo; Berb; Bry; Cocl; Con; Cyc; Ign; Lil-t; *Nat-m*; Nat-s; Plat; Pul; Rhus-t; *Sep*; SUL; Tarx; *Val.*
   AMEL: *Ars*; BELL; Colch; Led; Pho; Ran-b; Scil; Sul-io.
   Erect
      • **AMEL:** Ars; Bell; Cedr; *Dios*; Kali-p.
      • **Impossible:** Aeth; Cocl; Hydroc; Kali-br.
         - falls, after: Arg-n.

STANDING
   Eyes closed, with agg: Arg-n; Calad; Iodf; Lathy.
   Inability to remain: Chin-s.
   Legs keeps wide apart, when: Pho; Pic-ac; Terb.
   Tip toe, on agg: Cocl.
STAPHYLOMA: Ap; *Euphor*; Pul.
STARE, staring: See under EYES.
STARTLED easily: See FRIGHTENED easily.
STARTS: See JERKS.
   Easily: Med; Saba; Zin.
   Involuntarily, violent: Stro.
   Noise, least, from: Ant-c; Sil.
   Pain agg: Arg-n; Lyc.
   Sleep, in: See SLEEP, jerks during.
   Touch, on: Kali-c; Mag-c.
   Triples, at: Bor; Ther.
      • Unexpected, from: Arn.
Starve, he Must: Kali-m.
STARVING: Ign.
STEALS money: Calc.
   Necessity, without: Art-v; Cur; Nux-v; Tarn.
STEAM
   AGG: Kali-bi.
   AMEL: Ars-s-fl; Lyss.
STEPPING
   Backwards: See Gait.
   Downstairs agg: Stram.
      • High, steps, from agg: Phyt.
   Hard agg: See JARRING agg.
   High: See GAIT.
   Persons are, as if: Alo.

STERILITY: See under FEMALES, affections.

STERNUM
Abdomen, to: Stic.
Back to: Kali-bi; Kali-io; Merc-sul.
Caries: Con.
Close, too, to back: Cina.
Cold: Cam; *Ran-b*.
Coughing agg: *Bry*; *Caus*; Kali-bi.
Exostoses: Merc-c.
Formication: Ran-sc.
Itching, lungs in, behind+: Iod.
Pressure, behind: Pho-ac.
Spine, to: Con; Stic.
Stone in middle, as if +: Arg-n.
Throbbing: Lach; Sil.
- **Abdomen, to:** Stic.

Twisting: Pho-ac.
Under: Am-c; Aur; Calc; *Caus*; Cham; Gel; Iod; Pho; Rhus-t; *Rum*; Sang.
- **Aching:** Manc; *Rum*.
- **Axilla, to:** Kali-n.
- **Burning:** Sang.
- **Food has lodged, as if:** Led; Lyc.
- **Heaviness (crushing weight):** Aur.
  - ascending agg: Aur.
- **Lump:** Aur; Bur-p; Chin; Echi; Gel; *Pho*; Pul; Sil.
- **Rawness:** Kali-bi.
- **Sore:** Ran-sc.
- **Ulcer, as if:** Psor.

Warts, on: Nit-ac.

STERTOR: Op.
STICKY, stringy, pasty: See DISCHARGES.
STIFFENING OUT (of body):
Cam; Cham; *Cina*; Cup; *Ign*; *Ip*; Just; Pho; Stram.

STIFFNESS, rigidity: Aesc+;
Ap; Bell; Bry; *Caus*; Chel; *Cic*; Cimi; Dros; Dul; *Guai*; Ign; Kalm; Lach; Led; Lyc; *Med*; Nux-v; Old+; Onos; Phys+; Rat; RHUS-T; Sec; *Sep*; Sil; Stic; *Sul*; Sul-ac; Terb.
Cramp, from: Sele; Ver-a.
Move, cannot: Spo.
Pain agg: Nit-ac; Onos.
Painless: Old.
Paralytic: Lith; Old; *Rut*.

STIFLING: See PAIN, strangling.
STINGING: See PAIN, stinging.
Bees, as if: Ap; Gel.
STINGS (of bees, insects): Ap; Hypr; Latro; Led; Pulex; Urt.
STITCHES: See PAIN, stitching.
Painful: Stap.
Sides, in: See SIDE.

STOMACH
Affections in general: Aeth; Arg-n; ARS; Bry; *Calc*; Carb-v; *Chin*; Colo; Ip; Lach; LYC; NUX-V; PHO; PUL; Sep; Sil; *Sul*; Ver-a.
Acidity, hyper, alternating with hypo: Chin-ar.
Alternating with
- **Head or face:** Bism.
- **Skin:** Grap.

STOMACH

Anxiety
- Emotions, felt in: *Ars*; Colo; IGN; Kali-c; Mez; Nat-m; *Tarn*.
- Head, rising, into: Nat-m.

Atrophy: Bism; Kre; Ox-ac.

Axilla and upper arm, to: Am-m.

Backward: Berb; Bism; Con; Kali-c; Sul.
- Bending amel+: Bism.
- Reverse, or: Berb.
- Shoulders, between: *Bell*.

Behind: Arn; Cact; Ham; Kali-c; Stram.

Bitter, something, as if in: Cup.

Breathing deep
- Agg: Arg-n; Caus; Pul.
- Amel: Rum.

Bubbling: Caus; Lyss.

Burning: Am-m+; ARS; *Canth*; Caps; *Carb-v*; *Cic*; Colch; Merc-c; Pho; Ran-b; Rob; SEC; Sep; SUL; *Ver-a*.
- Breathing, deep agg: Calad.
- Painful+: Kali-io.
- Spot: Gymn.

Cancer: Am-m; Ars+; Bism; Cadm; Carb-ac; Carb-an; Con; Hyds; Kre+; Lach; *Lyc*; *Pho*.

Carrying, burdens agg: Cadm.

Chest, to: Kali-c; Nux-v.

Churning, in: Lyc.

Coldness (See Abdomen): Ars; Cam; Caps; Chin; Cist; Clem+; Lyc; Meny; Ol-an.
- Cold, drinks, after: Chin; Elap.
  - water, as from: Caps; Grat.

STOMACH, coldness
- Eating, before and after: Cist.
- Fruits, afte: Elap.
- Icy: Aco; Caps; *Caus*; Colch; Pho.
  - lump: Bov.
  - oesophagus, to: Meny.
  - pain, with: Colch.
  - rubbing and pressure amel: Carb-an.
  - sweat, with: Zin-io.

Contracted: Ars; Carb-v; Cup.

Cramp, constrictional squeezing: Asaf: Chel; Grap; Kre; Rat; Rob.
- Fluid passing through intestines, as if, with: Mill.

Craving at, before menses: Spo.

Cutting: Dios; Rat.

Death like sensation: Ars; *Cup*.

Digestion disordered: See INDIGESTION.

Distended (See ABDOMEN): Cic; Rat.

Drinks agg: Apoc; Rhod.

Dryness, in: Calad.

Eating amel (See ABDOMEN): *Chel*; *Grap*; Hep; Petr.
- Every bite, hurts: Ars; Calc-p.
- Too much agg: Ant-c; Cof; Ip; *Pul*.

Empty, hollow, sinking, weak feeling: Ant-c; Ant-t; Carb-an; Cocl; DIG; *Hell*; *Hyds*; *Ign*; *Ip*; Lac-c; *Lob*; Merc; Murx; *Nux-v*; PHO; *Pod*; Pul; SEP; *Stan*; Stap; SUL; Sul-ac; *Tab*; Tell; Tril; Ver-a; *Zin*.

STOMACH, empty feeling
- At 9-10 A.M.: Hep.
- At 11 A.M.: Ign; Petr; Pho; Sep; *Sul.*
  - amel: Dig.
- Brandy amel+: Old.
- Deep breath amel+: Ign.
- Eating
  - after: Grat; Old; Sars.
  - not amel by: Carb-an; Cina; Ign; Lach; Lyc; Mur-ac; Pho; Sep; Ver-a.
- Epilepsy, before: *Hyo.*
- Extending to heart: *Lob.*
- Fasting, as from: Sars.
- Food
  - loathing of, with: Hyds.
  - thought of, from: Sep.
- Headache, during: Sep.
- Heart weak or dilated, with: Chlo-hyd.
- Hunger; without: Lach.
- Milk, sips in, amel: Diph.
- Nausea, during: Pho.
- No desire to eat+: Am-m.
- Nursing, after: *Carb-an*; Old.
- Pressure agg: Merc.
- Stools, after: Mur-ac+; Sul-ac.
- Talking agg: Rum.
- Urination after: Apoc.
- Walking, fast amel: Myr.

Enlarged: Bar-c; Sil.

Epileptic aura: Calc; Cic; Nux-v; Sil; Sul.
- Extending to head: *Calc.*

Extending, to: Bism; Colch; Dul; Kali-bi; Lapp.

Fasting and eating, after agg: Bar-c.

STOMACH
Fever agg: Ip; Ver-v.

Flames, as of: Manc.

Floating in, water, as if: Abro.

Fluttering, in: Calad.

Fullness: *Carb-v*; Caus; *Chin*; *Kali-c*; LYC; Nux-m; Pho; SUL.
- Full of
  - dry food, as if: Cadm.
  - water, as if: *Kali-c*; Ol-an.

Gnawing: Aesc+; Am-m; Arg-m; Cina; Colo; Lith; Sep; Stan.
- Drinking hot water amel+: Lyc.
- Eating amel: Anac; Kali-p; Lach; Lith.
- Returns, few hours after: Lach.
- Temple (L): with: Lith.

Griping: See Cramps.

Gout, alternating, with: *Ant-c*; Nux-m.

Gurgling: Cup.

Drinking
- when: Cup; Hyd-ac.
- after: Pho.

Hanging down, as if: Bism+; Hep; Ign; Ip; Pho; Stap.
- Stools, after: Amb.

Hard
- Body, rolling about: Lil-t.
- Spot, painful, at: Kre.

Head, to: Calc.

Heat, flushes of: Ars; Bry; Nux-v.

Heavy weight, oppression: Bry; Chin; Kali-c; Lyc; Nux-v; Pic-ac; Pul+; Sul.
- Back, of: Ham.
- Cold drink, from: Rhod.

STOMACH, heavy
- Eating, after: Hep; Kali-bi.
- Eructation amel+: Par.
- Loose: Grat.
- Night, at: Kali-m.
- Spot, one, in: Bism.
- Stone, as from+: Par; Pul.

Horrible feeling in A.M. in drunkards: *Asar.*

Icy: See COLDNESS, Icy.
- water agg: Caus.

Injury, after: Nux-v.

Inflammation: See GASTRITIS.

Lifting, heavy agg: Bor.

Limbs, to: Kali-c.

Lump
- Ball etc. as if in: Ab-n; Arn; Bell; Bov; Lob; Nux-m; Osm; *Pul*; Sanic.
- Hard: Nux-m.
- Hot, burning: Bell.
- Icy: Bov.
- Rising up into throat: Lach; Senec.
- Sharp; Hyds.

Lying
- Amel: Grap.
- Side, on amel: Lyc.
- Left amel: Scil.
- Legs drawn up, with amel: Chel.

Milk
- Amel: Grap; Merc; Merc-cy; Mez; Rut.
- Cold agg+: Kali-io.
- Desire, for+: Sabal.

Over loading agg: *Nux-v*; Stap.
- As if+: Ant-c.

STOMACH

Passes or pressed against spine, as if: Arn; Ver-v.

Piles, operation, after: Croc.

Plug: Chel.

Raw: Carb-v; *Nux-v.*

Reflexes, from: Ol-an.

Replete, as if: Merc.

Rolling, over in: Pho.

Scraping, in: Ars; Pul.

Shoulder, right, to: Sang.

Sour, acidity (See SOUR): *Calc*; Caps; Carb-v; Chin; Kob; *Lyc*; *Mag-c*; Nat-m; *Nat-p*; *Nux-v*; *Pul*; Rob; Sep; Sul; Sul-ac.
- Alternating with decreased: Calc-ar.

Spine, to: Arn; Ver-v.

Spot, in: Arg-n; Bar-c; Bism; Kali-bi; Lyc.

Squeezing, in: Rob.

Stitching: Ars.
- Motion agg *Bry*; Pul; Spig.

Stones in, as if: Ant-t; Ars; Bar-c; Bry; Calc; Cocl; Manc; Naj; Nux-m; Nux-v; Osm.
- Cold: Sil.
- Eating amel: Ptel.
- Eructations amel: *Bar-c*; Par.
- Pressure, as from: Aesc+; Bro+; Cham+; Scil.
- Rubbing together: Cocl.
- Sharp, as if: Hyds.

Stools
- Agg: Amb; Pul; Sul-ac.
- Amel: Chel.

Summer agg: Guai.

STOMACH

Swimming, in water, as if: See Floating.

Talking, sensitive, to: Caus; Hell; Kali-c; Rum.

Tension: Carb-v; Lyc; Nux-v; Rut; Stan.
- Milk amel: *Rut.*

Throbbing, pulsations: Aco; Ant-t; *Calc*; Chin; Cic; Glo; Kali-c; Nat-m; Ol-an; *Nux-v*; Pho; PUL; *Sep*; Sil.
- Back, of: Kali-c.
- Eating agg: Sele.
- Eructation amel: Sep.

Trembling, quivering: Calc; Iod; Nux-v; Pho; Sang.
- Extends all over body: Lyc.

Twisting, rising to throat: Sep.

Ulcers: Hyds; Kali-bi; Lyc; Pho; Ran-b; Symp.
- Cancer+: Acet-ac; Carb-v; Crot-h.

Upside, down: *Aeth.*

Upward, from: Kali-m; Pho.

Urination agg: Laur.

Uterus, reflex from: Bor.

Vomiting
- Agg: Sep.
- Amel: Hyo.

Walking agg: Hep.

Warm, something rises up, causing suffocation: Val.

Water, as of: Ol-an.

Wine amel+: Aco.

Worm, crawling up throat: Zin.
- Morning, in+: Cocl.

STOMACH

Yawning
- Agg: *Ars*; Phyt.
- Amel: Lyc; Nat-m.

STOMATITIS: See MOUTH, aphthae.

STONE CUTTER'S PTHISIS: Calc; Lyc; Sil.

STOOL

Before AGG: Alo; Calc; Dul; Merc; *Nux-v*; Sul; *Ver-a*.

During AGG: Ars; Cham; *Merc*; Nit-ac; Nux-v; Pul; Sep; Sil; Spig; *Sul*; Ver-a.

After AGG: *Caus*; Merc; *Merc-c*; Nit-ac; Nux-v; *Pho*; Pod; Sele; Sil; Sul.

From AGG: Dios; Merc; *Merc-c*; Paeon.

AMEL: Bor; Colo; Gamb; *Nat-s*; *Nux-v*; Ox-ac; Pall; Pho-ac; Rhus-t.

Loose AMEL: Abro; Nat-s; *Zin.*

Pressing at AGG: Agar; Bell; Carb-an; Ign; Nux-v; Pul; Rat; Rhus-t; Sep; Tell.
- Leans far back, for: Med.

STOOLS

Acrid: Arn; *Ars*; Carb-v; Chin; Colch; Gamb; Ign; Iris; MERC; Nat-m; *Pul*; Rhe; Scop; SUL; Ver-a.
- Hair, destroys: Coll.

Ashy: See White.

Bad odour, foul, putrid: *Ars*; Asaf; Bap; Benz-ac; Bor; Calc-f; *Carb-v*; Chin; Grap; Kali-p; Nux-v; *Pod*; *Psor*; Pul; Sil; Stram; Sul; Sul-ac; Tub.

STOOLS, bad odour
- Cheese, rotten: *Bry*; *Hep*; Sanic.
- Eggs, rotten: Ascl; Cham; Psor.
- Penetrating: *Pod*; *Psor*; Stram.
- Sour: See Sour.

Balls, like: See Sheep dung.

Bilious: Cham; Crot-h; *Iris*; *Merc*; Nat-s; Pod; *Pul*; Sang; *Ver-a*.
- Warm drinks agg: Flu-ac.

Black: *Ars*; Coll; *Lapt*; Merc; Merc-c; Plb; *Op*; Stram; Sul-ac; *Thu*; VER-A.
- Foul: Chio; Crot-h; Lept.
- Tarry: Chio; Lept; Phys; Ptel.

Bladder symptoms, with: Merc-c.

Blood only (See HAEMORRHAGE): Aco; Alu; Erig; Ham; Merc-c; Rhus-t; Tril.

Bloody: Alu; Ars; *Canth*; Caps; Chin; Colch; Colo; Elap; *Ham*; Ip; Jal; Merc; MERC-C; NUX-V; PHO; Pul; Rhus-t; Sec; Senec; Terb.
- Clots: Cadm.
  - bright: Alu.
- End, at: Daph.
- Tarry: Ham.
  - frothy: Elap.
- Water: Fer-p; Merc-c; Pho; *Rhus-t*.

Blue: Bap; Colch; Pho.

Breakfast agg: Nat-s; Thu.

Bright: Sul-io.

Brown: Arg-n; Ars; *Bry*; Grap; Ip; Kre; Lyc; Merc; Nux-v; *Psor*; *Rhe*; Scil; Sec; Tub; Ver-a.
- Gushes: Ast-r; Kali-bi.

STOOLS

Burning, hot: Alo; *Ars*; Ascl; Bell; Bry; Caps; Cham; Gamb; IRIS; Kali-p; *Merc-c*; Pic-ac; Pod; Saba; Scop; Strop; Sul.

Changeable: Cham; Dul; Pul; Sanic+; Sul.

Chill, with: Ars; Colo; Lac-c; Merc; *Pul*; Sul; Ver-a.

Chopped, hacked: Aco; *Cham*; Nat-p; Sul-ac.
- Eggs, like: Merc; Pul.

Clayey: Chel; Chio.

Cold: Con; Cub; Lyc.

Colds agg: Calc; Rum; Tub.

Colours, several: Aesc; Colch; Euon; Kali-p; Menis; Sul; Zin-cy.

Constipated: See CONSTIPATION.

Corn meal, like+: Aru-t.

Crumbling: *Am-m*; *Mag-m*; Merc; *Nat-m*; Sanic.

Curdled, cheesy: Calend; Iod; Tab; Val.
- Screaming, with: Val.

Dark: Alu; Bap; Chin; Grap; Kali-n; Scil; Stram.

Diaper, running through: Benz-ac; *Pod*.

Difficult: See CONSTIPATION, inactivity from.

Dirty water, muddy: Ars; Bro; Fer-p; Jal; Lept; Ox-ac; Pho-ac; Pod.
- White: Pho-ac.

Dry: *Bry*; Lac-d; Lyc; *Nat-m*; Nit-ac; Nux-v; Op; Pho; Sil; Zin.
- Hard, and+: Ascl.

STOOLS

Dysenteric: See DYSENTERY.
Fatty: See Oily.
Filaments, like hair: Sele.
Flaky: Ver-a.
Flat: Merc; *Pul*; Sul; Ver-a.
Flatulent, gassy, noisy, spluttering: Agar; Alo; Apoc; *Arg-n*; Colo; Crot-t; Fer; Gamb; *Ign*; *Nat-s*; Nux-m; Strop; Thu; Thyr; Tub.
Flatus passing, on, agg: Alo; Ars-io; Caus; Mur-ac; Nat-p; Old; Pho-ac; Pod; Ver-a.
Floats: See Scum floating.
Flocculent: Kali-m.
Foamy, frothy: Arn; *Colo*; Form; Iod; *Kali-bi*; *Mag-c*; *Merc*; *Pod*; Rhus-t; Saba; Scil; *Sul*.
- Bloody, black: Elap.
- Fluent Coryza, with: Calc; Canth; Cham; Chin; Colo; Iod; Lach; Mag-c; Merc; Op; Rhus-t; Rut; Sul; Sul-ac.
- Gushing: Chin; Crot-t; Elat.

Foul: See Bad odour.
Frequent: Aco; Ars; Ascl; Calc; Caps; *Cham*; Elat; Kali-io; Merc; MERC-C; NUX-V; Pho; POD; Ver-a.
- Bloody water: *Fer-p*.
- But scanty: Ars; Merc; Nux-v.
- Causing unfitness for work: Ascl.
- Normal: Psor.

Gelatinous: *Alo*; Asar; Colch; Colo; Hell; Kali-bi; Mag-c; Rhus-t.
Glistening: Alo; Alu; Calc; Caus; Mez.

STOOLS, glistening

- Particles: Cina; Mez; Pho.

Granular, sandy: Ap; Arg-m; Bell; Cup; Hyds; Lac-c; Lyc; Mang; Mez; *Pho*; Plb; Pod; Sars; Zin.
Gray: See White.
Green (See GREEN): Colo; Crot-t; Gamb; Grat; Merc-c; Nat-m; Pod; *Rhe*; Sec; Sul-ac.
- Dark: Ars.
- Grass: Aco; ANT-T; ARG-N; Calc-p; Cham; *Ip*; Iris; *Mag-c*; Merc; Merc-d; Thu.
  - mucus stains skin around anus and scrotum, coppery: Cinb.
- Scum: Ascl; Bry; Grat; *Mag-c*; Merc; Sanic.
- Tea: Gel.
- Turns: Arg-n; Bor; Calc-f; Nat-s; Psor; Rhe; Sanic.
  - blue: Calc-p; Pho.
  - yellow: Ip.
- Water: Cup; Kali-br.

Gurgles, pops out: Alo; Crot-h; Gamb; Grat; Jat; Pod; Thu.
Gushing, pouring: Alo; Apoc; Ast-r; Bry; Calc-f; *Crot-t*; Cup; Elat; Fer; Gamb; Grat; *Jat*; Kali-bi; Nat-c; Nat-m; POD; Psor; Sang; *Sec*; *Ver-a*.
- All at once in somewhat prolonged effort: *Gamb*.
- Torrent, in: Nat-c.

Hacked: See Chopped.
Hard: *Alu*; Alum; BRY; Calc; Card-m; Coll; GRAP; Lach; Mag-m; *Nat-m*; *Nit-ac*; Nux-v; Op; Pho; *Plb*; Sele; Sep; *Sil*;

STOOLS, hard ..
    Stan; Stro; Sul; Ver-a; Verb; Zin.
  - First, then fluid: *Bov*; *Calc*; *Lyc*; Nat-m; Sul-ac.
    - black, then white and soft: Aesc.
  - Menses, during: Ap.
  - Thin first, then: Euphor.

Head washing agg: Tarn.

Heavy: Sanic.

Holds, back: Nit-ac; Sil; Sul; Thu.

Hot: See Burning.

Impacted: Calc; Nat-m; Sanic; Sele; Sep; Sil.

Involuntary, hurried: ALO; Ap; ARN; Bar-c; Bell; *Gel*; *Hyo*; *Mur-ac*; Nat-m; Nat-p; Old; Op; *Pho*; *Pho-ac*; Pod; Pyro+; Rhus-t; Sec; Stram; *Sul*; Tab; Thu; *Ver-a*.
  - Although solid: *Alo*; Ars; Caus; Colo; *Hyo*.
  - Bloody: Hyo.
  - Convulsions, during: Cup.
  - Coughing, when: Pho; Scil; Sul.
  - Flatus, every time, with: Old; Pho-ac.
  - Foetus, movement from: Pho-ac.
  - Fright, from: Op.
  - Headache, with: Mos.
  - Laughing on: Sul.
  - Lying when: Ox-ac.
  - Moved, when (Children): Pho-ac.
  - Sleep, during: Arn; Bry; Con; Mos; *Pod*; *Psor*.

STOOLS, involuntary
  - Sneezing, on: See Coughing.
  - Stooping: Rut.
  - Urine and: Ail; *Mur-ac*.
  - Urinating, when: *Alo*; Alu; Ap; Hyo; Mur-ac; Scil.
  - Vomiting, during: Arg-n; Ars.
  - Walking, while: Alo.
  - Yellow, watery: Hyo.

Knotty, lumpy: See Sheep dung, like.

Large caliber: Alum; BRY; Calc; Elat; *Grap*; *Kali-c*; Kali-s; Lac-d; Lept; *Lyc*; Mag-m; Mez; Nat-s; Nux-v; SANIC; Sep; Sul; *Ver-a*.
  - Burnt, as if: Bry.
  - Hard: Bry; Lac-d.

Mealy: Pod; Stro.

Meat water, like: Canth; Pho; Pod; Rhus-t.

Membranous: See Shreddy.

Menses agg: See DIARROEA.

Milk agg: Nat-c; Sep.

Milky: Calc; Chel; Chin; Dig; Merc; Pod; Sanic; Tab.

Misshapen, angular, square, etc: Nat-m; Plb; Sanic; Sele; Sep.

Molasses, like: Ip.

Mucus: Arg-n; ARS; Asar; Bor; CAPS; CHAM; *Colch*; Coll; Gamb; GRAP; *Hell*; Ip; Kali-m; Kali-s; *Merc*; *Merc-c*; *Nux-v*; *Pho*; PUL; Rhe; Rhus-t; Solid; Spig; SUL; Ver-a.
  - Balls, of: Ip.
  - Bloody: Colch; *Merc*; *Merc-c*; Nat-c; Nux-v; Pod.

STOOLS, mucus
- Coated: Am-m; Cham; *Grap*; Hyds; Nat-m; Pul.
- Copious: Terb.
  - involuntary: Solid.
- Green: Aco; *Arg-n*; Ars; Castr; Cham; Dul; *Gamb*; Iris; Laur; Mag-c; MERC; Merc-c; Pul.
- Jelly, like: Asar; Colch; Hell; Sep.
- Lumps, of: Alo; Cop; Grap; Ip; Mag-c; Pho; Spig.
- Offensive: Sep.
- Only: Ant-c; Asaf.
- Stools, after: Bry; Sep; Thu.
- Tenacious: Asar; Canth; Hell.
- Transperant: Bor; Colch; Hell.
- White: Bor; Kali-chl; Nat-m.
  - milky: Kali-chl.
- Yellow: Asar; Kali-s.

Muddy: See Dirty water.
Mushy: Bry; Chin; Nit-ac; Onos; Pho; Pul; Rhus-t; *Sul.*
- Yellow: Bry.

Musty: Colo.
Narrow, long: See Slender.
Nervous: See under DIARRHOEA.
Nightly: See under DIARRHOEA.
Noisy: See Flatulent.
Noon, at: Radm.
Odourless: Ap; Kali-bi; Pho-ac; Ver-a.
Oily, fatty: Ascl; Caus; Dul; Iod; Iris; *Mag-c*; Nat-s; Pho; Pic-ac; Tarn+; Thu.
Orange, tomato sauce like: Ap; Nat-c.

STOOLS
Pain, long after: See under RECTUM.
Pasty: See Sticky.
Purulent: Arn; Merc; Pul.
Putty like: Dig; Plat.
Receding: See CONSTIPATION, stool recedes.
Red: Chel; Lyc; Merc; RHUS-T; Sul.
Removed, must be: See CONSTIPATION.
Retained: *Cocl*; Sil; *Stram.*
- Pain from: Sil.
Rice water: Ars; *Cam*; Cup-ar; Jat; Pho-ac; *Ver-a.*
Rumbling, with: Colo; Strop.
Sago-like: Colch; Pho.
Sand, in: See Stool, granular.
Scanty: Am-m; Merc; Nux-v; Plb; Sil; Sul.
Scraping of intestine, like: Canth; Colch; Colo.
Scum floating: Ascl; *Bry*; Colch; Grat; MAG-C; Saba; Sal-ac; Sanic.
Sheep dung: *Alu*; *Alum*; *Chel*; *Grap*; Hyds; Lyc; Mag-c; MAG-M; *Merc*; *Nat-m*; Nit-ac; OP; PLB; Pyro; Sanic; Sep; Sil; Stan; Stro; *Sul*; Syph; Thu; Verb.
- Chalky: Bell; Calc.
- Green: Chin; Stan.
- Tallow, like: Mag-c.
Shreddy: Arg-n; Canth; Carb-ac; Colch; Colo; Merc-c.
Shooting: See Gushing.

STOOLS

Slender, narrow: Bor; Caus; Grap; Mur-ac; *Pho*; Sul.
Soft: See Mushy.
- First part, then hard: Nux-v.

Sour: *Calc*; Colo; Dul; Grap; Hep; Jal; Mag-c; Merc; Nat-p; Rhe; Sul.
- Milk, like: Tab.

Spraying: Thu.
Standing amel: Alu; Caus.
Starch, like: Arg-n; Bor.
Sticky, pasty: Bry; Chel; Colo; Crot-t; Kali-bi; Lach; Merc; Merc-c; *Plat*; Pod; Rhe; Rhus-t; Sul.
Stringy, tough: Colch; Grap+; Lept; *Pho*.
Suds, like: Benz-ac; Colch; Elat; Glo; Iod; Sul.
Sweetish, odour: Mos.
Tarry: See Black.
Tearing anus: Mez; Nat-m.
- Though, soft: Nit-ac.

Undigested: *Ars*; Bry; CALC; Calc-p; CHIN; Chio; *Fer*; *Grap*; Mag-m; *Old*; *Pho*; Pho-ac; Pod.
- Brown: Kre; Psor.
- Milk: Mag-c.
- One day, before, of: Old.

Urinous, pungent odour: Benz-ac.
Watery, thin: Ant-c; Apoc; Asaf; Benz-ac; Calc; Calc-p; Chin; Cina; Colch; *Colo*; Dul; Gamb; Hell; *Iris*; Jal; Kali-p; Kre; Nat-s; Old; Pho; Pic-ac; Pod; Rhus-t; Sec; Sul; Thu; Tub.
- Black: Ars.

STOOLS, watery

- Bloody: See under Bloody.
- Brown: Ars; Ast-r; *Grap*; Kali-bi.
- Green: Cham; *Grat*.
- Jaundice, with: Berb.
- Lumpy, and: Ant-c; Lyc; Sanic.
  - black, with: Thu.
- Muddy: Lept.
- Rice Water: See Rice water.
- Yellow: Dul; *Gamb*; Grat; Old; *Pod*; Stro; Thu.

Waxy: Kali-bi; Lept.
Wheyey: Cup; Iod.
White, gray, ashy: Ars; Benz-ac; Calc; Canth; Chel; Cina; Dig; Kali-c; Lach; *Merc*; Nat-m; Op; Pho; Pho-ac; *Pod*; Pul; Stil; Tarx; Urt.
- Chalk, like: Calc; Pod; Sanic.
  - curdy: Calend.
- Egg white, like boiled: Urt.
- Glassy: Ars-io.
- Parts, in: Pho.
- Putty like: Mag-c.

Yellow: Apoc; Ars; Colo; Crot-t; Merc; *Pod*.
- Bright: Aeth; Alo; Chel; Colch; Gel; *Kali-p*; *Nux-m*; *Pho*; Pho-ac; Pod; Sul-ac; Sul-io.
- Green+: Aeth.
- Saffron, like: Sul-ac.
- Whitish: Pho-ac.

STOOP

Inability, to: Bor.
- Coccyx, fall on, from: Hypr.

Shouldered: Sul; Tub.

STOOPING
AGG: Aesc; Agar; *Am-c*; Bell; BRY; *Calc*; Caus; *Lyc*; *Mang*; Merc; Nux-v; Pul; Ran-b; Sep; Sil; *Spig*; *Sul*; Tell; Ther; *Val*.
AMEL: Cina; COLCH; Con; HYO; Ign; *Iris*; Pul; Ran-b.
Easy, stretching difficult: Nat-m.
Prolonged AGG: Asar; Bov; Caus; Hep; Plat.

STORMS
AGG (See CHANGE of temperature agg): Hyd-ac.
After AGG: Calc-p; Rhus-r.
Before AGG: *Elap*; Med; Rhod; Rhus-t; Sul-io.

STOVE HEAT amel: See under HEAT.
STRABISMUS: See EYES squint.
STRAINING: See Pain, pressing.
STRAINS: See SPRAINS.
STRANGE
Does, thing: Arg-n; Cact; Sep.
Everything, seems (See BEWILDERED): Cic; *Med*; Plat; Val; Tub.
- **Disagreeable, and:** Val.
- **Terrible, and:** Cic; Plat.

Notions, pregnancy, during: Lyss.
Positions, in amel: See ATTITUDE BIZARRE.

STRANGER
Among, as if: Ast-r.
One were, as if: Val.
Presence of, in
- **AGG (See COMPANY agg):** Amb; *Bar-c*; Carb-v; Caus;

STRANGER, presence, agg..
Lyc; Petr; Pho; SEP; STRAM; Tarn; Thu.
- **menses, during:** Con.

AMEL: Thu.

STRANGLING SENSATION:
Sul; Val.
Sleep, falling to, on: Val.

STRANGURY: See URINATION, difficult.
STREAKS: See PAIN, linear, RED and SKIN.

STRENGTH
Changing suddenly: Tarn.
Sensation, of: See VIGOUR.
Sinking, suddenly+: Grap.

STREPTOCOCCUS INFECTION:
Ail; Arn; Sul-ac.

STRETCH, impulse to: *Alu*;
Am-c; *Ars*; Bry; Carb-v; CAUS; Cham; Grap; Guai+; Lyc; Mar-v; Meph+; NUX-V; Pul; Rhus-t; Rut; Scil; Zin.
- **Abdominal troubles, in:** Plb.
- **Chill, with:** Eup-p; Fer-p; Nat-s.
- **Drowsiness, with:** Pod.
- **Enough, cannot:** Grap.
- **Hiccough, with:** Amy-n.
- **Hours, for:** Amy-n; Plb.
- **Urination, before:** Pul.
- **Yawning, with:** Amy-n.

STRETCHES, twists, turns (See STIFFENING OUT):
Alu; *Bell*; *Calc*; Chel; *Chin*; Colo; Ign; Mar-v; Nux-v; Plb; *Rhus-t*; Sul.
Convulsions, before: Calc.
Cough after: Merc.

STRETCHING
  Extending limbs agg and amel: See under BENDING.
  Forcible amel: Sec.
  Parts agg: Stap.

STRICTURE: Canth; Cic; *Clem*; Con; Flu-ac; Guai; *Merc*; Nit-ac; Nux-v; Petr; Pul; Rhus-t; Sil; Sul-io.
  Dilatation, after: Con; Mag-m.
  Inflammation, after: Rhus-t.

STRIKES: Arg-m; *Bell*; *Cham*; *Cina*; Hyo; Kali-c; Lyss+; Plb+; Stram; Tarn.

STRINGY: See DISCHARGES, Sticky.

STROPHULUS: See under SKIN.

STUBBING TOE agg: Colch.

STUBBORN, OBSTINATE: Agar; *Alu*; Anac; Ant-c; Ant-t; Arg-n; Aru-t; *Bell*; BRY; *Calc*; *Cham*; Chin; Cina; *Hell*; Kre; NUX-V; Sanic; Sil; Tarn.
  Menses, before: Cham.

STUDY (See MENTAL EXERTION) **AGG:** Ars-io; Mag-p.

STUFFED UP: Anac; Coc-c; Med; Spo.

STUMBLING (See JARRING) **AGG:** Bry; Caus.

STUMPS painful: See PAIN, stumps in.

STUNNED, stupefaction: See DULL.

STUNNING: Flu-ac.

STUPID: See Childish.

STYES: See under EYELIDS.

SUBARACHNOID: Gel.

SUBINVOLUTION: See under UTERUS.

SUBSULTUS TENDINUM: See under TWITCHINGS.

SUCKLING: See under CHILDREN.
  Agg: See under MAMMAE.

SUDDEN EFFECTS, symptoms: Aco; Ap; Ars; *Bell*; Colo; Con; Cup; Hyd-ac; Lyc; Mag-c; Mag-p; *Mez*; Nat-s; Pho; Radm; Tab; Tarn; Tarn-c; Val; Ver-a.
  Changing about: Amb; Berb; Cimi; Dios; Val.

SUFFOCATION: See RESPIRATION, difficult.

SUICIDAL DISPOSITION, weary of life: Ant-c; ARS; AUR; Aur-m; Chin; Dros; Lach; Meli; Merc; Naj; Nat-m; *Nat-s*; Nit-ac; *Nux-v*; *Pho*; Psor; Pul; Sul; Thu; Tub.
  Blood, seeing on: Alu.
  Brooding: Naj.
  By dagger: Ars; Bell; Nux-v.
  By drowning: Dros; Hyo; Rhus-t; Sec; Sil+; Sul.
  By hanging: Ars; Bell.
  By poison: Ars; Bell; Pul.
  By shooting: Anac; Ant-c; Nat-s.
  By starving: Merc.
  Cars, under: Ars; Kali-br; Lach.
  Eroto mania, in: Orig.
  Height leaping, from: Arg-n; Gel; Iod; Lach; Sul.
  Homesickness, from: Caps.
  Knife, seeing on: Alu.
  Love disappointment, from: Bell; Caus; Stap.

SUICIDAL DISPOSITION
Menses, during: Merc.
Music, from: Nat-c.
Pain, from: *Aur*; Nux-v.
Weeping amel: Merc; Pho.

SULCI, membranes of: Kali-bi.

SULLEN: See Morose.

SUMMER
AGG: (hot weather agg): Aeth; Ant-c; Bell; Bry; Carb-v; Cup; Dul; *Flu-ac*; Gel; *Glo*; Grat; Iris; *Kali-bi*; Lach; Nat-c; Nat-m; POD; Rhe; Sele; Ver-a.
AMEL: Alu; Aur-m; Calc-p; Fer; Sil.
Over coat, wears in: Hep.

SUNBURN: See under BURNS.

SUN
Heat, exposure to
- AGG (See heat of fire agg): Cact; Cadm; Cocl; Kob; Murx.
- AMEL: Anac; Cinb; Con; Crot-h; Iod; Kali-m; Pic-ac; Plat; Rhod; *Stro*; Tarn.

Light
- AGG: *Ant-c*; Bell; Euphr; *Glo*; Kali-bi; Lith; *Nat-c*; Pru-sp+; Sele.
- Blinds: Lith.
- AMEL: Rhod; Thu.

Pains: See DIRECTIONS, increasing gradually.
Rise, after AGG: Cham; Nux-v.
Sleeping, in AGG: Aco.

SUNSET
AGG: Aur; Kre; *Merc*; Phyt; *Syph*.
AMEL: Coca; Lil-t; Med; Sele.
To sunrise AGG: Colch; *Syph*.

SUNSTROKE (See also HEAT exhaustion): Aco; Ant-c; Arg-m+; *Bell*; Cact; Cam; *Gel*; *Glo*; Hyo; Lach; Nat-c; Nux-v; Op; Stram; Ther; Ver-v.
Effects, chronic: Nat-c.

SUPERSTITIOUS: *Con*; Zin.

SUPPORT AMEL: Fer; Kali-c; Lil-t; Nat-c; Nat-m; Pho-ac; Sep.

SUPPRESSIONS (See DISCHARGES amel): Mez; Stram; Thu; Ver-a.

SUPPURATION: See ABSCESS, and PUS.
Stubborn: Kali-bi; Nit-ac; *Sil.*

SURGINGS: See WAVES.

SURPRISE
Agg: Gel.
Pleasant agg: Cof.
Unpleasant+: Gel.

SUSPENDED: See HANGING down, as if.

SUSPENSE agg: Arg-n.

SUSPICIOUS distrustful: Aco; Anac; Ars; Aur; BAR-C; Bry; *Calc*; Cann; CAUS; CIC; Cimi; Crot-h; Dig; *Hyo*; Kali-br; *Lach*; LYC; Merc; Nat-s; Nux-v; PUL; Rhus-t; Sec; Stram; Sul; Thyr.
Foolishly: Ap.
Looks on all sides: Kali-br.
People are talking about her: Bar-c; Hyo; Ign; Pall; Stap.
Walking, while: Anac.

SUTURES: See Fontanelles under CHILDREN.
Painful: Stap.

SWALLOW

Constant disposition to: Bell; *Caus*; Con+; Cub; Grap; Lach; Merc; Merc-c; Saba; Senec; Sep.

Choking, from: *Grap*; Lyc; Merc; *Merc-c*; Sep.
- With: Bell.

Drink must, to: Bar-c; *Bell*; *Cact*; Calad; Guai; Kali-c; Nat-c; Nat-m.

Eating amel: Caus; *Merc-c*.

Excitement agg: Stap.

Foreign body, as from: Ant-c.

Hastily, anger with: Anac.

Involuntarily: Cina; Mur-ac; *Sep*; Stap.

Lump, large, as of a, from: Cep.

Sleep, in: Calc; Cina.

Sour, bitter fluid, vertigo with: Caul.

Speaking, while: *Cic*; Stap; Thu.

Walking in wind, while: Con.

SWALLOWING

AGG (also painful, difficult): Am-c; Ap; Bar-c; *Bell*; Bro; Bry; Canth; Caus; Chin; Cina; Cocl; *Gel*; Grap; Hep; Hyd-ac; *Hyo*; Kali-c; Lac-c; LACH; Laur; Lyss; Meph; Merc; Merc-c; Merc-i-f; *Nit-ac*; Nux-m; Nux-v; Pho; Phyt; Plb; *Rhus-t*; *Stram*; Sul; Sul-io.

After AGG: Cadm; Vinc.

AMEL: Alu; Amb; Arn; *Caps*; IGN; Lach; Led; Mang; Mez; Nux-v; Pul; *Rhus-t*; Saba; Spo; Zin.

Chorea, in: Art-v.

Continuous AMEL: Ign.

Empty
- AGG: *Bar-c*; Bell; Bry; Cocl; Grap; Hep; *Kali-c*; LACH; Merc; Merc-c; *Merc-i-r*; Nux-v; Pul; Rhus-t; Saba; Sul; Tell.
- AMEL: Alu; Ip.
- Eating drinking amel: Ol-an; Tell.

Eyes open, while, during coma: Terb.

Food, goes wrong way, while: *Anac*; Caus; Hyo; Kali-c; Lach; *Meph*; Nat-m; Op.
- Large piece of, as if: Cep; Phys.
- Pushed up, when: Fer-io.
- Stops, and while: Con.
- Turns like cork-screw+: Elap.
- Warm
  - agg: Gel.
  - amel+: Hyo.

Hasty: Anac.
- AGG: Ars; *Nit-ac*; Nux-v; *Sil*.

Head, bends forwards and lifts his knees up, while: Bell.

Impeded: Nat-s.

Liquids
- AGG: Arg-n; Ars; BELL; Bro; *Canth*; Chin; *Crot-t*; Ign; LACH; Lyss; Merc; *Merc-c*; Nux-v; *Pho*; Stram; Ver-a.
- AMEL: Alu; Nit-ac; Nux-v.
- Cold agg: Kali-c.
- Hot agg: Phyt.
- Warm amel: Alu; Kali-c; Nux-v.

SWALLOWING

Lump, painful, swallow cannot+: Gel.

Neck, twists to get it down: Kali-m.

Noisy: Arn; *Ars*; Caus; Cina; Cocl; Cup; Gel; Hell; Hyd-ac; Lach; *Laur*; *Pho*; Thu.

Painful: Ant-t+; Ars; Bell; Canth; Lac-c; *Lach*; Merc-c; *Phyt*; Sil+; Sul+; Sul-io.
- Nose to ears: Elap.

Painless: Ap; Carb-ac.

Paralytic: Caps.

Pungent, acrid things AGG: Lach.

Small morsel, at a time: Alu.

Solids
- AGG: Alu; Ant-t; Ap; *Bap*; *Bar-c*; Crot-h; Kali-c; Lac-c; Merc-i-r; Plb; Sil.
- AMEL: Bro; Fer; *Hyo*; *Ign*; Kali-bi; Lach; Merc-cy; Rhus-t; Sanic.
- Lying down, when agg: Cham.
- Reach a certain point, and are violently rejected: Nat-m.

Sour agg: Ap.

Sweets
- AGG: Bad; Lach; Sang; *Spo*.
- AMEL: Ars.

Strangling: Ant-t; Dig.

Won't go down: Bar-c; Calc; Grap; *Hyo*; Lac-c; Lyc; Naj; Nit-ac; Sep; Stram.
- Even a teaspoonful: Lyc; *Nit-ac*.
- nausea, as from: Arn.

SWASHING: See SPLASHING.

SWAYING

Agg: See CAR SICKNESS, and ROCKING.

As if: See VERTIGO, swinging.

SWEAT

In general, easy tendency, to: Agar; Ant-t; *Calc*; Calc-s; Carb-v; *Chin*; *Fer*; *Grap*; Hep; Ip; *Jab*; Kali-c; Kali-s; Lach; *Lyc*; Med; Merc; Merc-cy; *Nat-c*; Nat-m; Nit-ac; *Nux-v*; Op; Ox-ac+; *Pho*; *Pho-ac*; Psor; Samb; *Sep*; Sil; Stan; *Sul*; Tub; *Ver-a*.

AGG (sweats without relief): Ars; BELL; Benz-ac; *Caus*; Cham; Chel; Chin; Dig; Form; Hep; MERC; *Nux-v*; *Op*; Pho; Pho-ac; *Pyro*; *Rhus-t*; *Sep*; *Stram*; *Sul*; Tarn-c; Til; Tub; Ver-a.

After AGG: Chin; Pho-ac; Sep.

AMEL: (See DISCHARGES amel): Bap; *Bry*; Canth; Cham; *Cup*; Eup-p; *Gel*; Iod; *Nat-m*; Psor; Rhus-t; Tarn.
- Headache, except: Eup-p.

Absent (See SKIN, dry): *Bell*; Bry; Calc; CHAM; CHIN; Colch; Colo; *Dul*; Lach; Psor; RHUS-T; Scil; *Sil*; SUL; *Stram*.

Acrid: Cham; Flu-ac; Tarn.

Affected parts, on: Amb; Ant-t; Cocl; Flu-ac; Kali-c; Merc; *Rhus-t*; Sil; Tarn-c.

Alternating, sides on: Agar.

Anger, from: Sep.

Aromatic: Benz-ac.

Awake, only while: SAMB; Sep.

SWEAT

Bloody: Crot-h; Lach; Nux-m.
Burning: See Hot.
- With: Mez; *Nat-c.*

Cannot: Apoc.
Chill
- Alternating, with: Ars; Chin; Mez; Nux-v; Spig.
- Followed, by: Carb-v; Hep; Nux-v.
- With: Tab.

Clammy: Ars; Cam; Cham; Cup; Fer; Fer-p; *Lyc*; *Merc*; *Pho*; Pho-ac; Tub; Ver-a; *Ver-v.*

Coition, after: Grap; Nat-c; Sep.

Cold: Am-c; *Ant-t*; *Ars*; *Cam*; CARB-V; Castr; *Chin*; Cocl; Cup; Dros; Fer; Hep; Ip; Lyc; *Merc*; Merc-c; *Sec*; Sep; Tab; Ther; Tub; VER-A; Ver-v.
- AMEL: Nux-v.
- Clammy, haemorrhage, with: Chin.
- Convulsions, with: Stram.
- Cough
  - during: Ant-t; Ver-a.
  - after: Dros.
- Easily, excited: Ther.
- Exertion, slight, mental or physical: Hep; Sep.
- Loquacity, after: Cup.
- Mania, with: Stram.
- Nausea, with: Ant-t; Lob; Ver-a.
- Palpitation, with: Am-c.
- Stools, during: Plb.
- Sudden, attacks of: Crot-h; Tab.
- Urination, after: Bell.

SWEAT

Colds, from: Nit-ac.
Colliquative: Agar; Ant-t; Ascl; Chin; *Jab.*
Coma, with: Benz-ac.
Company agg: Thu.
Coughing agg: Ars; Calc-s; *Carb-v*; HEP; Pho; Samb; Sep; *Tub.*
Covers, heat amel (uncovering intolerance of): *Clem*; Grap; Hep; Nat-c; NUX-V; Rhus-t; *Samb*; *Stro.*
Critical: Pyro.
Debilitating: Bry; Calc-p; Cam; Carb-an; Chin; Chin-s; Fer; Iod; Merc; Nit-ac; Pho; Psor; Samb; Sep; Tub.
- Delivery, after: Samb.
- Fever; after: Castr.
- Foul; Croc.
- Spinal injuries, from: Nit-ac.

Diarrhoea, with: Aco; Ascl; *Ver-a.*
Dyspnoea, with: Ars; Carb-v.
Eating
- Agg: Benz-ac; Carb-an; Carb-v; Cham; Nat-m; Nit-ac; Sul-ac.
- Amel: Lach.
- Food, warm agg: Pho; Sul-ac.

Egg, rotten like, smell: Stap.
Emission, after: Calc; Sep.
Emotion, after: Phys; Rhus-t; Sep.
Every thing, excites: Berb.
Exertion, slight, from: Aeth; Caus.
Exhausting: See Debilitating.

SWEAT

Eyes, closing, on: Bry; *Con*; Lach.

Face, except: Rhus-t; Sec.

Flatus, passing, while: Kali-bi.

Flies, attracting: Calad.

Fright, from: Anac; *Op*.

Gushing: Amy-n; Ap; *Bell*; *Colch*; Ip; Jab; Lach; Merc-cy; Nat-c; Pho; Samb; Tab; Thu; *Val*.
- Alternating, with dry hot skin: Ap.
- Company agg: Thu.
- Influenza, after+: Amy-n.
- Suddenly: Val.

Head except: Rhus-t; Samb; Thu.

Heart symptoms, with: Spo.

Hot, burning: Aco; BELL; CHAM; Con; *Ign*; *Ip*; Nat-c; Nux-v; OP; Psor; *Saba*; Sang; *Sep*; *Stan*; *Stram*; Til; Vio-t.
- Unconsciousness, with: Calc; Sep.

Itching, causing: Cham; Op; Rhus-t.

Lying on right side agg: Lach.

Menses agg: *Grap*; Nux-v; Ver-a.

Mice, like odour: Sil.

More pain, more: Cham; Til.

Motion agg: *Chin*; Hep; Merc; Merc-c; Psor; Sep; Stan; Ver-a.

Musk, like odour: Ap; Mos; Sul.

Musty: Cimex; Ol-an; Psor; Pul; Stan; Thu; Thyr.

Neck, about: Lach.

Nervous (See fright from): Jab; Rhus-t; Sep.

SWEAT

Night, at: Agar; Ars; *Calc*; Carb-an; Carb-v; Caus; Con; *Hep*; *Kali-c*; Kali-s; Lach; *Merc*; Merc-c; *Petr*; Pul; *Pru-sp*; *Samb*; Sep; *Sil*; Stro; Sul; Tarx; Thu.
- Climacteric: Stro.
- Phthisis of: See under NIGHT.

Offensive, foetid, putrid: Arn; *Bap*; *Bar-c*; Carb-an; Carb-v; Con; Croc; Grap; Hep; Led; *Merc*; Merc-c; Nit-ac; Nux-v; *Petr*; Psor; Pul; Sec; Sep; Sil; *Stap*; *Sul*; Thu; Vario.
- Coughing, after: Hep.

Oily, greasy: Bry; Chin; Flu-ac; Mag-c; *Merc*; Stram; Thu; Thyr.

Onions, garlic like: Art-v; Bov; Kali-p; Lach; Lyc; Thu.
- Convulsions, after: Art-v.

Pain
- Agg: *Cham*; Lach; *Merc*; Nat-c; Pul; *Rhus-t*; Sep; TIL.
- After: Chel.

Painful parts, on: Kali-c.

Palpitation, with: Calc.

Partial, single parts: Ap; Bar-c; CALC; Carb-v; Caus; Guai; Ign; Merc-c; Mez; Nux-v; Pho; *Pul*; Sele; SEP; *Sil*; *Sul*; *Thu*; Ver-a.
- Front of the body: Arg-m; Cocl; Pho; Sele.
- Lower part of the body: Croc.
- Parts
  - lain on: Chin; Nit-ac.
  - not lain, on: Aco; *Benz*; Nux-v; Thu.

SWEAT, partial
- Upper part: Asar; Calc; Kali-c; Op; Par; Sil; Spig; Tub.

Profuse, drenching: Bell; Benz-ac; Calc-hyp; *Carb-an*; Caus; CHIN; Coca; Guai; Hep; Jab; *Pho-ac*; Psor; Sele; *Sil*; Sul-ac; Tarn; Thyr; Til; Tub.
- Delivery, after: Samb.
- Diarrhoea, chronic, in: Tub.
- Fainting, with: Hyds.
- Mania, with: Stram.
- Many symptoms with: Samb.
- Nausea, with: Lob.

Prolonged, long lasting: Caus; Fer; Hep; Merc; Samb.

Pungent: Flu-ac; Thu.

Red: Lach; Nux-m.

Relief, without: See Sweat agg.

Rheumatism, with: Ascl.

Room, in: Ip; Pul.

Sadness, from: Calc-p.

Salty deposit: Nat-m; Sele.

Scanty: Alu; Grap; Sang.

Sensation, as if about to sweat but no moisture appears: Ign; Stan.

Shivering, with: Nux-v.
- Slight, after: Both.

Sitting, while: Ars.

Sleep
- During: Bell; Cham; Chel; Chin; Con; Hyo; Mez; Lach; Plat; Pul; Rhus-t; Sele; Sil; Thu; Til.
- Deep, in: Pul.
  - waking, from: Rum.
- Eyes closing on, even, when: Carb-an; CON.

SWEAT, sleep
- Falling, on: Ars; Merc; Mur-ac; Sul; Tarx; Thu.

Spasms, during: Bell; *Buf*.

Spots, in: Merc; Petr; Tell.

Staining the linen: Bell; Lach; Mag-c; Thu.
- Bloody Red: Lach; Nux-m.
- White: Sele.
- Yellow: Bell; *Carb-an*; *Grap*; LACH; MERC; *Sele*; Thu; Tub.

Steaming: Psor.

Sticky: Kali-bi; Lyc.

Stiffens
- Hair: Sele.
- Linen: Merc; Nat-m; Sele.

Stools
- Before agg: Merc; Tromb.
- During agg: Merc; Ver-a.
- After agg: Caus; Nat-c; Plb.

Strangers, in presence of: *Bar-c*; Sep.

Sudden: Carb-v; Crot-h; Ip; *Tab*.
- And disappearing suddenly: *Bell*; Colch.
- Chill, with: Tab.

Suppressed AGG: Aco; *Bell*; *Bry*; Calc; CHAM; CHIN; Colch; *Colo*; *Dul*; LACH; Psor; RHUS-T; Sep; *Sil*; Stram; SUL.

Sweetish: Calad; Merc; Thu.

Uncovering amel: Cham; Led; Lyc; Sec.

Unilateral, one sided: Bar-c; Jab; NUX-V; Petr; Pul; *Sul*; Thu.
- Right: Pho; Pul.
- Left: *Bar-c*; Chin; *Pul*.

SWEAT

Urination, after: Merc.
Urinous: Canth; Colo; Nit-ac.
Vinegar, smell, of: Iris.
Waking, on: Dros; Par; *Samb*; Sep; Sul.
Walking amel: Pul; Thu.
Warm amel: Aco.
Wash cannot: Mag-c; Merc.
Washing amel: Thu.
Writing, while: Hep; Kali-c; Psor; *Sep*; Sul; Tub.

SWEETISH: Thu.

SWEETS, body were made of: Merc.

SWELLED as if: See ENLARGED, as if.

SWELLING: Aco; *Ap*; Ars; Bar-c; Bell; *Bry*; Calc; Cham; Grap; Hep; *Lach*; Led; Lyc; MERC; Nit-ac; Nux-v; Pho; *Pul*; *Rhus-t*; SIL; SUL.

Absent in affected or inflamed parts: Ars; Cam; Carb-v; Con; Laur; Op; Pho-ac; Sul.
Baggy: Ap; Ars; Kali-c.
Body, whole of, as if: Buf.
Chronic: Cist.
Cold: Asaf; *Cocl*; Con; *Dul*; Merc; Sul.
Cordlike: Dul; Iod; Rhus-t.
Dark red: Asaf.
Glands, of: See under GLANDS.
Glandular: Lap-alb.
Hard: Ars; Bell; Chin; Con; Hep; Iod; Lach; Merc; Pul; Rhus-t; Sil; Spo; *Tarn-c*.
• Here and there: Pho.
Menses, during: Kali-c; Lac-c.
Nodes, like: Bry; Nit-ac.
Pale: Bar-c; *Bry*; Lach; Lyc; Rhus-t; *Sul*.
Receding: Ars; Calc; Hep; Kre; Lach; Lyc; Merc; Sep; Sil.
Red, shiny: Sabi.
Saccular: Ap; Ars; Kali-c; Rhus-t.
Vascular: Lyc.

SWIMMING

Or falling into water AGG: Ant-c; Bels.
While agg: Cocl.

SWINGING AGG: See CAR-SICKNESS and ROCKING.

• As if: See under VERTIGO.

SYCOSIS (See GONORRHOEA): Ap; Arg-m; Arg-n; Ars; Calc; Grap; Kali-io; Kali-s; Kalm; MED; Merc; NAT-S; *Nit-ac*; Pho-ac; Pul; Saba; Sabi; *Sars*; Sele; *Sep*; Stap; Sul; THU.

Suppressed: Merc; Nit-ac; Stap; Thu.

SYMMETRICAL: Arn; Kali-io; Lac-d; Syph; Thyr.

SYMPATHETIC: Caus; Ign; Nat-m; Nux-v; *Pho*.

SYMPATHY

AGG: Ars; *Bell*; *Calc*; IGN; Kali-s; *Nat-m*; *Plat*; Sabal; Sep; *Sil*.
AMEL: Asaf; Pho; *Pul*.
Bars, against friend: Arg-m.
Resents: Cof; Syph.

SYMPTOMS

Alternate: See ALTERNATING Effects.

SYMPTOMS

Begin on one side; go to other and there agg: See under PAIN.

Better, worse and without any cause: Alu; Psor.

Broods over his own: Sabal.

Change
- Constantly: Berb; Croc; Sang; Tub.
- Places, suddenly: Amb; Berb.

Diverse, many: Agar; Kali-io; Merc; Syph; Tub.

Every, is a settled disease: Lac-c.

Group, recur (See RELAPSES): Anac; Caus; Cham; Cocl; Cup; Plb; Sil.
- Alternating: Cimi.

Magnifies, her: Asaf; Buf; Cham.

Or sensations, appear on side lain on, not lain on etc: See under DIRECTONS.

Thinking, of agg: See THINKING of it agg.

SYNALGIAS (sexual): Ap; Tarn.

SYNCOPE: See FAINTING.

SYNOVITIS: See under JOINTS.

Crepitation: Nat-p.

SYPHILIS: Asaf; *Aur*; *Carb-an*; *Cinb*; *Iod*; Kali-bi; *Kali-io*; Kali-s; MERC; Merc-c; Merc-i-f; Merc-i-r; *Nit-ac*; *Phyt*; Sars; Sil; Still; Syph; Thu.

Fear of+: Hyo.

Infants of: Bad.

TABES DORSALIS: See LOCOMOTOR ATAXIA.

TACHYCARDIA: See PULSE rapid.

TACITURN silent, reticent: Ant-c+; Ars; Aur; *Bell*; Bry; Carb-an; Caus; Cocl; Glo; Hell; *Ign*; Mag-c+; Mez; MUR-AC; Pho; PHO-AC; Plat; Plb; *Pul*; Stan; Thu; *Ver-a*; ZIN.

Alternating with
- Mania+: Ver-a.
- Quarrelsomeness: Con.

TALK

Cannot (See VOICE lost): Dig; Pho; Stan; Sul.
- Weeping, without: Med.

Desire, to: Arg-m; Arg-n; Stic.

Hearing others AGG: Amb; Am-c; ARS; Cact; Chin; *Hyo*; Mag-m; *Mang*; Mez; *Nat-c*; *Nux-v*; Rhus-t; *Sep*; Sil; Stram; *Ver-a*; Zin.

Must: Frax; Stic.

Same over and over again: Med.

TALKING

Agg: See SPEAKING agg.

Others, about her: *Bar-c*; Hyo; Ign; Pall; Stan; Stap.

Painful: Cep.

Pleasure, takes in his own: Nat-m; Par; Stram.

Unpleasant things of AGG: Calc; Cic; Mar-v.

TALKS

Always about her pain: *Mag-p*.

Changes, subjects rapidly+: Agar.

Dead people, with: *Calc-sil*; Hyo.

Excitedly: Mos.

TALKS

Fast: Bell; Calc-hyp; Thu.
Faults, of others about: Ver-a.
Himself, to: Ant-t; Aur; Chlo-hyd; Hyo; Kali-bi; Mag-p; Mos; Pyro.
- Gesticulates, and: Mos.
- Loudly: Nux-m.

Incoherently+: Agar.
Nonsense, then angry, if not understood: Buf.
Nose through (children) with open mouth: Bar-m; Lac-c.
Persons, imaginary, with: Chlo-hyd; Hyo.
Senseless: Anac.
Sleep, in: Ars+; Bar-c; *Bell*; Carb-an; Cina; *Kali-c*; Lach; Nux-v; Pul; Pyro; Sil; Sul.
- Eyes open, with: Diph.
- Loudly: Nux-m; Sep; Sil+; Sul.
- Old men: Bar-c.

Spirits, with: Nit-ac.
Through him, other persons as if: Alu; Cann.
Troubles, of her: Arg-n; Asaf; Mag-p; Nux-v; Zin.
Verses, in: Agar+; Ant-c+; Nat-c.
Voice low, soft, in: Vio-o.

TALL: Calc-p; Mag-p; Pho.
TAPE WORMS: See WORMS.
TARRY: See DISCHARGES, MENSES and STOOLS.
TARSI (edges of eyelids): Bor; Merc; PUL; Stap; *Sul*; Val.

Blue: Bad; Bov; Phyt.
Burning: Ars; Euphr.

TARSI

Eczema: Bacil; Tub.
Inflammed: Clem; Grap; Mag-m; Petr; Pul; Sanic; Sul.
Itching: Calc; Pul; Saba; Stap.
Pustules: Ant-c.
Red: *Ars*; *Euphr*; Grap; Merc; Pul; Saba; Sep; SUL.
Scaly: Ars; *Grap*; Mag-m; Med; Merc; *Sep*.
Thick, swelled: Alu; Calc; *Euphr*; Grap; Hep; Merc; Pul; Tell.
Tumours: Mar-v; Sep.
Ulcers, on: Clem; Sanic.

TASTE

Acute: Chin; Cof; Nat-c.
After taste of food eaten: Ant-c; Caus; Dios; Nat-m; *Pho*; *Pho-ac*; Pul; Sil.
Alkaline: Kalm.
Altered, in general: Chin; *Pul*; Rhus-t.
Aromatic: Glo.
Astringent: Alu; Arg-n; Ars; Chio; Grap; Hyd-ac; *Merc-c*; Pho.
Bad, foul, repulsive, nauseous: Anac; *Arn*; Calc; Caps; Grap; *Merc*; Nat-s; NUX-V; PUL; Psor; *Rhus-t*; Stap; Sul; Syph; Vario.
- Coition, after: Dig.
- Eating
  - after: Lyc.
  - amel: Lil-t.
  - impossible: Myr.
- Epilepsy, before: Syph.
- Everything, to: Pod.

TASTE, bad
- Fever, during: *Arn*; Ars; Pul.
- Sweets, from: Lac-c.
- Menses, during: Kali-c.
- Morning, in: Ars; Bry; Calc-p; Nat-s; NUX-V; PUL.
- Waking, on: Val.
- Water, to: Aco; Ap; Ars; Aur; Bell; Bur-p; Fer; *Kali-bi*; *Nat-m*; *Pul*; Sil.

Banana, like: Mag-p.
Beer, like honey+: Mur-ac.
Bitter: Aco; Ant-c; *Ars*; BRY; Carb-v; Cham; Chel; *Chin*; Colo; *Lyc*; *Merc*; Nat-c; Nat-m; *Nat-s*; NUX-V; Pho+; Pod; PUL; Sep; Solid; Sul; Tarn+; Ver-a.
- Bread, to: Pul; Rhus-t+; Scil+.
- Butter, to: Chin; Pul; Rhus-t.
- Coffee, to: Sabi.
- Continuous: Colo; Solid.
- Drinking
  - agg: Ars; Bry; Chin; *Kre*; Pul.
  - amel: *Bry*; Psor.
- Eating agg: Ars; Pul.
- Everything, even saliva: Bor; Kre.
  - except water: *Aco*; *Stan*.
- Food, to: Chin; Iod; Nat-c; *Pul*; Rhe; Stram+.
  - but not drinks: Iod.
  - swallowing, when: Kre.
- Head ache, with: Calc-p.
- Menses, at: Calc-p; Caul.
- Milk, to: Sabi.
- Morning: *Cham*; *Pul*.
  - waking, on: Helo; Kali-io; Sul.

TASTE, bitter
- Night, at: Solid.
- Plums, to: Iod.
- Smoking
  - agg: Cocl; Pul.
  - amel: Aran.
- Sour: Arg-n; Asar; Cup; Lyc; Merc; *Nux-v*; Pho; Sep; Stan.
  - milk after: Amb.
- Sweet things, sugar: Rhe; Sang.
- Thirst, with+: Pic-ac.
- Tongue, cold with: Kali-m.
- Water, to: ARS; Calc-p; Chin; *Chin-ar*; Ver-a.

Bloody: Am-c; Ars; Bell; Fer; Ham; Ip; Lil-t; Nat-c; Pul.
- Coughing agg: *Bell*; Kali-bi; *Rhus-t*.
- Pregnancy, during: Zin.

Chalky: Nux-m.
Cheesy: Aeth; Lyc; Sep.
Coughing agg: Lach; Nux-v; Sang.
Dulled, flat, insipid watery: Anac; *Bry*; Chin; Ign; Merc; *Pul*; Stap.
- Everything to+: Mos.
- Food, to: Cup; Stro.
- Water, to: Aco.

Earthy: Fer; Ip; Nux-m; *Pul*.
Eggs, like rotten: *Arn*; Bur-p; Grap; *Merc*; *Mur-ac*; Pho-ac+; Psor.
- Coughing, when: Sep.

Every thing, inclination, to: Bell.
Fishy: Sep.

TASTE

Flat: See Dulled.

Greasy, fatty: *Alu*; Asaf; Caus; Iris; Kali-p; Mang; Petr; Pul; Tril; Val.

Herby: Nux-v; Pho-ac; Rhus-t; Sars.
- Food, to: Stram.

Illusions, of: Val.

Inky: Calc.

Insipid: See Dulled.

Lost, wanting: Anac; *Bell*; Cyc; Hyo; Mag-m; NAT-M; Pho; Pod; *Pul*; Sil.
- Cold
  - during: Nat-m; Pul.
  - after: Mag-m.
- Food, to: Hell; Nat-m; Pul.
- Salt, to: *Calc*; Canth.

Metallic, coppery: Bism+; Cimi+; *Cocl*; Cup; Hyd-ac; Iod; Kali-bi; MERC; *Nat-c*; Nux-v; Radm+; *Rhus-t*; *Seneg*; Thyr; Vario; Zin-chr.
- Tip, at: Thyr.

Milky: Aur; Pho.

Musty: Led; Lyc; Mar-v; Stap.
- Coughing, when: Led.

Oily: See Greasy.

Onions, like: Aeth.

Palatable, extremely+: Cann.

Peppermint, like: Ver-a.

Peppery: Echi; Hyds; Lach; Mez; Radm; Sul; Xanth.

Perfume, like: Bell; Cham; Coc-c; Glo.
- Water, to: Med.

Perverted: Mag-m; Nat-c.

Pussy: Hyd-ac.

Rancid: Alu; Carb-v; Cham; Kali-io; Mur-ac; Syph; Thu; *Val*.
- Drink and food, after: Kali-io.
- Sweet agg: Lac-c.

Salty: *Ars*; Chin; Con; Cyc; Kali-io; Lyc; *Merc*; Merc-c; Nat-m; Pho; Pul; *Sep*.
- Every thing: Sep.
- Food only, tastes natural: *Lac-c*.
- Food
  - not enough: Calc; Cocl.
  - too: Cep+; Chin; Cyc; Pul.
- Sour: Cup; Lach.
- Sweet: Croc; Pho.
  - water, to: Bro.

Sawdust like: Cor-r.

Semen, odour like: Ver-v.

Slimy: Kali-bi; Merc; *Pul*; Val.

Sour: *Arg-n*; Bell; Bism+; CALC; Chin; Grap; Ign; Kob; LYC; *Mag-c*; Nat-c; NUX-V; *Ox-ac*; *Pho*; Pul; Rhe; Rob; Stan; Sul; Tarx; Zin-val.
- Drinking, after: Nux-v.
- Every thing: Pod.
- Food, to: *Am-c*; Calc; Caps; Lyc; Mur-ac.
- Meat, to: Lapp.
- Milk
  - after: Amb; Pho; Sul.
  - to: Calad.
- Putrid, or+: Pod.
- Salty: Cup; Lach.
- Sweets, after: Calc.

Straw, like: Cor-r; Stram; Sul.

TASTE

Sweet: Bism+; Calad; Cup; Dul; Iris; Lil-t; Merc; Pho; Plb; *Pul*; Pyro; Saba; Scil; Sele+; Stan; Sul; Thu.
- Beer+: Cor-r.
- Bread, to: Cor-r; Merc.
- Butter, to: Mur-ac; Ran-b.
- Coughing, when: Pho.
- Every thing: Mur-ac; Phel.
- Food, to: Scil.
- Hunger, with: Nit-ac.
- Metallic+: Coc-c.
- Morning, in: Aeth; Ars.
- Mouth, back of: Lil-t.
- Salivation, with: Dig.
- Tobacco smoking, after: Dig.
- Tongue, tip, on: Plat.
- Water, to: Form.

Urinous: Psor; Seneg.
Watery: See Dulled.
Woody: Rut.

TEARING: See under PAIN.

TEARS: See LACHRYMATION.

Things, himself, etc: *Bell*; Cann; Kali-p; Sec; *Stram*; Tarn; Ver-a.

TEETH: ACO; *Ant-c*; Bell; Bry; *Calc*; Calc-p; *Caus*; CHAM; Chin; Cof; Kre; *Lach*; MERC; Mez; Nux-v; Plant; Pod; PUL; *Rhus-t*; SEP; Sil; Spig; STAP; *Sul*.

Right: Bell; Flu-ac; Stap.
Left: Caus; Cham; Clem; Euphor; Mez; Sep; Sul; *Thu*.

Alternating
- Between upper and lower: Aco; Laur; Nat-m; Pul; Rat; Rhod.

TEETH, alternating
- Sides: Amb; Am-m; Caps; Chel; Iod; Kali-n; Lyc; Psor; *Pul*; Stram; Sul; *Zin*.

Changing about: Bry; Cyc; Hyo; Hypr; Kali-bi; Kali-c; Mag-c; Mang; Nat-m; Nux-m; Pru-sp; Pul; Rhod; Sil; Thu.

Radiating: MERC.

Row in a whole: Ars; Aur; Carb-v; Glo; Lach; Mag-c; Mag-p; *Merc*; Nat-m; *Nux-v*; Psor; Sep; Spig; *Stap*; Zin.

Upper: Am-c; *Aran*; Bell; Carb-v; Chin; Kre.

Lower: Bell; Canth; *Cham*; Nat-c; Plb; Stap.

Canine: Calc; Nux-v; Sep; Sul-ac.

Incisors: *Colch*; Sul.
- Behind: Pho.

Molars: Bry; *Kre*; Stap; Zin.

Roots: Mag-c.

Abscessed, roots: Calc; *Hep*; Kre; Pho; SIL; Stap.

Acids
- Agg: Arg-n; Mur-ac.
- Amel: Pul.

Air, cold
- Agg: Calc; Caus; Cham; Merc; Rat; Sul; Tub.
- Amel: Clem; Mez; Nat-s; Nux-v; *Pul*; Sele.

Alternating, breast (L) with: Kali-c.

Beer amel: Cam.

Biting
- Agg: Am-c; Mez; Sep.
- Amel: Bell; Caus; Chin; Mur-ac; Ol-an; *Phyt*; *Pod*; Pru-sp.

TEETH, biting
- Mouth, empty, with: Cocl.
- Suddenly, involuntarily: Ap.

Black: Chin; Flu-ac; Kre; *Merc*; STAP.
- Spots, in: Kre; Scil.

Blowing nose agg: Thu.

Blunt: Am-c; Mez; Ran-sc; Rob; Sul-ac.

Brushing agg: Bry; Coc-c; *Lach*; Stap.

Bursting: Sabi.

Caries: See Decay.

Chatter: Lach; Nux-v; Radm.
- Coldness, internal with: Radm.
- Fear, from: Elap.
- Nervous: Kali-p.
- Sleep, in: Pul.
- Speak, on attempting to: Cocl.
- Trembling, inward with: Ant-t.

Cheek, rubbing amel: *Merc*; Pho.

Clench, inclination, to: Hyo; Lyc; Merc-i-f; *Phyt*; Pod.

Coated, as if: Colch; Dios; *Pho*.

Coition
- Agg: Daph.
- Amel: Cam.

Cold: Carb-v; Mez; Nit-ac; Pho-ac; Rhe; Spig; Sele.
- Air, coming from, as if: Rat.
- Edge, at: Gamb.
- Tips: Ol-an.

Cold things
- Agg: Ant-c; Arg-n; Hep; *Kali-c*; Lach; Merc-i-f; *Nat-m*; Rhod; *Rhus-t*; Sep; Stap; Thu.
  - not cold drinks: Con.

TEETH, cold things
- Amel: Bism; *Bry*; Chim; Clem; *Cof*; Fer; Nat-s; *Pul*.
- Hot, or agg: Carb-v; Merc; Merc-i-f; Lach; Syph.
- Rinsing with water amel: Rum.

Colds agg: Mag-c; Sep.

Crawling: Bar-c; Cham.

Crumbling: Euphor; Med; Plant; Stap; Thu.

Cupped, children, in: Syph.

Decay, caries, hollow: Ant-c; Bell; Bor; *Calc*; Cham; Euphor; Flu-ac; *Kre*; Lach; Merc; Mez; Nat-c; Plb; Sep; Sil; *Stap*; Syph.
- Children, in: Calc-p; *Kre*; Stap.
- Diabetes, in: Sul-ac.
- Gums, edge at: Syph; Thu.
- Long too, as if: Hep.
- Rapid: Flu-ac; *Kre*; Sep.
- Roots, at: Flu-ac; Thu.
- Sides: Mez; Stap; Thu.

Dental
- Extraction
  - convulsions after+: Buf.
  - persistent bleeding+: Pho.
- Operations after: Alum; *Arn*; Calend; Ham; Merc-i-f; Nux-v; Stap; Tril.

Dwarfed: Syph.

Eating
- Agg: Ant-c; Chim; Kali-c; Merc; Stap.
- Amel: Cham; Ign; Ip; Plant+; *Rhod*; Spig.
- Dinner amel: Rum.

TEETH

Edge on: Calc; Chio; Dig; Grat+; Iris; Lyc; Merc-i-f; Rob; Sul-ac.

Elongated, as if: Alu; Ant-t; Ars+; Berb; Caus; Cham; Colo+; Lach; Mag-c; Merc; Merc-i-f; Mez; Plant+; Sil+.
- Dull, and: Mez.

Enamel, deficient: *Calc-f*; Flu-ac; Sil.

Exertion agg: Chin.

Extending to ear or face: Alu; Ant-c; Cham; Kali-bi; Lach; Mang; *Merc*; Mez; Plant; Pul; Rhod.
- Finger tips, to: Cof.

Fistula: Caus+; Flu-ac; Nat-m; Stap.

Food, touch, on agg: Mag-m.

Fruits agg: Nat-c; Nat-s.

Grinding: Ap; *Ars*; BELL; Cic; *Cina*; Crot-h; Cup; Hell; Hyo; Lyc; *Phyt*; Pod; Sul; Ver-a; Zin.
- Convulsions, during: Buf; Cof; Hyo.
- Frightful: Plb.
- Sleep, in: Ars; Bell; Calc; Cann; CINA; Ign; Tub.
  - sitting posture, in: Ant-c.

Heavy: Flu-ac; Ver-a.

Hollow: See Decay.

Hot things agg: Calc; Dros.

Ice water amel: Clem; Cof; Fer.

Into, pains go: Chin; Fer; Kali-bi; Merc; Mez; Stap; Thu.

Itching: Kali-c.

Jammed: Lach; Merc-i-f; Tub.

Jerking: Calc; Cham; Euphr; Ip; *Merc*; Pul; Rhod.
- Tobacco chewing, smoking on: Bry.

Large, too: Berb; Calc; Sil.

Long too: See Elongated.

Loose: Am-c; Bor; Bry; Calc-f; Carb-an; Carb-v; *Caus*; HYO; MERC; *Merc-c*; *Nit-ac*; Nux-v; Psor; Rhus-t; Sil; Zin.

Lying
- Agg: Aran; Benz-ac; Rat; Sep.
- Amel: Spig.
- Painful side on amel: Hypr.

Menses agg: Bar-c; Calc; *Carb-v*; *Cham*; Cof; Lach; Sep; Stap.
- Before agg: Ant-c.

Music agg: Pho-ac.

Night agg: *Cham*; *Grap*; *Lyc*; Mag-c; MERC; Rat; Sul.

Noise agg: Cof; Plant; Ther.

Numb: Chin; Dul; *Pho*; Plat; Rhus-t.

Oily, as if: Aesc.

Out of place, as if: Syph.

Pain ceases suddenly agg 2 or 3 hours after: Rhod.

Pegged: Kre.

Picking
- Agg: Pul; Sang.
- Amel: Bell; Cep; Pho-ac.

Pregnancy agg: Chin; Kali-bi; *Kre*; Lyss; Mag-c; Nux-m; *Sep*.

Pressure
- Cold hand, of amel: Rhus-t.
- Hard amel: Stap.

TEETH

Pulled, as if: Calc; Chim; Mez; Nux-m; Pru-sp; Rhus-t.
- Cold water amel+: Chim.

Quivering: Phys.

Radiating pain: Kali-bi; MERC; Mez; Nux-v; Stap.
- Glands, swelled with: Kali-bi.

Rough: Phys.

Saliva flows, during pain: Cham; Dul; Merc; Nat-m+.

Salty things
- Agg: Carb-v.
- Amel: *Carb-an*; Mag-c.

Screwed together, as if: Euphor; Stro+.

Sensitive, tender: Gel; Lach; Sul.

Serrated: Med.

Smoking
- Agg: Bry; Clem.
- Amel: Bor; Spig.

Smooth, as if: Aesc; Colch; Dios; Pho; Sul-io.

Soft, feel: Calc-p; Caus; Med; Nit-ac; Sul-io.

Sordes, on: Ail; Ars; Bap; Bry; Chin; Hyo; *Pho*; *Pho-ac*; *Rhus-t.*
- Black: *Chin*; Con; *Flu-ac.*
- Brown: Bap.
- Slimy: Rhus-t.

Sticky: Arg-m; Crot-h; Lach; Psor; Sang; Syph.

Sucking
- Agg: Bov; Carb-v; Chin; Mang; Nux-m.
- Amel: Cep; Clem.
- In air amel: Mez.

Suckling when agg: *Chin*.

TEETH

Sweets agg: Merc-i-f; Mur-ac; Nat-c.

Tartar: Ars; Ascl; Bacil; Calc-ren; Calend; Carb-s; Chin; Epip; Merc; Plb; Thu.

Tea agg: Sele.

Temples, to: Merc; Mez.

Tension, in: Pul.

Touch of
- Food agg: Mag-m.
- Tongue agg: *Ant-c*; Merc; Mez.

Warm, as if: Flu-ac.

Wisdom teeth, eruption from agg: Calc; Flu-ac; Mag-c; Sil.

Worm, in: Syph.
- Wriggling+: Kali-io.

Yellow: Cep; Iod; Lyc; Med; Merc; Sil; Thu.

TEMPERATURE

Change of agg: See CHANGE OF TEMPERATURE agg.

Extremes of AGG: Ant-c; Carb-v; Caus; Ip; Lach; Sul-ac; Syph.

TEMPLES: *Anac*; *Arg-m*; BELL; CHIN; Cyc; Glo; Kali-c; Kre; Lyc; Nux-m; Par; Pho-ac; Plat; *Pul*; Rhus-t; Sabi; Thu; Verb; Zin.

Biting, chewing agg: Zin.

Blow, on: Lyc; Plat; Sul-ac.

Bolt passed through, as if: Ham.

Burning: Colo; Lyc; Mez; *Pho*.

Cold: Berb.

Coughing
- Agg: Lyc.
- Holds, while: Petr.

TEMPLES
Crushed, as if+: Pho-ac.
Cutting+: Nat-p.
Empty sensation: Cyc.
Finger tips, pressing, as if: Epip.
Hammering (L): Ham.
Heavy: Zin.
Menses agg+: Lyc.
Neck and face, to: Tarn.
Plug, driven in, as if+: Sul-ac.
Screwed, together+: Lyc.
Shocks, blows: See Blow.
Squeezed in visc, as if+: Dios.
Stomach pain, with: Lith.
Temple, to: Chin.
Throbbing: Aur; *Bell*; Glo; Zin-chr.
Twitch: Chin; Psor; Spig.
Veins: Ars; Cup; Flu-ac; Glo; Ham; Pul; Sang; Vip; Zin.
 • Swollen: Ars; Cub; Glo; Sang.
Wet weather agg: Bor.

TEMPESTUOUS ACTION: *Aco*; Glo; Tab.

TENACIOUS: See DISCHARGES, sticky.

TENDER: See DELICATE and PAIN, bruised.

TENDO ACHILLES: Anac; Benz-ac; Kali-bi; *Mur-ac*; Sep; Val; *Zin*.
Contracted: Cimi.
Cramp: Caus.
Painful: Benz-ac; Kali-bi.
 • Stepping, on: Rhod.
 • Swelled: Kali-bi.
Short, as if: Dios.

TENDO ACHILLES
Stiff: Cimi; Sul.
 • Walking, when: Ant-t.
Walking agg: Am-m; Ant-t; Cinb; Colch.

TENDONS: See FIBROUS TISSUE.
Crackling, in: Kali-m.
Flexure: Rut.
Injured: Anac.
Jerking, in: Sul-ac.
Pains, in: Rhus-t; Sabi.
Sheath, of: Bry; Iod; Rhus-t.
Swollen, hard: Calc-f.
Tense, short: Am-m; Caus; Dios; Grap; Guai; Nat-m; Ol-j.

TENESMUS: See PAIN, pressing down.

TENSION, tightness: Am-m; Asaf; Bar-c; Bell; *Bry*; Cact; Caus; Colo; Con; Kali-m; Lyc; Mag-p; Mos+; *Nat-m*; Nux-v; Par; PHO; Plat; PUL; Ran-b; RHUS-T; Senec; Sep; Stro; Sul; Verb; Vio-o; Visc.
All over body: Ars; Bar-c; Cact; Grap; Sul.

TERROR: Aco; Spo; Stram; Tarn.
Sudden: Glo.

TESTES: Arg-m; Arn; *Aur*; Clem; Iod; Merc; Nux-v; *Pul*; Rhod; Rhus-t; Sep; Spo; Stap.
Alternately: Berb; Rhod.
Atrophy: Ant-c; Iod; Kali-io; Sabal.
 • Sexual excess, after: Stap.
Bruised: Thu.
Burning, heat: Nit-ac; Nux-v; Pul.

TESTES

Cancer: Spo.
Coition agg: Mag-m; Pho-ac.
Cold: *Agn*; Merc.
Cramp: Psor.
- Emission, after: Caps.

Crushed: Arg-m; Ox-ac; *Rhod*.
Drawn up: See Retraction.
Enlarged, swelled: Bro; *Clem*; Dul; Mez; *Pul*; Rhod; Spo.
- Alternately: Ol-an.
- Pain, griping with: Dul.
- Sexual passion, unrequited, from: Iod.

Hanging low: Calc; Clem; Pul; Pyro; Sul.
- Right: Crot-t.

Indurated: Aur; Bro+; *Clem*; CON; Iod; Med; *Rhod*; Sil; *Spo*; Sul+.
- Jarring, slight agg: Bro.
- Painless: Bro.
- Small: Iod; Pul; Sil; Spo; Tub.

Inflammed (orchitis): *Aco*; Arn; Bap; *Clem:* Con; Ham; PUL; Rhod; Rhus-t; Spo.
- Epididymis: Pul; Rhod; Spo.
- Mumps, after: Jab; Plb; *Pul*.
- Sitting on cold pavement from: Pul.

Neuralgia: Berb; Ham; Zin.
- Nausea, with: Ham.
- Supro-orbital pain, with: Lycps.

Nodules: Psor; Syph.
Pulled up: Arg-n; Berb; Cic.
- As if: Ol-an.

Pressing: Caus; Pul; Zin.
Pressure of clothing agg: Arg-n.

TESTES

Retraction: Arg-n; Aur; Berb+; Cic; Clem; Ol-an; Plb; Rhod; Sabal; Zin.
- External ring, to: Cic.
- Left: Crot-t.
- Painful: Sabal.

Sexual excitement, suppressed, agg: Mag-m.
Softening: Caps; Sul-io.
Squeezing: Spo.
Stitching: Caus; Spo.
Throbbing: Ox-ac; Spo.
Tubercles: Iod; Pul; Sil; Spo; Tub.
Tumour: See SARCOCELE.
- Indolent: Tarn.

Undescended in children: Thyr.
Undeveloped in pining boys: Aur.
Urinating
- Agg: Polyg.
- Amel: Kob.

Walking agg: Zin.

TETANUS: Bell; Cic; Cocl; Cup; Hyd-ac; Hyo; Hypr; Ign; Nux-v; Op; Passif; Petr; Stram; Stry; Tab; Ver-v.

Lasting for days: Latro.
Tobacco swallowing, from: Ip.

TETANY: Calc; Cocl; Grap; Lyc; Merc; Plb; Sec; Sol-n.

Cold agg+: Thyr.

TETTER: See ERUPTIONS.

THICK, thickness: See DISCHARGES, Thick.

THIGHS: Ars; Chin; Clem; Guai; *Merc*; *Nat-m*; Phyt; Plb; Pyro; Sep.

Anterior: Anac; Bels; Cimi; Spo; Xanth.
- Cramps, before menses: Dict; Xanth.
- Weak: Lapp.

Inner: Petr; Rhod; Stan; Sul.
- Red and swollen: Stram.

Middle, knee to: Ind.

Outer: Caus; Helo; *Pho-ac*; Phyt.

Posterior (See SCIATICA): Colo; Gnap; Mang; *Rhus-t*; Sul; Zin.

Bandaged: Plat.

Blue: Bism.

Boils: Hyo; Ign.

Bones painful: Euphor; Guai; Rut.
- Dislocated, as if while sitting: Ip.

Broken, as if: Rut; Sul; Tub.

Change of weather agg: Phyt.

Cold: Berb; Spo.
- Colic, with: Calc.
- Menses, after: Coll; Colch.

Contraction: Rhus-t.
- Walking, while: *Nux-v*.

Cramps: Ant-t; Chel; Colo; *Cup*; Meny; Naj; Sul.
- Sitting agg: Mag-m; Meny.

Crossing agg: Agar.

Drops of water flowing down+: Aco.

Emaciation: Calc; Nit-ac; Sele.

Excoriation, easy on walking: Aeth.

Formication: Guai; Nat-c; Pall; *Sec*.

THIGHS

Itching: Bar-c; Calc; Sul; Zin+.

Menses agg: Mag-m; Meny; Xanth.

Painful: Anac; Plb; Pyro; Rhus-t.

Pains, into: Cham; *Stap*; Xanth.
- Ovaries settling in+: Sabal.

Pulsation (R): Ver-v.

Racking, violent in marrow: Naj.

Shocks: Agar.

Short, as if: Guai; Kre.

Sitting agg: Lyc; Mag-m; Pyro.

Stools agg: Rhus-t.

Sweat: Amb; Ars; Thu.
- Cold: Caps; Merc; Sep; Spo.

Tension: Am-m; Caus; Guai; Mag-m; Pul.
- Sitting amel: Guai.

Tingling: Merc.

Twitching: Kali-c; Kali-m.

Urination agg: Berb.

Water, warm, running down: Bor.

Weak: Cocl; Con; Eup-p; *Gel*; Lapp; *Mur-ac*; Nat-s; Stan; Urt.

THIN: See DISCHARGES, watery.

THINGS LOOK STRANGE: See STRANGE and BEWILDERED.

THINKING

Agg: Par.

About his own wrongs agg: Iod.

Bad act, has comitted, as if: Cyc.

Difficult: *Anac*; Bap; Berb; Con; *Gel*; *Lyc*; Nat-c; NUX-M;

THINKING, difficult ..
  NUX-V; Old; *Op*; *Pho*; PHO-AC; Pic-ac; Sep; Zin.
Disease, is incurable: Cact; Lac-c; Lil-t.
Duty, her, not done: Cyc.
Everyone is looking at her: Meli.
Fluids of agg: Lyss.
Himself, too little: Kob; Lac-c.
His own sufferings, of: Sabal.
Of it AGG: *Amb*; Arg-n; Aur; Bar-c; Calc-p; Caus; Colch; Gel; Helo; Lycps; Med; Nat-s; *Nit-ac*; Nux-m; *Ox-ac*; *Saba*; Spig; Spo; Sumb; Thyr; Tub.
  AMEL: *Cam*; *Cic*; Hell.
THINNESS, spare habit: Amb; Arg-n; Calc-p; Kre; Mag-p; Nat-m; Nit-ac; Nux-m; Nux-v; Pho; Psor; Rat; Sanic; Sars; Sec; Sul.
THIRST: Acet-ac; ACO; Arg-n; *Arn*; ARS; *Bell*; BRY; *Calc*; Calc-s; *Caps*; Caus; CHAM; CHIN; *Cina*; Croc; *Dig*; Eup-p; Hell; Iod; *Lyc*; MERC; NAT-M; Op; *Pho*; RHUS-T; Sec; *Sep*; *Sil*; STRAM; SUL; Tarn; VER-A.
Alternating, with aversion to drink: Berb.
Beer, for+: Petr.
But drinks
  • **Aversion, to:** Ars; *Hell*; Nux-v; *Stram*.
  • **Causes shuddering+:** Caps.
  • **Fears to:** Lach.
Chill
  • **Before:** Ars; Carb-v; *Chin*; *Eup-p*; Pul.

THIRST, chill
  • **During:** Ap; Arn; BRY; *Caps*; Cina; Eup-p; IGN; NAT-M; Nux-v; Pyro; Sep; Sil; Tub; Ver-a.
  • **After:** Ars; Chin; Dros; Pul.
Cold drinks, for: Aco; ARS; Bism; Bry; Calc; Chin; Diph; Dul+; Merc-c; PHO; Rhus-t; Thyr+; VER-A.
  • **Coldness of body, with:** Carb-v.
  • **Icy:** Mag-p+; *Pho*; Rut.
  • **Night, at:** Calc.
Consumption, in: Nit-ac.
Headache, with: Mag-m; Pulex+.
Heat, during: Aco; Ars; Bell; Bry; Eup-p; Nat-m; Nux-v; Tub.
Knows not for what, all drinks are offensive: Arn.
Large quantity, for: Ars; *Bry*; Lil-t; Nat-m; Pho; Sul; Ver-a.
  • **Long intervals, at:** *Bry*.
  • **Often+:** Coc-c.
Little and often, for: Aco; Ant-t; Ap; ARS; Bell; Chin; Hyo; *Lyc*; Rhus-t.
Morning: Nit-ac.
Mouth
  • **Bitter, with:** Con; Pic-ac.
  • **Heat, in+:** Hypr.
Much, eats little: Dig; Sep; Sul.
Nightly: Calc; Cham; Sil.
Pains, with: Cham; Nat-c.
Stools, after: Caps.
Sweat, with: Ars; Chin; Nat-m; Stram; Ver-a.

THIRST

Symptoms, severe, before: Lil-t.

Unquenchable+: Jat; Sec.

Vertigo, with: Ox-ac.

Violent, burning: Acet-ac; *Aco*; *Ars*; Bry; Colo; Cup; Eup-p; Merc; Merc-c; Nux-v; Pho; Pyro; Saba; Tarn; VER-A.

THIRSTLESS, aversion to water, drinks: Aco+; Aeth; Ant-t; AP; Bell; Canth; *Chin*; Colch; Fer; GEL; *Hell*; Hyo; Ign; Ip; Meny; NUX-M; Pho-ac; PUL; *Saba*; Sele; Sep; STRAM.

For days: Calad.

Heat, during: *Ap*; Carb-v; Cham; Cina; *Gel*; Hell; Ign; Ip; Nux-m; *Pul*; Saba; Sep.

THOUGHT

Buried, in: Carb-an; *Hell*; *Mez*; *Nux-m*; *Sul*.
- As to what would become of him: Nat-m.

Horrid: Psor.

Menses, during: Mur-ac.

Strange, pregnancy during: Lyss.

Unpleasant subject, fixed on+: Cocl.

Vanishing, of: Manc; Nit-ac+; Ol-an+.

THREAD sensation (See PAIN fine, and HAIR): Lach; Osm; Plat; Saba; *Val*.

Stretched, head to arm etc.: Lach.

THREATENING: Hep; Stram; Tarn.

THROAT (including inner mouth): *Ap*; Arg-n; Aru-t; *Bar-c*; BELL; Caus; Gel; *Hep*; *Kali-bi*; Lac-c; LACH; *Lyc*; MERC; *Merc-c*; Merc-cy; *Merc-i-f*; *Merc-i-r*; *Nit-ac*; Nux-v; *Pho*; Phyt; Pul; *Rhus-t*; Sul.

Right: Agar; Am-c; *Ap*; *Bell*; Bry; Carb-ac; *Ign*; Kali-m; Kre; LYC; *Merc*; Merc-d; *Merc-i-f*; Phyt; Sang; Stan; Sul; Syph; Tarn.
- To left: Ap; BELL; Calc; Caus; LYC; MERC-I-F; Pho; Saba; Sang; Sul-ac; Syph.

Left: Calc; Caus; Crot-h; Diph; Fer; Hep; Kali-c; Lac-c; LACH; Mar-v; Merc-c; Merc-i-r; Naj; Petr; Pho-ac; *Rhus-t*; Saba; *Sep*; *Sil*; Til.
- In A.M.: Cimi; Rhus-t.
- To right: Calc; LACH; Merc-i-r; RHUS-T; Saba; Stan.

Air
- Feels cold: Ol-an.
- Amel: Diph.

Alternating sides: *Alu*; Arn; Cocl; Colo; LAC-C; Pod; Pul; Sul.

Back, of: Aco; Cocl; Kali-c; *Merc*; Nit-ac; Rhus-t.

Angina (simple sore throat): Aco; Arg-n; Bap; Bell; Ign; Lach; Lyc; Merc; Merc-c; Merc-i-f; Pho; Rhus-t; Sep; Sil; Sul-ac.
- Chilliness, with: Mag-p.
- Colds agg: Sil.

THROAT, angina
- Diphtheria, after: Phyt.
- Morning, in: Rhus-t.
- Nervous: Mag-p.
- Operation, after: Fer-p.
- Singers: Fer-p.
- Smokers: Caps.
- Speakers: Coll; Kali-io.
- Winter agg: Mez.

Apple core, choke pear etc. as if: Aral; Merc; Nit-ac; Pall; *Phyt*; Plant; Ver-a.

Bitter: Chin; Con; Kre; *Pho*; Sil; Spo; Ver-a.
- Food, swallowing, on: Kre.

Boiling water rising in, as if: Stram.

Burning, heat, in: Aco; ARS; *Aru-t*; Canth; Caps; Caus; Cub+; Euphr; Iris; Lac-c; Lach; Lyc; Mez; MERC-C; Nux-v; Oenan; Petr; *Pho*; Phyt; Ran-b; *Sang*; *Sul*; *Ver-a*.
- Air cold amel: Sang.
- Eating, drinking when: Par.
- Pepper, like: Radm.
- Swallowing
  - compels: Strop.
  - when: Ars; *Bar-c*; Hep.
- Sweets agg: Sang.
- Vapour, hot, as of: Merc.

Chest, to: Sang.

Choking, constriction, spasm, narrow as if: Alu; Arg-m; Bap; BELL; Cact; Canth; *Caus*; *Cham*; *Hyo*; IGN; Lac-c; LACH; *Laur*; *Lyc*; Lycps; Merc-c; Merc-i-r; Mos; NAJ; Nux-v; Pho; *Plb*; Rum; *Spo*; Stram; Strop; *Sul*; *Sumb*; VER-A.

THROAT, choking
- Ascends speaking when: Manc.
- Bending head backwards, amel: Hep; Lach.
- Breathing, when: Chel.
- Contraction of fingers and toes, alternating with: Asaf.
- Cough, inclination, with: Cocl.
- Eat, when attempting to: Zin-val.
- Goitre, from: Grap.
  - exophthalmus, with: Meph.
- Hawking, when: Amb; *Arg-n*; Nux-v.
- Large morsel, as if from: Chel.
- Sleep, during: Lach; Spo; Val.
- Speaking when: Manc.
- Swallowing: Grap; Lyc; Mur-ac; Pul; *Stram*.
  - compels him to retch, while: *Grap*; Merc-c.
  - food: Carb-v; *Pul*.
  - hasty, as from: Chel.
  - liquid, drops of, when: Merc-c.
  - lump, as from, on empty: Grap.
  - urging to, with: Caps.
- Valve rolling and closing, as from: Fer.
- Walking
  - while: Nat-s.
  - amel: Dros.
- Warm drinks amel: Calc-f.
- Water, from: Bap; Bell; Canth; Hyo; Nat-m; Stram; Sumb.

THROAT, choking
- Word, every uttered with: Dros.
- Writing, while: Bar-c.

Closed, as if: Calc-f; Carb-v.
- Something by, preventing speech: Nat-p.

Clothes agg: *Kali-c*; *Lach*.
Clutches, at: Bell.
Coated feeling: Carb-v; *Pul*.
Cold
- Agg: Alu; *Ars*; Hep; Lac-c; Lob; LYC; Manc; Merc-i-r; Nux-v; Rhus-t; Saba; Sil; Syph.
- Amel (Heat agg): *Ap*; Arg-n; Calc; Diph; Ign; Kali-m; *Lach*; Merc-c; Merc-d; Merc-i-f; Pho; Phyt; Sang.
- Air
  - penetrating, as if: Ol-an.
  - wants: Diph.
- Drinks, seem warm: Nat-m.
- Warm, or amel: Lac-c.

Coldness: Cep; Cist; Kali-chl; Lyc; Ol-an.
- Peppermint, like: Sanic; Ver-a.

Colds agg: Bell; Cist; *Dul*; Lach; *Merc*; *Nux-v*.
Constriction: See Choking.
Coppery: Kali-bi; *Merc*.
Cotton, as if, in: Pho.
Coughing agg: Arg-m; Aru-t; Caps; Cist; Ol-an.
Cramps: Gel; Grap; Sars.
Crawling: *Carb-v*; *Kali-c*; Kali-m; Lach.
Cutting: Manc; Merc-c; Nit-ac.

THROAT, cutting
- Cold drinks agg: Manc.

Dark: Aesc; Ail; Arg-n; Bap; Crot-h; *Lach*; *Phyt*.
- Red: Arg-n; Bap; Cham; Merc-i-r.

Drinking
- Amel: Tell.
- Sips, in amel: Cist.
- water runs out, seems+: Ver-a.

Dry: Aco; *Aesc*; BELL; *Bry*; Calc; Caus; *Lyc*; *Merc*; *Mur-ac*; *Nat-m*; Nux-m; Petr; Pho; Pho-ac; Pul; Rhus-t; Saba; Sang; *Sep*; Stic; *Stram*; *Sul*; Sul-io; Thyr; *Ver-a*; Ver-v.
- But no thirst: See MOUTH.
- Singer's: Sang.
- Spot: Cist.
- Stiff, and+: Onos.
- Swallows, saliva constantly+: Cub.
- Thirst, with: Stram.

Ear, extending to: Gel+; Guai; Hep; Kali-bi; Kali-m; Lach; Merc; Merc-c; Merc-d; Phys+; Phyt; Sang; Stap.
- Yawning, on: Hep.

Eating amel: Benz-ac; Tell.
Empty: See Hollow.
Enlarged, as if: Sanic.
Eructation agg: Phys.
Exertion agg: Caus; Lac-c.
Fissures, cracks: Aru-t; Bell; Elap; Kali-bi.
Food lodges in swallowing when: Arg-n; Ars; Bar-c; Caus; Chin; Grap; Ign; Kali-c; *Lyc*; *Nat-m*; PUL; Sul.

THROAT

THROAT, food lodges
- As if+: Pall.
- Returns through nose: Aru-t; *Cocl*; Gel; Hyo; Lach; *Lyc*; Merc; Op; *Pho*; Sil; Sul-ac.

Foreign body, as if, in: Ant-c; Aral.

Full: Arn.
- Speaking agg: Iod.

Glistening, glazed: Ap; Kali-bi; LAC-C; Nat-m+; Petr; Pho; Stram.

Grasps, the: *Aco*; Aru-t; Asaf; Cep; Dros; Iod; *Naj*; Pho.

Gray: Phyt.

Hair in (See HAIR, sensation and THREAD sensation): Kali-bi; Saba; Sil; Sul; Val.
- Back of: Coc-c.

Hanging, loose, as if, in: Alu; Berb; Iod; *Lach*; Merc; *Pho*; Plat; Saba; Sul; Val.
- Hyoid bone, near: Pall.

Hawks: See HAWKING.

Hollow, empty: Calc-p; Flu-ac; Iris; Lach; Lob; Phyt; Rum; Sanic; Xanth.
- Swallowing, on: Lyc.

Hot something rises, in: Caps; *Merc*.
- Fright from, anxiety with: Hypr.

Inflamed: Aco; Alu; Am-m; Ap; Arg-n; Bap; *Bar-c*; Bell; Bro; Bry; *Caps*; Cham; Chin; Cocl; Cof; Dul; Fer-p; HEP; Ign; *Lach*; Lyc; Mang; *Merc*; Nit-ac; Pho; Pul; *Rhus-t*; Petr; Sul; Sul-ac; Ver-a.
- Painless: Bap.

THROAT

Irritation agg: Coc-c.

Itching: Ap; Aru-t; Caus; Con; Nux-v.
- Coughing, when: Zin-io.

Lifting agg: Caus; *Sil*.

Lump, ball, plug, globus: Asaf; Coc-c+; Hep; IGN; *Lach*; *Lob*; *Lyc*; Naj; Nat-m; Par; Psor; *Pul*; Saba; Sep; Ust.
- Coughing
  - agg: Lach.
  - amel: Kali-c.
- Eructation amel: Mag-m.
- Hard: Nux-m.
- Hawks: Merc-i-r.
- Hot: Lach; Phyt.
- Left side: Lach; Sil.
- Rises and is swallowed again: Alo; Asaf; Bar-c; *Calc*; Cam; Chel; Con; Kali-c; Lac-c; *Lach*; Lil-t; Plb; Spo; *Rum*.
- Rolling, and: Fer.
- Sleep, in: Lach; Nux-v.
- Soft: Lach.
- Something, in: Merc.
- Soreness, with: Nat-m.
- Speech, preventing: Nat-p.
- Sticks, and: Lyc.
- Swallowed, as if: Phys.
- Swallowing
  - empty agg: Fer; Grap.
  - impeding: Lob.

Lying on back amel: Lach; Spo.

Menses, during agg: See MENSES, throat agg.

Morsel, as if, in: Saba.

Mouldy, taste, in: Mar-v.

THROAT

Mucous, constant, in+: Eucal.
- Glairy+: Pall.

Narrow, as if: See Choking.

Neck and shoulders, to: Kali-bi.

Nose, ascending into: *Bro*; Lac-c; Merc; Sep.

Numb: Bap.

Odour, from: Petr.

Open, wide, as if: Bar-m.

Painful; See Angina and Raw.

Paralysis: See SWALLOWING, noisy.

Pepper, as if, in: Radm.

Pressure toward: Asaf.

Puffy: Arg-n; Lac-ac; Phyt.

Purple: Ap.

Raw, sore: *Arg-m*; *Arg-n*; ARU-T; Bap; *Bell*; Calc; Carb-v; Caus; Chin; Ign; Lach; *Lyc*; Merc; Merc-c; *Nit-ac*; NUX-V; *Pho*; Radm.
- Clergyman's: Alu; Aru-t.
- Onions from: Alu.
- Streak: Ol-an.

Rough, scraping: Anac; Arg-m; *Chin*; Mez; *Nux-v*; Sul; Ver-a.
- Sing, attempting to, on: Agar.
- Talking agg: Seneg.

Sipping water amel: Cist.

Skin, hanging, as if: Saba.

Slimy: Am-m+; Bell; Caps; Chel; *Lach*; Merc; Petr; PUL.

Smokers of: Arg-n; Caps+; Nat-m.

Smoking agg: Caps; Coc-c; Tarx.

Sneezing agg: Hypr; *Pho*; Poth.

THROAT

Soppy: Sul-ac.

Sore: See Angina, and Raw.

Spasms: See Choking.

Speaking
- Agg: Aco; Alu; Bar-c; Bry; Dul; Ign; *Kali-io*; Mang; Merc; Pho; Rhus-t; Sul.
- Amel: Hep.

Splinter, stick, as of a: Alu; *Arg-n*; *Hep*; Ign; Kali-c; Nat-m; *Nit-ac*; *Phyt*; Sul; Thyr.
- Across: Thyr.
- Breathing agg: Arg-m.
- Eructation agg: Arg-n.
- Neck, moving agg: Arg-n.
- Speaking agg: Mag-c.
- Swallowing
  - agg: Arg-n; Mag-c.
  - amel: Kali-bi.

Spongy: Cist.

Spot, dry, sore etc.: Ap; Caus; Cimi; *Cist*; Con; Crot-h; *Hep*; *Hyo*; Lac-c; LACH; Lith; Merc-cy; *Nat-m*; Nit-ac; *Pho*; Phyt; *Sil*.

Sticks, full of+: Alu.

Sticky, clammy, pasty: Aesc; Bap; Chel; KALI-BI; *Lach*; Myr; Pho-ac; Pul; Sec; Sul-ac.

Stiff, rigidity: Chel; Lach; Merc-i-r; *Rhus-t*.

Stooping agg: Caus.

Sweet
- Agg: Bad; Lach; Sang; Spo.
- Amel: Ars.

Swelled: Ail; AP; Hep; *Lach*; MERC; Merc-c; Nux-v; Phyt; Spo.

THROAT, swelled
- As if: Lach; Pul.

Taste in: Nux-v; Sil.
- Bitter, low down: Kre.
- Coughing agg: See Hawking.
- Eating agg: Hell.
- Hawking agg: Mar-v; Nux-v.
- Mouldy: Mar-v.

Tension: Merc; Merc-i-f; Rhus-t; Senec.
- Yawning agg: Arg-m.

Thread, hanging as if: Coc-c; Pulex+; Saba; Val.
- Salivation, with: Val.
- Vomiting, with: Val.

Tickling (See itching internal): Stic.
- Coughing agg: Zin-io.
- Lachrymation, with: Cocl.
- Lungs, down: Ver-a.

Tongue protruding agg: Kali-bi+; Saba.

Turning about, in: Lach.

Ulcers: Ap; *Ars*; Bap; Hep; Kali-bi; Kali-io; Lach; Merc; *Merc-c*; Mur-ac; *Nit-ac*; Nux-v; Rhus-t; Sul-ac; THU.

Upward through or from: Aco; Ars; BRO; Calc; Carb-v; Fer; Kali-bi; *Kali-c*; Lac-c; *Lyc*; Merc; Nat-m; Nux-v; Pho; *Sep*.

Vapour, in: Ap; Fer; Ol-an; Sul.
- Coughing, when: Ol-an.
- Sulphur, as of+: Pul.

Vesicles, full of: Canth.

Voice, overuse agg: Bar-c.

Wash leather: Phyt.

Weak: Lac-c; Stan.

White washed: Sul-ac.

THROAT
Winter agg: Mez.

Worm, wriggling in: Hypr; Pul.

Yawning
- Agg: Arg-m; Arg-n; Nat-c; Zin.
- Amel: Manc.

THROAT EXTERNAL: Bell; Lyc.

Right: Caus; Flu-ac; Lyc; Merc; Nat-c; Nat-m; Nit-ac; Sil.

Left: Asaf; Calc; Con; Sul.

Alternating sides: Am-m; Calc-p.

Carotid arteries, throbbing of: Aur; *Bell*; Cact; Chin; Glo; Pru-sp; Spig; Ver-v.

Clothing agg: See Sensitive.

Cold: Spo.
- Wind blowing on, as if: Old.

Constriction: Lach; Stram.

Glands: Am-m; *Bar-c*; Bell; Bro; Calc; Calc-f; Calc-io; Calc-p; *Cham*; Grap; Hep; *Ign*; *Iod*; Lach; Lyc; Nat-m; Rhus-t; Spo; Stap; Sul; Vip; Zin-io.
- Air passing through, breathing on, as if: Spo.
- Right: Ars; Kali-c; *Merc*; Nit-ac; Sil; Zin-io.

Itching: Alu.

Larynx, motion of: Stram.

Numb: Spo.

Red: Bell; Grap; Sul; Ver-a.

Sensitive to touch, pressure, clothes: Ant-t; Ap; Bap; Crot-h; Crot-t; Lac-c; LACH; Merc-c; Nux-v.

Swallowing agg: Zin.

Sweat: Mang; Rhus-t; Stan.

THROAT EXTERNAL
Swelling: Lyc; Rhus-t; Tarn.
- Goitre like: Vip.
- Speaking loudly, when: Iod.

Tension: Nux-m.
Tumours: Bar-c; Bro.
Twitch: Agar.
Uncovering AGG: Hep; Kali-c; Nux-v; Rhus-t; Scil; Sil; Zin.

THROAT PIT:
Ap; Arg-m; *Cham*; Chlor; Hep; Kali-bi; Pho; *Rum*; Sang; *Sep*; Zin-chr.

Constriction: *Bro*.
Crawling, formication, causing cough: Sang.
Fullness: Lach.
Irritation: Ign; Rum; Sang.
Lump, in: Lob.
Painful: Caus; Lach.
- Hawking, when: Caus.

Pressure: *Bro*; Calc; *Lach*.
Sore: Ap; Arg-n.
- Back, of: Lach.

Stitching: Spo.
Swollen: Lach.

THROBBING: See PULSATION.
THROMBOSIS:
Ap; Arn; Ars; Both; Ham; Lach.

THROWS things away:
Agar; Cina; Colo; Dul; Kre; *Stap*; Tarn; Thu; Tub.

Bugs, in handfuls: Ars.

THRUSTS, stings, as of:
Ap; Arn; Cina; Plat; Rut; Sul-ac; Thu.

THUMBS
Aching: Sang.
Ball, with: Sang.
Bent, backwards: Cam; Lyc; Merc.
Clenched: Cup; Hyo; Merc.
- Convulsions, with+: Stan.
- Palms, into: Hell.

Cramp
- Contraction, index finger with: Cyc.
- writing, when: Mur-ac.

Lame: Calc-s.
Painful: Anac; Kre; Manc; Ox-ac.
Sprained, as if: Grap; Pru-sp.
Stiff: Kre.
- Writing, while: Kali-c.

Sucking: Calc-p; Nat-m; Sil.
Swelling: Sang.
Ulcer, turning yellow: Kali-io.
Up, arms to shoulder: Cedr; Naj.

THUNDERSTORMS
AGG (See CHANGE OF TEMPERATURE agg): Nat-c; Nat-p; *Pho*; Psor; Rhod; Syph.
AMEL: Rhus-r.

THYROID: See GOITRE.
Dysfunction: Calc.
Pinched, as if: Nat-ar.

TIBIAE:
Agar; *Asaf*; Calc; Carb-v; Cinb; Lach; Merc; Mez; *Pho*; Phyt; Pul; Stil.

Burning: Zin.
Caries: Sil.
Cold: Mos.
Coppery, spots: Nit-ac.
Exostosis: Merc-c; Nit-ac.
Lying agg: Pul.

TIBIAE

Node: Calc-f; Cinb+; Sul-io.

Osteo sarcoma, in middle: Syph.

Pain, in: Cast-eq+; *Lach*; Pho; Phyt; Stil; Sul-io.
- Digging: Mang.
- Spots: Amb.
- Stretching, while: Aur.
- Throat, with: Lach.

Periosteum+: Mang.

Spongy: Guai.

Sticking: Pul.

Syphilitic: Merc; Phyt; Stil; Sul-io.

Ulcer, on: Flu-ac.

TIC: Arg-n; Ars; Hyo; Laur; Lyc; Ran-b; Sep; Tarn; Zin.

TICKLING: See ITCHING, internal.

Amel: Sep.

TIGHTNESS: See TENSION.

TIME agg and amel

Morning
- AGG (4 A.M. to 9 A.M.): Agar; AM-M; ANT-T; Arg-m; Ars-io; AUR; Bor; Bov; *Bry*; CALC; Calc-p; Cann; Carb-an; *Carb-v*; Castr; Cham; CHEL; Cina; Con; *Croc*; Echi; Elap; Hep; *Ign*; Kali-bi; Kali-c; Kali-n; LACH; Naj; Nat-m; *Nat-s*; *Nit-ac*; NUX-V; Onos; Petr; PHO; Pho-ac; *Pod*; Pul; *Rhod*; RHUS-T; Rum; Saba; SCIL; *Sep*; Spig; SUL; *Val*.
- AMEL: Chel; Merc; Zin.

TIME, morning
- Bed, in AGG: Alo; *Amb*; *Am-m*; Bry; Con; *Kali-c*; *Lyc*; *Nux-v*; Pho; Sep; *Sul*.
- Evening, and AGG: Alu; Bov; *Calc*; Caus; Coc-c; *Grap*; *Kali-c*; Lach; *Lyc*; PHO; Psor; *Rhus-t*; Sang; SEP; *Stram*; *Stro*; *Thu*; Ver-a.
- One day, evening, next day: Eup-p; Lac-c.
- 6 A.M. AGG: Alo; *Alu*; Arn; Bov; Fer; *Hep*; Lyc; *Nux-v*; Sil; Sul; VER-A.
- 7 A.M. AGG: *Eup-p*; Hep; Nat-c; *Nux-v*; *Pod*; Sep.
- 8 A.M.
  - AGG: *Eup-p*; Nux-v.
  - to 12 Noon AGG: Cact; *Chin-s*; *Eup-p*; *Gel*; Nat-c; NAT-M; Nux-v; Pho; Saba; Sep; Stan; Sul.
- 9 A.M.
  - AGG: Bry; *Eup-p*; Kali-bi; Kali-c; Lac-c; Nat-m; Nat-s; Nux-v; Sep; Sul-ac; *Verb*.
  - to 4 P.M. AGG: Verb.

Forenoon
- AGG (9 A.M. to 12 Noon: Arg-m; CANN; Carb-v; Guai; Hep; Laur; NAT-C; *Nat-m*; Nux-m; *Pod*; Ran-b; Rhus-t; SABA; SEP; Sil; STAN; SUL; Sul-ac; Val; Vio-t.
- AMEL: Alu; Lil-t; *Lyc*.
- 10 A.M.
  - AGG: *Ars*; *Bor*; Chin; Chin-s; *Eup-p*; GEL; *Iod*; Med; NAT-M; Petr; *Pho*; *Rhus-t*; Sep; Sil; *Stan*; *Sul*; Thu.

TIME, forenoon, 10 a.m.
- to 3 P.M. AGG: Chin-s; Nat-m; Tub.
- 11 A.M. AGG: Ars; Asaf; Bap; *Cact*; *Chin-s*; Cocl; *Gel*; *Hyds*; Hyo; Ip; *Lach*; Mag-p; Nat-c; NAT-M; Nat-p; *Nux-v*; *Pho*; *Pul*; *Rhus-t*; *Sep*; *Stan*; SUL; *Zin*.
- 12 Noon
  - AGG: Ant-c; *Arg-m*; Chel; Chin; Elap; *Eup-p*; Gel; Kali-c; Lach; *Nat-m*; *Nux-v*; Pho; *Sil*; Spig; Stram; *Sul*; Val; Verb.
  - to 4 P.M. AGG: Alu; Ars; Bell; Lach; Lyc; Pul; *Sil*; Thu; Zin.
    Eating, after AMEL: *Chel*.
  - to midnight AGG: Lach.

Afternoon
- AGG (12 Noon to 6 P.M.): Agar; Alo; ALU; Amb; Ant-c; AP; Asaf; BELL; Bry; Chel; Chin; Cimi; Colo; *Dig*; Hell; *Ign*; *Kali-n*; LYC; PUL; *Rhus-t*; Sep; *Sil*; *Sul*; *Thu*; ZIN.
- AMEL: Cinb; Gel; Nat-s; Phyt; Rhus-t; Sep.
- 1 P.M. AGG: *Ars*; Cact; Chel; Cina; Grat; Kali-c; *Lach*; Pho; *Pul*.
- 2 P.M. AGG: Ars; Chel; *Eup-p*; *Fer*; Gel; *Lach*; Mag-p; Nit-ac; *Pul*.
- 3 P.M.
  - AGG: Ant-t; *Ap*; *Ars*; Asaf; BELL; Cedr; Chel; *Chin-s*; Con; Samb; Sang; *Stap*; *Thu*.

TIME, afternoon, 3 p.m.
- to 5 P.M. AGG: Sep.
- 4 P.M.
  - AGG: *Aesc*; *Anac*; *Ap*; Ars; Cact; Caus; *Cedr*; *Chel*; Chin-s; *Colo*; *Gel*; Hell; Ip; LYC; Mang; Nat-s; Nit-ac; Nux-m; *Nux-v*; *Pul*; Rhus-t; Sul; Verb.
  - to 8 P.M. AGG: *Ap*; *Caus*; Colo; Hell; Hyo; LYC; Nit-ac; Nux-m; Pho; Plat; *Pul*; *Rhus-t*; Saba; Sep; *Sul*; Zin.
  - to day light AGG: Syph.
- 5 P.M. AGG: Alu; Bov; Caus; Cedr; *Chin*; Colo; Con; *Gel*; Hep; Hypr; *Kali-c*; *Lyc*; Nat-m; *Nux-v*; *Pul*; *Rhus-t*; Sul; THU; Tub; Val.

Evening
- AGG: (6 P.M. to 9 P.M.): ACO; Alu; Amb; *Am-c*; *Ant-c*; *Ant-t*; Arg-n; *Arn*; Ars; BELL; *Bry*; Calc; *Caps*; Carb-an; Carb-v; *Caus*; Cep; Cham; *Colch*; CYC; EUPHR; Flu-ac; *Hell*; *Hyo*; KALI-N; Kali-s; Lach; LYC; *Mag-c*; MENY; *Merc*; *Mez*; Nat-p; NIT-AC; *Pho*; Pho-ac; PLAT; *Plb*; PUL; *Ran-sc*; *Rum*; Rut; SEP; Sil; *Stan*; STRO; SUL; Sul-ac; Syph; Val; *Zin*.
- AMEL: Alu; *Aur*; Bor; Med; Sep.
- Mid-night, until AGG: Anac; Bro.
- 6 *P.M.*
  - AGG: Ant-t; *Cedr*; *Hep*;

TIME, evening, 6 p.m. ..
    Kali-c; Nat-m; NUX-V; Petr; Pul; Rhus-t; Sep; Sil; Sumb.
  - to 4 A.M.: Guai.
  - to 6 A.M.: Kre.
- 7 P.M. AGG: Alu; Bov; Cedr; Chin-s; Fer; Gamb; Gel; Hep; Ip; Lyc; Nat-m; Nat-s; Nux-v; Petr; Pul; Pyro; Rhus-t; Sep; Sul; Tarn.
- 8 P.M.
  - AGG: Alu; Bov; Caus; Cof; Elap; Hep; Mag-c; Merc; Pho; Rhus-t; SUL.
  - to 12 midnight AGG: Arg-n; Bov; BRY; Carb-v; Gel; Lyc; Mur-ac; Pho; Pul; Rum; Stan; Sul.

Night
- AGG (9 P.M. to 4 A.M.): ACO; Arg-n; Arn; ARS; Ars-io; Bell; Calc; Calc-p; Calc-s; Carb-an; CHAM; CHIN; Cimi; Cof; COLCH; Con; Cyc; Dul; FER; GRAP; HEP; Hyo; Iod; Ip; Jal; Kali-bi; Kali-c; KALI-IO; Lach; Lil-t; MAG-C; Mag-m; Mang; Meph; MERC; NIT-AC; Pho; PLB; PSOR; Pul; Rhus-t; Rum; Sep; SIL; STRO; SUL; SYPH; Tell; ZIN.
- 9 P.M. AGG: Ars; Bov; BRY; Gel; Merc.
- 10 P.M. AGG: Ars; Bov; CHIN-S; Grap; Ign; Lach; Petr.
- 11 P.M.
  - AGG: Aral; Ars; Bell; CACT;

TIME, night, 11 p.m. ..
    Calc; Carb-an; Rum; Sul.
  - AMEL: Bor.
- 12 Midnight
  - AGG: Aco; Arg-n; ARS; Calc; Calad; Canth; Caus; Chin; Dig; Dros; Fer; Kali-c; Lach; Lyc; Mag-m; Mur-ac; Nat-m; Nux-m; Op; Pho; Rhus-t; Samb; Stram; Sul; Ver-a.
  - After AMEL: Anac; Form: LYC; Ran-sc.
  - To 4 A.M. AGG: Am-c; Ars; Caus; Cedr; Dros; Kali-bi; Lach; Nat-m; Nux-v; POD; Rum; Sul; Ver-a.
  - To Noon
    AGG: Ars.
    AMEL: Pul.
- 1 A.M. AGG: ARS; Carb-v; Mag-m; Pul.
- 2 A.M. AGG: ARS; Benz-ac; Canth; Caus; Como; Dros; Fer; Grap; Hep; Iris; Kali-ar; KALI-BI; Kali-c; Kali-p; Lach; Lachn; Lyc; Mag-c; Mez; Nat-m; Nat-s; Nit-ac; Ptel; Pul; Rum; Sars; Sil; Spig; Sul.
- 3 A.M. AGG: Am-c; Am-m; Ant-t; Ars; Bry; Calc; Canth; Cedr; Chin; Fer; Iris; KALI-C; Kali-n; Mag-c; Nat-m; Nux-v; Pod; Psor; Rhus-t; Sele; Sep; Sil; Sul; Thu.
- 4 A.M.
  - AGG: Alu; Am-m; Anac; Ap; Arn; Bor; Caus; Cedr;

TIME, night, 4 a.m. ..
Chel; Colo; *Con*; Fer; *Ign*; Kali-c; *Lyc*; *Mur-ac*; *Nat-c*; Nit-ac; NUX-V; *Pod*; *Pul*; Radm; Sep; Sil; Stan; *Sul*; Ver-a.
- to 8 A.M. AGG: Alu; Arn; Aur; Bry; Chel; *Eup-p*; Hep; Kali-bi; Lach; *Nat-m*; Nux-v; POD; Rum; *Sul*; Ver-a.
- to 4 P.M. AGG: Kali-c.
• 5 A.M. AGG: Alo; Ap; CHIN; Dros; *Kali-c*; Kali-io; *Nat-m*; Nat-p; Pho-ac; Rum; Sep; Sil; *Sul*.

TIME SENSE CHANGED: Alu; Cann; Lach; Merc.

Passes
• Too quickly: *Cocl*; Ther.
• Too slowly: Alu; Amb; Arg-m+; Arg-n; Cann; Glo; Med; Merc+; Nux-m; Nux-v; Pall.

TIMID: See SHY.

TINGLING (See ITCHING internal): Aco; Kalm; Sec.

Pain, after: Sec.

TINNITUS: See HEARING, illusory noises and MENIERE'S DISEASE.

Vertigo then: Chin.

TIRED: See WEAKNESS.

Acts, as if born: Onos.

Always, women+: Alet.

Of Life: See DEATH, desires and SUICIDAL DISPOSITION.

TO AND FRO: See ALTERNATIONS.

TOBACCO

AGG: Ars; Ars-io; *Cam*; Gel; *Ign*; Nux-v; Pho; Plant; *Pul*; Radm; Sele; Spig; Spo; Stap; Strop; Ver-a.

AMEL: Aran; *Hep*; Naj; Plat; Sep; Stro; Tarn.

Aversion, to: See AVERSIONS.

Bitter taste+: Cocl.

Chewing AGG: *Ars*; Lyc; Plant; Ver-a.

Disgust for, produces+: Plant.

Smoke agg+: Aco; Cic.

Smokers agg: Sec.

Smoking, when breaking off: Calad.

TOES: *Arn*; *Caus*; *Grap*; Plat; Pul; Ran-sc; Sabi; *Sul*; Thu.

Balls, of: Berb; Led; Petr; Pul; Spig.
• Painful: Med.

Bend, while walking: Bad; Lyc.

Bluish: Sec.

Broken: Cocl; Lach.

Burning: Ap; Tarx.

Cold: Abro.

Corns: See Callosities.

Cracked: Saba; Sars.
• Between: Saba; Sil.
• Under: Saba.

Cramps: Calc; Caus; Cup-ac; Pho; Ver-a; Zin-chr.
• Dysmenorrhoea, alternating with: Dios.

Drawn
• Down: Ars; Colch; Cup; Hyo.
• Up: Cam; Cic; Lach.

Eczema with loss of nails: Bor.

TOES

Enlarged, as if: Ap; Laur.
Glistening: Sabi.
Gout: See GOUT.
Great (toe): Arn; Asaf; Caus; Kali-c; Nat-s; Plat; Radm; Sabi; Sil; Zin.
- Felon: Caus.
- Inflamed: Sabi.
- Needles, at: Ran-sc.
- Numb: Ars; Calc; Cham; Nat-s.
- Swelled: Led; Sabi.

Hips, to: Pall
Inflamed: Sil.
Instep, to: Anac.
Jerking: Agar; Calc; Merc.
Joints: Aur; Caus; Kali-c; Led; Mar-v; Sabi; Sep; Sul; *Zin*.
Nails (See NAILS): Grap; Saba.
- Under: Ant-c; Flu-ac; Grap; Mar-v.
  - pricking: Elap.

Numb: Abro; Grap; Pho; Sec.
- Extending to other parts: Thal.

Painful: Phyt; Rhod.
Prickling: Abro.
Red: Sabi.
Soreness, between: Nat-m.
Spasms: *Chel*; Cup; Sec; Zin.
- Stairs, ascending, on: Hyo.
- Walking, on: Hyo.

Spread apart: Glo.
Stubbing agg: Colch.
Swelled: Grap.
- As if: Zin.

Thighs, to: Nux-v; Thal.

TOES

Tips, of: Kali-c; Thu.
- Aching: Zin.
- Blisters: Nat-c.
- Formication: Thu.
- Painful: Kali-c; Zin.
- Wind blowing through, as if: Cup.

Tremor: Arn; Mag-c.
Ulcers on: Sil.
Vesicles: Sec.
White, becomes from sweat: Grap.

TONGUE: Bell; Hyo; *Merc*; Mur-ac; Nux-v; *Pho*; *Plb*; *Pul*.

Across: Acet-ac; Asar; Kali-p; Kob; LACH; Merc.
Aphthae: *Bor*; Carb-v; Kali-chl; Merc; Mur-ac; Sul; Thu.
Atrophy: Mur-ac.
Bites: *Buf*; Dios; *Ign*; Thu; Vip.
- Sleep, in: Cic; Pho-ac.
- Talking, while: Hyo.
- Tip, of: Ther.

Black: Arn+; Ars; Carb-v; *Chin*; Crot-h; Dig; Gymn; Hyo; Lept; Lyc+; *Merc*; Op+; *Pho*; Radm.
- Centre, down: Lept.
- Gangrenous: Bism.

Bleached, as if+: Bor; Sec.
Bleeding: Aru-t; Bor; Sec.
Blue: Ant-t; *Ars*; *Dig*; Gymn; *Mur-ac*.
- White: Ars; *Gymn*+.

Broad: Mag-m; Merc; Nat-m; Pul.
- As if: Nat-m; Par; Plb; Pul.

Burning, burnt etc: Aco; Adon; Aesc+; Ap; Ars; Bap+; Bell;

TONGUE, burning..
Calc-p; Colo+; Hyds; Ign; *Iris*; Kali-io; Mag-m; Mur-ac; Nat-s; Ol-an+; Phys+; Plat; Pod; Ptel; *Pul*; Saba; Sang; Sanic; Ver-v.
• Stomach, to: Bro; Mez.
Cancer: Kali-cy; Mur-ac.
Catches teeth, on protruding: Ap; Hyo; LACH.
Centre, down (strips): Ant-t; *Arn*; Ars; *Bap*; Caus; Iris; Lach; Malan; Merc-c; *Pho*; Pyro; *Rhus-t*; VER-V.
• Furrow: Nit-ac.
• Pea like elevation: Castr.
Clean: Cina; Dig; Hyo; Ip; Mag-p; Sec.
• Menses, during: Sep.
• Urine, profuse, when: Solid.
Coated: Bell; *Bry*; Chin; Merc; *Nux-v*; Pho; Pul.
• Diagonally: Rhus-t.
• Edges clean with: Arg-n.
• Green, base at: Caps.
  - salivation, with: Nit-ac.
• One side: Daph; Mez; Rhus-t.
• White: ANT-C; Ant-t; *Ars*; *Bell*; Bism; Bry; Calc; *Chin*; Hyds+; Hyo; Kali-bi; *Kali-m*; Merc; Nit-ac; Pho; *Pul*; *Sul*; Tarx.
  - centre: Petr.
• Yellow: Bry; Chel; Chin; Hyds; Kali-p; *Mag-m*; Merc; Nux-m; Ol-j+; Pul+; Rhus-t; Spig.
  - edges indented,with: Chel; Hyds.
  - greenish: Chio.
  - moist, filmy: Merc-i-f; Nat-p+.

TONGUE, coated
  - mustard were spread on, as if: Kali-p; Pod.
  - patchy: Lil-t.
Cold: Cam; Carb-v; Cist; Iris; Kali-chl; Naj; Ver-a.
Contracted: Carb-v; Merc-c.
• Cylindrical: Cina.
Control, loss of: Aesc.
Cracks, fissures: Ail; Ars; *Aru-t*; BELL; Benz-ac+; Bor; Flu-ac; *Hyo*; Iod+; KALI-BI; Kali-io; Lyc; *Nit-ac*; *Pho*; RHUS-T; Sec+; Spig; Sul.
• Across: Kob.
• Bleeding: Aru-t.
• Centre: Nit-ac; Syph.
• Directions, in all: Flu-ac; Nit-ac.
• Middle of+: Mez.
• Peeling, off: Ran-sc.
Cramp: See Spasm.
Crawling: Plat; Sec.
Cutting, before asthma: Bor.
Diagonally: Rhus-t.
Dirty: Cean; Chin; Hyds+; Nat-s.
Distorted: Con.
Dotted: Ant-t; Bell; Grap; Stram.
Drawn
• Backward: Tarn.
• Up: Chio.
Dry: *Ars*; BELL; Bor; *Bry*; Calc; Hell; Hyo; Lyc+; Nux-m; Pho; RHUS-T; Sul.
• As if: Nat-m; Nux-m.
• Brown+: Ail.
• Half: Bell; Sang.
• Middle: Ant-t.
Ecchymoses: Pho.

TONGUE

Edges, of: Ap; Nat-m; Phyt.
- **Aphthae:** Arg-n.
- **Beads, foam, on:** Am-c; Ap; Iod; *Nat-m*; Pho.
- **Dark, streaked:** Petr.
- **Indented:** Ant-t; Chel.
- **Needles, at:** Nux-v.
- **Painful, sore:** Ap; Zin.
- **Red:** *Ars*; Bell; Bry; *Chel*; MERC; Sul.
  - centre: Rhus-t.
  - tip, and: Ap; Sul.
- **Turned up:** Sanic.
- **Ulcer**
  - right: Sil; Thu.
  - left: Ap.
- **Vesicles, on:** Am-c; *Ap*; Lach; Nat-m; Pho.
  - white: Thu.

Eruptions, on: Nat-m; Sars; Zin.
- **Psoriasis:** Cast-eq.
- **Ringworm:** Nat-m; Sanic.

Filmy: Merc-i-f.
Flabby: Cam; Dig+; Hyds; Merc; Pod; Sanic+.
Formication: See Crawling.
Fur thick white+: Guai.
- **Dots+:** *Grap*.

Furrow across: Merc.
- **Centre:** Nit-ac.

Furry: Merc.
Glistening: Ap; Ars; Cist; *Kali-bi*; Lach; Pho; Sul-io; Terb.
Gray: Chel; Kali-c; Kali-m.
Greenish at base+: Caps.
Hair, on: All-s; Kali-bi; Nat-m; Nat-p; *Sil*.
- **Reading while:** All-s.

TONGUE

Hangs out of mouth: Ap; Stram.
Heavy: Bell; *Gel*; Glo; Kali-bi; Lach; Lyc; Mur-ac; Nat-c; Nat-m; Nux-m; Nux-v.
Hypertrophy, of: Iod.
Indented: *Ars*; Bor; *Chel*; *Hyds*; Kali-io; Mag-m; MERC; *Pod*; Pul; *Rhus-t*; Stram; Syph+.
Induration: Hyds; Hyo; Merc-d; Nux-m.
- **Knotty:** Carb-an.

Inflamed: Aco; *Ap*; Bell; *Crot-h*; Lach; MERC; Merc-c.
Jerking, in: Cham.
Large, as if: Par.
Leather like
- **Burnt:** Hyo.
- **Hard:** Aur.

Lolling: See Oscillating.
Long, as if: Aeth; Mur-ac.
Lumps, hard: Mur-ac.
Mapped: See Patchy.
Motion of, difficult: See under Protruded.
- **Lapping:** Buf.

Neuralgia: Ap; Crot-t; Kali-ar; Mang.
Nodes, on: Iod; Mang; Mur-ac.
Numb: Aco; Echi; GEL; Hell; Nat-m; *Nux-m*; Old; Pul.
- **One side:** Nat-m.
  - vertigo, with: Agar.

Oily, greasy: Iris; Phys.
Oscillating: Hell; Hyo; Lach+; Lyc.
- **Spasms, during:** Sil.

Painful: See Sore.

TONGUE

Palate, sticks to: Bry; Kali-p; Nux-m; Sanic.

Papillae, showing (strawberry): Arg-n; Ars; Aru-t+; *Bell*; Caus; Kali-bi; Terb.

Paralysis: Bar-c; CAUS; *Gel*; Hyo; Lach; *Op*; *Plb*; Sec+.
- Creeping: Kali-p.

Patchy, mapped, spots: *Ars*; Dul; Hyds; Kali-bi; Lach; Merc; *Merc-c*; NAT-M; *Nit-ac*; Ran-sc; *Rhus-t*; Sep; Syph; *Tarx*; Tub.

Pea like bodies, with red centre: Castr.

Pointed: Chel; Ip; Lach; Petr.

Prickling, under: Lyss.

Protruded: Ap; Bell; Crot-h; Cup; Phyt; Vario; Vip.
- Brain affections, in: Ap; Hyd-ac.
- Cannot be+: Merc-c.
- Difficulty, with: Ap; Caus; Gel; Hyo; Lach; Myg; Pho.
  - drawing, in: Hyo.
  - jerk, with: Kali-br.
  - sore throat, with: Saba.
- Pain, then+: Kali-bi.
- Rapidly, darting in and out like a snake: *Cup*; Lach; Lyc; Merc; Vip.
- Side, right: Crot-h; Op.
- Sleep, in: Vario.
- To keep it cool: Sanic.

Protruding
- AGG: Cocl; Cist; *Kali-bi*; *Phyt*; Syph.
- AMEL: Med.

Puckered, as if: Ars.

Puffy: Bor.

Rattles: Hyo.

Raw: Carb-v; *Nux-v*; Sil.

Red: Ant-t; AP; *Ars*; Bell; Hyo; *Kali-bi*; Lach; Merc; *Pho*; Rhus-t; Sang.
- Base at: Bry.
- Centre, along: Ver-v.
- Cracked, in dysentery: Kali-bi.
- Dots, fine: Stram.
- Fiery: Ap; Pyro; Sang.
- Stiff, painful; moving when: Merc-i-r.
- Streak, centre down: Caus; Ver-v.
  - middle: Ant-t; Cham; Pho-ac.
- Stripe down centre, widens at tip: Calad.

Root, of: Bap; Kali-bi; Kali-io; Lach; Nat-s; Phyt.
- Burning: Med.
- Green: Caps; Chio.
  - yellow: Nat-s.
- Swelling: Caus.
- Tension: Kali-io.
- Tickling: Stan.
- White: Kali-m; Nat-m; Sep.
- Yellow: Merc-i-f; *Nat-p*; Nat-s; Phyt.

Rough: Aru-t; Pod.

Sandy: Ap; Cist.

Scalloped: Mag-m.

Shrunken: Mur-ac.

Side, one: Bell; *Calc*; Lob; Mez; Nat-m; RHUS-T; Sang; Sil; Thu.

Skin, covered with, as if: Rhus-t.

TONGUE

Slimy: Eucal; *Pul.*
Smooth, glazed: Ap; Lach; Pyro; Sul-io; Terb; Tub.
Soft: Merc; Rhus-t; Stram.
Sore, painful: Agar; Calc; Caps; Carb-v; Ign; *Nit-ac*; Pul; Saba; Sep.
• Root at, when yawning: Lach.
• Spots, on: *Agar*; Ant-c; Sil; Tarx.
Spasms: Arg-n; Cocl; Con; Lyc; Syph.
• Causing embarassment of speech: Rut.
Spongy+: Benz-ac.
Stiff: Anac; Ap; *Bell*; Hyo; Lac-c; Merc-i-r; Mur-ac; Nat-m; RHUS-T.
Stitching: Merc.
Strawberry: See Papillae Showing.
Stripe: See under Red.
Swelled: Aco; Anac; *Ap*; Ars; Bell; Canth; Caus; Crot-h; Dul; Hyds+; Lyc; *Merc*; Polyg; Zin.
• Small, round, in middle: Dros.
Tearing: Merc.
Thick, as if: Bap; Gel.
Tickling: Alu; Stan.
Tip, of: Kali-c; *Rhus-t*; Sul; Thyr; Zin.
• Burns like pepper+: Coc-c.
• Burnt: Calc; Caps; Chin; Colo; Nat-s; Psor; Terb.
• Clean, white at back+: Hypr.
• Cracked: Lach.
• Needle pricks: Merc.

TONGUE, tip of
• Pimple, painful: Buf.
• Pricking+: Radm.
• Red: Arg-n; *Ars*; Ip; Merc-i-r; *Phyt*; RHUS-T; *Sul*.
 - painful: Arg-n.
 - triangle: Arg-n; *Rhus-t*; Sep.
• Spot, dark red: Diph.
• Sweet: Plat.
• Vesicles: Ap; Caus; Kali-c; Lyc; Nat-c.
Tremulous: Agar; Ap; Cam; Canth; Gel; Hell; *Lach*; Lyc; *Merc*; Pho; Plb; Sul.
• Protruding, when: Bell; Gel; Hell; Hyo; *Lach*; Plb.
Tumour, were forming: Kali-m.
Twitching: Castr; Glo; Sec; Sul.
Ulcerated: Arg-n; *Bap*; Carb-v; Kali-io; MERC; Psor.
• Jagged+: Cund.
• Yellow: Hell.
Under: Flu-ac; Grap; *Lyc*; Nat-c; *Sanic*.
Veins, distended: Dig; Thu.
Warm, as if: Cimi.
Warts, on: Aur.
Weak: Bar-c; Caus; Con.
White: See Coated.
Wood, made of, as if: Ap.
Wrinkled: Calc-p; Merc-i-r; Pho; Sul-ac.
Yellow: See Coated.
TONSILS: Bap; *Bar-c*; BELL; Calc; *Calc-p*; Guai; Hep; Lac-c; LACH; Lyc; *Merc*; Merc-d; MERC-I-F; MERC-I-R; NIT-AC; Pho; *Phyt*; Sil; Sul; Tub.

TONSILS

Chamois skin, wash leather: Phyt; *Rhus-t.*

Chronicity: Bar-c; Bar-m; Bro; Hep; Kali-io; Lyc; Mez; Nat-m; Sul-io; Thu.
- Hardness of hearing with+: Hep.

Crypts, greyish white: Calc-io; *Ign.*
- Mucus plug of, constantly form: Calc-f.

Enlarged: BAR-C; *Bar-m*; CALC-F; CALC-IO; CALC-P; Con; Ign; *Lach*; *Lyc*; Merc; Merc-i-f; *Merc-i-r*; Nit-ac; Stap; Syph: *Tub.*
- Coryza, after: Saba.
- Deafness with, children+: Kali-bi.
- Mouth, opening agg: Calc-p.
- Pus, plugs of, with: Calc-f.

Foul: Ail; Bap; *Lach*; Lyc; Merc; Nit-ac.

Glisten: Ap; Lac-c.

Gray: Kali-m; Merc-cy.

Indurated: Alu; *Bar-c*; *Bar-m*; Phyt.

Lacunar: Ail; Merc-i-f+.

Menses, at agg: Lac-c.

Pricking, pin, as of+: Sil.

Recurrent: Guai; Phyt.

Red
- Bright: Aco; *Bell*; Phyt.
- Dark: Aesc; Bap; Carb-ac; *Lach.*

Suppurating (quinsy): Bar-m; Bell; Guai; HEP; Lach; *Lyc*; *Merc*; Nat-m; Phyt+; Psor; SIL; *Tarn.*

TONSILS, suppurating
- Chronic: *Bar-c.*

Throbbing, in: Am-m; Phyt.

Ulcers (See THROAT): Ail.
- Behind: Ars; Merc.

TOPER (See FOOD & DRINKS, alcoholic drink agg): Caps; Ran-b; Sele; Stram; Sul-ac.

Abstaining, after agg: Calc-ar.

TORMENTS everybody with her complaints: *Zin.*

TORN

Loose, as if: See under BONES.

Off, as if+: Ap.

Out, feeling: Alu; Bry; Calc; Elap; *Pru-sp*; Rhus-t.

Pieces, to: See SHATTERED.

TORPID: Asaf; Dros; Kali-s; Led; Nat-m; Nux-m; Op; Sil.

TORTICOLLIS: See NECK, wry.

TOSSING about: See under RESTLESSNESS.

Convulsions, during: Bar-m.

Suddenly: Chin.

TOUCH

Agg: See SENSITIVE, and TOUCHY.

AMEL: *Asaf*; *Bism*; *Calc*; *Cyc*; Grap; *Mur-ac*; Pall; Sang; Spig; Stap; Tarx; *Thu.*

Each other (of arms, fingers etc.) AGG: Lac-c; Psor; Sanic.

Hair, even of a: Ap.

Pain amel but appears somewhere else: Asaf; Sang; Stap.

Sense of, disturbed: Par.

Slight AGG: Aco; Ap; *Bell*; *Chin*; Ign; LACH; Merc; *Nit-ac*; *Nux-v.*

TOUCH, slight
- Hard pressure AMEL: Bell; *Castr*; *Chin*; Ign; *Lach*; *Nux-v*; Plb; Psor.

Things impulse, to: Bell; Lycps; Sul; *Thu*.
- Inability to do so: Sul.

TOUCHED when agg: See under FEAR.

TOUCHING anything
AGG: Cham.
AMEL: Spig.
Cold things, AGG: *Hep*; Mang; Merc; Nat-m; *Rhus-t*; *Sil*.
Warm things AGG: Sul.

TOUCHY (mentally and physically): Aco; Ant-c; Ant-t; Cham; Cimi; CINA+; Hep; Pul+; Sanic.

TOURIST: Coca; *Plat*.

TOUSY, dishevelled: Bor; Flu-ac+; Med; Sul.

TOXAEMIA: See BLOOD SEPSIS.
Pregnancy, of: See under PREGNANCY.

TRACHEA: See LARYNX.

TRAIN SICKNESS: See CAR SICKNESS.

TRANQUIL: See PLACID.

TRAUMATISM: See INJURIES and SHOCKS.

TRAVEL
Desire, to: *Calc-p*; Iod; Lyss; Tub.
Ill effects, of+: Ars.
- Far away places+: Merc.

TREMBLING, tremors: Amb; Agar; Anac; Ant-t; ARG-N; *Ars*; CALC; *Cic*; *Cimi*; Cocl; Con; GEL; Grap; Hyo; IOD; Jab; Kalm; *Lach*; Lil-t; Lycps; Med; MERC; Mos; Naj; NUX-V; Ol-an; *Op*; Phys; *Plat*; *Pul*; RHUS-T; Saba; Sang; Stan; Stap; *Stram*; Stro; Sul; Sul-ac; Tab; Ther; Tub; Ver-v; *Zin*.

Air, open amel: Clem.
All over: Bro; Visc.
Amorous, caressing during: Caps.
Anger, from: Nit-ac; Ran-b.
Anxiety, with+: Samb.
As if: Seneg.
Burns, after: Calc.
Cold drinks, amel: Pho.
Concomitant, as a: Calc-p.
Convulsions, before: Abs; Ver-v.
Coughing agg: Cup; Just; Pho.
Delirium, with: Aco; Ap; Ars; Bell; Bry; Calc; Chin; Hyo; Ign; Nat-m; Op; Phys; Plat; *Pul*; Rhus-t; Saba; Samb; Stram; Sul; Ver-a; Ver-v.
Direction, downward: Iod; Merc.
- Upward: Sil; Spig.

Electric shock, through body, with: Buf.
Emotions, from: *Cocl*; Mar-v; Plb; Psor; *Stap*.
Exertion, slight, from: Anac.
Exophthalmos, with: Meph.
Fear, from: Elap.
Hands and feet+: Ap; Ox-ac.

TREMBLING

Headache, with: Bor.
Here and there: Ver-v.
Hungry, when: Alu; Crot-h; Sul; Zin.
Intentional: Arg-n; *Cocl*; *Kali-br*; Rhus-t; *Sec*; Zin.
Internally: Calc; Caul; Diph; Grap; *Hep*; Iod; Mar-v; Med; Rhus-t; Stan; Stap; SUL-AC.
• Excitement agg: Mar-v.
Lower part: Amb.
Meeting friends, when: Tarn.
Motion, slow agg: Stan.
Music, from: Alo; *Amb*; Thu.
Nervous: Cimi; Cof; Gel; Lil-t; Mag-p; Pho; *Stap*; Stram.
Noise, sudden, from: Alo; Kali-ar.
Nursing, infant, after: Old.
Pains agg: Cocl; *Nat-c*; Plat; Pul; Zin.
Paralyzed part: CAUS; Merc; Nux-m; Plb.
Periodical: Arg-n.
Senile: Bar-c; Con.
Shivering, with: Cina.
Side lain on: Cimi; Clem.
Smoking, from: Hep; Kali-c; Nat-m; Nit-ac; Sep.
Spasmodic: Ign; Nux-v; Saba.
Stool, after: Ars; CON.
Sweat, with: Jab; Merc.
Thunderstorm, from+: Nat-p.
Touch, unexpected: Cocl; Kali-ar.
Urinating when: Gel.
Voluptuous: Calc.

TREMBLING

Waking, on: Merc; Tarn; Ver-a.
Walk
• On Attempting to: Cup-ar.
• While: Stan.
Writing, while: Pho; Sil.
TRENCH MOUTH: Merc-c.
TRICKLING, dropping or flowing as of water: Arg-n; Buf; *Cann*; Caus; Glo; Grap; Kali-bi; Lap-alb; Nat-m; Petros; Pho; Rhus-t; Sep; Stan; Sumb; Tarn; *Thu*; Ver-a; Vario.
Affected part, on: Arg-n.
Hot: Hep; Sep; Stan; Sul; Sumb.
TRICKY: Cup.
TRIFLES (mental symptoms) AGG: *Ars*; CHAM; Cina; Cof; Dros; Hep; *Ign*; Nit-ac; NUX-V; SIL; Thu.
Seem imporant: Ars; Calc; Caus; Con; *Grap*; *Hep*; Ign; Nat-m; *Nux-v*; Sil; Thu.
TRISMUS: See JAWS, locked.
TUBE METALLIC: Merc-c.
Hot water, running through, as if, pain during: Terb.
TUBERCULOSIS: See CONSUMPTION.
TUMID: See PUFFINESS.
TUMOURS: See GROWTH NEW.
TUNE OUT OF+: Nux-v.
TURGIDITY (See also PUFFINESS): Am-m; *Ap*; ARS; BELL; *Bry*; Cham; Kali-c; *Lyc*; Merc; *Nux-v*; Op; Pho; *Rhut-t*; Stram.

TURNING
Around AGG: Calc; *Ip*; Kali-c; Par.
Affected part, AMEL: Bell.
- Left to right amel: Lach; Pho.
- Right to left agg: Scop; Sul.

Over: See under BED and ROLLING.
Rapidly, as if: Mos.
Right, to AGG: Carb-v; Spig.
- Before he can rise: Kali-c.
- Walking, when: Helod.

Sideways AGG: Bell; Calc; Kali-c; Nat-m.
Something by limps AMEL: *Sep*.

TWILIGHT
AGG: *Ars*; Berb; CALC; Caus; Nat-s; Pho; Plat; PUL; *Rhus-t*.
AMEL: Bry; Meny; *Pho*; Plat+; Seneg; Tab.
Sees things, in: Berb.

TWINGES nips: See PAIN, twinging.

TWISTING: Ars; Bell; Calc; Cina; Colo; Dios; Elap; Ign; *Nux-v*; Pul; Rhus-t; *Sil*; VER-A.

TWITCHING (See CONVULSIONS): Agar; Amb; Asaf; Cina; Gel; Hyo; Ign; Iod; Kali-c; Laur; Mez; Mos; Nat-c; Saba; Sec; Stram; Strop; Tarn; Zin.
Coldness, with: Amb.
Convulsions, before: Ast-r.
One side, other side lame: Ap.
Painful: Agar; Meny.
- After: Sec.
- With: Meny.

TWITCHING
Paralysed parts, of: Arg-n; Merc; Pho; Sec; Stram.
Sleep, during: Ars+; Bar-c; Op; Sul+.
Subsultus tendinum: Ars; *Hyo*; *Iod*; Lyc; Mur-ac; Pho; Pho-ac; *Zin*.

TYMPANUM: See under EAR.

TYPHOID (See BLOOD SEPSIS):
Ars; Bap; Bell; *Bry*; Kali-c; Mur-ac; Op; Pho; Pho-ac; Pyro+; *Rhus-t*; Sul; Tarx.
Aborting: Bap; Pyro.
Vaccination, ill effects+: Bap.

TYPHUS fever: Ars.

UGLY (in behaviour): Bry; Buf; *Cham*; Cina; *Nux-v*.

ULCERS: *Arg-n*; ARS; Ars-io; *Asaf*; Calc; Calc-s; Carb-v; Caus; *Hep*; *Kali-bi*; Kali-chl; Kali-s; *Lach*; *Lyc*; MERC; *Nit-ac*; Pho; Pho-ac; Phyt; PUL; Rhus-t; Sep; SIL; *Sul*; Sul-io; Syph; Vip+.

Areola, edges, margins, with: Ars; Asaf; Hep; Lach; Lyc; Merc; *Pul*; *Sil*.
- Dark: Aesc; *Lach*.
- Elevated: Ars; Asaf; *Merc*; *Sil*.
  - indurated, and: Ars; Lyc; Sil.
- Eruptions, pimples etc. in: Carb-v; *Hep*; Lach.
- Fungoid: Lach.
- Hanging, over: Kali-bi.
- Hard: Flu-ac; Grap; Pul; Sil.
  - red: Pul.
- Sensitive: Asaf.
- Shiny: Pul.

ULCERS

ULCERS, areola
- Small ulcers, over: Calc; Hep; Mez; Pho; Rhus-t.
- Zigzag, irregular margins, with: *Merc*; Nit-ac; *Pho-ac*.

Atonic, indolent, painless: *Ars*; Carb-v; Con; Hep; Hyds; *Lach*; LYC; Op; PHO-AC; Sec; *Sil*; *Sul*.
- Tumours, removal after: Hyds.

Bed sores: See under BED.

Black: Anthx; Ars; Bism; Carb-v; Kali-ar; Lach; Lyc; Sec.

Bleeding: Arn; Ars; Bur-p; Carb-v; Hep; *Lach*; Lyc; Merc; Nit-ac; *Pho*; Pho-ac; Sul-ac.
- Menses, during: Pho.

Bloody water, from: Carb-ac; Kali-ar; Rhus-t.

Bluish: Ars; Asaf; Crot-h; *Lach*; Mur-ac; Sil; Tarn-c; Thu; Vip.

Boils, around: Hep.

Break and heal, recur: Carb-v; Kre; Vip.

Burning: Anthx; *Ars*; Carb-v; Caus; Kali-ar; Lyc; Merc; Plb; Pul; Rhus-t; *Sil*; Sul.

Cancerous+: Aur.

Coition agg: Kre.

Cold feeling, in: Ars; *Bry*; Rhus-t; Sil.

Cutting: Bell; Kali-ar; Merc.

Deep, perforating: Ars; *Calc*; Calc-s; KALI-BI; Kali-c; Lach; Merc; Merc-c; Mez; *Mur-ac*; *Nit-ac*; *Pul*; Radm; Ran-b; Rat; *Sil*; Sul; Tarn.
- Hard and+: Mez.

ULCERS

Dirty: Lach; Merc; Nit-ac.

Dotted: Arg-n; Ars; Kali-bi; Med.

Dropsical persons, in: Ars; Grap; Hell; Lyc; Merc; Rhus-t; Scil; Sul.

Dry, hard: Mang.

Flowing: Kali-ar; Kali-s; Nat-s; *Rhus-t*; Zin-s.
- Yellow water: Kali-s.

Heat
- Agg (cold application amel): Cham; Flu-ac; *Led*; Lyc; *Pul*.
- Amel: Ars; Clem; Con; HEP; *Lach*; Rhus-t; *Sil*; Syph.

Honeycombed: Cinb.

Indolent: See Atonic.

Injury, slight, after: Mang.

Irregular: Ars; Kali-bi; Merc; Phyt; Sars; Sil.

Itching: Kali-ar.

Maggots, with: Saba; Sil.

Mustard poultice, from: Calc-p.

Offensive, foul: Carb-v; Hep; Kali-ar; Mur-ac; Sec; Sil.
- Asafoetida like+: Carb-v.

Painful: Ars; Bell; Carb-v; Grap; Hep; Sabi; Sil.

Painless: See Atonic.

Phagedinic+: Cist.

Pimples, around: Hep.

Pulsation: Hep.
- Walking, when: Mur-ac.

Rapid, malignant: Arg-n; *Ars*; Carb-an; *Carb-v*; Caus; Chel; Hyds; Lyc; Merc; *Merc-c*; NIT-AC; Petr; Ran-b; Ran-sc; *Sil*; Thu.
- Borders, blue with: Mang.

ULCERS
Round, punched: Kali-bi; Merc; Phyt.
Scooped, out: Vario.
Senile: Tarn-c.
Sensitive, touch causes convulsions: Stap.
Shallow, flat, superficial: ARS; Hyds; LACH; *Lyc*; Merc; *Nit-ac*; Thu.
• **Climaxis, at:** Polyg.
Shoes, pressure, from: Bor; Paeon.
Small: See Dotted.
Spongy: Sil.
Suppressed: Clem; Lach; Sul.
Swelled: Lyc; *Merc*; Pul; *Rhus-t*; Sep; *Sil*; Sul.
Syphilitic: Ars; Asaf; *Iod*; Kali-io; Merc; Merc-c; *Nit-ac*; Phyt; Thu.
Tumours, removal after: Hyds.
Varicose: See BLOOD VESSELS, distended.

ULNAR NERVE along: Aran; Hypr; Kalm; Pod; Rhus-t; Tub.

UMBILICUS: See NAVEL.

UNATTRACTIVE, things seem: Chin.

UNCERTAIN+: Merc.
Execution, of: Med.
Gait etc.: Con.

UNCIVIL: See UGLY.

UNCLEAN: See DIRTY Habits.
Odour, body, of: Guai.

UNCONSCIOUS, insensible
(See Numbness): Aco; Ars; Bar-c; *Bap*; BELL; *Cam*; Cocl;

UNCONSCIOUS ..
Cup; Hell; Hyd-ac; HYO; Ign; Lach; Mos; Nat-m; Nux-m; OP; PHO-AC; Pul; STRAM.
Becoming, as if: Cup.
Blood, sight of: Nux-m.
Coition, after: Agar; Dig.
Convulsions, after: *Buf*; Cic; Oenan; Stan+.
• **Prolonged:** Bell.
Emotions, from: Cof; Ign; Lach.
Eyes
• **Closing, on:** Ant-t; Cann.
• **Open, with:** See Coma, Vigil.
Fever, during: Ap; Arn; Mur-ac; Nat-m; Op.
Frequent spells: Ars.
Menses
• **During:** Lach.
• **Suppressed, from:** Nux-m.
Odours from: *Nux-v*; Pho.
Pain, during: Hep; Nux-m; Val.
Parturition, during: Cimi; Cof; *Nux-v*; Pul; Sec.
Pregnancy, during: Nux-m; Nux-v; Sec.
Prolonged: *Cic*; *Gel*; Hyd-ac; Laur.
Rubbing soles amel: Chel.
Sudden: Canth; Cocl; Kali-c.
Swallow, inability, to: Amy-n.
Talking, while: Lyc.
Trance, as if, in: *Lach*; Laur.
Transcient: Ign; Pul.

UNCOUTH: Bar-c; Caps.

UNCOVERING
AGG: See HEAT amel and WIND, draft agg.

UNCOVERING
AMEL: See COLD amel.
Chest AMEL: Sars.
Least AGG: Hep; Nux-v; Rhus-t; Sil.
Neck AMEL: Sars.
Wants, in sleep: Plat.

UNDRESSING
Agg: See under ITCHING, and WIND agg.
Air, open in AGG: Pho.

UNDULATIONS (See WAVES):
Asaf; Grap; Nux-v; Rhod; Sep; Strop; Zin-io.

UNEASY FEELING:
Aeth; Ascl; Cedr; Cup; Dros; Grap; Guai; Sep; Stan; Val; Ver-v.
Knows not what to do, with himself: Stan.
Sexual desire, with: Ant-c.

UNHAPPY: See SADNESS.
UNLUCKY: Ver-a.
UNREAL, everything seems:
Alu; Cann; Cocl; *Med*.
Like a dream+: Anac.

UNPLEASANT THINGS, dwells on+: Benz-ac.
UNRULY+: Am-c.
UNSOCIAL: Anac; *Syph*.
UNSTEADY
As if: *Agar*; Arg-n; Bar-c; Caus; Cic; Cocl; Kali-br; Lil-t; Nat-c; Sec; Stan; *Sul*.
Look, eyes roll vacantly+: Lach.

UNSUCCESSFUL, thinks himself: Naj; Sul.
UNTIDY: *Sul*.

UNUSUAL THINGS, from any agg+: Amb.
UP AND DOWN: See DIRECTIONS.
UPPER LIMBS: See ARMS.
URAEMIA:
Ap; Ars; Aru-t+; *Bap*; *Bell*; *Canth*; Hell; Hyo; *Op*; Pic-ac; Plb; Senec; *Stram*; Terb+; Urt; Ver-v.

URETERS:
Ap; *Bell*; *Berb*; Canth; Carb-an; *Lyc*; Oci-c; Par; Polyg; *Sars*; Sep; Terb; Ver-a.
Burning: Terb.
Cramp: Nit-ac; Polyg.
Cutting: Bell; Berb; Carb-an; Lyc; Par-b; Polyg; Sars; Ver-a; Ver-v.
Inflammation+: Canth.
Sore: Ap; Berb; Oci-c.
Vomiting, with: *Oci-c*.

URETHRA:
Arg-n; *Cann*; *Canth*; Caps; Clem; Lyc; Merc; Pho; Pul; Sul; Thu.
Abdomen, to: Sars.
Abscess: Canth; Pul; Rhus-t.
Bleeds: Merc-c.
- **Coition, during:** Caus.
- **Gonorrhoea, suppressed after:** *Pul*.
- **Paraplegia, with:** Lyc.
- **Stools, during:** *Lyc*; Pul.
- **Urine, first part, with:** Con.
- **Urination, after:** Hep; Merc-c; Pul; Sars; Thu.
  - Bladder pain, with: Ant-t.

Burning: Aco; Ars; Berb; Cam; Cann; *Canth*; Merc; *Merc-c*; Nux-v; Pru-sp; Sil; Sul; Thu.
- **Coition agg:** Agar; Canth; Clem; Sep; *Sul*.

URETHRA, burning
- Emission, during: Ant-c; *Sul.*
- Erection, with: Canth; Nit-ac.
- Flatus passing agg: Lyc; Mang.
- Stools, during: Colo.
- Urination
  - before: Bor; Cann; Canth; Caps.
  - during: Nat-c; Uran-n.
  - after agg: Merc.
  - amel: Berb; Bry; *Merc*; Stap.
  - at the end of agg: Clem; Nat-c.
  - coition, after: Caus.

Caruncle: Arg-n; Ars; *Cann*; Hep; Nit-ac; Sul; Sul-io.

Clogged: Merc; Sep.

Cold drop of urine, passing as if: Agar.

Cramp: Canth; Chin; Clem.

Crawling: Fer-io; Lyc; Petros; Pho-ac.

Cutting: Arg-n; Calc-p; *Canth*; Con; Thu.
- Glans penis, grasping amel: Canth.
- Seminal discharge, on: Con.
- Urination
  - during: Ant-t+; Canth; Con.
  - after: Canth; Nat-m.

Discharge
- Acrid: Arg-n; Merc-c.
- Bloody: Calc; Canth; Sil+.
- Cream, like: Caps.
- Foetid: Benz-ac; Carb-v; Hep; Sil.

URETHRA, discharge
- Gleety: Agn; Alu; Alum; Benz-ac; Kali-chl; Kali-io; Nat-m; Petros; Sele; Sep; Sul; Thu.
- Milky white, stools after: Iod.
- Mucous: Elap; Sep.
- Night, at: Sep.
- Painless: Fer; Nat-s; Thu.
- Persists: Alu; Arg-m; Kali-bi; Pho; Sul.
  - urinating after: Sars.
- Thin: Lyc; Nat-m; Nit-ac; Pho; Psor; Sul; *Thu.*
- Yellow: Alu; Arg-n; Merc; Pul; Sep; Thu.
  - stains: Alu; Nat-m; Psor.

Dragging: Til.

Drawing: Flu-ac; Merc.

Drops
- Biting, forcing its way out: Sele.
- Few pass out as if+: Amb.
- One remained, after urination: Kali-bi.
- Rolling continuously as if: Lact-v; Sele; Stap.

Flatus, passing agg: Mang.

Heavy: Eup-p; Saba; Til.

Hot wire, in: Nit-ac.

Indurated: Arg-n; Clem; Hypr; Merc-i-r.
- Whip cord like: Clem.

Itching: Merc-c; Nux-v; Rhus-t; Sil; *Sul.*

Jerking: Alu; Cann; Lyc; Petr; Pho; Sars; Thu.

Knot, ball, as if, in: Arg-n.
- Rolling through: Lach.

URETHRA
Narrow, as if: Arg-n.
Nodes, in: Bov.
Numb: Arg-n; *Caus*; Kali-br; *Mag-m*.
Open, as if: Cop.
Pulsation: Merc-c.
Riding agg: Stap.
Running out something, after emission: Dig.
Stinging: Sabal.
- **Flatus pasing on:** Mang.

Straw thrust back and forth, as if: Dig.
Stricture: Canth; Cic; *Clem*; Nat-s; Nit-ac; PETR; Pul; Sul-io.
- **Dilatation, after:** Mag-m.
- **Drunkards:** Op; Sec.
- **Gonorrhoea, after:** Sul-io.
- **Spasmodic:** Nux-v.

Tingling: Clem; Petros.
Trickling: Arg-n; Kali-bi; Petros; Stap; Thu.
Tumour, small, in: Lach.
Twitching: Cann; Canth; Pho.
Ulcers: Merc-c; Nit-ac.
Uneasy feeling: Cedr.
Urinating amel: *Merc*; Stap.
Walking agg: Stap.
URGING (See PAIN, pressing): *Canth*; Lil-t; *Merc-c*; Sabi.
URIC ACID DIATHESIS, lithemia (See URINE, red sediment): Benz-ac+; Berb; Bur-p; Coc-c; *Lyc*; Nat-s; Sars+; Sep; Thu; Urt.

URINARY ORGANS in general:
Aco; AP; Arn; Ars; Bell; *Berb*; Calc; Cam; Cann; CANTH; *Caus*; Dul; Fer; Hell; Hep; Hyo; Lyc; *Merc*; *Merc-c*; Nat-m; Nit-ac; *Nux-v*; Op; Par-b; Pho; Pho-ac; Polyg; PUL; Rhus-t; Sars; Scil; Stap+; Sul; *Terb*; Til; Thu; Val; Ver-a.

Rheumatic symptoms, alternating, with: Benz-ac.

URINATION
Before AGG (crying etc): Aco; *Bor*; Canth; *Colo*; *Lyc*; NUX-V; PUL; Sanic; Sars.

At start of AGG: *Aco*; Canth; Clem; *Merc*.

During AGG: Aesc; Alo; Berb; *Cann*; *Canth*; *Hep*; Lil-t; *Lyc*; MERC; Nux-v; *Pho-ac*; PUL; *Sep*; Sul; THU.

At close of AGG: *Canth*; Equi; Merc-c; Mez; Nat-m; Sars.

After AGG: Cann; *Canth*; *Colo*; Equis; *Hep*; Med; Merc; MERC-C; *Nat-m*; Petros; Stap; THU.

AMEL: Chin-s; *Gel*; *Ign*; Lith; Lyc; Pho-ac; Sang; Sil; Ver-a.

Abortion, after agg: Rhe.

Cutting: Canth; Sep.

Desire, morbid urging: Ant-t; Ap; Arg-n; Bell; Berb; *Bry*; Cam; Cann; CANTH; *Caus*; Chin; Ip; Kali-c; Lil-t; MERC-C; Nat-m; NUX-V; *Pho-ac*; *Pul*; *Sabi*; *Sars*; Scil; Sep; *Stap*; SUL; Thu.
- **Absent in pregnancy+:** Hyo.
- **Clots, bloody from vagina**
  - amel: Coc-c.
  - with: Chim.

URINATION, desire
- Coition, after: Nat-p.
- Diarrhoea, during: Ap; Ars; Canth; *Merc-c*.
- Fever, during: Ant-t; *Ap*; Bell; Pul.
- Fruitless, ineffectual: Arn; *Ars*; *Canth*; Caps+; Caus; Chim; *Dig*; Hell; Hyo; MERC-C; Nit-ac; NUX-V; Op; Pho; Pho-ac; Pul; *Sars*; Stram.
- Heart, affections, with: Dig.
- Labour, after: Op; *Stap*.
- Lifting weight, on: Bry.
- Married women, newly: *Stap*.
- Menses, before: *Kali-io*; Sars.
- More urine, more urge+: Colch.
- Night: Dig; Lyc; Sabal; Sil; Sul.
- Pain, from: Terb.
- Prolapsus of uterus, from: *Lil-t*; Sep.
- Rectum, as if ball in, with: Lil-t.
- Restricted
  - causes pain: Petr.
  - cannot, pain after+: Rut.
  - if, then desire ceases: Sanic.
- Stools, before: Rhe.
- Thinking of it agg: Ox-ac; Oxytr.

Difficult, painful, dysuria, strangury: Aco; Arg-n; Ars; Bell; *Cann*; CANTH; Caps+; *Cham*; Cop; Dig; Dul+; Erig; Hyo; *Lil-t*; Lyc; MERC-C; NUX-V; Op; Par-b; Petros; Plb; *Pru-sp*; *Pul*; Sabal; Sars; *Stap*; *Sul*; Terb.

URINATION, difficult
- Alcoholic drinks, from: Nux-m.
- Attempting to urinate, on: Plb.
- Dances around the room, in agony: *Ap*; Cann; *Canth*; Petros.
- Delivery, after: Ap; Equi.
- Dentition, during: Erig.
- Dribbling, with: Bur-p.
- Dysentery, in: Arn.
- Dysmenorrhoea, with: Nux-m; Senec; Ver-v.
- Enuresis, alternating, with: Gel.
- Erection, then: Radm.
- Feet, wet from: Cep.
- Forceps delivery after: Bur-p.
- Headache, with (children): Con; Senec.
- Hysterical: Nux-m.
- Lying amel: Kre.
- Menses before: Sars.
- Neuralgic: Pru-sp.
- Pregnancy, during: Equi; Eup-pur; Pho-ac; Plb; Stap.
- Presence of others, in: *Amb*; Hep; Mur-ac; Nat-m; Tarn.
- Prostate, enlargment, with: Ap; Med; Petros.
- Renal colic, with: Coc-c.
- Riding on rough ground, from: Eup-pur.
- Spasmodic+: Vib.
- Utrine profuse with: Equi.
- Uterine
  - complaints, with: Nux-m.
  - displacement, with: Senec.
- Women, plethoric, in: Chim.

Double up, must, to urinate+: Pru-sp.

URINATION

Dribbling: CANTH; Caus; *Clem*; Dig; Kali-m; Lil-t; Merc; *Merc-c*; Nux-v; Pic-ac; Plb; Polyg; *Pul*; Sele; Stap; *Sul*; Tab; Terb.
- As if, rest agg: Sep.
- Forceps delivery, after: Bur-p.
- Involuntary: Arn; Canth; Caus; Clem; Sele.
  - angry, when: Pul.
- Labour, after: Arn; Tril.
- Prostate enlarged, with: Nux-v.
- Retention, with: Caus; Nux-v.
- Seat, rising from, when: Spig.
- Senile: Bar-c; Cep; Cic; Con; Equi; Nux-v.
- Sitting, while: Merc-c; Sars.
- Spurts, in, then: Bur-p; Caps.
- Stools
  - during: Colo.
  - after: Nat-c; Sele.
- Urination, after: Cann; Clem; Hep; Sele.
- Walking, when: Sele.
- Women, in winter, agg: Rhus-t.

Drinking, after: Ap; Arg-n; Caps+; *Fer-p*; *Samb*; Sars.

Dysuria: See Difficult.

Feeble, slow, weak: *Alu*; Arg-n; *Arn*; *Caus*; Clem; Hell; HEP; *Lyc*; Merc; Merc-c; Mur-ac; Nat-m; Op; Rhus-t; *Sars*; *Sep*; Sul; Thu.
- Copious, but: Plb.
- Difficulty in breathing and heart symptoms, with: *Laur*.
- Drops vertically: Arg-n; Caus; Gel; *Hep*.
  - violent pain, in bladder, with: Calc-p.

URINATION

Frequent: Alu; Ap; *Arg-m*; Arg-n; *Bar-c*; Calc; Canth; *Caus*; *Grap*; Hyo; Ign; Kali-io; Kali-n; Kre; *Lyc*; Mang; MERC; MERC-C; NUX-V; Psor; Pul; *Rhus-t*; *Scil*; *Stap*; *Sul*; Thu; Vib.
- Constipation, with: Sars.
- Day time: Kre; Rhus-t.
  - night, and: Merc.
- Every 10 to 15 minutes: Bor.
- Haemorrhage, with: Vib.
- Headache, with: Vib.
- Hour, every: Calc-ar.
- Hysterical: Gel.
- Menses, during: Hyo; Vib.
- Night more, than day: Thu.
- Pain, with: Thu.
- Pregnancy, during+: Pod.
- Prostate affections, in: Ap; Fer-pic; Sabal; Stap; Ther.
- Riding in carriage amel: Lyc.
- Urine, scanty with: Hell.

Hurried, sudden, irresistible: Arn; Bry; Canth; Clem; KRE; Nux-v; Petros; Pho; Pho-ac; *Pul*; Rum; Sanic; Scil; SEP; SUL; Thu.
- Water, hearing running or putting hands, in: Canth; *Lyss*; Sul.

Inability to pass, during pain: Con.

Infrequent, seldom: Ap; *Canth*; Lac-c; Lob; Nux-v; Op; Scil.
- Daytime: Bor; Lyc; Ther.
  - Twice, but scanty: Pyro.
- Once a day but profuse: Lac-c; Syph.
  - difficultly, with: Lac-c.

URINATION

Interrupted, intermittent: Agar; Ant-c; Ap; Carb-an; Caus; *Clem*; *Con*; Gel; Hep; Kali-c; Kali-p+; Led; Lyc; Op; Sabal; Sars; Sul; Thu.
- Coition, after: Pho-ac.
- Priapism, with: Ant-c.
- Spurts in, swelled prostate with cutting pain: *Pul.*
- Strains a few drops, then full flow follows: Clem.
- Suddenly, pain followed by: Pulex.

Involuntary: Ail; Ap; Ars; Ars-io; Bell; CAUS; Dul; *Fer*; *Hyo*; Lyc; Nat-m; Nux-m; Pho; Psor; *Pul*; *Rhus-t*; Sabal; Sec; Sep; Stap; Uran-n+.
- Bed, in: See BED wetting.
- Bladder feels empty, when: Helo.
- Coition, fright, from: Lyc.
- Constipation, with: Tarn.
- Convulsions, during: Buf; Caus; Cup; Hyo; Plb; Zin.
- Coughing, on: Ant-c; Ap; CAUS; Kali-c; Kre+; Mur-ac; *Nat-m*; Nux-v; PHO; *Pul*; Scil; Sep; Sul; Tarn; Thu+; Ver-a; Verb; Vib; Zin+.
  - night, at: Colch.
  - pregnant, women: Cocl.
- Day time
  - only: *Fer*; Flu-ac.
  - and night: Arg-n; Ars; Caus.
- Desire, if restricted: Pul; Sul; Thu.
- Dreams of urination with: Kre; Seneg; Sep.

URINATION, involuntary
- Effort on, no urination flow: Gel.
- Exertion agg: Bry.
- Flatus passing, when: Mur-ac; Pul; Sul.
- Fright, from: Op; Sep.
- Hurry, in, when: Lac-d.
- Inattention, from: Sep.
- Laughing, when: *Caus*; Nat-m; Nux-v; Pul; *Sep*.
- Lying agg: Bels; *Kre*; Lach; Lyc; Pic-ac; *Pul*; Uva.
- Menses, during: Hyo.
- Noise, sudden: Pul; Sep.
- Old people, in: Alo; Carb-ac; Cic; Iod; Sec.
- Parturition after: Arn; *Ars.*
- Pregnancy during: *Ars*; Nat-m; *Pul;* Sep; Syph.
- Prostate enargement with: Iod.
- Putting hands in cold water: Kre.
- Riding
  - agg: Lac-d; Thu.
  - amel: Lyc.
- Rising from seat agg: *Mag-c*; Petr; Spig.
- Running, while: Arn; Bry; Lac-d.
- Sitting
  - agg: Caus; Nat-m; *Pul*; Rhus-t; Sars.
  - amel: Zin.
- Sleepy, when: Bell.
- Sneezing, when (See coughing): Alet; *Caus*; Pho-ac; Pul+; Zin+.
- Standing, when: Bell; Fer.

URINATION, involuntary
- Stools, after: Mur-ac; Zin.
- Sudden movement, from: Fer.
- Surprise, pleasurable agg: Pul.
- Train catching, while: Lac-d.
- Uterus, prolapsed, from: Fer-io.
- Walking
  - while: Fer; Lac-d; Mag-c; Nat-m; Pul; Vib; Zin+.
  - amel: Rhus-t.
  - fast agg: Alet.
  - yet attempting to, when standing still, nothing passes: Mag-m.

Jets, in: See Spurts, in.

Menses
- Before agg+: Kali-io.
- Urging+: Sars.

Nervous: Cimi; *Ign*; Vib.

Nightly: Calc-f; Hyo; *Lyc*; *Rhus-t*; Spig; Sul; Ther; Uran-n.

Odd position, in: Zin.

Painful: See Difficult.

Pains agg: Calc; *Gel*; Terb; Thu.

Profuse, copious, polyuria: See URINE, profuse.
- Amel: Gel; Ign; Meli; Sang; Solid.
- Alternating with scanty urine: See URINE, profuse.

Retarded, must wait for urine to start: See Feeble.
- Bending backwards, amel: Alu.
- Doubling up amel: Canth; Pru-sp.
- Dribbling with: Alu.
- Hearing, water running amel: Lyss.

URINATION, retarted
- Lying amel: Kre.
- Odd position, in amel: Zin.
- Presence of others, in agg: *Amb*; Hep; Mur-ac; *Nat-m*; Tarn.
- Pressing
  - hard or straining at stool amel: *Alo*; *Alu*; Caus; Hep; Lil-t; Mag-m; *Mur-ac*; Op; Tub.
  - more, less it flows: *Kali-c*.
  - prostatic affections in: Ap.
  - so hard that anus protrudes: MUR-AC.
- Sitting
  - agg: Pul; Sars.
  - amel: Caus; Zin.
- Spasm of sphincter, from: *Op*.
- Standing
  - amel: Alu; Caus; Con; Hypr; *Sars*; Syph.
  - day time agg, but flows freely at night: Sars.
  - on cold pavements agg: Carb-v.
  - with feet wide apart body inclined forward, amel: Chim.
- Stooping amel: Canth; Par-b; Pru-sp.

Sensation, without: Alu; Arg-n; *Caus*; Kali-br; *Mag-m*.

Slow: See Feeble.

Spurts, in: Bur-p; Clem; Con; Tub.

Stools, only with: Alo; Ap; Mur-ac.

Stops and starts: See Interrupted.

URINATION
Stream
- Forcible: Cic; Nux-v.
- Forked: Arg-n; Merc-c; Pru-sp; Thu.
- Slender: *Clem*; *Cop*; Eup-pur; Grap; Nit-ac; Ol-an; Stap.
  - thread, like: Pru-sp.
- Spray, like: Kre.
- Twisted: Sul-io.

Uneasy feeling: Cedr; Ver-v.

Unsatisfactory, imcomplete: Ars; Caus; Clem; *Hep*; Lach; Mag-m; Sele.

Urging to stool, with: *Nux-v.*

Weakness, after: See Under WEAKNESS.

White at close: Pho-ac; Sars.

URINE
Altered in general: Pul; Sep; Sul.

Acrid: Arn; Benz-ac; *Hep*; Laur; Lyc; Med; *Merc*; Merc-c; *Pul*; Sul; Urt.

Albuminous: See ALBUMINURIA.

Alkaline: Bap; Carb-ac.

Ammoniacal, strong odour: *Asaf*; Benz-ac; *Iod*; Med; *Mos*; Nit-ac; Pho; Pic-ac; Stro.
- Menses, during: Nit-ac.

Aromatic: Eup-pur; Fer-io; Onos; Terb.

Bile, containing: Cean; *Chio*.

Biting: Sele.

Black: Ap; Ars; Carb-ac; *Colch*; Kali-c; *Lach*; Merc-c; *Terb*.
- Dung mixed, as if +: Ars.
- Inky: *Colch*.

Bloody (See HAEMATURIA and HAEMORRHAGE)**:** *Arn*; Ars; Ip; Merc-c; *Pho*; Sec; Scil; Senec; *Terb*.
- Backache with: Kali-bi.
- Clots: Chim.
- Constipation, with: Lyc.
- Cramps in bladder, after: Mez.
- Cutting in abdomen and urethra, with: Ip.
- First part: Con.
- Last part: Ant-t; *Hep*; Mez; Pul; Sars; Zin.
- Menses suppressed, with: Nux-v.
- Paraplegia, with: Lyc.
- Pathologial cause, without: Bell.
- Piles, suppressed, from: Nux-v.
- Sexual excess, after: Pho.
- Spine, shivering along with: Nit-ac.
- Urination
  - after: *Hep*; Thu.
  - frequent with: Ham.
  - urging, with: Sabi.

Bluish: Nit-ac.

Briny odour: See Fishy.

Brown: Arn; Ars; Benz-ac; Bry; Canth; Chel; Merc-c; Sep.

Burning: See Hot.

Cat's like, smell: Vio-t.

Cloudy: Ap; Berb; Bry; Canth; Carb-v; Chel; Chin; CINA; Con; Grap; MERC; Myr; *Pho*; Pho-ac; *Saba*; Sep; Sul.
- Fever, during: Pho.

URINE, cloudy
- Sweat, with: Ip; Merc; Pho.
- Turning: Bell; Berb; BRY; *Cham*; Chel; Chin; Grap; Lyc; *Pho-ac*; Terb.

Cold: Agar; *Nit-ac*.

Dark: Aco; Ant-t; Ap; Bell; Benz-ac; *Bry*; Calc; Chel; Colch; Lach; *Merc*; Sele; Sep; Solid; Terb; Ver-a.
- Flecks, in: Hell.

Drop, remains after urination: Kali-bi; Mag-m+.

Fishy odour: Ol-an; Sanic; Uran-n.

Flocculent: Berb; CANTH; *Mez*; Sars.

Flows in drops, then spurts in: Caps.

Frothy: Aur; Cean; Cep; *Chel*; *Kali-c*; *Lach*; Lyc; Scop; Sele; Seneg; *Spo*; Syph; Thu.

Foul, offensive: Ap; Arn; Bap; *Benz-ac*; Calc; Carb-v; DUL; Kre+; Nit-ac; *Pul*; SEP; Solid; Sul; Tarn; Thu.
- Dark red, at night, normal during day: Mos.
- Profuse: Rhod.
- Putrid: Hyds.

Garlicky: Cup-ar; Pho.

Gassy: Sars.

Greenish: Cam; Carb-ac; Cean; Merc-c; Ol-an; Ver-a.
- Red sediment, with: Mag-s.

Heavy: Bur-p; Coc-c.

Horse's Like: Benz-ac; Nat-c; Nit-ac.

Hot, burning: Alo; Ap; *Ars*;

URINE, hot ..
BELL; *Benz-ac*; Bor; Cam; *Cann*; *Canth*; Cub; *Hep*; Lil-t; Med; *Merc*; *Merc-c*; Nat-c; Nat-s; Nit-ac; Nux-v; Senec; Sep; Sul; Thu; Uva.
- Constipation, with: Fer.
- Coryza, fluent, with: Ran-sc.
- Menorrhagia, with: Fer.
- Urination before and after: Seneg.

Indican containing: Nit-ac; Nux-m; Pic-ac.

Itching, causing: Merc; Urt.

Less than drinks: Kre; Lith; Raph.

Milky: Ap; Aur; CINA; Hep; Kali-bi; Kali-p; Lapp; Lil-t; Lyc; *Pho-ac*; Vio-o; Visc.
- Blood, with: Kali-bi.
- Frequent+: Iod.
- Hydrocephalus, in: *Ap*.
- Menses, before: Pho-ac.
- Stools, after: Iod.
- Turns: Cina.
- Urination, at close of: Carb-v; Pho-ac; Sars; Sep.

More than drinks: *Ap*; Bell; Colo; Lac-ac; *Merc*; Nux-v; *Pho-ac*.

Muddy: Aesc; Kali-c; Nat-m; Rhus-t.

Musk like: Oci-c.

Odourless: Cedr; Spo.

Oily: Chin-s; Merc-c.

Onions, smell, like: Gamb.

Orange coloured: Lept.

Oxalic acid containing (oxaluria): Berb; Caus; Kali-s;

URINE, oxalic acid ..
  Nat-p; Nat-s; Nit-ac+; *Nit-m-ac*; Ox-ac; Terb.
 Pale, colourless: Cann; *Con*; Gel; Kali-c; Nat-m; PHO-AC; Sep; Stro.
 Pellicle, cuticle, on: Colo; *Par*; Pho; Psor; Pul; Sep.
  • Iridescent: Cep; Par; Pho.
  • Oily: Adon+; Crot-t; Iod; Pho; Sumb.
  • Red: Mez.
 Phosphates, containing: Alfa; Benz-ac; Calc-p; Lapp; Nit-ac+; Pho; *Pho-ac*; Pic-ac; Solid; Stan.
 Profuse, copious, increased (polyuria): Acet-ac; Alo; *Arg-m*; Arg-n; Cann; Cep; Cimi; Gel; Kre; Lac-c; Led; *Lyc*; Lycps; Merc; Mos; *Mur-ac*; Nat-c; Nat-s; Ol-an; *Pho*; *Pho-ac*; Plant; Pul; *Rhus-t*; *Scil*; Scop; *Spig*; Sul; Thu; Uran-n; Val; *Verb*; Vib.
  • Burning and backache+: Ant-c.
  • Concomitant, as a: Vip.
  • Coryza, with: Sep.
  • Dropsy, in: Scil.
  • Frequent, and+: Iod.
  • Haemorrhage, with: Calc; Gel; Ign; Lach; Mos; Sars; Stram; Sul; Vib.
  • Headache, with: Iris; Lac-d; Mos; Ol-an; Vib.
  • Heat of body, with: Samb.
  • Hysterical: Ol-an.
  • Menses, with: Cham; Hyo; Med; *Pho-ac*; Phyt; Vib.

URINE, profuse
  • Nervousness, with+: Fer.
  • Pain, during: Arg-m; Lac-d.
  • Scanty and alternately: Bell; *Berb*; Dig; Eup-p; Gel; Nit-ac; Senec.
 Purulent: Arn; Bap; Canth; Clem; Polyg; Sul-io; Uva.
  • Urination after: Hep.
 Raspberry, smell like: Sul-io.
 Recedes: Pru-sp.
 Red: Arn; Ars; Benz-ac; Berb; Bry; Canth; Chel; Lept; Lob; Merc-c; Sep; Stram.
  • Dark: Phyt.
 Residual: Dig.
 Retained (in bladder): ACO; Am-c; *Ap*; *Arn*; *Ars*; Bell; *Cam*; CANTH; Caus; Con; Erig; Gel; Hell; *Hep*; *Hyo*; LYC; Nux-v; *Op*; Par-b; Pul; Tarn; *Terb*.
  • As if, after urination: Berb; Hep.
  • Birth, at: *Aco*; Ap.
  • Cholera in: Cam; Canth; Carb-v; *Ver-a*.
  • Cold and wet exposure, from: *Aco*; *Dul*; Gel; Rhus-t.
  • Colic, during: Colo; *Plb*.
  • Confinement
   - during: Plb.
   - after: Ars; Bell; *Caus*; Equi; Hyo; Op.
  • Dribbling, with: Alu; *Caus*; Gel; *Nux-v*.
  • Dysentery, in: Arn.
  • Exertion, after: *Arn*; *Caps*; *Rhus-t*.
  • Fever, during: Fer-p; Op.
  • Fright, from: Aco; Op.

URINE, retained
- Hysteria, in: Ign; *Zin*.
- Illness acute, in, (fever etc.): Fer-p; Lyc; Op.
- Infants: Benz-ac.
  - nursing, angry on nurse: Op.
- Locomotor ataxia, in: Arg-n.
- Menses, during: Kali-bi.
- Music amel: Tarn.
- New born+: *Aco*; Ap.
- Old men: Solid.
- Operations, after: Caus.
- Overdistension, with: Hell.
- Painful: Canth; Caus; Nux-v.
- Painless: Nit-ac.
- Paraplegia, with: Apoc.
- Pavement, cold, standing on: Carb-v.
- Pregnancy during: Equi.
- Presence of others, in: NAT-M.
- Prostate enlargement, with: Chim; Dig; Stap.
- Sleepiness, with: Terb.
- Spasm, neck of bladder+: Op.
- Urging
  - unsuccessful+: Sec.
  - without: *Ars*; *Caus*; Pho; Plb.
- Water, noise from amel: Hyo; Lyss; Tarn; Zin.
- Whistling amel: Cyc; Tarn.

Saccharine: See DIABETES mellitus.

Saffron, like: Form; Oci-c.

Salts, deficient in: Led.

Sandy: Am-c; Benz-ac; Coc-c; *Led*; LYC; Pho; *Sars*; *Sele*; *Sep*; Sil; Sul-io; Tarn; Zin.
- Brown: Sul-io.
- Sticky: Pyro; Tub.

URINE, sandy
- Turbid: Chim.
- White: Berb; Calc; Grap; Kre; *Pho*; RHUS-T; Sars; Sep.
- Yellow: Cimi; Pho; Sep; Zin.

Scanty: AP; *Ars*; Aru-t; Bry; CANTH; *Colch*; Con; *Dig*; Dul; *Grap*; HELL; Hyo+; Hypr; Kali-n; Led; Lil-t; Lyc; Merc; Merc-c; Nat-s; Nit-ac; *Op*; Pho; Plb; Polyg; Pul; Rhus-t; *Rut*; Sars; Sele; *Sep*; Solid; *Stap*; Sul; Sul-io; Terb; Til; Ver-a.
- Agg: Benz-ac; Oci-c; Solid.
- Fever, during: Ap; Pul.
- Frequent and: Meny; Merc; Ol-an.
- Headache, then: Iod; Ol-an.
- Menses
  - before: *Ap*; Sil.
  - during: Nat-m.
- Nervous women: Agar.
- Thirst, with: Lith.

Sediment: Amb; Canth; Colo; *Lyc*; Merc; Pho-ac; Pul; Sars; *Sep*; Val; Zin.
- Adherent: Ap; Colo; Fer; Pho; Polyg; *Pul;* Pyro; SEP; Tub.
- Black: Colch; Lach; Terb.
- Bloody: Canth; Chim; Pho-ac; Pul; Sep.
- Branny: Ant-t; Merc; Pho; Val.
- Brick dust: See Red.
- Brown: *Amb*; Ap; Arn; Lach.
- Cheesy: *Pho*; Pho-ac; Sars; Sec.
- Clayey, earthy: Berb; Zin.
- Cloudy: Berb; Pho-ac.
- Coffee ground: Ap; Hell; Terb.

URINE, sediment
- Flaky, flocculent: Berb; Canth; *Mez*; Sars; Zin.
- Gelatinous: Berb; Colo.
- Gravel: Lyc; Polyg; Sars; Sep.
- Limy: Sabal.
- Mealy: Ant-t; Ap; Berb; Calc; Chin; Grap; Merc; Nat-m; Pho; Pho-ac; Sul.
- Mucous: Benz-ac; *Berb*; Chim; Equi; Merc-c; Nat-m; Par-b; *Pul*; Sars; Sep; Terb.
  - uterine displacement with: Senec.
- Muddy: Terb.
- Red, brick dust: Arn; Ars; Bry; *Canth*; Chin; Dig; Kali-c; Lob; LYC; Merc-c; *Nat-m*; Par-b; Pho; PUL; Sele; Senec; SEP; Tarn; *Val.*
  - peppery: Iod.
  - rosy: Am-ph.
  - thick: Kali-c.

Shreddy: Seneg.

Sour: Coc-c; Grap; Petr; *Sep*; Solid.
- Whooping cough, during: Amb.

Specific gravity
- Decreased: Merc-c; Pho; *Plb*.
- Increased (See Diabetes mellitus): Arn; Chio; Colch.

Stains diaper
- Brown: Benz-ac.
- Red: Sanic.
- Yellow: Phyt.
  - dark: Chel.

Suppressed: ACO; *Ap*; *Arn*; *Ars*; Cam; CANTH; Carb-v; Lach; Laur; Lob; LYC; Pul; Sec; Solid; STRAM; Urt+; Ver-a.

URINE, suppressed
- Cholera, in: *Ars*; Carb-v; Cup.
- Concussion of spine, from: Arn; Tarn.
- Convulsions, with: *Cup*; Stram.
- Dentition, during: Terb.
- Fever, during: Arn; Ars; Bell; Cact; Hyo; Op; Stram.
  - typhoid, after: Zing.
- Infants, in: Chim.
- Menses, during: Kali-bi.
- Spine, concussion, from: Arn; Tarn.
- Unconsciousness, during: Dig; Plb.

Sweetish odour: Arg-m; Eup-pur+; Nux-m; Terb.

Thick: Berb; Coc-c; Merc-c; Nux-v; Raph; Sep; Ver-a.

Valerian like: Murx.

Violet, odour like: Cam; Cop; Eucal+; Lact-v; Nux-m; Osm+; Terb; Thyr.

Viscid: *Colo*; Nat-s; Sep.

Watery: Gel; Ign; Mur-ac; Sep; Scil.
  - dung mixed, with: Ars.

White: See Milky.

Yellow: Aur; Berb; Card-m; Lach; Sep.
- Beer like+: Chel.
- Dark: Sang.

URINOUS ODOUR (of breath, secretions etc.): Benz-ac; Canth; *Colo*; Nat-m; Nit-ac; Ol-an; Sec; Urt.

URTICARIA, hives, wheals: Ant-c; AP; Ars; CALC; Calc-s; Caus; Chlo-hyd; Cop; *Dul*; Grap;

URTICARIA

Hep; Lach; Led; Mez; Nat-m; Pho; Polyg; RHUS-T; Sep; Sil; Sul; *Urt.*

Alternating, with
- Asthma: Calad.
- Rheumatism: Urt.

Ascarides, with: Urt.
Bathing agg: Bov.
Change of weather agg: Ap.
Chill, during: Ap; Ars; *Nat-m*; *Rhus-t.*
Chronic: *Lyc*; Strop.
- Children, in: Cop.
- Recurring: Hep.

Cold
- Air
  - agg: Nit-ac; *Rhus-t*; Sep.
  - amel: Calc; Dul.
- Bath agg: Calc-p.
- Drinks agg: Bell.

Colds agg: *Dul.*
Diarrhoea, with: Bov; Pul.
Evening agg: Kre; Nux-v.
Exercise, warmth of
- Agg: Con; *Nat-m*; Psor; *Urt.*
- Amel: Hep; Sep.

Fever, during: Ap; Cop; Ign; Rhus-t.
Fish
- Agg: Ars.
- Shell: Terb: Urt.

Flat, plaques, in: Form; Lob.
Giant: Ap; Kali-io.
Itching without: Uva.
Liver symptoms, with: Canc-fl; Myr; Ptel.
Meat agg: *Ant-c.*

URTICARIA

Menses
- Agg: Dul; Kali-c.
- After agg: Kre.
- Delayed agg: Pul.
- Profuse, with: Bov.

Morning, awakening, on: Bov.
Nausea, after: Sang.
Night agg: Chlo-hyd.
Nodular: Sul-ac.
Palpitation, with: Bov.
Pinworm, with: Urt.
Purple: Chin-s.
Receding: Strop.
Respiration difficult, with: Ap.
Rheumatism
- With: Rhus-t; Urt.
- Alternating with+: Urt.

Rubbing amel: Elat.
Scratching agg: Dul; Lach; Mez; Rhus-t.
Shuddering, with: Ap-g.
Suppressed agg: Urt.
Undressing agg: Pul.
Warmth amel: Lyc.
White: Nat-m.
- Apex: *Ant-c*; Pul.

Yearly, same season: Urt.

UTERUS: Arn; *Bell*; Castr; Caul; Cham; Cimi; Kali-c; Mag-m; Pall; Plat; *Pul*; Sabi; Sec; Sep; Ust+; Vib.

Anteversion: See Displacement.
Ascending agg: Plat.
Atony: Cimi.
Ball: Ust.
- Hot, ascends to throat: Raph.

UTERUS

Bearing down pains (See FEMALE ORGANS): Frax; Pall.
- Child nurses, when: Ust.
- Colds agg: Hyo.
- Sweat, hot with: Til.

Bending double amel: Cact; Cimi; *Nux-v*.

Bloated, wind in, as if+: Pho-ac.

Burning: Calc-ar+; Lach; Nux-v; Sep; Tarn; Terb.
- Limbs, pain alternating with: Rhod.
- Parturition, after: Rhod.

Bursting, something, in: Elap.

Cancer: Alum; ARS; Ars-io; Aur; Bell; Calc-ar+; Carb-an; Chin; Clem; *Con*; Grap; Hyds; Iod; *Kre*; *Lach*; Lyc; Mag-m; Merc; Murx; Pho; Plat; Sabi; Sars; Sec; *Sep*; Sil; Tarn; *Thu*.

Cause of many symptoms+: Caul.

Clutched and released as if: Sep.

Cold: Petr.

Colds agg: Hyo.

Consciousness, of: Helo; Lyss; Murx.

Cramp: Cocl; Pul.

Curetting, after: Bur-p; Kali-c; Nit-ac.

Cutting: *Bell*; Cocl; Con; Ip; Pall; *Pul*; Sul.
- Stools amel: Pall.

Displacement of (anteversion, retroversion): Ab-c+; Bell; Calc; Caul+; Eupi; Fer-io; Frax; Grap+; Helo; Lach; Lapp; Lil-t; Lyss+; Nat-m; Sep.

Distended, as if, filled with wind: Pho-ac.

Drop out, would: Crot-h.

Dropsy (hydrometra): Hell; Lyc.
- Limbs, piercing pain in: Hell.

Enlarged: Aur; Calc-io; *Con*; Helo; Lyc; Mag-m; Plat; Plb; *Sep*; Ust.

Full, as if: Alo; Bell; Helo.

Gnawing: Thyr.

Heart, alternating with: Lil-t.

Heavy: Calc-p; *Chin*; *Gel*; Helo; Pall; Pul; *Sep*.
- Hysteria, after: Elap.
- Leucorrhoea, with: Cimi.

Hour-glass contraction: Bell; Sec.

Hydrometra: See Dropsy.

Hypertrophy: Calc; Ust.

Induration: Aur.
- Abortions, after repeated: Aur.

Inert: Alet; Caul; Caus+; Cimi; Goss; Helo; Kali-c; Plb; Sabi; Sec; Sep.

Infantile: Bar-c; Calc-p; Fer; Helo; Iod; Pho; Senec; Thyr.

Inflamed: Ap; Ars; *Bell*; Canth; Lac-c; Lach; Lyc; Pul; *Rhus-t*; Sabi; *Sec*; *Sep*; Terb; Vib.
- Puerperal: Til.

Jerking: Ast-r.

Knotted, as if: Ust.

Lying agg: Amb.
- Back on amel: Onos.

Motions, in: Tarn.
- Foetus, as of a: Nat-c; Tarn.

Numb: Phys.

UTERUS

Nursing agg: Arn; *Cham*; Sil.
Open, as if: Lach.
Os rigid: See under CERVIX.
Painful: Bell; Colo; Helo; Ign; Lach; Murx; Nux-v; Pod; Pul.
Pessaries, after agg: Terb.
Prolapse (See PROLAPSE): Am-m+; Arg-m; Arg-n; Aur; Cimi; Coll; Fer-io; Frax; Helo; Lapp; Lil-t; *Pall*; *Plat*; Psor; Pul; Rhus-t; Senec; Sep.
• Coition
  - agg: Nat-c.
  - amel: Merc.
• Confinement, after: Helo; Pod; Rhus-t.
• Diarrhoea, from: Petr.
• Electric shock, down the thigh: Grap.
• Forceps delivery, after: Sec.
• Fright, from: Gel; OP.
• Head holding, and straining amel: Pyro.
• Hot weather in: Kali-bi.
• Lifting agg: Aur; Calc; Nux-v; Pod; Rhus-t.
• Lumbar backache, with: Nat-m.
• Lying
  - amel: Nat-m; Sep.
  - back on, amel: Nat-m; Onos.
• Menses
  - during: *Pul*; *Sep*.
  - after: Ip.
• Morning, in: Bell; NAT-M; Sep.
• Standing agg: Lapp.
• Stools
  - agg: Calc-p; Con; *Pod*; Psor; Stan.

UTERUS, prolapse, stools
  - straining at agg: Nux-v; Pod.
• Urination
  - dribbling with: Fer-io.
  - during: Calc-p.
  - foul, with: Benz-ac.
• Walking agg: Lapp.
• Weakness from: Sul-ac.
Pulsation, in: Bell; Cact.
Pyometra: Lach; Merc; *Pul*; *Sep*.
Reaching high with arms agg: Aur; Grap; Sul+.
Reflex symptoms from: Bell; Cimi; Goss; Helo; Kali-c; Lil-t; Plat.
Septic: See PUERPERAL SEPSIS.
Sharp pain: *Aco*; Con.
Soft, softening of: Op.
• As if: Ab-c.
Sore: Arn; Aur; Bell; Bry; *Gel*; Lach; Lapp; *Murx*; *Til*; Ust; Ver-v.
• Coition, during: *Pul*.
• Riding in carriage agg: Arg-m.
• Squeezed, as if: Bels; Gel; Kali-io.
  - menses, during: Kali-io.
Spasms, menses without: Kali-c.
Stitching: Aco; Bell; Con; Sep.
Subinvolution: *Arn*; Cimi; *Frax*; *Helo*; Kali-br; Pul; SEP; Sul.
• Abortion, after: Psor.
Swelled: Aur; Calc-io; Con; Lap-alb; Lyc; Plat; Sec; Sep.
Thighs
• Anterior, to: Vib.
• Down+: Ust.

UTERUS
Throat, to: Gel.
Tilted to
- Right: Murx; Pul.
- Left: Sep.

Tumours: See FIBROIDS.
Ulcer: Carb-an; Hyds; Kre; Ust.
- Abortions, from: Aur.

Undeveloped: Plb.
Undressing amel: Onos.
Weak, as if during stool and urination: Calc-p.

UVULA: *Ap*; Kali-bi; Merc; *Merc-c*; Phyt.
Bleeding: Lac-c.
Coughing agg: Ham.
Dripping: Aral; Cep; Hyds; Kali-bi; Merc-c; Spig.
Elongated, flaccid: Alu; Bar-m; Caps; Cof; Crot-t; *Hyo*; Kali-io; Lach; Pho; *Sul*.
- As if: Coc-c; Croc; Dul.
- Hawking constant from: Coc-c.
- Pressing on something hard: Caps.

Hanging to
- One side: Lach.
- Right: Ap; Nat-m.

Itching: Saba.
Oedema: *Ap*; Kali-bi; Merc-c; Phyt; Rhus-t.
Painful: Ap; Sang.
Relaxed as if: Kali-bi.
- Bladder like+: Kali-bi.

Sensitive: Clem; Sul.
Stiff: Crot-h.

UVULA
Swelled: Ap; Caps; Iod+; Kali-io; Merc-c; Pho; Sil.
Ulcers: Kali-bi; *Merc-c*.
- Eating: Hep.

White, shrivelled, and: Carb-ac.

VACCINATION, ill effects of
AGG: Ant-t; *Ars*; Hep; Kali-m; MALAND; Mez+; Sars; SIL; SUL; THU; Vacci; Vario.

VACILLATING: See IRRESOLUTE.

VAGINA: Berb; Calc; Fer; Kali-c; Lyc; Merc; Pul; *Sep*; Sul.
Aphthae: Caul.
Bloody water, from: Nit-ac.
Burning: Berb; Nit-ac; Pulex; Sul; Tarn.
- Coition, after: Lyc; Lyss.
- Hour, fixed, at: Chel.

Cancer: KRE.
Cold: Grap; Nat-m; Sec.
- Icy: Bor-ac.

Constriction: See Spasms.
Contraction: Kre; Sep.
Cotton ball, as if in: Pulex.
Cutting: Sil.
- Coition, during: Berb.
- Urination agg: Sil.

Cysts: Lyc; Pul; *Sil*.
- Serous: Rhod.

Damp: See Moist.
Discharge suppressed agg: Bur-p.
Dry: Fer-p; Grap; Lyc; Nat-m; Tarn; Zin-chr.
- Menses, after: Sep.
- Uneasy sensation, with: Zin-chr.

VAGINA

Enlarged, as if: Sanic.
Excoriation: Kali-bi.
Fistula: Carb-v.
Flatus from (physometra): *Bro*; Lac-c; *Lyc*; Nux-m; Nux-v; Pho-ac; Sang; Tarn.
- Abdomen, distended with: Sang.

Gangrene, after prolapse: Sul-ac.
Heavy, after hysteria: Elap.
Hot: Fer-p; Grap; Sec; Tarn.
Induration, painful: Chin.
Insensitive, during coition: See Numb.
Itching: Calad; Carb-ac; Cof; Hydroc; *Kre*; Med; Nit-ac; Plat; *Sep*; Stap; Sul; Tarn; Thu.
- Coition, after: Nit-ac.
- Deep in: Con.
- Pregnancy, during: Sabi.
- Rubbing agg: Med.
- Sexual excitement, with: Canth.
- Urinating, when: Kre.
- Warm bathing amel: Med.

Jerking in, upwards, morning: Sep.
Large, as if: Sanic.
Moist, as if: Ast-r; Eup-pur; Petr.
- Ease, feeling of, with: Ast-r.

Mucous flow, from sexual excitement: Senec.
Nodules, in: Agar.
Numb: Berb; Bro; Pho; Sep.
- Coition, during: Fer; Kali-br; Pho.

VAGINA

Orange coloured fluid from: Kali-p.
Painful: See Sensitive.
Pressing, upward, sitting on: Fer-io.
Prolapse: Bur-p; Fer+; Plat; Pod; Psor; *Sep*.
- Weakness, from: Sul-ac.

Pulsation: Alu; Merc.
Raw, sore: Berb; Fer; Kre; Lyss; Sul+; Tarn.
- Menses, during: Kali-c.

Scratching agg: Tarn.
- Until it bleeds: Sec.

Sensitive: Calc; Kre; Lyss; Plat; Stap; Thu.
- Coition agg: Hyds; Sul; Thu.
- Urinating agg: Coc-c.

Shooting up: Rhus-t; Sabi; Sep.
Sitting agg: Stap.
Spasms (vaginismus): Bell; *Cact*; Caul; Mag-p; Plat; *Plb*; Sep.
- Coition agg: *Cact*; Gel; Plat.

Stitches: Kre.
Swollen: Nit-ac.
Tears: Sec.
Ulceration: Mez.
Urinating agg: Sil.
Vegetation, granular: Stap.

VAGINISMUS: See VAGINA, spasms.

VALVE, leaf, skin as of a: Alu; Ant-t; *Bar-c*; Fer; Iod; Kali-c; Kali-io; Lach; Mang; *Pho*; Saba; *Spo*; Thu.

VALVULAR disease: See HEART, valves.

VANITY: See PRIDE.

VAPOUR, smoke, fumes as of: Ap; ARS; Bar-c; Bro; *Chin*; Ign; Lyc; *Pul*; *Ver-a*.
  Hot, through all orifices: Flu-ac.
  • Head, rising to: Buf.

VARICELLA: See CHIKENPOX.

VARICOCELE (See BLOOD VESSELS, distended): Coll; Fer-p; Flu-ac; Ham; Pul.
  Strain, after: Rut.

VARICOSES: See BLOOD VESSELS, distended.

VARIOLA: See SMALL-POX.

VARNISH like: Euphr; Grap; Nat-m; Petr; *Rhus-t*; Thu.

VAULTS agg: See DAMPNESS and CELLARS agg.

VEINS
  Broken: Card-m.
  Hard, knotty: Ham; Nux-v.
  Hot water, as if, in: Syph.
  Sore: *Ham*; Pul.
  Thrombosed, hard: Card-m; Flu-ac.
  Whipcord, like: Calc-hyp.

VENOSITY: Carb-v; Pul; Sul.

VERMIN: Stap.

VERTEBRA
  Absent, as if: Mag-p; Psor.
  Cracking, in: Nat-c; Ol-an; Sul.
  • Cervical: Cocl.
  Dorsal, upper: Kalm.
  • Last: Zin.
  Gliding, over each other, as if: Ant-t; Sul.
  Heat agg: Agar.

VERTEBRA
  Loose, as if: Calc.
  Slipping (See DISLOCATION easy): Sanic; Sul.
  Tumour: Lach; Tarn.

VERTEX: *Cact*; Calc; *Calc-p*; Carb-an; Caus; Cimi; Cup; Glo; Hypr; *Lach*; Lyc; Meny; *Nit-ac*; Pho; Pho-ac; RAN-SC; *Sil*; SUL; VER-A; Ver-v.
  Aching: Ign.
  • Eyes, between and : Ver-v.
  Across (ear to ear): Chel; Kali-m; Naj; Nit-ac; Pall; Phys; Sabal; Sil.
  Breathing deep agg: Anac.
  Burning, heat: Calc; Frax; Glo; *Grap*; Lach; SUL.
  • Grief, after: Calc; Pho.
  • Spot: Arn.
  Bursting: Carb-an; Cimi; Sanic+; *Sil*; Syph+.
  • Eating amel: Carb-an.
  Cold: *Calc*; *Calc-p*; Naj; *Sep*; VER-A.
  • Agg: Naj.
  • Icy+: *Calc*.
  • Lump, as if+: *Ver-a*.
  Congestion: Cinb.
  Coughing agg: Anac.
  Cracking, in: Cof.
  Crawling: Cup.
  Dry: Ars; Frax.
  Fly off, as if: *Bap*; Bur-p; Cann; *Cimi*; Iris; *Syph*; Xanth.
  • Air, cold, letting in: Cimi.
  Heavy: See Pressure.
  Hot, as if+: Tarx.

VERTEX

Itches, during headache: Ver-a.
Jaws, to: Lach.
Lying agg: Manc.
Menses agg: Fer-p.
Night
- Agg: Laur.
- Amel: Mag-c.

Numb: Glo; Mez; Plat.
Open and shut+: *Cann.*
Pressure, heavy, crushing: Alo; Ap; Bell; CACT; Cimi; Fer-p; Glo; Hypr; *Lach*; Lapp; *Lyc*; MENY; NAT-M; PALL; *Pho-ac*; Plb; Sil; Stan; Sul; Zin; Zin-chr.
- Agg: *Chin*; Lach; Phys; Ther.
- Amel: Cact.

Sides down: Fer-p; Hypr.
Sleep amel: Calc.
Sore, painful: Chin; Nit-ac; Sul.
Stooping agg: Meny.
Sweat, pricking during each meal: Cep.
Tension: Lob.
Throbbing: Bry; Caus; Cocl; Lach; Pho; *Sil*; Sul; Syph; Visc.
- Sudden: Visc.

VERTIGO: Aco; Agar; Ail; Ap; Arg-m; BELL; BRY; *Calc*; *Chel*; Chin-s; *Cocl*; *Con*; *Cup*; *Cyc*; Dig; Dul; Fer; Gel; Lyc; *Nat-m*; *Nux-m*; NUX-V; Onos; Op; *Petr*; PHO; PUL; *Rhus-t*; Sang; Sec; Sep; *Sil*; *Sul*; Tab; Zin-io.

AGG, during: *Aco*; *Calc*; Cyc; Fer; GEL; NUX-V; *Pho*; Pul; *Stram.*

VERTIGO

Air, open agg+: Cyc.
Ascending
- An eminence agg: Bor; *Calc*; Sul.
- Stairs agg: *Calc*; Kali-bi.
  - descending, and: Phys.

Aural: Aur; Bry; Chin; Nat-sal; Sil.
- Noises in ear, with: Iris.

Bending, backward amel: Ol-an.
Blood, rushing to the head with: Bell; Dig; Glo; Hell; Merc; Ver-v.
Blowing nose agg: Codei; Culex; *Sep.*
Breathing, deep agg: Anac; Cact.
Burdens, carrying on head agg: Tarn.
Chill, with: Cocl.
Coition, after: Bov; Pho-ac; Sep.
Cold
- Application amel: Nat-m.
- Drinks, from: Colch.

Constipation agg: Calc-p.
Coloured light agg: Art-v.
Coughing agg: Anac; Ant-t; Cof; Kali-bi; Mos.
Crossing
- Bridge agg: Bar-c; Bro; Lyss.
- Running water agg: Arg-m; Bell; Bro+; Fer; Hyo; Lyss; Sul.

Dark, in: Alu; Arg-n; Kali-io; Pic-ac; Stram.
Deafness, with: Merc-c.

VERTIGO
Descending
- Agg: Bor; Con; Fer; Gel; Plat; Sanic; Tarn; Vib.
- Spire: Sil.

Drawn up and pitched forward as if: Calc; Euon.
Drinking agg: Crot-t.
Drunk, as if: See Intoxicated.
Eating amel: Alu; Cocl; Dul; Nux-v; Saba.
Emissions, after: Bov; Caus; Nat-c; Sars.
Epileptic: Arg-n; Ars; *Hyo*; Sil; Tarn; Visc.
- After: Calc.

Erection agg: Tarn.
Exertion
- Agg: Cact.
- Amel: Pho.
- Violent agg: Mill.

Eyelids, twitching with: Chin-s.
Eyes
- Closing
  - agg: Ap+; Arg-n; Arn; Calad; Chel; Lach; Nat-m; Sil; Stram; *Ther*; Thu.
  - amel: Lol-t; Tab; Ver-v+.
  - opening, or: Alu.
- Focus, out of, when: Alu.
- Glassy+: Pho-ac.
- Opening amel+: Alum.
- Wiping amel: Alu.

Faint like: Bry; Cocl; Nux-v; Ther.
Falls
- Backward: Chin; Spig; *Rhus-t.*
- Forward: Nat-m; Rhus-t.
- Left, to: *Nat-m*; Sil.

VERTIGO, falls
- Right, to: Calc; Caus; Sil; Zin.
- Sideways, Benz-ac+; Calc; Cocl; Nux-v.

Fasting agg: Sul-io.
Female symptoms, with: Cyc.
Fevers, with: Carb-v; Cocl; Kali-c; Pul.
- All stages+: Eucal.

Flickers, before eyes, with: Aran.
Flowers, smell, from: Hyo.
Forehead, felt in: Arn; Croc; Euon; Gel; Pho; Sul.
Fright, after: Op.
Fulness and aching in vertex with: *Cimi.*
Gas light agg: Caus.
Hair binding agg: Sul-io.
Hands raising, above head: Onos.
Headache
- With: Ap; Bell; Calc; Con; Croc; Fer; Iod; Lac-c; Lil-t; Nux-v; Onos; Sil; Stro; Sul+.
- Before: Calc; Plat; Plb; Til.

Head
- Bent, backwards+: Stram.
- Big, feels during: Kob.
- Holding still amel: Con.
- Injury, from: Op.
- Lightness, of+: Op.
- Pushed, forward, as if: Fer-p.
- Resting amel+: Ver-v.
- Scratching agg: Calc.
- Sinks, forward: Cup.
- Sweat amel+: Nat-s.

VERTIGO, head

- Turning, quickly agg: Adon+; Colo.

Heart symptoms, with: Kali-c; Lach; Pho; Ver-a.

Heels, turning on, quickly amel: Stap.

Height, falling from as if: Caus; Gel; Mos+.

High celled room, in: Cup-ar.

Intoxicated, as if: Gel; NUX-V; Pul.

Kneading, motion on agg: Sanic.

Kneeling agg: Mag-c; Ther.

Lie down, must: *Cocl*; Nat-s; *Pho*; *Pul*; Spig.

Lifting
- Head from pillow+: Ant-t.
- Weight, on: Pul.

Lightning, from: Crot-h.

Looking
- Anything turning+: Lyc.
- Fixedly, at an object+: Old.
- One object at agg: Lach.
- Running water at agg: Arg-m; Bro; *Fer*; *Ver-a*.
- Sideways, agg: Thu.
- Up agg: Caus; Chin-ar; Grap+; Kali-p; Sang+; Sil; Thu.

Lying
- Agg: Ap; Calad; *Con*; Kali-m; Pul; Rhod.
- Back, on agg: Merc.
- Left side on agg: Iod; Lac-d; Onos; Pho; Sil; Zin-io.
- Right Side, on agg: Eup-p; Gel; Mur-ac; Rhus-t.

VERTIGO

Menses
- Affections, with: Caus+; Cyc.
- Before and during+: Sul-io.
- Profuse, with: Calc; Ust.
- Suppressed, from: Sabi.

Mental exertion
- Agg: Nat-c.
- Amel: Pho.

Motion (of head etc.)
- Agg: *Bry*; CON; Dig; Kali-br; Lil-t.
- Least agg+: Thu.
- Rapid agg: Sang.
- Shaking agg: Hep.

Nausea and vomiting, with: *Chin-s*; Cocl; Fer; Lapp; Lob; Petr; Sele; *Ther*.

Night, at: Tarn.

Noise agg: Ther.

Nose bleed, follows+: Carb-an.

Objects
- Seem far off+: Stan.
- Whirl around each other, as if: Saba.

Occiput, felt in: Bry; Carb-v; Con; *Gel*; PETR; *Sil*; Ver-a; Zin.

Pain
- Agg: Cimi.
- Before: Ran-b.

Palpitation, with: See HEART, palpitation.

Paralysis, before: Old.

Periodical: Cocl; *Nat-m*; *Pho*.

Pitched, forward, as if: Euon.

Pregnancy, during: Alet; Gel; *Nat-m*.

Pulse, slow, with: Ther.

VERTIGO

Railway travelling agg: Kali-io.

Reading
- Agg: All-s; Grap; Merc-i-f.
- Aloud agg: Par.
- Walking, while amel: Am-c.

Reeling (See REELING): Arg-n; Bell; *Gel*; Lol-t; Nux-v; *Pho*; Rhus-t.
- Amel: Carb-an.
- Coition, after: Bov.

Riding in carriage
- Agg: Hep.
- Amel+: Nit-ac.

Ringing in ears, with+: Lith; Pho-ac.

Rising
- From bed, raising up agg: Adon+; BRY; Chel; Cocl; Merc-i-f; Nat-m; Nux-v; Pho; *Phyt*; Ver-v; Vib.
- Hand above head, on: Onos.

Rocked, as if: See Swinging, as if.

Rocking amel: Sec.

Room and bed spin around+: Cadm.

Scratching agg: Calc.

Senile: Amb; Arn; Bar-c; Bels; Bry; Con; Cup; Op; Rhus-t.

Sewing agg: Grap.

Shaving agg: Carb-an.

Sitting
- Agg: Ap; Meph+; *Pho*; PUL; Sul.
- Amel: Cyc+; Lac-d.

Sleep
- During, at night: Caus.
- Falling on: Tell.

Sleepiness, with: Aeth; Gel; Laur; *Nit-ac*; Nux-m; *Sil*; Zin.

Smoking agg: Gel; Nat-m; Nux-v; Tab.

Seezing agg: Ap; Nux-v; Seneg.

Sour, fluid gulping, with: Caul.

Sparks, before eyes+: Ign.

Spasms,
- Before: See EPILEPTIC.
- Muscles of, with: Cic.

Standing amel: Nux-v; Pho-ac.

Stars white, before eyes, with: Alu; Ant-t.

Stomach pain, with: Cic.

Stools
- Agg: Kob.
- Amel: Cup; Pho; Zin.

Stooping
- Agg: Anac; Caus+; Meph+; Sul+; Ther+.
- Amel: Carb-an; Petr.
- Rising from: Anac; Saba; Sil.

Stupefaction, with: Aur; Calc; Zin.

Summer agg: Psor.

Sun facing agg: Agar; Glo; Kali-p; Nat-c.

Sweat
- With: Merc-c; Tab; Ver-a.
- Amel: Nat-s.

Swinging, swimming
- As if: Calad; *Merc*; Ox-ac; Petr; *Sul*; Thu.
- Left, to: Eup-p.
- Lying down, on: Ox-ac.
- Swimming vision, with: Strop.

VERTIGO, swinging
- Waking, on: Pho.

Syphilitic: AUR.

Talking agg: Alu; Cham.

Tea
- Agg: *Nat-m*; *Sep*.
- Amel: Glo.

Throat, choking, with: Iber.

Tinnitus,
- With (See MENIERS DISEASE): *Chin-s*; Iris.
- After: Chin.

Touch agg: Cup.

Trembling, with: Crot-h; Gel; Zin.
- Internal: Cup.

Turning
- As if in circle: Arn; Bry; *Con*; Cyc; Nux-v; Pho; *Pul*; Rhus-t.
- Agg: Con; Hyds; Old.
- Amel: Stap.
- Heels on amel: Stap.
- Right
  - agg: Lach.
  - amel+: Alum.
- Then headache: Rhus-t.

Turns in circle, as if: Bell; Berb; *Calc*; Caus.

Unconsciousness, followed by: Sil.

Urination urging, when: Hypr.

Vertex, felt in: Calc; Chel; Lyss; Med; Scop.

Violent: Meph.

Vision affections, with: *Cyc*; Fer; GEL; Nux-v; Strop.

Vomiting amel: Eup-p; Nat-s; Op.

VERTIGO

Wakes with, night at: Saba.

Walking
- Agg+: Anac.
- Air open, in agg: Lach.
- Darkness in agg: Stram.

Walls, falling on her, as if: Arg-n; Saba.

Weakness, with: Aeth+; Colch; Echi; Sele.

Whirling: See Turns in circle, as if.

Window
- Looking out of agg: Ox-ac.
- Standing near agg: Nat-m.

Wine agg: Nat-c.

Writing, while: Grap; Kali-bi; Sep.

VESICLES: See Under ERUPTIONS.

VEXATION: See ANGER

Agg: See MORITIFICATION, agg.

VIBRATIONS, fluttering: Am-c; Bell; Bro; Carb-v; Cimi; *Glo*; Meli; Meph; Old; Op; *Sang*; Sep; Sul.

AGG: Colch.

Lying down, as: Clem.

Stepping, on: Arn.

VICARIOUS: See DISCHARGES and MENSES.

VIGOUR

Increased, during convulsions: Agar.

Sense, of: Cof; Nat-p; Op; Pho; Psor.

VINEGAR application of, amel: Meli.

VIOLENT

VIOLENT: See PAIN, tearing.

Effects: *Aco*; Alu; Anac; *Ars*; BELL; Bry; Canth; Carb-v; CHAM; Cup; Glo; Hep; *Hyo*; Ign; Iod; *Lach*; *Lyss*; Merc; Merc-c; Mez; NUX-V; Ox-ac; Spig; STRAM; Sul; *Tarn*; *Ver-a.*

VISE: See COMPRESSION.

VISION

Affections of, in general: Arg-n; Aur; BELL; *Con*; *Cyc*; *Gel*; *Hyo*; Jab; *Lyc*; NAT-M; Nux-v; Op; *Pho*; Pul; Rut; Sep; *Sil*; *Stram*; SUL.

Accommodation disturbed: Phys.

Acute: Bell; Buf; Chin; Hyo; Nux-v.
- Night at, hysteria in: Fer.

Amaurosis: See Paralysis of optic nerve.

Animals, bugs etc. sees: Cimi; *Hyo*; *Stram*.
- Snakes: Arg-n; *Gel.*

Asthenopia: Croc; Fer; *Jab*; *Nat-m*; *Rut*; Seneg.

Astigmatism: Gel; *Lil-t*; Phys; *Tub*.

Black, sudden blind spells: BELL; Caps; Cic; *Con*; Cyc; Glo; Grap; Hyo; Merc; *Nat-m*; Old; *Pho*; *Pul*; Sep; Sil; *Stram*; Sul.
- Menses, during: Grap; Pul; Sep.
- Periodical: Iris.

Blindness, loss of vision (See also paralysis of optic nerve): Aco; Con; HYO; Merc; Op; *Pul*; *Sil*; STRAM; Syph.

VISION, blindness
- Alcohol, from: Terb.
- Cause, without: Tab.
- Colour: Bell; Carb-s; Chlo-hyd; Cina; Onos; *Sant.*
- Day+: Lyc.
- Epistaxis, with: Ox-ac.
- Eyes
  - inflammation, from: Manc.
  - over use, from: Crot-h.
- Fainting, suddenly, after: Plb.
- Grief, from: Crot-h.
- Headache
  - with: Caus.
  - after: Sil.
- Hydrocephalus, in: Apoc.
- Hysterical: Pho; Plat; Sep.
- Lightning, from: Pho.
- Masturbation, from: Pho-ac.
- Menses
  - before: Dict.
  - amel: Sep.
- Nausea, with: Sep.
- Optic nerve, atrophy from: Syph.
- Periodical: Merc.
- Progressive central scotoma with: Carb-s; Iodf; Plb; Tab; Thyr.
- Reading, while: Pho.
- Retinal haemorrhage, from: Both; Crot-h.
- Retro-bulbar neuritis from: Chin-s; Iodf.
- Stools, amel: Ap.
- Stooping agg: Fer-p.
- Sun, lying in, from: Con.
- Tobacco, from: Pho.
- Vertigo with: Bell; Gel; *Nux-v.*

VISION, blindness
- White objects, looking steadily at: Tab.

Blue: Aur; Cina; Crot-c; Lyc; Tril; *Zin-chr*.

Circles: See Rings.

Coughing agg: Ign; Kali-m.

Crossed: Con; Kali-bi.
- Looking, one eye, with amel: Kali-bi.

Dark: Psor; Stram; Sul.

Dazzled, bright: Bar-c; Con; Dros; *Kali-c*; Nat-c; *Sil*.

Dim, blurred: Agar; Aur; Bell; Calc; CANN; CAUS; Chin; Con; Cyc; EUPHR; Gel; *Hep*; Lach; Lyc; Merc; Nat-m; Nit-ac; *Op*; *Pho*; Pho-ac; PUL; Rut; Sep; SIL; Sul.
- Looking sideways amel: Chin-s.
- Luminosities, after: Ther.
- Reading, after+: Colch.
- Twilight amel: Bry; Lyc.

Diplopia: AUR; Bell; *Cic*; Cyc; GEL; HYO; Med; *Nat-m*; *Nit-ac*; Pho; Pul; Stram; Sul; Ver-a; Ver-v.
- Bending head backwards amel: Seneg.
- Blowing nose, on: Caus.
- Deafness, alternating with: Cic.
- Diphtheria, after: Lach.
- Heart, affections with: Lach.
- Horizontal: *Nit-ac*; Old.
- Looking
  - right to, amel: Caus.
  - sideways agg: Gel.

VISION, diplopia
- Lying amel: Spo.
- Masturbation, from: Cina; Sep.
- Measles, after: Caus; *Kali-c*.
- Nausea, with: Crot-t.
- Pregnancy, during: Gel.
- Rubbling eye amel: Carb-an.
- Sexual excess, from: Sep.
- Uterine affections, from: Sep.
- Vertical: Atrop; Kali-bi; Lith; Rhus-t; Seneg; Stram; Syph.
  - menses, during: Lith.
- Vertigo agg: Bell; Old.
- Writing agg: Grap.

Distances, misjudging, of: Cann; Carb-an; Onos; Stram.

Downcast: Kali-c; Stan; Ver-a.

Drops, before: Kali-c.

Errors of: Spig.
- Difficult to fit glasses: Spig.

Exertion, physical amel: Aur.

Eyes
- Closing agg: Bell; Bry; *Calc*; Pho; Thu; Ver-v.
- Using one amel: Kali-bi; Pho; Phys.

Fantastic apparitions: Bell; Stram; Ver-a.
- Terrifying, in twilight, children+: Berb.

Far sight (hypermetropia): Arg-n; *Calc*; Nat-m; SEP; SIL.

Field of: Flu-ac; Hep; Mang; Pho; Thu.
- One half: Hep.
- See objects, besides: Calc; Cam; Cann; Colo; Grap; Ign; Lac-c; Nux-m; Nux-v; Stram; Thu.

VISION

Fiery, bright: *Bell*; Cinb; Hyo; *Kali-c*; *Pho*; *Spig*; Sul.

Fingers: Psor.

Fixed, absence of: Spig.

Flickering; flames; flashes, fiery: BELL; Coca; Cyc; *Grap*; Hyo; Ign; *Kali-c*; Lach; Nat-m; *Pho*; Sep; *Spig*; Sul.
- Borders black, with: Cimi.
- Coughing on: Ign.

Flies: See Muscae volitantes.

Foggy: See Misty.

Foundry, working in agg: Merc.

Fringe, as of: Con.

Glimmering, glittering: Cyc+; *Grap*; Iod; Lach; Nux-v; Ol-an; Pho; Strop; Syph; Ther.
- Needles: Cyc.
- Stooping, on: Ther.

Green: Ars; Cina; Dig; Osm; Pho; Phyt; Sant; Stram; Vario.
- Rising on: Vario.
- Spot, dark, in: Stro.

Hair as of a: Euphr; Lach; Plant.

Halo around the light: Bell; Chim+; Lach; Osm; PHO; Pul; *Sul*.

Headache
- Before agg: Gel; Glo; Grap; Iris; KALI-BI; Lach; *Nat-m*; Pho; Pod; PSOR; *Sep*; Sil; Sul; Ther; *Tub*.
- During agg: Bell; Iris; Pho-ac; Pod; *Pul*; Zin.
- After agg: Caus; Con; *Lach*; Pho; Sil; *Sul*.

VISION

Hemiopia: Ars; Aur; Chio; Cyc+; Lach; Lith; *Lyc*; Mur-ac; NAT-M; Tub.
- Right half, lost: Calc; Cocl; *Lith*; Lyc.
- Left half lost: Calc; Cic; Nat-c.
- Headache, then: Nat-m.
- Horizontal: *Ars*; Aur; Tub.
- Lower, lost: Aur; Sul.
- Menses, during: Lith.
- Pregnancy, during: Ran-b.
- Upper, lost: Ars; Aur; Cam; Dig.
- Vertical: Caus; *Lith*; Lyc; Mur-ac; Nat-m.

Illusions of
- In general: Bry; *Hyo*; Op; Sec; Sep; Spig; *Stram*; Thu; Val+; Ver-a.
- Operations, after: Stro.
- Same person front and behind+: Euphor.

Imaginary, on closing eyes: See Eyes closing agg.

Letters
- Appear
  - dancing: Bell; Lyss.
    disappear when reading: Cic; Cocl.
  - double, when writing: Grap.
  - red: Pho.
  - smaller+: Glo.
- Run together: Bur-p; Cann; Fer; Grap; *Nat-m*; Rut; *Sil*; Stap; Stram.

Light
- Agg: Hyo.
- Amel: Gel; Stram.
- Artifical agg: Aur; Lyc; Nat-m.

VISION

Lightning: Kali-c; Nat-c; Pho; Spig.

Looking with one eye amel: See Eyes using one.

Luminous
- Dark, in: Val.
- Operations, after: Zin.

Menses
- Before agg: Dict.
- During agg: Cyc; Grap; Pul; Sep.

Mirage: Lyc.

Misty: Ars; *Calc*; *Caus*; *Croc*; Cyc; Gel; Meny; Merc; PHO; Pul; Sul; Zin.
- Luminous yellow, quivering: Kali-c.
- Seminal emissions, after: Sars.

Muscae volitantes: Agar; Chin; Cocl; Merc; Nat-m; Pho; Phys; Sep; *Sil*; *Stram*; Sul.
- Right: Chin-s; Cimi; Sele; *Sil*.
- Left: Agar; Calc; *Caus*; Merc; *Sul*.
- Brown: Agar.
- White: Jab; Ust.

Near sight (myopia): Con; Lil-t; Nit-ac; *Pho*; Pho-ac; Phys; *Pul*.
- Head, turns sideways to see clearly: Lil-t.

Nebulous+: Mill.

Objects appear
- Black: Caps; Stram.
- Blood, covered with: Stro.
- Blue: Tril.
- Borders, coloured, with: Hyo.
- Bright: Hyo; Nat-c; Val.
  - dark room, in: Val.

VISION, objects appear
- Crooked, distorted: Bell; Buf; Nux-m; Stram.
- Distant: Anac; Carb-an; Gel; Ox-ac; Stan; Stram; Sul.
  - yawning, when: Cep.
- Fade away, then reappear: Gel.
- Glisten: Ol-an.
- Half in light, half in dark: Glo.
- High, lean forward and about to fall: Arn.
- Inverted: Bell; Kali-c.
- Large: Berb; Caus; Euphor; Hep; *Hyo*; Laur; Nat-m; *Nux-m*; Onos; Ox-ac; Pho.
  - linear: Ox-ac.
- Move in circle, on closing eyes: Hep.
  - to and fro: Cic.
  - to right: Nat-sal.
- Moving, dancing: *Arg-n*; *Bell*; Cic; Cocl; Con; Glo; Psor.
  - colours, changing: Stro.
- Nearer: Bov.
  - distant seem, yawning on: Cep.
  - each other, to: Nux-m.
  - eyes, to: Val.
- Persons are, as if: Bell; Calc; Nat-p; Stram.
- Round, pass before eyes while lying: Caus.
- Run together: Berb; Sil.
- Shade, as if, in: Seneg.
- Small: Med; Merc-c; Plat; Stram+.
- Tremble, then get dark+: Psor.

VISION, objects appear
- Turning in circle, as if: Chel; Cyc; Nat-m.
- Vibrating: Carb-v.
  - dark, become, then: Psor.
- Whirl, each other, around: Saba.
- White: Chlo-hyd; Grat.

Pale: *Sil.*

Paralysis of optic nerve: *Bell*; Bov; *Caus*; Con; GEL; Hyo; Kali-io; Nat-m; PHO; *Pul*; *Sec*; *Sil*; *Stram*; Sul.

Perceptive power, lost: Kali-p.

Photopsies: See Illusions.

Presbyopia: See Far sight.

Purple: *Ver-v.*

Rain through, looking, as if: Nat-m.

Rainbow: Bell; Bry; Con; Pho-ac.

Red: BELL; Con; Hep; Hyo; *Pho*; Rut; Sul; *Ver-v.*
- Night, at: Cedr.
- Spot: Ver-v.

Rings: Calc; Calc-p; Carb-v; Elap; Kali-c; Psor.
- Turning: Kali-c.

Scintillations: See Sparks.

Shade amel: Con; Pho.

Shadows: Rut; Seneg.
- One side of object: Calc.

Sitting erect agg: Kalm.

Snow, exposure to, agg: *Aco*; Cic.

Sparks: *Bell*; *Chin*; Kali-m; Lyc; Sec; Sep.
- Blowing nose, on: Nat-s.
- Dark, in: Bar-c; Bell; Pho.

VISION, spark
- Eyes closing, on: Hyds.
- Headache, during: Chel; *Mag-p.*
- White: Alu.
- Winking, on: Caus.

Spots, spotted: Am-m; Cyc; *Kali-c*; PHO; Sil; Sul.
- Fiery and: Elap.
- Green, dark in: Stro.
- Sewing, after: Am-c.
- White: Jab.

Stooping agg: Fer-p; Elap; Ther.

Striped: *Con*; Sep; Sul; Thu.
- Green: Thu.

Triplopia: *Bell*; Con; Sec.

Veil, as of a (See Misty): Pho; Sep+.

Violet: Cina.

Wavering: Morph; Nat-m; Ver-v; Zin-chr.

Weak: ANAC; BELL; *Chin*; Con; Nat-m; Op; Pho; Rut; Seneg.
- Coition, after: Kali-c.
- Headache, with: Zin.
- Masturbation, from: Cina.

White: Chlo-hyd; Grat.

Yellow: Alu; Calend; Canth; Cina; Dig; Sep.
- Attacks on blindness, after: Bell.
- Day during: Cedr.

Zigzag: Con; Grap; Lach; Lyc; *Nat-m*; Pho; Sep; Sul-io.

VITREOUS OPACITY, diffusion:
Gel; Ham; Hep; Kali-io; Merc-c; Merc-i-r; Seneg; Sul; Thu.

Turbid: Choles; *Kali-io*; Pho; Pru-sp; *Seneg*; Sul.

VIVACITY: See CHEERFUL.

VOCAL CORDS: See under LARYNX.

VOICE (See also SPEAKING, speech): Aco; *Bell*; Bro; Canth; Carb-v; *Caus*; DROS; Hep; *Iod*; Mang; *Merc*; PHO; Pul; Spo; Stan; *Stram*; Ver-a.

Altered: Ox-ac.

Barking: *Bell*; *Canth*; Lyc; Spo; Stram.

Breaks, cracks, fails, changes key: Ant-c; Aru-t; Bell; Con; Grap; Sep; Spo; Stram.
- Suddenly, in higher tones: Stram.

Changeable: Arg-m; Ars; *Aru-t*; Fer; Mang; Seneg.
- Boys and girls, in: Mang.

Colds agg: Carb-v; Caus; Mang; Merc; Pho; Sele.

Control, lacks, using amel: Grap.

Creaky: Sec.

Croaking: Aco; *Stram*.

Crowing: Spo; Stram.

Deep: Carb-v; Dros; Stan.

Distant, seems: Sabal.

Echoes in ear: Caus; Pho.

Exertion agg: Arn.

Hissing: Nux-v; Pho.

Hoarse, croupy: *Aco*; Arg-m; Arg-n; Ars-io; Aru-t; BELL; *Bro*; Bry; *Calc*; Caps; CARB-V; CAUS; *Cep*; Cham; DROS; *Hep*; IOD; *Kali-bi*; Kali-m; *Lach*; MANG; *Merc*; Nat-m; PHO; Sele; SPO; Stan; Stram; *Sul*; Tell; Verb.
- Breathing cold air agg: Cup.

VOICE, hoarse
- Children, in: Cham.
- Choking: Iod.
- Chronic: Mang; Sil.
- Colds, from: Arn; Ip; Sele.
- Cold water bath, from: Ant-c.
- Coughing and expectoration amel: Mang; Stan.
- Diptheria, after: Phyt.
- Evening: *Carb-v*; Caus; *Pho*; Rum.
- Exertion agg: Arn.
- Heart complaints, with: Hyd-ac; Nux-m; Ox-ac.
- Heated, if agg: Bro.
- Larynx, burning in+: Am-m.
- Laughing, when: Calc-f.
- Leucorrhoea, with: Nat-s.
- Menses agg: Gel; Grap; Lac-c; Spo; Syph.
- Morning: Calc; Calc-p; CAUS; *Mang*; Pho; *Sul*.
  - evening, and: Caus.
- Painful: Iod.
- Painless: Calc+: Ip.
- Periodical, painless: Par.
- Reading or reciting aloud agg: Calc-f; Seneg.
- Sexual loss agg: Seneg.
- Singers: Caps; Hep.
- Smoking amel: Mang.
- Sneezing amel: Kre.
- Speakers: Caps; Caus.
- Stooping agg: Caus.
- Talking
  - agg+: Coca.
  - amel: Caus; Grap; Tub.
  - painful: Merc-cy.
- Walking against the wind agg: Euphr; *Nux-m*.

VOICE, hoarse
- Wet getting, from: Arn; Merc-i-r.

Hollow: Bell; *Dros*; *Spo*; Stan; *Ver-a*.
Human agg: Mur-ac.
Husky: *Dros*; Grap+; Merc; *Pho*.
Indistinct: *Bro*; CAUS; Lyc.
Lost, aphonia: Alum; *Am-caus*; *Ant-c*; Arg-m; Arg-n; Ars-io: Bro; CARB-V; *Caus*; Colch+; Hep; Kali-bi; Kali-p; Mang; Ox-ac; *Pho*; Phyt; Stram; Ver-a.
- Chronic: Phyt.
- Colds agg: Alu.
- Cough, with: Mang.
- Epilepsy, before: Calc-ar.
- Exertion agg: *Carb-v*.
- Menses
  - before: Syph.
  - during: Gel.
- Over-heating, from: Ant-c.
- Paralytic: Bar-c; Caus; Kali-p; Ox-ac.
- Singers: Arg-m+; ARG-N; CAUS; Mang; Sele.
  - periodically: Cup.
- Sudden: Alu; Bell; *Caus*.
- Tongue affections without: Both.

Loud: Hyo; Nux-m.
Low: Canth; Hep; Ox-ac; Ver-a.
Male agg: Bar-c; *Nit-ac*.
Nasal: Bell; *Kali-bi*; Lyc; Pho-ac; STAP.
Over use, talking, singing agg: Ant-c+; Arg-m; *Arg-n*; *Aru-t*; Caps; Caus; Fer-p; *Grap*; Merc; RHUS-T; *Sele*; Seneg; Stan.

VOICE
Rough: Bell; Carb-v; Hyo; Kali-bi; *Pho*; Pul.
- Overuse from+: Ant-t.

Screeching: Samb.
Shrill: Aco; Samb; Spo; Stram.
Slow: Ars; Pho; Thu.
Speaking through full mouth, as if: Nux-v.
Stammering: See SPEECH.
Toneless, loss of timbre: *Dros*; Stram.
Tremulous: Merc.
Trumpet, like: Verb.
Unsteady: Seneg.
Using amel: Ant-t; Caus; Grap.
Weak: Alu; Ant-t; Canth; Carb-an; Cocl; Hep; Spo; *Stan*; *Ver-a*.
- Menses, during: Plb.

VOICES HEARS: See IMAGINATIONS, voices of.

VOMITING (remedies in general)
Aco; Aeth; Ant-c; *Ant-t*; Ap; APOC; Arn; ARS; *Bry*; Cadm; Carb-an+; *Cham*; *Cina*; Colch; *Cup*; *Fer*; IP; Iris; Kre; *Lob*; NUX-V; Op; Pho; Plb; *Pul*; *Sil*; Strop; *Sul*; Tab; VER-A; *Ver-v*.

AGG: Aeth; *Ars*; CUP; Dros; *Ip*; Old; *Pul*; Sil; *Sul*.
AMEL: Ant-t; Coc-c; Dig; Eup-p; Kali-bi; Nux-v; *Sang*; Sanic; Sec; Tab; Xanth.
Acrid, scalding: Chio; *Iris*; Kali-c; Kali-m; *Kre*; Lyc; Med; Rob; *Sang*; Sul.
Albuminous, glairy: Jat; Kali-bi.

VOMITING

Anxious: Ars; Tab.
At once: Apoc; Ars; Cadm; Zin.
Bed, after going, to: *Tarn.*
Bilious (See YELLOWNESS): Bism; Flu-ac; Ip; IRIS; Lept; Nat-s; Op; *Sang*; Ver-a.
- Amel: Card-m; Eup-p; Sang.
- Cramps, with: Cham.
- Eating, after: Bism.
- Errors of diet, from: Flu-ac.
- Stooping, on: Ip.

Bitter: Bry; Chio; Eup-p; *Iris*; Kali-bi; *Nux-v*; Pho; Pic-ac+; Sang.
- Drinks, after: Eup-p.
- Greenish, after cold drinks: Rhod.
- Water: Lac-d+; Mag-c.

Black: ARS; *Cadm*; Kre; Mez; NUX-V; Pho; Ver-a.
Blood: Arn; Cact; Cadm; *Carb-v*; *Chin*; *Crot-h*; Fer; *Ham*; *Ip*; Pho; Sabi; Sec.
- At the close of: Ver-a.
- Infants: Lyc.
- Menses, instead of, in girls: Ham.
- Splenic affections, from: Card-m.
- Topers in: Alum.

Bluish: Kali-c.
Brain affections, in: Bell; Glo; Kali-io; Plb.
Brown: Ars; Bism; Bry; Carb-v; Mez; Nat-s; Plb; Rhus-t.
Burning, hot (See Acrid): Mez; Pod.
Cancer, from: Carb-ac; Kre.

VOMITING

Chill
- During: Eup-p.
- After: Eup-p; Lyc; Nat-m.

Coffee grounds: Cadm; Con; Echi; Mez; Pho; Pyro.
Coition, after: Mos; Saba; Sil.
Colic, with: Hyo.
Consumption, in: Kali-br; Kre.
Continuous: Ars; Hell; Ip; Merc; Plb; Pyro; Syph.
Convulsions
- Alternating with: Cic.
- Before: Hyd-ac.
- With: Ant-c; Hyo.

Convulsive: *Bism*; Cup.
Coughing
- With: See under COUGH.
- After: Sul-ac.

Curds: Aeth; Calc; Nat-p; Sanic; Sil; Val.
- Sour: Calc; Nat-p.

Cyclic, infants, in: Cup-ar; Iris; Kre; Merc-d.
Death, desires, during: Phyt.
Delayed, after a while: Bism; PHO.
Difficult: *Ant-t*; Ars.
Drinking
- Agg: *Ant-c*; *Ars*; Bry; Kali-bi; Pho; Sil; Tab; Ver-a.
- Cold amel: Cup; Pho; Pul.
- Every: Apoc.
- Immediately after, even smallest quantity: *Ars*; *Bism*; *Bry*; *Cadm*; Cina; Pho; Pyro; Ver-a; Ver-v; Zin.
- Warm after: Bry.
- Water, from: Sars.

VOMITING, drinking
- When it becomes warm, after a while: Kali-bi; PHO; *Pyro*.

Easy: Apoc; *Ars*; Bap; *Cham*; Fer; Ip; Jat; Phyt+; Sec+.

Eating
- After: Kali-br.
- Amel: Ant-t; Nux-v; Pul.

Emotions, from: Kali-br.

Eructation, with: Mur-ac.
- Recur, as if would, with: Goss.
- Sour, with: Nit-ac.

Exhausting: Aeth; Ant-t; Cadm+; Pod; Ver-a; Ver-v.

Faecal: Op; Plb; Pyro; Raph; Rhus-t; Tab.

Fearful: Ant-c.

Fever, during: Ant-t; Bap; Eup-p; Nat-m.

Fluids, only: Ars; Bism.

Food
- Every kind of+: Acet-ac.
- Odour, from: Stan.

Forcible: Aco; Ant-t; Apoc; Con; Nux-v; Petr; Ver-a; Ver-v.
- Eating, shortly after: Sanic.
- Sudden: Ant-t; Kali-bi; Kali-chl; Pic-ac.
  - fever, with: Bap.

Frequent: *Ars*; *Chin*; Con.

Frothy: Aeth; ARG-N; Ars; *Kre*; Led; Mag-c; Nat-c; Pho; Sil; *Ver-a*.
- Hot: Pod.

Greasy, oily: Iod; Mez; Nux-v.

Green: *Ars*; Bell; Cham; *Chel*; Cimi; Eup-p; *Ip*; Merc-d; NAT-S; Stram; *Ver-a*.

VOMITING, green
- Bitter, cold drinks, after: Rhod.
- Black: Hell; Mar-v.
  - olive: Carb-ac.

Hawking mucus, in the moring: Bry; Calc-p; Euphr; Nux-v.

Headache, with: Bry; Caus; *Chel*; Cocl; IP; *Iris*; Meli; NUX-V; PUL; Sang; Sep; Ver-a.

Hiccough, after: Jat.

Hot water amel: Ars; Chel; Sul-ac.

Hunger, with: Ver-a.

Hysterical: Kali-br.

Incessant, without food connection: Lac-d.

Ingesta, food of: Ars; *Bry*; Chin; *Cina*; Eup-p; FER; *Ign*; Kre; Lyc; NUX-V; Pho; PUL; Sang; *Sil*; *Sul*; Ver-a.
- Colic, abdominal followed by: Manc.
- Long after meals: Aeth; Ars-io; *Fer*; Kre; Plat; Pul; Sabi; Sang.
  - whooping cough, in: Meph.
- Milk, except: Hyds.
- Night, at: Kali-c.
- Smallest quantity: Ver-v.
- Water
  - bitter: Lac-d.
  - except: Hyds.
  - then: Pul.

Lifting agg: Sil.

Liquids, only: See Fluids.

Lying on
- Back agg: Rhus-t.

VOMITING, lying on
- Left side agg: Sul-ac.
- Right side
  - agg: Crot-h.
  - amel: Ant-t.

Menses
- During: Am-m; Apoc; Kali-c; Lach; Pul.
- After: Crot-h.

Midnight, after+: Fer.

Milk: Aeth; Calc; Mag-c; Pod; Sanic; Sil; Val; Vario.
- Mother's: Sil.
  - anger, after: Val.
- Peristently: Calc-p; Pho-ac.
- Undigested: Mag-c.

Milky: *Sep.*

Month, every: Crot-h.

More than he drinks: Kali-bi.

Morning: Caps; Cup; Grap+; Hep.
- Early: Stan.
- Sickness, during menses+: Grap.

Motion, least agg: Tab.

Mouth, rinsing on: Sep.

Mucous: Arg-n; *Dros*; *Ip*; Kali-bi; Nux-v; Pho; PUL; Sul-ac; Ver-a.
- Amel: Nat-m.
- Bloody: Merc-c.
- Green: Kali-chl; Plb.
- Sour: Kali-c.
- Watery, mass of: Guai.

Nausea, without: Ant-c; Apoc; Arn; Ars; Chel; Fer+; Kali-bi; Lyc; Phyt+; *Ver-v*; Zin.

Neuralgia, with: Aran.

Night, at: Kali-c.

Obstinate, for days: Oenan.

VOMITING

Offensive: Ars; Nux-v; *Sep.*
- Fluid: Abro.

Operations on abdomen, after: Bism; Cep; *Nux-v*; *Pho*; Stap.

Painful: Ars; *Ver-a.*

Periodical: Cup; Iris; Plb.

Peritonitis, in: Op.

Pessary in vagina, from: Nux-m.

Pregnancy agg: Alet; Anac; Asar; Chel; Cocl; *Cyc*; Fer+; Goss; Ign; *Ip*; Jab; *Kre*; Lac-d; LOB; MED; Nat-s; Nux-m; *Nux-v*; Psor; Sep; Sul; Symp; Tab; Thyr+.
- Obstinate: Alet+; Jab; Psor.

Pressure on spine and neck, from: Cimi.

Projectile: See Forcible.

Purging, with: Aeth; Ant-t; Ap; Arg-n; ARS; Asar; Bor; Cam; Cham; Colch; Cup; Ip; *Iris*; Merc; Pho; *Pod*; Sec; Seneg; Sul; Sul-ac; VER-A; Ver-v.
- Bilious: Eup-p.
- Blood: Erig.
  - black: Ars.
- Fright, from: Op.
- Headache with: Grap.
- Menses, during: Am-m.
- Urination, and: Crot-h.

Relief, without: Ant-c.

Renal origin, from: Senec.

Respiratory symptoms, with: Lob.

Rice
- After: Tell.
- Water: Cup; Kali-bi; Ver-a.

Salty: Benz-ac; Iod; Nat-s.

VOMITING

Scratching, when: Ip.
Septic: Bap; Crot-h; Lach; Vip.
Shievering, with: Dul.
Sleep, then: *Aeth*; Ant-t; Cup; Nat-m; Sanic+.
Solids only: Arn; Bry; Cup; Fer; Sep; Ver-a.
Sour: Calc; Caus; Chio; Iris; Lac-d; Lyc; Mag-c; Med; Nat-p; Nux-v; Pho; Psor; Pul; Rhe; Rob; Sul; Sul-ac; Tab; Ver-a.
- Chill, fever, during: Lyc.
- Water: Con.

Stains, black: Arg-n.
Stomach, from, full, after interval of days: *Bism*; Grat.
Stools
- During: Arg-m; Ox-ac.
- After: Aeth.
- Straining from: Ther.

Stooping agg: Cic; *Ip*.
Stringy: Croc; Cor-r; Cup; Kali-bi.
Sudden, projectile: Ant-t; Kali-bi; Kali-chl; Pic-ac.
Sugar amel: Op.
Swallow
- Attempting, on: Merc-c.
- Empty agg: Grap.

Sweat, cold with: Ars; Cup-ar; Tab; *Ver-a*.
Sweetish: Iris; *Kre*; Plb; *Tub*.
Syncope, with: Cocl.
Talking, loudly, when: Cocl.
Teeth, sets on edge: Chio; Rob.
Thirst, with: Ars; Canth.

VOMITING

Tumours, cerebral, from: Coc-c; Cocl.
Unconsciousness, during: Ars; Benz-n.
Uncovering abdomen, amel+: Tab.
Uraemic: Apoc; Ars; Samb; Scop; Senec.
Urine, of: Op.
Urticaria, suppressed from: Urt.
Uterine: Caul; Kre; Lil-t; Senec.
Vertigo during+: Nux-v; Tab; Ver-a.
Violent: Ant-t; Ars; Canth; Colch; Crot-t; Cup; Kali-bi; *Nux-v*; Pho; Phyt; Stan; Tab; *Ver-a*.
- Death, desires: Phyt.
- Nausea, without+: Ver-v.
- Sitting up, on: Sil.

Water
- Cold amel: *Cup*; Pho; Pul.
- Except: Hyds.
- Sight of (must close eyes while bathing): Lyss; Pho.

Watery: Ars; *Bry*; Caus; Dros; Iris; Rob; Tab; VER-A.
- Greenish: Old.
- Sweetish: Iris.
- Then food: Iod; Nux-v.

Wine amel: Kalm.
Worms: Cina; Saba; Sang.
Yellow: Pho; Ver-a.
- Bright: Kali-bi.

VORACITY: See APPETITE, increased, ravenous.

VULNERABLE: See SKIN, heal won't.
VULVA (labia): Sep; Thu.
  Abscess: Hep; Lach; Merc; *Pul*; Sep.
  Apthous: Helo.
  Cheesy deposits, on: Helo.
  Dry: Tarn.
  • Menses, after: Sep.
  Eczema, around+: Grap.
  Eruptions: Sep.
  • Herpetic: Nat-s.
  Holds: Lil-t; Sanic.
  Hot: Carb-v; Tarn.
  Itching: Amb; *Calad*; Carb-v; Coll; Helo; Senec; Sil; Stap; Sul; Tarn.
  • Burning: Calad; Kali-io; Senec; Sul; Urt.
  • Leucorrhoea, with: Fago; Hyds.
  • Pinworms, from: Calad.
  • Sexual excitement, with: Kali-bi.
  • Urinating, when: Amb; Kre.
  Oozing, constant, from: Aur.
  Open: Bov; Sabal; Sec; Sep.
  Painful, menses, during: Rhus-t.
  Raw: Tarn.
  Sensitive, sore: Carb-v; Coc-c; Plat; Stap; Sul; Tarn.
  Sitting agg: Berb; Kre; Stap; Sul.
  Swelled: Carb-v; Hep; Pul; Senec; Sep.
  • As if: Colch; Coll.
  • Intense itching+: Rhus-t.
  • Pregnancy, during: Pod.

VULVA
  Wet, as if: Eup-pur; Petr.
WAKING: See AWAKES.
  Agg: See AWAKENING, after.
WALKING
  Agg and amel: See MOTION.
  Backward AGG: Mang.
  Bare feet, with AMEL: Psor.
  Bent AMEL: Am-m; Con; Pho; Sul.
  Bones of legs, on, as if: Cham.
  Bridge on narrow or over water AGG: Ang; *Bar-c*; *Fer*; Sul.
  Canal, by the side of AGG: Ang.
  Circle, in: Thu.
  Cotton on, as if: Onos.
  Crooked AMEL: Am-m.
  Dark, in AGG: Zin.
  Eyes, closed with
  • Agg: Alu; Arg-n; Calad; Iodf; Zin.
  • Amel: Con.
  Feet
  • Swing, half circle, in: Cic.
  • Swollen, as if, with: Helod.
  Floor, on: Ars; Cham.
  • Hand, wrings, and: Buf.
  Foot, left, cannot put on ground, when: Mag-c.
  Goes to one side: Amy-n.
  Ground
  • Level on agg: Ran-b; Ver-a.
  • Rough, on agg: Clem; Hyo; Lil-t.
  Hard pavement, on AGG: Ant-c; CON; *Hep*.

WALKING

Impulse to: Aco; Arg-n; *Ars*; *Bur-p*; Fer; Flu-ac; Kali-io; Lil-t; Lyc; Mag-c; Merc; Naj; Pho; Sep; Tarn; Thu; Val.

Inability, fall after: Arg-m.
- Pregnancy, during: Bels.

Involuntarily, quick steps with: Coca.

Knees
- Drawn up, involuntary when: Ign.
- On: Med.

Late learning: See CHILDREN, walk late.

Must (See Motion amel): Ars; Aur; Calc; Dig; Dios; Iod; Murx; Op; Paeon; Rut; Stro; Tarn.
- Night, at: Merc.

Needles, on, as if: Eupi; Rhus-t.

Peas, hard on, as if: Nux-m.

Pitches, forward, as if, on: Terb.

Side
- To one: Amy-n; Ver-v.
- Way AGG: Caus; Kali-c.

Sponge on, as if: Helod.

Sudden loss of strength+: Con.

Toes, on: Crot-h; Lathy.

Turns, right to, while: Helod.

Velvet, on, as if: Sec.

Wool on as if: Xanth.

WANDER home to home, desire+: Elat.

WANDERING: See PAIN, wandering.

WARM

Applications, warmth, poultice AGG (See also HEAT, agg): AP; BELL; Calc; *Carb-v*; Crot-h; Cup; Flu-ac; IOD; Kali-io; Kali-s; LACH; Led; Lil-t; Lyc; *Merc*; *Nat-m*; *Pul*; Sabi; Sanic; *Sec*; Spig; *Sul*.

Covers etc. AMEL (See also HEAT, amel): *Hep*; Ign; *Mag-c*; NUX-V; Pul; Rhus-t; *Samb*; Scil; *Sil*; *Stro*.

WARTS (See FUNGUS GROWTH)

Bleeding: Caus.

Flat: Berb; Caus; *Dul*; Merc-i-f; Rut.

Granular: Arg-n.

Horny: Ant-c; Sil.

Itching: Kali-c.

Large, soft: Mag-s; Dul.

Pedunculated: *Thu*.

Red: *Calc*; Nat-s; *Thu*.
- Body, all over: Nat-s.

Shooting: Bov.

Suppressed: Meny; Nit-ac; Stap; Thu.

Ulcerating: Caus; Hell.

WASH, impulse to: Psor; Syph.

WASHING: See BATHING.

Clothes agg: Pho; Ther.

Floor agg: Caus; Merc-i-r.

Head agg: Canth; Tarn; Zin-chr.

WATER

Agg: See DAMPNESS agg.

Bloody, meat washing: See DISCHARGES, meat water.

Cannot bear touch of it: Am-c

Chokes him: Stram.

WATER

Cold, too: Phys; Ther.

Dropping or flowing on part: See TRICKLING.

Falling or swimming, in agg: Ant-t; Bels.

Forcing its way, during pain as if: Coc-c.

Foul agg+: Crot-h.

Horror of, cold: Phys.

Hot, flowing on part: See under TRICKLING.

Looking, running water agg: See LOOKING moving objects agg.

Sight of, AGG: Bell; Bro; Canth; Lyss; Stram; Sul.
- Pregnancy, during: Pho.

Smells, like old musty rain water: Sanic.

Taste bad, putrid etc.: See under TASTE.
- Sweet: Form.

Thinking, of it agg: Ham.

WATERBRASH (See also raising mucus): Ars; Bar-c; BRY; CALC; Carb-v; Lyc; Mez; Nat-m; NUX-V; Par; Petr; PHO; Pul; Rob; Saba; Sang; Sep; Sil; Stap; Sul; Sul-ac.

Alternate day agg: Lyc.

Bitter
- Nausea, with+: Am-m.
- Sour, with stomach pain: Kre.

Burning: Sumb.

Chilliness, with: Sil.

Cold: Caus; Ver-a.

Convulsions, before: Hyd-ac.

WATERBRASH

Cough, after: Ab-n.

Headache, with: Mag-m.

Heat of body, with: Cic.

Lying down, on: Psor.

Menses, before: Nux-m; Pul.

Milk, from: Cup.

Night: Carb-v; Kali-c.

Pregnancy, during: Nat-m; Nux-m; Tab.

Salty: Carb-an; Caus.

Sensation, of: Kali-io.

Sudden: Bar-c.

Sweetish+: Ant-c.

Tobacco amel: Ol-an.

Tongue, brown, with: Sil.

WATERY: See DISCHARGES, watery, thin.

WAVERING: See IRRESOLUTION.

WAVES, ebullitions, fluctuations, orgasms: Am-m+; Amy-n; Aur; Bell; Calc; Fer; Gel; Glo; Kre; LACH; Lil-t; Lyc; MELI; Nux-v; Pho; Sang; SEP; Spo; Stro; Strop; Sul; Sul-ac.

Heat, of: See HEAT, flushes of.
- Pain, during: Cam.

WEAKNESS, enervation, prostration: Aco; Alu; Am-c; Anac; Ant-t; Ap; Arg-m; Arn; ARS; Bap; Bar-c; Bro; Bry; Calc; Calc-p; CARB-V; Caus; Chel; Chin; Cocl; Colch; Cup; Dig; Fer; GEL; Grap; Hep; Hyo; Ign; Iod; Ip; Kali-c; Kali-p; Kalm; Lach; Laur; Lyc; Med; Merc; Merc-c; Merc-cy; Mur-ac;

WEAKNESS ..

Nat-c; *Nat-m*; Nat-p; Nat-s; *Nit-ac*; *Nux-v*; PHO; *Pho-ac*; Pic-ac; Psor; Pyro; *Rhus-t*; Scil; Sec; *Sele*; *Sep*; *Sil*; Solid; *Spo*; *Stan*; *Stap*; *Sul*; Sul-ac; Sul-io; *Tab*; Tarn; Thyr; *Tub*; VER-A.

Acute diseases
- In: Aeth; Ail; Ant-t; Ap; Ars; Gel; Merc-cy; Mur-ac; Strop; *Tarn-c*; Ver-a.
- After: *Chin*; Meph; Psor; Sele; Ver-a.

Air open
- Agg: Plat; Spig.
- Amel: Con.
- Walking in
  - agg: Alu; Cocl; Rhus-t.
  - amel: Flu-ac; Kali-io; Sul.

Appetite, increase with: Sec.
Causeless: Psor.
Chest, starts in, as if: Seneg.
Coition after (males) AGG: *Calc*; Kali-p; Sele; Sil.
- Shuddering, with: Kali-c.
- Females: Berb; Sep.

Cough, after: Cor-r; Ver-a.
Die, as if, he would: *Ars*; Old; Vinc.
Early, rapid and: *Merc-cy*.
Easy: Cyc; Nat-m; Pic-ac; Sil.
Eating, after: Zin.
Emission agg: Dios; Kali-p; Kob; Lyc; Med; Nux-v; Pho; Pho-ac; Sil; Stap.
Epilepsy, after, one arm one leg+: Cadm; Pho.
Even cannot take food: Bar-c; Stan.

WEAKNESS

Excess, after any: Plb.
Exertion agg: Pho.
Going downstairs, then up+: Stan.
Head resting, closing eyes amel: Anac.
Heat, flushes of, after: Dig; Sep.
Indolence and luxury from (women): Helo.
Influenza, after: Abro; Con; Kali-p; Nat-sal+.
Injury, after: Acet-ac; Sul-ac.
Internally: See EMPTY.
Menses
- During: Carb-an; Cocl; Iod; Pic-ac; Sep.
- Amel: *Sep*.
- After agg: Alu; Am-c; Cimi; *Ip*.
- Scanty, with: Ip.

Mental and physical work from (women): Helo.
Morning: Ars; Carb-v; *Lach*; *Lyc*; Pho-ac; *Sep*; Stap.
- 11 A.M.: Pho; Sep; SUL; Zin.

Nausea, with: Ant-t.
Nursing
- Sick persons, after: Cimi; *Cocl*; Nit-ac.
- Women, in: Carb-an; *Chin*; *Pho-ac*.

Operations, after: Acet-ac; Hypr; Stro.
- Haemorrhage, severe, from: Stro.

Out of proportion, to disease: Ars; Sul-ac.

WEAKNESS

Pains from: Arg-m; *Ars*; Cham; Kali-p; Kalm; Pic-ac; Rhus-t; Ver-a.
Palpitation, after: Kali-c.
Paralytic: Ars; *Chin*; Cocl; *Fer*; Gel; Hell; Kali-c; Kali-p; Kalm; Mur-ac; Pho; Pho-ac; *Sul*; Ver-a.
• Pleurisy with: Saba.
• Sense of: Stro.
• Stiffness, with: Lith.
Periodical: *Arg-n.*
Rapid: *Ars*; *Bap*; Lyc; Sep; Tub; *Ver-a.*
Restless, and: Ars; Rhus-t; Zin.
Riding, from: Card-m.
Sadness, from: Calc-p; Ign; Pho-ac.
Scientific labour agg: Grap.
Sea bathing agg: Mag-m.
Sensitive, and: Terb.
Sickness, after: See Acute diseases, after.
Single parts in (See SINGLE PARTS, effects): Val.
Sinking, readily: *Merc.*
Speak, cannot, from: Cocl.
Stools
• After: *Ars*; Bism; Cocl; *Con*; Kali-p; *Merc*; Nat-s; Nit-ac; Pic-ac; Pho; Pod; Sec; Tub; Ver-a.
• Mucous, after: Bor.
Suckling, after: Carb-v.
Sudden (See COLLAPSE): Ars; Con; Crot-h; Grap; *Laur*; Pho; Ran-b; Sep.
• Vision, illusions of with: Sep.

WEAKNESS

Symptoms, few, with: Syph.
Takes, the voice away: Canth.
Talking agg: Alu; Stan; Sul.
Tremulous: Arg-n; Chin; Con; Hep; Nat-m; Old; Ol-an; Petr; Stan.
• Smoking, after: Hep.
Trifle causes, from: Am-c; Ars.
Unpleasant impressions, from: Pho.
Upper part of, with trembling of lower: Amb.
Urination after: *Ars*; Caus; Cimi; Fer; *Gel*; Nux-v; *Pho.*
Waking, on: Nux-v; Sep; Syph.
Walking
• Amel: *Rhus-t*; Rut; *Sul.*
• Air open in, after: Spo.
Worked, hard, as from: Ap.
WEALTHY, thinks he is: Cann; Pho; *Plat*; *Pyro*; *Sul*; Ver-a.

WEANING

Ill effects of: Bry; Cyc; Pul.
Eruptions, after: Dul.

WEARINESS (See WEAKNESS):
Cann; Croc; Pul.
Exertion, slight from: Bar-c.
Painful: Rut.
Sleepiness
• With: Ant-c.
• Eating, when: Kali-c.

WEATHER changes of agg: See CHANGE OF TEMPERATURE agg.
Hot AGG and AMEL: See SUMMER agg and amel.
Humid: See HUMID.

WEATHER

Rough, windy AGG: Rhod.

Wet
- AGG: See DAMPNESS agg.
- AMEL: See Air, clear, amel.

WEDGE: See PLUG.

WEEPING

AGG: *Arn*; *Bell*; Croc; Cup; *Hep*; Mar-v; Stan; Ver-a.

AMEL: Anac; Cimi; Cyc; Dig; *Grap*; *Lach*; Lyc; Med; Nit-ac; Plat; PUL; Tab.

WEEPS: *Aeth*; Ap; Aur; *Bell*; CACT; Calc; Caus; *Cham*; Cic; Cof; *Grap*; Ign; Kali-br; Lac-c; Lil-t; *Lyc*; Mag-m; Med; *Nat-m*; NUX-M; Pall; Pho; *Plat*; PUL; Rhus-t; *Sep*; Spo; *Sul*; Sul-ac; VER-A.

Alone, when: Con; Nat-m.

Aloud: Cup; Lyc.

Anger
- With: Ant-t; Ars; Sul; Zin.
- After: Nux-v; Plat.

Bitterly: Nat-m.

Cause, without: Ap; Cact; Grap; Nat-m; Pul; Rhus-t; Sul; Syph; Vio-o.
- Day and night: Ap.

Chill, during: Bell; Calc; Cham; Lyc; Pul; Vio-o.

Chorea, in: Caus.

Convulsive: Mag-p.
- Asthma with: Bov.

Coughing
- Before: See CRIES, cough agg.
- With: Spo.

Day, during: Stram.

Discontent, self, with: Nit-ac.

Disease, progressive, with: Aeth; Calad.

Dreams, in: Calc-f; Plant; Spo; Stram; Tarn.

Eating while: Carb-an.

Emotions, from: Ast-r; Kre; Naj.

Frequently+: Ust.

Heat, during: Aco; Bell; Pul; Spo.

Hopeless, from: Arg-n.

Immoderately: Fer.

Involuntarily: Croc; Ign; Mang; Nat-m; Plat; Pul; Rhus-t; Sep.

Inwardly+: Ign.

Lamenting, and: Cof.

Laughs, and, by turns: Ign; Sumb.

Lonely, feeling, from: Lith.

Looked at when: Nat-m.

Menses
- Before: Pho.
- During: Ars.

Music, from: Amb; Grap; Kre; Nat-c; Thu.

Nursing, while: Lac-c; Pul.

Pains
- With: Cof; Plat.
- After: Glo.

Palpitation, with: Pho.

Paralysis, in: Caus.

Piano, hearing on: Cep; *Nat-s*.

Pregnancy, during: Mag-c.

Questioned, when: Cimi.

Reading, when: *Crot-h*; Lach.

Sexual excitement, with: Ast-r; Stram.

WEEPING
Silently: Cyc.
Sits, and, for days: Amb.
Sleep
- **In:** Carb-an; Cham; Lyc; Nat-m; Nux-v; Stan.
- **Loudly:** Kali-io.
- **Waking, without:** Hyo.

Spasms, after: Alu; Caus.
Spells, of: Sep.
Spoken to, when: Cimi; Med; Nat-m; Plat; Stap.
Stools agg: Aeth; Bor; Cham.
Sweat, with: Bell; Cup; Lyc; Op; Spo.
Telling of her sickness, when: Kali-c; Med; *Pul*; Sep.
- **Over again, and:** Med.

Thanked when: LYC.
Trifles, at (in children): *Caus*; Nat-m.
Undresses, and: Thyr.

WEIGHT
As of a heavy: Aco; Ars; Bar-c; Bell; BRY; *Cact*; Dios; Elap; Lach; Nux-m; NUX-V; Petr; PHO; Pho-ac; *Pul*; Sep; Zin.
Cold: Agar.
Hanging to part, as if: Cur; Nit-ac; Rhod; Rut.
Tied up, to part, as if: Ver-a.

WELL
Feel, does not, but knows not why: Bro.
Says he is, when very sick: Ap; Arn; Ars; Cann; Cof; Iod; Op.
Unusally, then AGG: Bry; Nux-v; Pho; *Psor*; Sep.

WENS+: Bar-c.
WET agg: See DAMPNESS agg.
WETTING hands and feet agg: See COLD, single parts and FEET, wetting.
WHEALS: See URTICARIA.
WHEEZING: See RESPIRATION, whistling.
WHINING, whimpering: *Ant-t*; Ap; Aur; Carb-an; *Cham*; Cic; *Cina*; Merc; Pod; Pul; Senec.
Ailments, little, with: Tub.
Attacks of sickness, before: Ant-t.
Mood+: Bar-c.
Sleep, in: Pod; Rhe.
WHIRLING: See VERTIGO.
WHISPERS: Calc; Cup; Fer; Ign; Merc; Ol-an.
Ear in, as if: Anac.
Herself, to: Pyro.
Sleep, in: Pyro.
WHISTLES: Croc; Lach; Plat; Stram.
Fever, during: Caps.
Involuntary: Carb-an; Lyc.
Low, soft, voice: Vio-o.
WHITE, whiteness (of skin, discharges etc.): Ant-t; Ars; CALC; Carb-v; Chel; *Chin*; Cina; Dig; *Fer*; *Grap*; Kali-m; LAC-C; MERC; *Nat-m*; Pho; Pho-ac; *Pul*; Sep; Sul; *Ver-a*.
Chalky: Ant-c; Mez.
Milky: *Kali-m*.
Spots: Alu; *Ars*; Grap; Merc; Nat-c; Sep; SIL; SUL.
Loss of hair with: Psor.

WHITE
Swelling: See JOINTS, swelling, pale.
Turning: Sul-io.
- And insensible: Sul-io.
- Blue: Calc.
- Red: Hell.

WHITLOW: See FINGERS, felon.
WHIZZING: See HUMMING.
WHOOPING COUGH: See COUGH, whooping.

WIFE
Is faithless: Hyo; Stram.
Run away from him, will: Stap.

WILD FEELING: Amb; *Cimi*; Lil-t; Med.
WILD look+: Val.
WILFUL: See STUBBORN.
WILY: See TRICKY.

WIND, air, draft
AGG: *Aco*; Ars; *Bell*; Calc; Calc-p; Caps; Cham; *Chin*; Colch; Colo; *Hep*; Kali-c; Lach; Lyc; Mag-c; Mag-p; Med; Nux-m; *Nux-v*; Pho; Pho-ac; Pul; Rhe; *Rhod*; Rhus-t; Samb; Scil; Sele; SIL; Stro; SUL; Verb.
AMEL: Fer; Iod; Sec; Tub.
Blowing on part, as of a: See AIR, blowing on part.
North AGG: Ars; Asar; Carb-v; Caus; Hep; Nux-v; Sep; Spo; Zin.
Slight AGG: Caps.
Warm
- AGG: Sele.
- AMEL: Thu.

WINE agg: See FOOD & DRINKS, wine agg.

WINKING: See under EYES.

WINTER
AGG (See cold agg): *Ars*; *Aur*; Dul; Flu-ac; Hep; Kali-c; Kalm; Nux-v; Petr; Psor; Rhus-t.
AMEL: Sul-io.

WIPING AGG: Alo; *Grap*; Lach; Mur-ac.
AMEL (eyes): Alu; *Calc*; Cina; Croc; Cys; Euphr; *Nat-c*.

WITHERED, shrivelled: Ars; *Calc*; *Chin*; *Cocl*; Cup; *Iod*; Lyc; *Sec*; *Ver-a*.

WITTY: See JESTS.

WOMEN: See FEMALES AFFECTIONS of, and OLD MAIDS.
Aversion to: Dios; Lach; Pul.
Childless: Arg-n; Cocl.
Neurotic, high strung: Scut.
Unmarried+: Cocl; Sil.
Widows: Stap.

WOODEN feeling: Kali-n; Petr; Rhus-t; Thu.
WOOLENS AGG: Merc; Pho; *Psor*; Pul; Rhus-t; Sul.
WORD HUNTING: Arg-n; Arn; Lach; Pho-ac; *Plb*; Pho+; Thu.
Swallows: *Cic*; Stap; Thu.
WORK dislikes, dread of: See AVERSIONS, work and INDOLENT.

WORMS: Aco; Art-v; *Calc*; Chin; *Cina*; Cup-ox; Ign; Merc; Nat-p; *Saba*; *Sil*; *Spig*; Stan; *Sul*; Vio-o.
Fever, from: Cina.
Hook: Card-m; Chenop; Thymol.

WORMS

Pin, thread: Calc; Chin; Fer; Ign; *Mar-v*; Naph; Rat; Saba; Sul; Urt.

Tape: Calc; Grap; Plat; Pul; Saba; Sil; Sul.

WORN OUT+: Amb.

WORRY: See CARE and GRIEF.

Causeless: Petr.

WORTHLESS feels+: Anac.

WOUNDS: See INJURIES.

Atrophy, of: Form.

Bleed
- Edges closed from: *Mill.*
- Suppurate and: Pho.

Blue: Lyss.

Break and heal again (See ulcers): Carb-v; Pho.

Healing rapid, for: Manc.

Poisoned: Cist.

WRAPPED body etc. as if: Bar-c; Cact; Grap; Med; Nux-v; Sul.

WRAPPING: See COVERS.

WRAPS up, in summer: Hep; *Psor.*

WRETCHED: Tab.

WRIGGLES: Val.

WRINGING: See TWISTING.

WRINKLED: *Calc*; Cam; Pho-ac; Sars; *Sec*; Sep; Ver-a.

WRISTS: Bov; Calc; Caus; Kali-c; Rhus-t; Rut; Sabi; Sep; Sul.

Right: Ox-ac; Vio-o.

Aching, loss of power, with: Fer-p.

Burning: Nat-c.

Cold: Calc-f; Gel.
- Puerperal sepsis, in: Pul.

WRISTS

Contracted, as if: Bels.

Cracking: Arn; Con.

Ganglion: Benz-ac; Calc-f.

Grasping agg: Fer-p.

Knitting agg: Kali-c.

Menses agg: Nat-p.

Numb: Zin.

Paralysis: Plb.

Pins and needles: Colch.

Sore, bruised: Rhod.

Strained, as if: Ox-ac.

Turning agg: Merc-i-f.

Weak: Val.

Writing agg: Lyc; *Mag-p.*

WRITING agg: See FINGERS, writing, and working with.

Cramps, while: See FINGERS, cramps.

Mistakes, in: See MISTAKES.

WRONG

Cannot tell, what is: Thu.

Doing, something: Hell.

Everthing, seems: Naj.

Had done something: Cina+; Ign; *Nux-m*; Rut.

Position: See POSITION, wrong.

WRY NECK: See NECK, wry.

X-RAY burns: Calc-f; Pho; Radm.

YAWNING: Ant-t; Ars; CAUS; Chel; Cina; *Croc*; Grap; Hep; IGN; Kali-p; *Kre*; Lyc; Mag-p; Mang; NUX-V; *Op*; Pho; Plat; Pul; *Rhus-t*; Sul; Zin-val.

AGG: Alo; Am-m; Caus; *Cina*; IGN; Kali-c; *Kre*; NUX-V; *Rhus-t*; *Sars.*

YAWNING

AMEL: Berb; Chin-s; Croc; Guai; Stap.

Accompaniment, as an: Agar; Ant-t; Castr; Cina; Kali-c; Kre; Sars.
- Abdominal, symptoms, with: Castr.

Chill
- Before: Eup-p.
- With: *Eup-p*; *Nat-m*; Thu.

Coldness, with: Nat-c.

Coma, in: Amy-n.

Continuous+: Castr; Lathy.

Coughing
- While: Bell.
- After: Anac; *Ant-t*; Ip; Kre; Op.

Eating agg: Nat-s; Scil; Sul.

Eructations, with: Tell.

Evening: Arn.

Fever, during: Chin-s; *Rhus-t*.

Frequent: Chel; Grap; Sul.
- Listening to others, when: Caus; Lyss.

Girdle, sensation, with: Stan.

Headache, and: Form; Stap.

Hiccough, with: Amy-n; Cocl.

Hysterical: Kali-p; Tarn.

Incomplete, fruitless: Lach; Lyc.

Interrupted: Lyc.

Jaw, lower trembling, with: Old.

Laughter involuntary, followed by: Agar.

Menses
- Before: *Pul.*

YAWNING, menses
- During: Am-c; Carb-an.

Must, feels+: Guai.

Near objects, seem distant when: Cep.

Pains
- Before: Agar.
- With: Aran; Pho.

Paying, attention to others when: Caus; Lyss.

Profound, repeated+: Amy-n.

Respiratory affections, in: Bro.

Shuddering, with: Cina; Hyd-ac; Meny; Old.

Sleep, deep, in: All-s; Castr; Cep.

Sleepiness, without: Plat; Rhus-t.

Sleepy, and: Kali-n; Kre.
- Cough, after: Anac.

Spasmodic+: Cocl; Plat.

Spasms, before: Agar; Merc; Tarn.

Stretching
- Amel: Carb-v; Guai.
- And: Amy-n; Calc-p; Caus; Cham; Elat; Nux-v; Rhus-t; Stap.
- Indoor: Rut.
- Wretched feeling, with: Form.

Tears, with: Mag-p; Stap.

Violent: Hep; Ign; Mag-p; Plat; Rhus-t; Sil+; Stap.
- Repeated, coma in: Amy-n; Kali-c.

Walking in open air: Euphor.

YEARLY agg: See PERIODICITY, yearly.

YELLOW fever: See FEVER, yellow.

YELLOWNESS (of skin, discharges, etc.): Aco; *Ars*; *Ars-io*; Bry; Calc; Carb-an; Cham; CHEL; *Chin*; Con; Crot-h; Eup-p; Fer; Hep; *Hyds*; Iris; Kali-bi; Kali-c; Kali-s; *Lach*; LYC; MERC; Merc-i-f; Nat-s; Nit-ac; Nux-v; *Pho*; *Plb*; Pod; PUL; SEP; *Sul.*

   Golden, bright or orange: Aeth; Alo; Alu; Card-m; CHEL; Cina; Colch; Kali-c; *Kali-p*; *Merc*; NUX-M; Pho; Sang; SUL-AC.

YELLOWNESS

   Green: Ars-io; Mang; *Merc*; *Pul.*
- Turning: Con.

   Spots: Arn; Con; Fer; Petr; Pho; Sep; Sul.
- Summer, in: Chin-ar; *Chio.*
- Vexation, from: *Cham*; Kali-c; *Nat-s.*

   Sticky: Hyds; Kali-bi; Sumb.

ZEALOUS: Nux-v.

ZIGZAG: Calc; Rhod; Sars; Sul-io.

ZOSTER: See ERUPTIONS, zoster.

ZYGOMAE: See MALAR BONES.

Doctor Hahnemann's say on Mother Tincture and Dilutions

§ 123 Unadulterated Herbs
Each of these medicines must be taken in a perfectly simple, unadulterated form; the indigenous plants in the form of freshly expressed juice, mixed with a little alcohol to prevent it spoiling; exotic vegetable substances, however, in the form of powder, or

B. Jain assures herbs from original source of cultivation or reliable vendors.

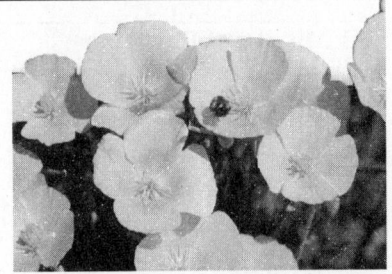

§ 264 Genuine Medicine
The true physician must be provided with genuine medicines of unimpaired strength, so that he may be able to rely upon their therapeutic powers; he must be able, himself, to judge of their genuineness.

At B.Jain we guarantee accurate herb and thus 100% accurate & pure Mother Tincture.

§ 268 Quality control to check genuinity of herb
The other exotic plants, barks, seeds and roots that cannot be obtained in the fresh state the sensible practitioner will never take in the pulverized form on trust, but will first convince himself of their genuineness in their crude, entire state before making any medicinal employment of them.[1]

[1] In order to preserve them in the form of powder, a precaution is requisite that has hitherto been usually neglected by druggists, and hence powders

B.Jain QC Department checks various parameters like TLC, UV, Infrared assuring genuinity of herbs and 100% accurate Mother Tincture.

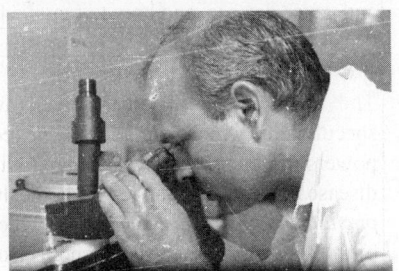

Homoeopathic Pharmacy Hahnemann's Way

MASTER HAHNEMANN was a person who envisioned an entire system of medicine and then fully developed it into a powerful and practical tool within the span of a single life. This system of medicine he named it as Homoeopathy. In his books at various places he tells us about the various important facts and his observations which he found were important and gave us the cardinal principles of homoeopathy.

§ 1 Mission of Physician

The physician's high and only mission is to restore the sick to health, to cure, as it is termed[1].

[1] His mission is not, however to construct so-called systems, by interweaving empty speculations and hypotheses concerning the internal essential nature of the vital processes and the mode in which disease originate in.

§ 3 Knowledge of Physician

If the physician clearly perceives what is to be cured in diseases, that is to say, in every individual case of disease *(knowledge of disease, indication)*, if he clearly perceives what is curative in medicines, that is to say, in each individual medicine *(knowledge of medicinal powers)*, and if he knows how to adapt, according to clearly defined principles, what is curative in medicine to what he has discovered to be undoubtedly morbid in the patient, so that the recovery must ensure - to adapt it, as well in respect to the suitability of the medicine most appropriate according to its mode of action to the case before him *(choice of the remedy, the medicine indicated)*, as also in respect to the exact mode of preparation and quantity of a required *(proper dose)*, and the proper period for repeating the dose; - if, finally, he knows the obstacles to recovery in each case and is aware how to remove them, so that the restoration may be permanent, then he understands how to treat judiciously and nationally, and he is a *true practitioner of the healing art.* [(4)]

§ 4 Physician as Preserver of health

He is likewise a preserver of health if he knows the things that derange health and cause disease, and how to remove them from persons in health.[(a)]

§ 6 Unprejudiced observed

The unprejudiced observer - well aware of the futility of transcendental speculations which can receive no confirmation from experience - be his powers of penetration ever so great, takes note of nothing in every individual disease, except the changes in the health of the body and of the mind *(morbid phenomena, accidents, symptoms)* which can be perceived externally by means of the senses; that is to say, he notices only the deviations from

§ 269 Dynamisation/Potentisation

In Sec. § 269 – Another paragraph with foot-notes is added in the Sixth Edition, as follows:

[This remarkable change in the qualities of natural bodies develops the latent, hitherto unperceived, as if slumbering[2] hidden, dynamic (§ 11) powers which influence the life principle, change the well-being of animal life[3]. This is effected by mechanical action upon their smallest particles by means of rubbing and shaking *and through the addition of an indifferent substance, dry or fluid are separated from each other.* This process is called dynamizing, potentizing (development of medicinal power) and the products are dynamizations[4] or potencies in different degrees.']

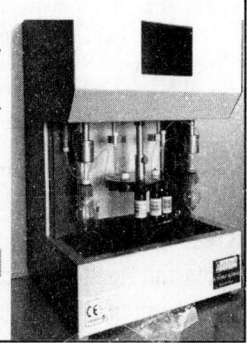

B. Jain latest K-Tronic potentiser for accuracy of potency (99.6% Accuracy) of B. Jain Liquid Dilutions

§ 270 Pure Alcohol

millionth part in powder form. For reasons given below (b) one grain of this powder is dissolved in 500 drops of a mixture of one part of alcohol and four parts of distilled water, of which one drop is put in a vial. To this are added 100 drops of pure alcohol[3] and given one hundred strong succussions with the hand against a hard but elastic body[4]. This is the medicine in the first degree of dynamization with which small sugar globules[5] may then be

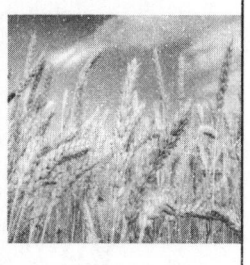

B. Jain uses Grain based ENA for MT and Dilutions which is purest form of alcohol is less bitter thus assuring pure vehicle.

§ 270 Highest Quality Globules

[3] The vial used for potentizing is filled two-thirds full.
[4] Perhaps on a leather – bound book.
[5] They are prepared, under supervision by the confectioner, from starch and sugar and the small globules freed from fine dusty parts by passing them through a sieve. Then they are put through a strainer that will permit only 100 to pass through weighing one grain, the most serviceable size for the needs of a homoeopathic physician.

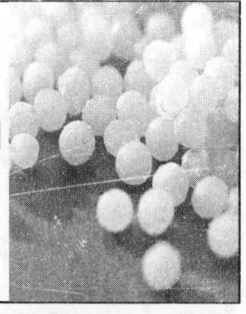

B. Jain uses pharma grade sugar for preparation of globules to assure unadulterated vehicle for you.

§ 271 Medicine preparation method should be reliable

['If the physician prepares his homoeopathic medicines himself, as he should reasonably do in order to save men from sickness,[2], he may use the fresh plant itself, as but little of the crude article is required,

[2] 'Until the State, in the future, after having attained insight into the indispensability of perfectly prepared homoeopathic medicines, will have them manufactured by a competent impartial person, in order to give them free of

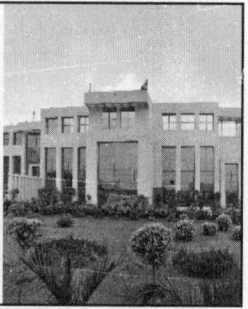

B. Jain has a GMP Certified manufacturing plant with two accrediation (India and Health Canada). B.Jain documents each and every steps followed in preparation of medicine to guarantee the reliability a homeopath needs.

Do You Have Access to all above?

If you want your medicines to comply to above standards

Ask for B. Jain Medicines

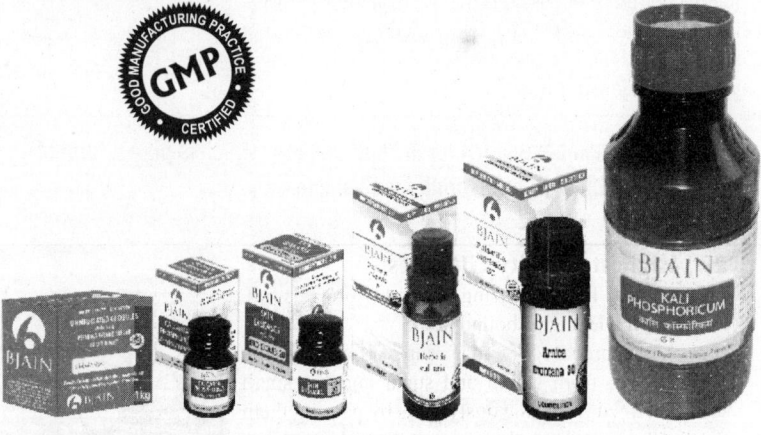

BJAIN Pharmaceuticals (P) Ltd.

Corporate Office: 1921/10, Chuna Mandi, Paharganj, New Delhi - 110055 (INDIA)
Factory Office: E-41/F, RIICO Industrial Area, Khushkhera, District Alwar, Bhiwadi - 301707, India
Tel. +91-11-45671000 Fax: +91-11-45671010 Email: pharma@bjain.com www.pharma.bjain.com